1003 Cecil, Apt. 11

Houston, Texas 77025

795- 4183

HEART-LUNG BYPASS

Principles and Techniques of Extracorporeal Circulation

PIERRE M. GALLETTI, M.D., Ph.D.

Assistant Professor of Physiology, Department of Physiology, Division of Basic Health Sciences, Schools of Medicine, Dentistry and Nursing, Emory University, Atlanta, Georgia

GERHARD A. BRECHER, M.D., Ph.D.

Professor and Chairman of Physiology, Department of Physiology, Division of Basic Health Sciences, Schools of Medicine, Dentistry and Nursing, Emory University, Atlanta, Georgia

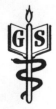

GRUNE & STRATTON

NEW YORK · LONDON

Grune & Stratton, Inc.
111 Fifth Avenue
New York, New York 10003

Library of Congress Catalog Card Number 61-17895
International Standard Book Number 0-8089-0146-x

Printed in the United States of America

Contents

Foreword

The recent astonishing advances in cardiovascular surgery have been the result of progress in many interrelated fields. The introduction and development of cardiac catheterization and angiocardiography have permitted more precise anatomic and functional diagnoses of surgically correctable cardiac lesions. There has been a great improvement in the science and art of anesthesiology, as well as in the pre- and postoperative care of surgical patients. The skill of the surgeon has kept pace with these advances and his orientation has become truly scientific.

The most recent breakthrough in the field of cardiovascular surgery has come with the introduction of the extracorporeal heart–lung circulation. This has revolutionized the approach to cardiovascular surgery and offered the opportunity to perform corrective procedures hitherto not even dreamed of. As a consequence, extracorporeal machines of diverse design have appeared in a veritable flood, and it has become difficult to keep pace with and to evaluate the various modifications. This in turn has tended to submerge the need for defining the fundamental principles that should govern their design and employment. In the excitement of developing the gadgetry, the fundamental concepts of physiology associated with the employment of an artificial lung, an artificial heart, an artificial circulation and massive blood exchange have not been fully evaluated. The present volume was written in an attempt to correct this deficit in knowledge. No better authors than Drs. Galletti and Brecher could have been selected for this task. Their fundamental grasp of the physiology involved and their extensive experience with the "artificial organs" used in heart–lung bypass make them eminently suited to bring this entire field into proper perspective.

They deal in this monograph with a careful critique of the available artificial machines, with the snares that beset their use and with guiding principles that need to be borne in mind constantly. The authors bring into proper focus that which is known and that which is still to be determined. The fact that they are not surgeons and not actively involved in the use of any one particular extracorporeal circulation scheme adds particular validity to their review and conclusions.

It has been a pleasure and an education to read this work in manuscript form. It is certain that careful study of this monograph will more than repay the reader for the time spent, whether he be a surgeon, an internist, a pediatrician, or a fundamental biologist who is involved in modern cardiovascular surgery. Considering the continuing rapid expansion of this field, the presentation is amazingly up-to-date.

Louis N. Katz, M.D.

Chicago, Illinois
September 26, 1961

Preface

This treatise brings together information about the technology and basic physiology of extracorporeal circulation. It is intended to serve as a textbook for physicians, nurses and technicians, as well as for biologic scientists and engineers, by presenting facts and concepts in a language understandable to all in these professions.

During the last decade the use of heart–lung bypass for human surgery has precipitated such rapid developments in techniques that it is very difficult to keep up with them. Pertinent publications are scattered throughout numerous journals in many countries and are not always easily available. This fact alone calls for an extensive review of the world literature. Lack of a suitable equipment review sometimes leads physicians and engineers to begin expensive developmental work without being aware of acceptable solutions already reached elsewhere. In addition, it is necessary to elucidate many complex technical problems, to unravel controversies and to unearth valuable biologic data which are buried in descriptions of obsolete methods. All these needs are particularly felt by the newcomer to the field of extracorporeal circulation who is often bewildered by the wealth and disorganization of the information.

In the Fall of 1959, a postgraduate course of lectures was given at Emory University as an introduction to the problems of artificial circulation. The organization of the book in fairly self-contained chapters is patterned after this lecture series. Besides an extensive review of the work of others, the text includes also experimental results from the laboratory of the authors. Part of the book deals with descriptions of materials, gas exchange devices and pumps. The importance of the physiologic interactions between the organism and the extracorporeal circuit is particularly stressed, because much of the success of any perfusion depends upon a clear understanding of these relations. As a result of obvious pressures, heart–lung bypass procedures were used for human surgery before enough of the essential background knowledge had been acquired. In recent years, much new information has been gained in the operating room. Now the time has come to give, in the light of basic physiologic principles, a systematic account of the empiric observations made since the advent of heart–lung bypass as a clinical procedure.

All illustrations are originals or simplified modifications of other drawings, in order to emphasize principles rather than details of construction. Photographs of equipment are omitted because they often fail to illustrate the salient points. To make this book useful as a reference text, an extensive bibliography of the world literature, limited to the technologic and physiologic aspects of extracorporeal circulation, is included. For brevity many aspects of extracorporeal circulation are presented in review form only. Not treated or mentioned only briefly are cross circulation, regional perfusion, isolated organ perfusion, external dialysis (artificial kidney), cross dialysis, transplantations and long range survival of organs. No emphasis is placed on the problems of clinical indications for heart–lung bypass or hypothermic perfusions. Details of surgical procedures are only discussed in so far as they relate to the perfusion techniques.

At the present stage of development, any attempt to organize the existing knowledge of extracorporeal circulation may appear premature and foolhardy. In presenting this book, the authors are not unaware of their own biases and limitations. Their efforts will be justified even if they result only in a better appraisal of the problems open to future research.

ACKNOWLEDGMENTS

A book of this sort could not see print without the contributions of numerous persons at various steps of completion. The greatest debt we owe to Dr. Carl J. Wiggers, who with his monumental knowledge of cardiovascular physiology helped with valuable suggestions and criticisms. Through his rich experience in cardiology, Dr. Louis N. Katz has contributed the most pertinent improvements to the final version of the manuscript. Parts of the manuscript have been reviewed by specialists in various areas: Mr. Silas A. Braley and Drs. Marion deV. Cotten, Rodney P. Gwinn, E. Converse Peirce and Peter A. Stewart. The content of many chapters has been influenced by research projects carried on in our laboratory by teams including Drs. Naci Bor, Dorothy Brinsfield, Leonide Goldstein and Max A. Hopf.

Most of the illustrations were conceived by the authors and superbly designed and executed by Miss Madeleine Hopf, Miss Ruth B. Geering, Mr. William C. McCracken and Mrs. Vera Townsend, with the aid of the Department of Medical Illustration at Emory University under Miss Kathleen Mackay.

To the staff of the A. W. Calhoun Medical Library under Miss Mildred Jordan, we are indebted for their untiring cooperation. Mrs. Sonia Galletti, Mr. James M. Alday and Mr. James Hazelwood assisted in establishing the bibliography. Miss Cecilia Colly carried the heavy secretarial load and we gratefully acknowledge her patience in preparing the manuscript. Mr. Murray Miller of Drexel Institute of Technology in Philadelphia helped us greatly through his editorial and stylic advice. We wish to express our sincere appreciation for the valuable support of the Life Insurance Medical Research Fund. Most of our own research incorporated in this book was made possible through the facilities at Emory University and supported by the National Heart Institute and the Georgia Heart Association. We gratefully acknowledge their help.

I. Introduction

The science of extracorporeal circulation is very young. Less than a decade has elapsed since the first heart–lung machines were successfully applied for the benefit of human patients. In the last few years, advances in biologic technology have climaxed in the design of such elaborate perfusion devices that the modest laboratory forerunners, which date back more than a century, are almost forgotten. This introduction will merely highlight a few of the numerous milestones lining the road to modern heart–lung machines, state the principal peculiarities of extracorporeal circulation and explain some terms commonly used in the field. Other historical details will be taken up in context with the subject matter treated in later chapters.

HISTORICAL MILESTONES

The concept of an artificial circulation was first promulgated by Le Gallois in 1813. He contended that life may be preserved by external perfusion in any portion of an organism even though separated from the rest of the body. This assertion followed experiments by Sténon, Bichat and a number of physiologists of the late eighteenth and early nineteenth century who observed that after apparent death, the vital properties of the brain, spinal cord, nerves and muscles could be restored temporarily by permitting blood to pass through the organs. In 1828, Kay showed that artificial circulation of venous blood was capable of re-establishing irritability in dying mammalian muscle. External perfusion of kidneys was first attempted in 1849 by Loebell in Carl Ludwig's laboratory. Brown-Séquard, between 1848 and 1858, demonstrated the necessity of oxygenating the blood used as a perfusate. "Red" incoagulable blood, obtained by whipping of "black" blood, was forced through arteries by means of a syringe. In this manner Brown-Séquard succeeded in maintaining some evidence of reflex nervous activity in isolated mammalian heads provided the perfusion was initiated promptly after decapitation of the animal. In experiments on the limbs of guillotined criminals he even used his own blood to demonstrate that muscles at the stage of rigor mortis, devoid of all signs of response to galvanic stimulation, could be reactivated by perfusion with oxygenated blood and kept responsive while the unperfused part of the body decayed.

In 1868, Ludwig and Schmidt described an apparatus by which arterial blood could be infused under constant pressure from a reservoir into an isolated surviving mammalian organ. Improvements in the oxygenation of the perfusate were reported from Schmiedeberg's laboratory by von Schröder (1882), who thought of bubbling air through the venous blood from the bottom of a bottle, thereby producing foam. The first artificial heart–lung machine in

1

which the oxygenation of the perfusate could be accomplished without interrupting blood flow was devised by von Frey and Gruber in 1885 (*see frontispiece*). For gas exchange, the blood was spread as a thin film exposed to oxygen over the inner wall of a slanted, rotating cylinder. Von Frey and Gruber provided special arrangements for blood gas analysis in the perfusion circuit. They were able to support quantitatively the visual evidence of reduction of the oxygenated hemoglobin in artificially perfused tissues, noted by earlier workers. The perennial interest of Ludwig's and Schmiedeberg's schools in mechanical perfusion devices culminated in 1895 when Jacobj described a method of gas exchange through an excised animal lung in which respiration was artificially maintained. Here, for the first time, the trauma inherent in direct contact of the blood with gas during the process of oxygenation could be prevented. The excellence of the lung for arterialization and detoxication of the blood in a perfusion circuit was established by constant improvements of the heart–lung preparations which flourished at the turn of the century (Otto Frank, Ernest Starling).

The mechanization of the pumping part of the circuit, although seemingly simpler to devise than that of the gas exchange function, lagged far behind. Constant pressure reservoirs set a definite time limit to the experiment. A distinct beneficial effect of fluctuations in the pressure supplied to the perfusion medium with the syringe injection method was first recognized by Ludwig and Schmidt (1868). Hamel (1888) devised an apparatus in which the movements of a pendulum periodically interrupted the flow to the tissues, thus converting a constant pressure into an intermittent one. Jacobj (1890) designed an elaborate perfusion apparatus in which pulsatile pressure was created by periodic and forcible compression of a rubber balloon placed on the arterial side of the circuit. Pulse pressure as a necessary factor in perfusion was emphasized by Hooker (1910). By means of a cam and sliding carriage, Hooker's pump yielded a pulsatile wave of pressure similar to the normal pulse and allowed alterations in the amplitude of the pulse pressure. Although even fancier devices are used nowadays to tackle the same problem, the beneficial effect of pulsatile flow in extracorporeal circulation is still a highly controversial subject.

The main objection to most types of perfusion apparatus was the necessity for a large supply of blood. In 1903 Brodie published an account of a pump oxygenator circuit which presented a considerable advantage over many of the types previously employed: it could perfuse an organ with no other blood than that obtained from the animal itself, thereby avoiding most of the difficulties resulting from use of artificial or heterologous perfusion media. Indeed, the injurious effects of foreign blood had been suspected since the time of Prevost and Dumas (1821), who noted abnormal reactions after transfusion when blood of another species was used. Although repeatedly shown to be harmful in its effects on tissues of another species, the blood of sheep, horses, or oxen was often used to prime extracorporeal circuits for dogs or cats. Martin (1881) in his experiments upon the isolated dog's heart employed calf's blood, but he mentions that in several instances this blood was toxic. Brodie (1903) reported that the heart perfused with foreign blood became irregular, and went into fibrillary twitchings from which it could not recover even when perfused with the animal's own blood. As the realization of the incompatibility of blood from different species became more prevalent at the beginning of this century, the use of heterologous blood in experimentation was progressively abandoned.

The long accepted procedure of defibrination of blood for perfusion experiments, regardless of its origin, greatly obscured the question of the toxicity of heterologous blood. Magendie (1838) had found defibrinated blood incapable of carrying on the normal function of the circulating medium after transfusion. He presented experimental data which indicated that the removal of fibrin gave rise to a serious and bloody transudate into the lungs and intestines so that death ensued. In the eyes of other workers, the weight of Magendie's name behind such a statement did much to discredit defibrination. Careful studies by Bischoff (1835), Panum (1864) and Ponfick (1875) failed to turn the weight of experimental evidence against a common belief in the extreme toxicity of defibrinated blood, even when used in transfusion between animals of the same species. The advent of modern anticoagulants such as heparin (McLean, 1916; Howell and Holt, 1918) finally pushed the problems of defibrinated blood into the background.

Looking critically at the drawbacks of the early perfusion experiments, Belt, Smith and Whipple (1920) summarized the factors whose variations might bring about injury to the organism: aeration, composition and temperature of the perfusion medium, interruption in the continuity of flow, mean infusion pressure and pulse pressure. Rather vividly they pointed out that "a perfusion experiment is no better than its weakest point," a statement which still holds for today's more sophisticated procedures. A disillusioning conclusion from one century of experience in the animal laboratory was expressed as late as 1954 by deBurgh Daly, whose own contribution to the understanding of perfusion effects has influenced a generation of physiologists: "The condition of the animal during perfusion is in all its main signs that of peripheral circulatory shock, and the condition becomes progressively worse in the later stages of perfusion."

The concept of extracorporeal circulation as an aid to cardiac surgery originated in 1937 with the now classic publication of Gibbon on artificial maintenance of the circulation during temporary occlusion of the pulmonary artery. Gibbon felt that a machine capable of performing the function of the heart and lungs would enable the surgeon to operate upon intracardiac abnormalities under direct vision in a relatively dry, bloodless field. Meanwhile the brain, the myocardium, the liver, the kidneys and other tissues would receive adequate flows of oxygenated blood from the artificial heart–lung machine. The pioneer work of Brukhonenko (1929a, b) with oxygenation in excised lungs had demonstrated that a dog's head severed from the body and artificially perfused would remain responsive for hours. Brukhonenko (1937, 1956) and Terebinskii (1940, 1950) applied the "autojector" for total body perfusion, mainly for the purpose of resuscitation of animals after apparent death. Bjørk (1948a) attempted to extend the time limit of circulatory arrest by artificial perfusion of the head with oxygenated blood. He obtained survivals, but in his opinion a heart–lung machine of much larger capacity was needed for whole body perfusion. A little later, it was discovered (Andreasen and Watson, 1952, 1953) that even a limited amount of flow, such as that furnished for instance by the amount of blood draining from the azygos vein during caval veins occlusion, would permit survival after a drastic reduction of body perfusion lasting up to 30 minutes. The principle that a small perfusion flow, directed mainly to the brain and to the heart, suffices to prevent irreparable damage (unfortunately called "azygos principle") was successfully applied in man by Lillehei and his group (1955).

Up to that time it was believed that open heart surgery at normal temperatures requires an arterial blood flow which approximates the cardiac output under resting conditions. The "azygos principle" of low flow perfusion opened the way for the use of oxygenators of limited capacity, far easier to conceive and to operate than high flow machines. The pioneer work of early designers like Bjørk and Crafoord (1948) and Senning (1952) in Sweden, Jongbloed (1949, 1951) and Kolff (1949) in Holland, Kunlin (1948) and Thomas (1948,

1950) in France, Dogliotti, (1951) Mondini (1948, 1949) and Tosatti (1949) in Italy, Tyrer (1952) in Australia, Melrose (1953) in England, Iankovskii (1939) and Vainrib (1956) in the USSR, Sakakibara (1957 a, b) in Japan, Gibbon (1937, 1939a, b), Clark and Gollan (1950), Dennis (1949, 1951), Karlson (1949, 1952) and many others in the United States was finally rewarded around 1955 by the clinical application of perfusion techniques for open heart surgery.

Why was the success of extracorporeal circulation delayed until recent years? What were the factors that finally permitted the break with the old, half-satisfactory procedures? No doubt the advancement of biologic technology removed a number of obstacles to the development of better machines. Heparin and protamine permitted control of the clotting mechanism. Plastic tubing and sheets, siliconized glass and highly polished stainless steel provided good approximations to the "physicochemically inert" container, while the availability of antifoaming substances solved the nightmare of those who for 80 years attempted the oxygenation of blood on the bubbling or foaming principle. With the modern surgical approach to extracorporeal circulation, the haphazard equipment of the physiologic laboratory—rubber tubes, glass containers, and brass cannulae—was discarded. Considerations of expenses and risk were appreciated in a new light. Knowledge of human blood incompatibilities and improved postoperative care for patients in hospitals opened a safe way to procedures which were difficult to carry out with the limited facilities of a physiologic laboratory.

Although invaluable information has been gained from the actual demonstration that temporary exclusion of the heart and lungs can be compatible with survival in human beings, overenthusiasm for clinical progress has resulted in a disorganized development. In the last ten years, the focus of interest among heart–lung machine investigators has shifted many times, from prevention of hemolysis to reliable control of the clotting mechanism and from adequate release of carbon dioxide to maintenance of body blood volume, as one by one technical problems have been empirically solved. The focus of "superstition" also has moved from time to time. Inadequacy of arterial blood re-entry through a femoral vessel, toxicity of the coronary blood, toxicity of high oxygen tensions, and the danger of combining heart–lung bypass and hypothermia have been, in turn, held responsible for perfusion failures which could not be rationally explained otherwise. These shifts of interest to different aspects of the perfusion procedures, as time goes on, point to the necessity of a formal and theoretic approach to the problems of extracorporeal circulation.

Summarizing

Over one hundred years of development of laboratory forerunners preceeded the heart–lung machines which are presently able to substitute temporarily for the cardio–pulmonary function. Early in the nineteenth century scientists were able to reinstate responses in isolated organs through perfusion with blood. Machines for continuous perfusion were developed toward the end of the nineteenth century. Understanding of blood incompatibility and coagulation processes had to be gained for the development of satisfactory blood handling techniques. The demonstration that a limited amount of flow suffices to prevent damage to vital organs ("azygos principle") gave the necessary impetus to the use of extracorporeal circulation in human surgery. Recent advances in biologic technology as well as empiric knowledge of the physiologic demands of the perfused organism also contributed to the success of present perfusion techniques.

EXTRACORPOREAL VERSUS NORMAL CIRCULATION

Before discussing specifically how mechanical devices can be substituted for the natural heart and lungs, the fundamental similarities and differences between normal and extracorporeal circulation of blood should be considered. As pointed out by Swan (1959) and Hudson (1959), ideal cardiopulmonary bypass—implying the delivery of the correct amount of appropriately oxygenated blood to the tissues of the whole body without any attendant or ensuing adverse physiologic effects—does not exist. Extracorporeal circulation, though intended to mimic normal circulation, falls short in many respects. Some basic differences are inherent to the procedure itself and concern alterations in the circulatory system which cannot be substantially overcome by future advance in knowledge or improvement in technique. Other features depend upon the elimination of neuroregulatory mechanisms when the heart and lungs are excluded from the key position they retain normally.

The primary purpose of the normal circulation is to supply the body tissue cells with nutrient materials and to remove the metabolic waste products. For the cells it probably makes no difference whether the force which permits the flow of blood to reach the capillaries is provided by the contraction of cardiac muscle fibers (fig. 1) or by a mechanical pump (fig. 2). It also makes no difference to the functioning of the body tissue cells whether oxygen, the most urgently needed substance for their metabolism, is obtained by a gas exchange process in the normal lungs (fig. 1) or in an artificial device (fig. 2). It may therefore be surmised that a well designed artificial heart–lung machine should be able to maintain undisturbed cell function throughout the organism. Undoubtedly such a statement represents an idealistic and oversimplified view. The most striking new circulatory conditions introduced by extracorporeal circulation are as follows:

(*1*) The necessity of tying snares around the cannulae located in the major central veins, in order to divert all the venous return towards the extracorporeal circuit, results in an almost complete separation of the superior and inferior caval beds. Hence, there is no possibility for equalization of venous pressures in these two territories and, under special conditions, wide differences between superior and inferior caval pressure may develop.

(*2*) Arterialized blood is infused into a peripheral artery through a centrally directed cannula. Thus, the blood flow in the aorta during extracorporeal circulation is, at least partially, reversed. The distribution of blood from an artery of small diameter towards vessels of larger size may have various consequences. The branches which leave the aorta at right angles are not likely to be affected by the reversal of aortic flow, whereas the ones which leave at more acute angles (like the mesenteric arteries) may lose some of their

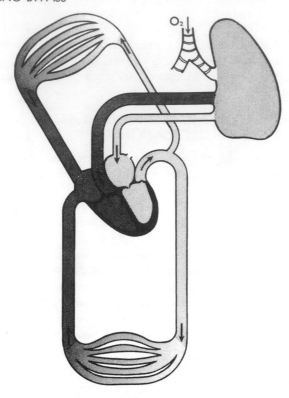

Fig. 1. Normal human circulatory system according to the concept of William Harvey. The venous blood (dark shading) enters the right heart cavities and is pumped to the lungs. There the blood is oxygenated (change in shade). After it has returned to the left heart, the arterial blood (light shading) is distributed to the tissues. While passing through the capillary beds of the body, the arterial blood gives up oxygen, picks up carbon dioxide, and thus, becomes again venous blood.

quota of blood flow on a purely directional basis. When the perfusion pressure is low, factors which control hindrance offered by the resistance vessels, such as critical closing pressure, and which differ in different parts of the vascular system, may deprive certain organs of blood flow, which in other portions of the circulation flow may be normal (Swan, 1959).

(3) Because of the ectopic origin of aortic flow, and of the mechanical characteristics of blood pumps, no way has yet been found to simulate the pulse of the normal heart in the central and peripheral vessels. In the normal circulation the aortic arch capacity is small, and much of the blood ejected by the left ventricle into the aorta has already flowed peripherally, possibly out of the arterial tree, by the time diastole begins. To the contrary, during artificial circulation, the volume of blood in the aorta is dynamically sustained by a mechanical pump which tends to replace the blood as it flows out of the arterial tree, and to keep the arterial pressure constant. These mechanical considerations are of little concern under most conditions. However, they must be weighed in case of aortic insufficiency. As observed by Clauss, et al., (1959), the maintenance of a continuous blood supply to the aorta favors regurgitant flow and hinders atrial drainage, because it cancels the safety factors which

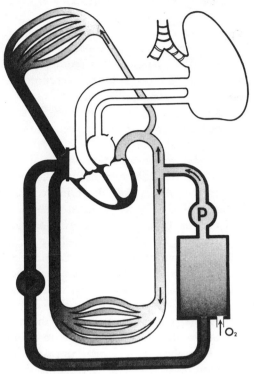

Fig. 2. Artificial maintenance of cardiorespiratory function, or "total heart–lung bypass." The entire systemic venous blood is prevented from entering the right heart cavities. Instead it is drained by a mechanical pump (P) into an artificial circuit outside the body, and oxygenated in an artificial gas exchange device (right lower part of figure). The arterialized blood is returned by another pump (P) to the systemic arterial system through a cannula in a branch of the aorta. It then perfuses the various capillary beds, but is prevented from entering the left heart cavities by the closed aortic valves. The extracorporeal circuits are represented by heavy lines. White areas in the figure are those excluded from the circulation and intended to be bloodless. Depending on the site of infusion, the direction of arterial blood flow may be reversed in some areas of the body (indicated by arrows).

would otherwise provide a low diastolic pressure in the aorta (Wiggers and Maltby, 1931).

(4) The blood is drained out of the organism and returned to it under a variety of pulsatile conditions, usually out of phase with the remaining cardiac action. This may jeopardize any sensing system concerned with phasic responses during the cardiac cycle, such as the aortic arch and carotid sinus baroreceptors.

(5) The body circulation is called upon to operate in the absence of reflexes which normally arise from receptors in the cardiac walls. The vascular isolation of the pulmonary bed may also elicit or obscure reflex mechanisms which normally affect the systemic circulation since excluded vascular beds keep their nervous supply intact. Little is known about pulmonary–systemic reflexes in the normal organism because of the complexity of the responses involved. Artificial separation of the two circulations, while providing better

defined conditions, may add to this complexity or even uncover unsuspected mechanisms.

(6) Similar considerations apply to reflexes elicited from regions of the systemic circulation. Splanchnic bed reflexes, coronary chemoreflexes and respiratory reflexes from the extremities or from the carotid sinus are some of the mechanisms possibly "jammed" by extracorporeal circulation.

(7) An extracorporeal circulation implies an extravascular route for the blood. Most of the circuits are open to the atmosphere at some point. Thus particular care must be exerted to prevent bacterial contamination and air embolism. Completely closed circuits minimize the risks. Yet attention is still required to prevent particulate embolism or cessation of flow.

(8) The necessity of using cannulae or catheters, the inner diameter of which is small as compared to the vessels they dwell in, results in high blood flow velocities and therefore, the possibility of local turbulence and irregularities of flow at the sites of venous drainage and arterial infusion.

(9) Outside of the organism, blood is propelled by pumps through tubes and containers of irregular diameter and shape. Laminar patterns of flow, which generally prevail in the normal circulation, are therefore unlikely in the extracorporeal circuit. In fact, blood appears there as a uniform random suspension of red cells in plasma rather than an ordered fluid, with a central core of erythrocytes and a plasma sleeve, as existing in living vessels.

(10) Little is known about the pattern of flow in an artificially perfused organism. If laminar flow should no longer prevail after blood re-enters the arterial system, assumptions about peripheral resistance based upon Poiseuille's law may have to be revised.

(11) Heart–lung bypass involves some degree of "overriding" of temperature regulation by the thermoregulatory centers. Heat removal is carried out mainly in the artificial circuit instead of through the skin and lungs. The thermoregulatory centers no longer control the blood flow and probably have little influence upon its distribution to various organs. On the other hand, external temperature changes, if desired, can be forcefully conducted into vital internal organs at a rate which cannot be achieved by any other technique.

(12) For the time being, all heart–lung bypass procedures in man and in animals have been done under anesthesia, and they will probably be carried out in the foreseeable future with at least some pain preventing agents. Therefore, it is important that great attention be given to the type of anesthesia and its disturbing effect on regulatory mechanisms.

Despite these shortcomings and the amazing lack of information on physiologic adaptation to extracorporeal circulation, efforts of recent years have been characterized by a conspicuous success in reducing the mortality rate from heart–lung bypass procedures. The main reason for this improvement is that the limits of tolerance have been found empirically. Since heart–lung bypass is primarily a "tool" for cardiac surgery, it is used for the shortest possible time, just to meet surgical demands, and is discontinued as soon as practicable. This attitude is bound to remain for many years to come. However, what is basically needed is a better knowledge of what happens in extracorporeal circulation. As already pointed out in 1953 by Andreasen and Watson, there may have been a "mistake in the selection of the primary question, where (the) mechanical aspect of the subject has been allowed to assume the exclusive attention of workers. . . . The really fundamental question is that concerned with discovering the reactions to be expected from this entirely new organism, or preparation: the animal living with its heart and lungs excluded." This is especially true if one has in mind the performance of long term perfusions, which could be of value in numerous clinical disorders

Summarizing

It probably makes little difference to the function of body cells whether oxygen and carbon dioxide are exchanged in a normal or an artificial lung and whether a heart or a mechanical pump provide the tissue perfusion. However, heart–lung bypass inherently differs from the normal circulation in the following respects: distribution of blood from ectopic sites, separation of superior and inferior cava venous beds, nonlaminar flow, high flow velocities and pressure gradients across cannulae, random mixing of blood cells, abrogation of internal temperature regulation, interference with organ to organ reflex regulating mechanisms and modification of circulatory and metabolic responses by anesthesia. Present success of heart–lung bypass is based more on empiric knowledge of the tolerance to bypass than on sound understanding of what physiologic alterations and adaptations occur in the organism. Primary consideration of the demands of the organism is mandatory for the development of long lasting perfusion procedures.

TERMINOLOGY

In the field of extracorporeal circulation, as in any new field with an upsurge of developmental ideas, the terminology is still unsettled. Some of the terms have arisen through an extension of words commonly used in related areas, some have been derived from Greek and Latin roots or are just new creations of "laboratory slang." Many are clear cut and understandable, whereas others are ill defined or poorly chosen. Since there is no sanctity to terms as such, one could be tempted to indict the less fortunate ones and replace them with new words. At the present stage, however, this would merely add to the confusion. Therefore we do not propose any new terminology. Only in the case of a few controversial expressions such as *inflow* and *outflow* are we using plain descriptive wording with unambiguous connotations.

In this chapter we are restricting ourselves to the definition of those conceptual and technical words which are specifically used in the field of extracorporeal circulation and are important for a general understanding of the subject matter. Other terms will be defined or described at their logical place in the individual chapters. No attempt is made to cover the basic terminology of hemodynamics. The reader unfamiliar with the language of physiology is referred to a textbook such as Wiggers (1949), Ruch-Fulton (1960), Guyton (1961) or Wright (1961). A valuable summary of concepts and notations of pressure and flow under conditions of cardiopulmonary bypass can be found in the report of the Committee on Definition and Conformity of Nomenclature and Measurements used in Studies on Extracorporeal Circulation (Allen, 1958 a, pp. 504–518).

Perfusion—A general term designating the flow of blood or of other fluids through circulatory channels in the tissues. Perfusion refers to the distribution of blood or other fluids from the arterial system to the tissues of either the entire body or of some specific organ or region. The energy which causes the perfusion medium to reach the capillaries may be provided by the heart action ("normal" or "physiologic perfusion") or by an external circuit ("external perfusion").

Extracorporeal Circulation—A general term used for an artificial system by which the entire circulation or part of it is transported outside the body. Extracorporeal circulation covers procedures as different as the perfusion of isolated organs, the shunting of blood from arteries to veins and vice versa, or the connection of a living organism to any kind of artificial device outside the body, as long as the blood drained from the organism is eventually returned to it.

Heart–Lung Bypass—A procedure in which blood passes from the central systemic veins to a large vessel in the systemic arterial tree without entering the heart cavities and the pulmonary vascular bed. Unless stated otherwise, heart–lung bypass means *total* bypass, i.e., the entire systemic venous blood is directed through channels outside the body so as to avoid the heart cavities and the pulmonary vascular bed. Heart–lung substitution is a necessary complement to heart–lung bypass. Looked upon from this point of view, the whole procedure of heart–lung bypass may be defined as a technique for maintaining,

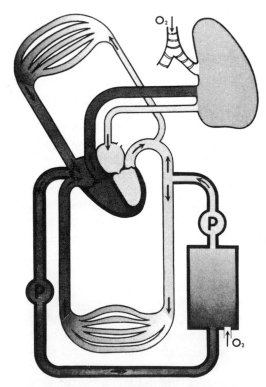

Fig. 3. Partial replacement of cardiopulmonary function, or "partial heart–lung bypass." The partition of the systemic venous blood into two different streams, one through the heart and pulmonary vascular bed, the other through the extracorporeal circuit, is indicated by the diverging arrowheads at the level of the right atrium. The extracorporeal circuit is the same as in fig. 2. Since part of the venous blood enters the right ventricle, is ejected through the pulmonary bed and flows as arterialized blood into the left cardiac chambers, the heart and lungs are still functional. Their blood flow is merely reduced.

with the help of mechanical pumps and gas exchange devices, normal hemodynamic and metabolic conditions in a living organism in the absence of cardiac and pulmonary function. The double concept of shunting of blood around the heart and lungs, and of mechanical substitution for these organs, is present in most of the uses of the expression heart–lung bypass (*see* fig. 2).

Heart–Lung Machines—A general term referring to various mechanical devices consisting of pumps and gas exchangers used as substitutes for the heart and lungs in an extracorporeal circuit.

Artificial Heart—A mechanical pump to replace the pumping action of the heart.

Artificial Lung—A mechanical gas exchange device to replace the gas exchange function of the lungs.

Gas Exchange Device—A mechanical device in which venous blood is exposed to a gas mixture rich in oxygen and arterialized by removal of CO_2 and binding of oxygen in approximately normal amounts. This term is synonymous with "artificial lung."

Pump Oxygenator—A synonym for "heart–lung machine", although pointing only to the propulsion and oxygenation of blood without reference to CO_2 removal.

Venous Drainage—A specific term used in reference to extracorporeal circulation procedures for designating the flow of blood from the systemic veins or from the right atrium into an external circuit (*see* left part of fig. 2). "Venous drainage" is a purely descriptive term to which we give preference over the frequently used term "inflow." In fact, "inflow" can be misleading since it depends on whether the perfused organism or the external machine are considered as the primary center of interest. It is worthy to recall that the term "inflow" for designating the transfer of blood from a living organism to an artificial device came to prominence at a stage when more attention was devoted to the technologic than to the biologic aspects of extracorporeal circulation procedures.

Arterial Infusion—A specific term used in extracorporeal circulation procedures to denote the flow of blood from an external circuit into the arterial tree (*see* right part of fig. 2). The term "outflow," frequently used for the passage of blood from the extracorporeal circuit into the arterial tree, is only meaningful if one looks upon the flow of blood from the heart–lung machine. It loses its meaning if one looks upon the flow from the point of view of the organism. "Arterial infusion," or occasionally as synonym "arterial reinfusion," is therefore given preference in this book as a simple, descriptive and noncontroversial term.

Partial Heart–Lung Bypass—A term referring to the situation in which only a part of the blood circulating within the organism is diverted into an extracorporeal circuit, whereas the other part follows the normal circulatory pathways (fig. 3). Through this procedure the systemic venous blood is partitioned: one portion flows as usual into the right ventricle and from there via the pulmonary circulation to the left heart and the systemic arteries, whereas the other portion is drained externally and infused directly into the systemic arterial bed, thus bypassing the heart and the lungs. The proportion of the blood flowing through the pulmonary circulation and through the extracorporeal circuit can be altered: if all the blood flows through the extracorporeal circuit, it is referred to as *total* heart–lung bypass, as defined above, whereas if some fraction of the venous return flows through the heart and lungs, the procedure is called *partial* heart–lung bypass. It is important to stress that the expression "partial heart–lung bypass" does not refer to the bypassing of a part of the body, e.g., lower or upper extremities, as the term might also be interpreted to imply (*see below*: Regional Perfusion).

Partial Perfusion—A specific term referring to a situation where only a part of the perfusing medium stems from the extracorporeal circuit whereas the other part originates from the ejection of the heart. Looked upon from the organism as a whole, "partial perfusion" can be synonymous with "partial heart–lung bypass." "Partial perfusion" points mainly to the condition in which the metabolic and hemodynamic support of the organism is carried simultaneously by the heart itself and by an external pump oxygenator. "Partial heart–lung bypass" stresses the diversion of some part of the venous return towards an external circuit.

Assisted Circulation—Any perfusion procedure aimed at supporting the circulation and/or the metabolism in the organism by mechanical means for temporary relief of the heart.

Isolation Perfusion or Regional Perfusion—A procedure in which one organ or an area of the organism is transiently deprived of its normal blood supply and perfused in a closed circuit by a mechanical pump oxygenator. Meanwhile the heart and lungs provide the circulation for the rest of the organism.

Separate Perfusion—Any artificial circulation procedure in which two or more organs or areas are simultaneously perfused by independent circuits, regardless of whether pumps, pump oxygenators or the heart ventricles are used for the propulsion of blood.

Right Heart Bypass—A procedure to channel the venous blood from the central veins directly into the pulmonary arterial bed by means of a pump. The purpose is to free the right ventricle and pulmonary outflow tract from all venous blood (see fig. 10).

Left Heart Bypass—A procedure to channel the oxygenated blood from the pulmonary veins directly into the systemic arterial tree by means of a pump. As a result, the left ventricle and the root of the aorta are free of blood (see fig. 11).

Endogenous Oxygenation—The oxygenation of venous blood, prior to its passage through the lungs, by injecting oxygen gas or oxygen releasing compounds directly into the venous system (see fig. 5).

Duration of Bypass—The overall period during which an extracorporeal circulation procedure is taking place. The procedure may refer to total heart–lung bypass or to partial heart–lung bypass. In order to be meaningful, the term should be qualified as to the duration of each phase of the bypass, from the beginning to the end of the procedure.

Priming Volume—Volume of blood or blood substitute necessary for filling the entire extracorporeal circuit to permit artificial perfusion at a minimal rate of flow.

Pump Oxygenator Priming Volume—Amount of blood necessary for priming the pump–oxygenator alone, regardless of the volume contained in collecting chambers, reservoirs, heat exchangers, filters or tubing.

Hold-up—Amount of blood which must be added to the priming volume in order to have just enough blood available in the gas exchange device at the highest flow rate anticipated.

Bypass Circulatory Volume—The sum of priming volume plus hold-up, or the volume of blood in the entire extracorporeal circuit when the heart–lung machine is fully supporting the circulation of the organism.

Stand-by Volume—The amount of blood which needs to be held in reserve for safe operation of the heart–lung machine.

It must be pointed out that this and the three preceeding definitions, taken from Allen (1958), are at variance with the meaning of "hold-up" in the valuable paper of Gimbel and Engelberg (1954). There hold-up is defined as "the entire blood volume within the oxygenator during its operation." This is the same as what is now generally called "bypass circulating volume." The distinction between priming volume, hold-up and bypass circulating volume is steadily losing its interest as more and more heart–lung machines are built in such a way that no variation in oxygenator blood content is permitted, regardless of flow.

Coronary Venous Return—Volume of blood drained from coronary veins and Thebesian vessels into the right heart cavities after complete occlusion of the caval veins. During cardiotomy this blood is removed by suction to provide a "dry" operative field.

Cardiotomy Venous Return—All blood, regardless of its origin, aspirated from the heart cavities during cardiotomy. It may include blood from coronary, Thebesian and bronchial vessels as well as blood flowing into the heart through ectopic vessels, defects or incompetent valves.

Cross-circulation—A general term indicating a heterogenous group of experimental and therapeutic procedures loosely linked by one common factor: that blood is exchanged between two organisms, or parts thereof (Andreasen, 1955). The terms of cross-circulation, cross-transfusion, cross-perfusion and donor–circulation are often applied indiscriminately to procedures of blood exchange, although the means of attaining this aim, and the purpose served by the exchange of blood, differ widely (fig. 4). When the connec-

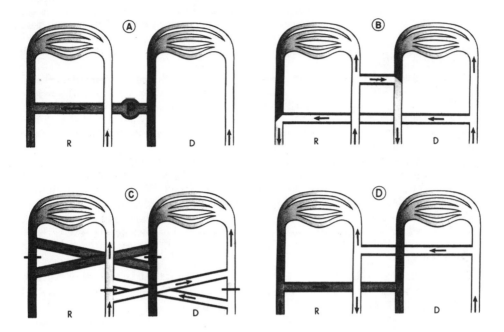

Fig. 4. Schemes of four different types of cross circulation procedures. Each inverted U symbolizes a major vascular bed with its arterial tree (light shading), capillary bed and venous tree (dark shading). The vascular beds of two different organisms, a donor (D) and a receiver (R) are placed side by side and linked by tubes (heavy lines).

A. Procedure for interchange of blood between two organisms. The blood is propelled from the vein of the donor (D) to the vein of the receiver (R) by means of a pump. In order to avoid large fluctuations in blood content either of organism D or R, the direction of flow is alternately reversed. The same aim can be achieved by using two vein-to-vein links in which the blood flows in opposite directions. This procedure could be properly called cross transfusion.

B. Procedure for interchange of blood between two organisms without mechanical pumps. The blood flows from the artery of the donor D into the vein of the receiver R, and from the artery of R into the vein of D. Since the flow in the shunt lines is partially dependent upon the arterial pressure, it is obvious that they are not necessarily equal or balanced. This procedure is usually called uncontrolled cross circulation. If pumps or flowmeters are introduced in the shunt lines in order to equalize the flows, the procedure is properly called controlled cross circulation.

C. Procedure for perfusion of a vascular bed of a first organism (R) by blood from another organism (D), while blood of the organism R is used for perfusing a vascular bed of D. To maintain complete separation of the blood of D and R, the venous trees are also cross linked. The purpose of this procedure is to perfuse under controlled conditions a vascular bed which is completely isolated but for its neural pathways, from the organism to which it belongs. In this way, neural and humoral stimuli can be studied independently. The preparation may be properly called crossperfusion.

D. A particular type of cross circulation in which arterial blood of one organism D fully supplies the vascular system of another organism R. Simultaneously the venous blood of the receiver R returns to the venous system of the donor D. This procedure is intended for fully supporting the circulation of the receiver by the cardiocirculatory system of the donor. In order to support simultaneously his own circulation and that of the receiver, the donor has to be of a larger size. This procedure is usually called donor circulation.

tions do not include external pumps or flowmeters, the procedure is often called uncontrolled, or direct, or free cross-circulation. If pumps or flowmeters are interposed in the flow lines for the purposes of volumetric control, the procedure is called controlled, or indirect cross-circulation. Strictly speaking, cross-circulation should apply only to procedures of blood exchange in which two organisms are linked artery to vein in both directions (fig. 4, B).

Donor-circulation—A special type of cross-circulation in which one organism (donor) continuously supplies arterial blood to the arterial system of the other (receiver). The venous blood of the receiver is simultaneously returned to the venous system of the donor (fig. 4, D). Through such arrangement the donor maintains the circulation of both organisms. The heart and lung of the receiver can then be temporarily excluded to permit cardiac surgery under conditions of total heart–lung bypass.

Cross Transfusion—An interchange of blood between two organisms connected vein to vein (fig. 4, A). Blood is propelled from one organism to the other in the desired direction by means of a pump. The flow direction is reversed as needed. The expression "reciprocal blood transfer" is frequently employed with a synonymous meaning.

Cross Perfusion—A physiologic preparation in which the cardiovascular system of a donor supplies an isolated vascular bed in the receiver, and conversely (fig. 4, C).

Summarizing

The terminology of heart–lung bypass is still in flux. It is too early to take issue on the definition of words. The following general expressions are described only for an understanding of the technical language employed in this book: perfusion, extracorporeal circulation, heart–lung bypass, heart–lung machine, artificial heart, artificial lung, gas exchange device, pump–oxygenator, partial heart–lung bypass, partial perfusion, assisted circulation, isolation perfusion, regional perfusion, separate perfusion, right heart bypass, left heart bypass, endogenous oxygenation, duration of bypass, priming volume, pump oxygenator priming volume, hold-up, bypass circulatory volume, standby volume, coronary venous return, cardiotomy venous return, cross-circulation, donor-circulation, cross-transfusion, cross-perfusion. The two controversial expressions *inflow* and *outflow* are circumvented by using the simple descriptive language: venous drainage and arterial infusion.

II. Methods of Substituting for Cardiopulmonary Function

Since the advent of perfusion techniques in the early nineteenth century, a number of methods have been devised for maintaining life in animals deprived of their cardio-respiratory system. Many of these heart–lung bypass procedures have culminated in actual application to human beings for therapeutic purposes. They will be reviewed in this chapter.

ENDOGENOUS OXYGENATION

Nysten (1811) was the first physiologist to attempt extrapulmonary oxygenation in animals deprived of their respiratory function (fig. 5). In unanesthetized dogs, breathing pure nitrogen, Nysten injected up to 200 ml of oxygen intravenously. He succeeded in prolonging the survival time from 4 to 12 minutes as compared to the control animals, and by pulmonary gas analysis obtained some evidence of absorption of the oxygen given. Nevertheless, no animal could be kept alive for any long period of time by intravenous oxygenation alone. The procedure came to be known as "endogenous oxygenation" because the binding of oxygen to hemoglobin, though not performed in the lungs, was still carried out within the body.

In 1902, Gaertner demonstrated that the continuous intravenous injection of limited amounts of pure, electrolytically prepared oxygen is perfectly compatible with life. He therefore suggested this method for complementary oxygenation when the lungs are unable to fulfill their function satisfactorily. Numerous investigators after him concluded that in animals oxygen can be administered safely intravenously in quantities ranging between 1 and 2 ml./Kg./min. Since the normal oxygen requirement is on the order of 6 to 7 ml./Kg./min., the injection of 1 ml./Kg./min. should theoretically raise the oxygen content of the venous blood by approximately 1 vol. percent, provided the oxygen so administered is readily and immediately available to the red cells. Bourne and Smith (1927) however, observed that in quantities theoretically sufficient to alleviate hypoxemia, intravenous oxygen elicits the signs of pulmonary embolism, namely cardiac irregularity, systemic hypotension, and finally, right heart failure. As a result, the hypoxemic condition becomes worse rather than better under the treatment. Dick (1939) and Ziegler (1941) confirmed these views. Dick also found in normal animals that the arterial oxygen saturation decreases almost immediately upon intravenous injection of oxygen, the right ventricular pressure increases and a reflex hyperventilation occurs, even when the aortic pressure does not change.

Another approach to intravenous oxygenation was proposed in 1935 by Singh. He placed animals in a high pressure chamber and found that at twice normal atmospheric pressure (1520 mm Hg) about 30 to 40 per cent of the oxygen required by a cat could be introduced intravenously without any harmful effect. At four times normal atmospheric pressure (3040 mm Hg) a dog was kept alive for 16 minutes without taking in any oxygen through the lungs. This survival time was barely longer than that achieved by Nysten at normal atmospheric pressure a century before. Later, Singh and Shah (1940) demon-

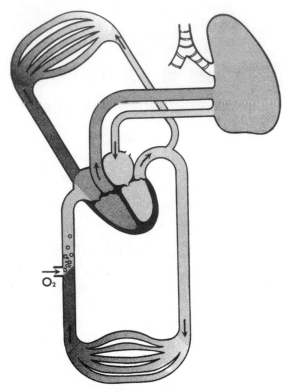

Fig. 5. Endogenous oxygenation. Oxygen is infused into a systemic vein, as indicated by the arrow and the bubbles in the inferior caval system. Venous blood (dark shading) is arterialized at the site of oxygen infusion (light shading). Mixing of this blood with venous blood from other parts of the body occurs in the right atrium. The right heart and pulmonary arterial tree are filled with partially arterialized blood (medium light shading).

strated that in man about 10 ml. of commercial oxygen or 20 ml. of pure, electrolytically prepared oxygen can be administered intravenously for 30 minutes without untoward effects. Used in critically ill patients, these amounts brought a distinct clinical improvement. Recently, Singh (1960) has taken advantage of hypothermia to increase the oxygen solubility in blood and simultaneously decrease the oxygen requirement during endogenous oxygenation.

It had been felt for a long time that a substantial improvement could be achieved if the size of the bubbles were reduced, so as to facilitate their absorption and decrease the risk of mechanical obstruction of the pulmonary vascular bed. In 1952 Lary devised a method by which minute oxygen bubbles could be injected into the venous circulation. With the aid of a wetting agent and heparin, bubbles were emitted from a porous filter into an artificial arteriovenous shunt. By this procedure dogs breathing pure nitrogen were kept alive for periods up to one hour. An attempt to use the organism as its own bubbling chamber under conditions of total heart–lung bypass was reported by Connolly, et al. (1958, b). These authors devised a special catheter which in the closed chest animal prevented any venous return to the right heart. They bubbled oxygen into the central veins and tried to drain the resulting foam into an extracorporeal circuit. The blood was then defoamed over silicone coated surfaces and reinjected continuously into the arterial tree. This ambitious goal met with only a partial success, owing mainly to the impairment of venous return and drainage by the foam.

In addition to the injection of gaseous oxygen into the veins, experiments have been performed using compounds which liberate free oxygen. Sodium peroxide solutions have been advocated for artificial oxygenation of the brain during circulatory arrest (Laewen and Sievers, 1910). Hydrogen peroxide may also release useful amounts of oxygen in the blood stream, though it was first reported to induce hypertension (Oliver and Murphy, 1920). In recent times intravenous oxygenation by hydrogen peroxide solutions has been revived by Abeatici, et al. (1958, 1959, a, b, c) and tested clinically. Species differences related to the amount of catalase present in the blood were uncovered. The procedure appeared to be of some help for additional oxygenation of patients suffering from gross reduction in their pulmonary function. However, the necessity of diluting the hydrogen peroxide with saline, in order to obtain a favorable gas exchange with the blood, precluded a prolonged use of this technique of oxygenation. Furthermore, it shared a drawback common to all techniques of endogenous oxygenation, namely that nothing is done about carbon dioxide elimination. One must therefore either rely on the lungs for increased CO_2 release, or face the difficulties associated with CO_2 retention.

Of experimental interest is the technique of "pervascular oxygenation" first described by Magnus (1902) and recently developed in Burns' laboratory: blood is removed from the vascular system and moist gaseous oxygen is simply injected in its place. Surprisingly enough, isolated organs can in this way be kept responsive for many hours. Since most tissues can utilize reserves of glycogen and fat, the distribution of oxygen alone meets their most urgent need. Evidence of oxygen utilization in carbohydrate metabolism has been furnished by Carter and Sabiston (1961). The problem of edema, which limits all long term perfusions, is at least partially solved. The amount of nutrients stored in the organs and the accumulation of metabolites are limiting factors (Mercker, 1959). This method of oxygenation was first used for supporting spinal cord (Bunzl, et al., 1954) or muscle (Burns, et al., 1958) preparations. It has been recently adapted to the isolated heart by Sabiston, et al. (1959), with maintenance of the heart beat up to 8 hours. Perfusion of the coronary arteries in situ with oxygen has been performed with later reversion to blood and reestablishment of the normal circulation. Retrograde perfusion of the heart through the coronary sinus is also efficient, but does not provide as strong a heart beat as coronary artery perfusion (Talbert et al., 1960). These studies indicate that oxygen perfused in the gaseous state can be utilized by the tissues. However, it is still too early to envision all the possible developments of this intriguing technique.

Summarizing

Many attempts have been made during the last 150 years to produce endogenous oxygenation of the blood by injecting oxygen directly into veins. Oxygen has been administered either in gaseous form or in solution of compounds such as hydrogen peroxide which readily release oxygen. Dogs breathing pure nitrogen were kept alive up to an hour by infusing minute oxygen bubbles into the venous circulation. Temporary beneficial effects of intravenous oxygen were also observed in human patients. Up to now, none of the procedures for endogenous oxygenation has proved efficient enough to replace pulmonary gas exchange completely.

CONTROLLED PERFUSION OF VITAL ORGANS

In view of the small amount of oxygen introduced by endogenous oxygenation, limitation of the perfusion of oxygenated blood to the most important organs, namely the brain and the heart, has been suggested. By appropriate cannulation, the brain or the heart can be vascularly isolated while remaining in situ. Their blood supply is secured by a pump from a reservoir bottle or from the arterial system of a donor while the systemic circulation is arrested. This technique has been conveniently named "controlled perfusion of vital organs" because the blood flow can be regulated in the absence of systemic circulation.

It has long been known that temporary arrest of the circulation is tolerated relatively well by most organs with the exception of the brain. In 1836, Cooper had observed that ligation of the carotid and vertebral arteries resulted in asphyxia and death within four to five minutes. However, if the arteries were only compressed and not divided, a release of the compression within this time limit permitted reestablishment of viable conditions. Brown-Séquard (1858) was actually the first to demonstrate directly that an isolated head could be maintained alive by arterial perfusion with oxygenated blood. Laewen and Sievers (1910) succeeded in having rabbits, whose heads had been vascularly isolated and perfused with oxygenated Ringer's solution, survive for five minutes. Tuffier (1920) suggested the injection of oxygenated Ringer's solution into the carotid artery to maintain cerebral circulation during cardiac surgery. In 1939 O'Shaughnessy also thought that the key to advance in cardiac surgery was the provision for an adequate cerebral blood flow while the heart was out of action. He succeeded in prolonging the duration of circulatory arrest up to 10 minutes by perfusing the brain with an oxygenated hemoglobin solution.

In studies initiated around 1935, Crafoord showed in dogs that the flow of blood to all organs except the brain could remain suspended for as long as 20 minutes with no sign of subsequent damage. Adequate cerebral circulation was maintained by anastomosing the carotid and jugular vessels to the corresponding vessels of another dog. In the same laboratory Bjørk (1948, a) attempted the perfusion of vascularly isolated dog heads with blood oxygenated by a mechanical gas exchange device. Using this technique brain perfusion through one of the common carotid arteries, the other being clamped, could be maintained for about 90 minutes with survival. However, it should be recalled that the vertebral arteries in the dog are large enough to provide adequate cerebral blood flow in the presence of bilateral carotid ligation. In Bjørk's experiments *complete* maintenance of the cerebral circulation by an artificial circuit, during total occlusion of all the vessels supplying the head, was usually not successful. Tosatti (1951) and Batezatti and Taddei (1953) had no greater success than Bjørk. Peniston and Richards (1955, b), however, reported a 50 per cent survival rate following brain perfusion by donor circulation. Parkins, et al., (1954), succeeded in preventing brain damage during circulatory arrest by perfusing the carotid arteries with cold blood, a procedure also used by Brockman and Fonkalsrud (1958) and Vishnefsky, et al., (1960).

The usefulness of isolated brain perfusion is often limited by the incidence of spontaneous ventricular fibrillation when the myocardium is not given enough oxygen to meet its own requirement. Although a myocardium deprived of oxygen may be revived after a far longer period than a brain (one hour or more), it is initially unable to support the circulation. The return to a normal state, with the heart acting as an efficient pump, may then require some external intervention, such as electrical defibrillation, cardiac massage and intraventricular injection of epinephrine. All of these procedures involve considerable hazard. Therefore artificial coronary perfusion has often been combined with artificial oxygenation of the brain in an attempt to extend the period of suspended systemic circulation (Kunlin, 1948; Burstein and Binet, 1950; Gaertner, et al., 1955; Massimo and Boffi, 1958). Such a procedure can be successful, particularly under hypothermic conditions, but dual perfusion of the brain and the heart necessitates complicated cannulations. Furthermore, the usefulness of the method is limited by the progressive ischemia of the spinal chord which occurs at normal body temperature when the descending aorta is not perfused for more than 15 to 20 minutes. In recent years the procedure of combined brain and coronary perfusion has been successfully employed in hypothermic patients by Kimoto, et al. (1956, 1960) and Sakakibara (1957).

Controlled perfusion of the vital organs under conditions of circulatory arrest has a major drawback. It necessarily involves an anaerobic environment for most of the body tissues. The amount of energy available does not then suffice to maintain function, except for a very short period. A minimal metabolic level may persist and preserve the *viability* of the cells, though not their specific *function*, depending upon their energy expenditure, energy reserves, rate of glycolysis, rate of phosphocreatin catabolism, and other factors. The notion of metabolism of preservation (*Erhaltungsumsatz*), introduced by Schneider and reviewed by him in 1959, explains the possible revival of organic function after long periods of tissue asphyxia. This concept implies the local accumulation of acid metabolites in the ischemic tissues (*see* Chapter XIV). Thus, when a normal arterial supply to the whole circulation is re-established, the temporarily stored end products of anaerobic metabolism are washed out and a tide of acid metabolites floods the heart and brain, endangering their performance at the time when it is most urgently needed. In fact, Schneider has shown that the period during which the brain can be revived after complete circulatory arrest is as long as 8 to 10 minutes. This period is reduced to four minutes when the whole body undergoes circulatory arrest, because the asphyxia associated with cardiac arrest makes it impossible for the circulatory system to recover its performance immediately. Therefore normal blood pressure levels cannot be reached during the first few minutes of recovery and eventually the survival time of the brain is encroached upon. A prolongation of the survival time of the whole organism can be obtained by adequate treatment of the transient cardiac failure during early recovery. Brockman and Jude (1960) have reached a similar conclusion.

In spite of their limited clinical applicability, the studies of circulatory arrest with simultaneous or subsequent perfusion of vital organs have exerted a remarkable impact on our physiological thinking. For years it has been accepted that the asphyxia which accompanies circulatory arrest exerts its deleterious effect *during* the period of suspended circulation. It now became increasingly evident that the damage actually occurs *afterwards*, and can be prevented or reversed by proper means such as artificial perfusion or therapeutic cooling.

This new physiologic concept which may modify the prevailing approach to a number of clinical situations has evolved from research in various areas, i.e., the work of Russian physiologists in resuscitation by artificial circulation, the relating of metabolic levels to the revival of organic function by the school of Schneider and the clinical demonstration that brain damage from otherwise lethal hypoxia can be prevented by lowering the temperature of the organism after the hypoxic period.

Summarizing

The brain, the heart and the spinal chord are the first organs to suffer from a lack of oxygen supply in case of circulatory arrest. Vascular isolation and temporary perfusion of vital organs in situ while the rest of the organism is left without circulation has been attempted repeatedly. Survival has been improved by combining controlled perfusion with local hypothermia. However, the drawback of perfusions limited to vital organs is that the other organs eventually suffer from lack of oxygen. This consideration limits severely the period of tolerance of the whole organism for the procedure.

DONOR CIRCULATION

Donor circulation is a special type of cross circulation which is of practical importance for heart–lung bypass (see fig. 4, D). Fredericq (1890) is credited with having introduced into physiology the techniques of cross circulation. He used paired dogs or rabbits and made glass connections from the proximal carotid artery of each animal to the distal carotid artery of the other. Hedon (1909, 1910) also cross circulated blood from the proximal to the distal carotid artery. He used for this procedure the Payr's cannula, a metal tube whose inner surface has been walled with a stretched segment of a fresh jugular vein. Thereby the blood did not come in contact with foreign substances, but only with the intima of blood vessels, so that the difficulties of clotting in the connecting circuit were temporarily overcome. Bazett and Quinby (1920) reported a method for cross circulating the entire cardiac output from one heart to another and vice-versa. They introduced scales to control the shift of blood from one animal to the other and found that: "The animal in better condition bleeds into the other", a phenomenon which has been rediscovered several times since. Nyiri (1926) and Thalimer, et al. (1938) used cross transfusion in attempts to lower the blood urea level of a nephrectomized dog paired with a normal partner. When the reciprocal blood transfer was performed at low flow rates, the procedure could be carried over long periods: Firor (1931) relates two instances in which the exchange of blood was maintained for more than 6 days. In intact, unanesthetized dogs, Egdahl (1955) achieved flows of 200-750 ml./min. for 6 to 24 hours without external regulation of flow. However, equal size of the connecting tubings and cannulae was found to be of paramount importance for balancing the blood flows between the two animals. Other investigators felt the necessity of some artificial regulation of flow and therefore introduced controlled cross-circulation techniques. Anrep (1925) observed that one animal bleeds into the other unless flows are equalized. He used a heart lung preparation which afforded complete control over flow and pressures to study the regulation of the circulation under more precisely known conditions. Pumps (Salisbury, 1949; Warden, et al., 1954, a, b), flowmeters (Little, et al., 1947; Brecher, et al., 1955), expansion collars around the connecting lines so as to regulate their diameter (Jones, et al., 1955), or zero reading scales (Peniston and Richards, 1955, a; Brecher, et al., 1955) served to assure the equality of flow in both lines from donor to recipient and back again from recipient to donor (*see* review of older literature in Wiggers, 1950). The procedure was repeatedly applied in man in attempts to clear through the kidneys and liver of a healthy donor a toxic substance formed or retained in the organism of his sick partner (Duncan, et al., 1940;

Vecchietti, 1948, 1953; Salisbury, et al., 1950, 1952). At present there is not much prospect for practical use of cross transfusion in humans because more convenient methods are available.

In order to apply the principle of controlled cross-circulation to man for the purpose of heart–lung bypass, a simple extracorporeal circuit is required (fig. 6). Blood from a peripheral artery of the donor (usually the femoral artery) is infused into the aorta of the recipient by means of a pump. After passage through the various capillary beds, the blood is collected from the superior and inferior caval veins of the recipients and returned through tubing to the donor's veins with the aid of a pump. Details of cannulations required for total heart–lung bypass and for left heart bypass have been adequately discussed by Southworth and Peirce (1952).

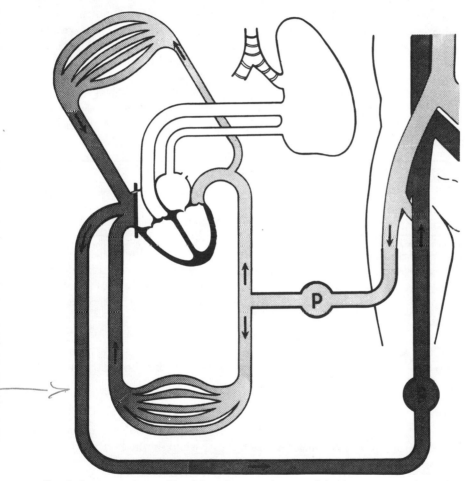

Fig. 6. Donor circulation. Blood from the arterial system of the donor is pumped into the arterial system of the receiver. Meanwhile, the blood accumulating in the venous system of the receiver is prevented from entering the right heart cavities, and directed towards the venous system of the donor. Thereby the heart and lungs of the receiver are excluded from the circulation. Since the donor must carry simultaneously his own circulation and that of the donor, the organisms must be different in size. An adult would usually act as a donor for a child.

It is obvious that such a system must be balanced so as to avoid exsanguination or overtransfusion of one member of the pair. Fluctuations in the recipient's venous return often limit the satisfactory control of a donor circulation. As already pointed out by Andreasen and Watson (1953) the venous return available from the recipient with the heart and lungs excluded is variable and unpredictable. Apparently neurogenic or chemogenic fluctuations in venomotor activity result in blood pooling in the peripheral parts of the circulatory system. When this occurs, or when the patient loses blood during the cardiotomy, the mechanical pump cannot remove enough blood from him and the two-way circulation becomes unbalanced. In order to make the venous blood flow back to the donor independent of fluctuations in the venous return from the recipient, it is best to drain the recipient's blood by gravity into a reservoir. From there it is pumped at a constant flow rate to the donor. This arrangement provides for the continuity of blood return to the donor in case of temporary decrease of the amount drained from the recipient. The rate of arterial infusion is then carefully gauged so as to be as close as possible to the rate of venous return, while remaining sufficient to maintain adequate brain and myocardial support in the patient.

Donor-circulation for the purpose of open heart surgery has been developed in the experimental laboratory by Kerr, et al. (1952), Southworth and Peirce (1952), Andreasen and Watson (1953), Warden et al. (1954, 1955c), Jones et al. (1955), Zacouto and Coraboeuf (1955) and Petrovskii and Solov'ev (1956). It has been used with conspicuous success for open heart surgery in humans (Lillehei, et al., 1955 a, b, c). Total heart–lung bypass has been achieved for periods of up to 40 minutes with perfusion of the patient's body at flow rates below normal but still adequate for survival. No complicated machinery or judgments are needed to maintain the patient's homeostasis since the donor's circulation warrants this complex control automatically. However, the small volumes of flow obtainable without overstressing the donor limit the usefulness of the procedure to relatively short periods. Acidosis due to insufficient perfusion of the recipient develops when the procedure is unduly prolonged. The hazard involved for the donor must also be considered. In these procedures, he is anesthetized and may become exsanguinated, unless the bidirectional flow is accurately balanced (Brecher, et al., 1955). The risks involved probably outweigh the benefits of homeostasis maintenance. Since the main function of the donor is to act as an oxygenator, donor circulation has been largely abandoned in favor of mechanical devices for gas exchanges.

Summarizing

Blood can be continuously exchanged between two animals or humans by linking their circulatory systems. This technique, when applied for the purpose of total heart–lung bypass is known as donor-circulation. It involves usually a large donor (adult) and a smaller recipient or patient (child). The venous blood from the patient is prevented from entering his heart and lungs, and diverted into the venous system of the donor. Simultaneously, the circulatory system of the donor provides arterial blood to perfuse the arterial tree of the patient. An important virtue of donor circulation is the maintenance by the donor of homeostasis in the recipient. One of the drawbacks lies in the danger that the donor may be unnoticeably exsanguinated if the two-way blood flow should become unbalanced.

RESERVOIR PERFUSION

The simplest of the methods permitting total cardio-pulmonary bypass utilizes continuous perfusion of the arterial system from a reservoir of oxygenated blood. To maintain the patient's blood volume constant, an equivalent quantity of venous blood is simultaneously removed from the superior and inferior caval veins (fig. 7). Two mechanical pumps or a single pump with dual action (Warden et al., 1955) serve to control the exchange between the patient and the arterial and venous reservoirs. Instead of pumping, gravity can also be used to infuse and collect the blood (Callaghan et al., 1955).

The application of reservoir perfusion to open heart surgery followed the demonstration that venous inflow into the heart can be arrested for 15 minutes provided a minimum of perfusion is maintained by arterial transfusion (Berkas, et al., 1954; Cookson and Costas-Durieux, 1954; Bjørk, 1956). In experimental work arterial blood is obtained directly from a donor animal, which can provide more than its own blood volume if it is given stored blood at the same time.

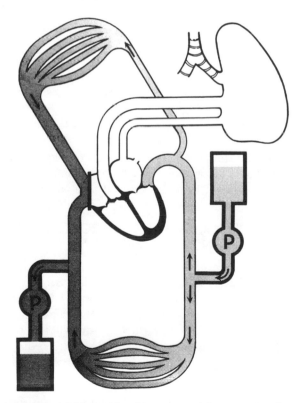

Fig. 7. Reservoir perfusion. Venous blood is prevented from entering the right heart cavities. Instead, it is drained by a mechanical pump into a venous reservoir. The arterial tree is perfused from a reservoir with arterialized blood collected prior to the procedure.

For human surgery blood is used that has been withdrawn from a vein of an extremity which has been heated to about 45° C. for 15 or 20 minutes (Warden, et al., 1955 b). Since under such conditions arterio-venous shunts open, this blood is almost as high in oxygen content as arterial blood. The venous blood can also be oxygenated in vitro, using special containers devised for the purpose (Brown, et al., 1956; Button, et al., 1957). Special care must then be taken to avoid bubble formation, and to remove any froth which may have formed before infusing the blood into the arterial system of the patient.

The limiting factor of reservoir perfusion is the amount of blood available. No matter how simple and safe, the reservoir perfusion puts the surgeon under the pressure of time and should be reserved for short operations in small infants: 10 liters of collected arterialized blood suffice to oxygenate an infant for only 20 minutes at a flow rate of 500 ml./min.

It is also possible to collect venous blood from the patient during the operation and to reoxygenate it outside of the body. This blood can then be used again for arterial transfusion. Under such conditions, the only limiting factor is the initial supply of oxygenated blood needed to sustain the patient until the first container of venous blood has been collected and oxygenated (Brown, et al., 1956). The amount of blood necessary to start this procedure is still considerable. It is larger than that necessary for most of the currently used heart–lung machines. Despite its intriguing simplicity "intermittent extracorporeal oxygenation" therefore offers no marked advantage over the use of a pump-oxygenator.

Summarizing

The vital functions of the organism have been successfully maintained by perfusing the systemic arterial tree from a reservoir of oxygenated blood while the venous blood is drained to the outside. Meanwhile operations can be performed on a heart that is temporarily excluded from the circulation. The duration of the perfusion is limited by the quantity of blood available and the necessary flow rate. The venous blood can be oxygenated in special collecting containers and then reinfused into the arterial tree to prolong the operation time.

HOMOLOGOUS AND HETEROLOGOUS LUNG OXYGENATION

The isolated lung of an animal, ventilated and perfused adequately, was among the first oxygenating devices proposed (fig. 8). With regard to the efficiency of gas exchange and the gentleness of blood handling, it still remains a standard for comparison of mechanical systems. The technique of extracorporeal gas exchange based upon the use of an isolated lung is known as "homologous" or "heterologous lung oxygenation", according to whether or not the isolated lung belongs to an animal of the same species as the one perfused.

Jacobj (1895) then working in Schmiedeberg's laboratory in Strassburg, was seemingly the first to devise an elaborate perfusion apparatus using extracorporeal lung oxygenation. By a suitable arrangement of stopcocks and connectors, the venous blood issuing from the organ studied was directed into an excised lung, came back oxygenated, and was re-used

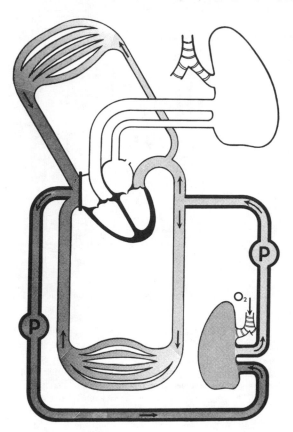

Fig. 8. Homologous or heterologous lung oxygenation. The arrangement of the circuit is the same as for total heart–lung bypass with a mechanical oxygenator (fig. 2), except that the isolated lung of another animal is used instead of the artificial gas exchange device. The foreign lung is ventilated with oxygen. Venous blood enters the lung through the pulmonary artery. Once arterialized the blood leaves from the pulmonary veins or left atrium and is pumped into the arterial tree of the perfused organism.

for continuous perfusion of the organ. To Brukhonenko should be given the credit of having developed the method to a point of perfection which permitted total body perfusion in dogs at flows up to 2.5 L/min. His heart–lung machine (the "autojector," fig. 9) first described in Russian, remained largely unmentioned in the Western literature, though accounts of its design and performance were available (Brukhonenko, 1929 a, b; Brukhonenko and Tchetchuline, 1929). Total heart–lung bypass with the autojector permitted maintaining the animals responsive for 2 to 3 hours. However, the Russian physiologists were strongly influenced by the eighteenth and nineteenth century controversies on the nature and conditions of "excitability." Henceforth, their main attention was focused on the resuscitation aspects of artificial circulation rather than on the conditions of artificial maintenance of respiration and circulation for cardiac surgery. Hemingway (1931) and Beland, et al. (1938) stressed the filtering capacity of an excised lung inserted in a perfusion circuit. Barcroft (1933) used it in the first important hemodynamic studies of the totally perfused organism. In a review of all perfusion techniques available at the time, Fleisch (1935) concluded that the homologous lung is the best oxygenator and described an ingenious device for automatically controlled perfusion of isolated organs

Where attempts at total heart–lung bypass were directed towards surgical application, Terebinskii (1940) and Tosatti (1949) felt the technique of homol-

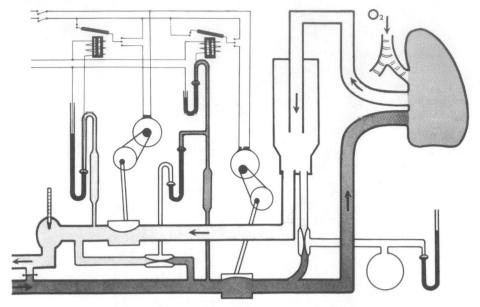

Fig. 9. "Autojector" of Brukhonenko (1929) employing the principle of homologous lung oxygenation for regional or total body perfusion. The venous blood is aspirated in the venous line by means of a diaphragm pump, and injected into the pulmonary artery of an isolated ventilated lung. The arterial blood drains from the pulmonary veins into a reservoir, from which it is injected under pressure into the perfused organ or organism. On the positive pressure side of each pump there are arterio-venous shunt lines which are controlled by external cuffs under a known pressure. If the organism or the lung oppose too much resistance to perfusion, blood flows through the shunt. Conversely, if there is not enough venous return from the perfused organism, leading to venous collapse, blood will be aspirated from the arterial line into the venous lines. Electromagnets are used in conjunction with level sensing devices in order to arrest the pumps when pressures prevailing in the circuit are too high. (Redrawn from Brukhonenko, 1929a)

ogous lung oxygenation to be far superior to mechanical devices. Groups led by Potts (Potts, et al., 1951; 1952; Fisher, et al., 1952), Wesolowski (Sugarman, et al., 1951; Wesolowski, et al., 1952) and Mustard (Mustard, et al., 1952; Mustard, 1955) reported successful maintenance of life by the combination of a homologous lung with a mechanical heart while cardiac operations were performed in the experimental animal. Most of the early difficulties were caused by unpredictable deterioration of the lung performance during the course of perfusion. Campbell, et al. (1955) drew attention to some points essential to the maintenance of the preparation: patency of the pulmonary veins so as to assure free drainage, a compression chamber for depulsation in the pulmonary artery limb of the circuit, and care with the ventilatory mechanics of the isolated lung or lobe. Even with these precautions pulmonary edema frequently resulted within one hour. In our experience the onset of pulmonary edema could be much delayed by the use of intermittent positive-negative pressure respiration, so as to decrease the mean pulmonary arterial pressure without diminishing the blood flow rate.

The procedure of heterologous lung oxygenation has been applied in human surgery. Mustard (1955), Campbell, et al. (1956), and Guasp, et al. (1956) used dog or monkey lungs meticulously washed by perfusing them with dextran. However, the need of a circuit as complex as that for an artificial heart–lung machine, the irregular performance of the lung oxygenator and worst of all, the danger of infection with microorganisms normally present in animal tissues seemed to preclude the general use of animal lungs in human surgery. In the experimental laboratory this technique remains the cheapest and most readily available method of oxygenation. The preparations proposed by Edwards (1957) and Waldhausen, et al. (1957) are actually the best. With the lungs remaining in the chest and the inflow and outflow cannulae introduced through the ventricles, the delicate lung structures are optimally protected from undue trauma. The homologous lung preparation is also better suited than most artificial lungs for the purpose of measuring gas exchange directly.

Summarizing

Lungs of the same species (homologous lungs) and those of species other than the perfused organism (heterologous lungs) have been used for oxygenating blood. The patient's venous blood enters the isolated lung via the pulmonary artery. Arterialized blood is collected from the pulmonary veins for infusion into the patient's arterial tree. Danger of early edema formation in the isolated lung and of infection of the patient by microorganisms, which cannot be eradicated from the animal lung, limits this method in human surgery. However, it is still widely employed in the experimental laboratory.

RIGHT HEART BYPASS

In view of the difficulties encountered in artificial oxygenation of blood, several workers attempted in the early 1950's cardiac surgery using the patient's own lungs for gas exchange. One of the methods devised consisted of side-tracking the venous blood around the right heart cavities and infusing it with a pump into the pulmonary artery (fig. 10). The technique of right heart bypass, first described by Dusser de Barenne (1919), was applied by Sewell and Glenn (1950) and Leeds, et al. (1950, 1951) for supporting the pulmonary circulation during a period of functional exclusion of the right ventricle. The venous blood was withdrawn from the superior and inferior caval veins and infused by a pump into a lobar branch of the right pulmonary artery through a cannula directed centrally. In that way, only a small part of the lung parenchyma was isolated from the circulation, while most of its surface served for gas exchange. The right ventricle and, upon clamping, the root of the pulmonary artery were free of blood, creating ideal conditions for pulmonary valvular surgery.

The circuit required for such a procedure was remarkably simple and its priming volume small. The qualities of the lung as a large oxygenator, a filter and a bubble trap are unsurpassed. The difficulties resided in the cannulation of the thin-walled pulmonary blood vessels and in the possible occurrence of vasospastic phenomena in the perfused lung, resulting in a decreased efficiency of gas transfer or even in pulmonary edema. Dodrill, et al. (1952a) observed that reduction of the normal tension on the right atrial wall during right heart bypass reflexly initiated a slowing of the heart and a decrease in systemic arterial pressure due to peripheral vasodilation. However, the effect was rarely so pronounced as to interfere with the perfusion of the coronary vessels which supplied the still actively pumping left ventricle, and the systemic circulation was not greatly endangered. The technique of right heart bypass was also studied in the experimental laboratory by Provenzale and Tonelli (1951) and Felipozzi, et al. (1957). Wesolowski, et al. (1953b) demonstrated that the efficiency of pulmonary gas exchange is independent of the pulsatile or non-pulsatile nature of blood flow. The performance characteristics of the right heart bypass preparation in terms of hemodynamics have been recently discussed by Grodins, et al. (1960). Dodrill, et al. (1953) were seemingly the first to apply the procedure clinically for the correction of congenital pulmonary stenosis. Right heart bypass has not gained widespread acceptance owing to the scarcity of cases in which it can safely be employed.

Summarizing

In bypassing the right heart, blood is withdrawn from the central veins and pumped mechanically into the pulmonary artery so that the normal lung provides oxygenation. Surgery on the right heart and pulmonary outflow tract has been successfully performed during such shunting. Pulmonary edema and difficulties in the cannulation of pulmonary vessels are occasionally encountered and limit the practicality of this method.

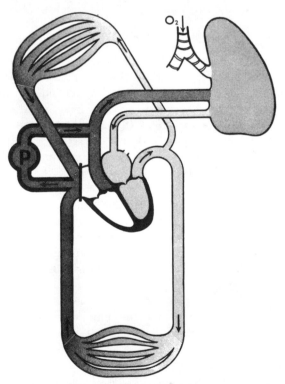

Fig. 10. Right heart bypass. Venous blood is prevented from entering the right heart cavities. Instead it is channeled by a mechanical pump (P) into the pulmonary artery, from which it follows its normal course through the lungs. The right heart cavities are intended to be bloodless (white area).

LEFT HEART BYPASS

Artificial circuits for bypassing the left heart cavities have been developed using a similar approach to that for bypassing the right heart cavities (Sirak, et al., 1950; Burstein and Binet, 1950; Wesolowski and Welch, 1951; Dodrill, et al., 1952; Schebitz, et al. 1954). Blood already arterialized in the lungs is drained from the pulmonary veins or the left atrium and delivered under pressure into a peripheral artery, thereby excluding the left ventricle and the aortic root from the circulation (fig. 11).

The major technical difficulty of left heart bypass resides in the collection of the pulmonary venous blood. Open gravity drainage of the left atrium is preferred by Austen and Shaw (1960) and Snyder, et al. (1960), because the anatomic structures concerned are very thin and collapse readily when suction is applied for the drainage of blood. Furthermore, the left atrium, which can be considered as a large collecting vein, is connected to the left ventricle in such a way that blood is easily lost through the mitral orifice. This difficulty may be overcome by an expanding mechanical diaphragm which occludes the mitral ring (Sirak, et al., 1950). It can also be avoided by direct cannulation of the left pulmonary veins, after the right pulmonary artery has been clamped so as to channel all the pulmonary blood flow through the left lung alone (Kantrowitz, et al., 1950, 1951; Clowes, 1951, 1952; Provenzale and

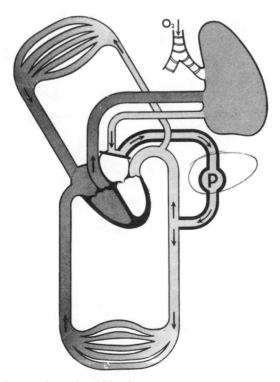

Fig. 11. Left heart bypass. Arterialized blood returning from the lungs is prevented from entering the left heart chambers. Instead it is collected and infused into the arterial tree by a mechanical pump (P). Depending on the site of infusion, the direction of arterial blood flow may be reversed in some areas of the body (indicated by arrows). The left heart cavities are intended to be bloodless.

Tonelli, 1951). In view of the extreme efficiency of gas transfer across the pulmonary membrane, Peirce and Southworth (1953) have directed the entire pulmonary artery flow exclusively into the left lower lobe, and collected the blood from the left lower pulmonary veins into a small elastic reservoir which supplied the pump. In this procedure, no trauma of major consequence should be inflicted to pulmonary structures since the gas exchanging lobe is simply removed after the bypass.

Other hemodynamic problems are involved when the circulation is maintained with an extracorporeal left ventricle. According to Dodrill, et al. (1952), the removal of the normal distension of the left atrium and ventricle by the suction of the pump does not initiate any reflex effect upon the circulation, as compared to the effects produced by right heart bypass. Observations by Rose, et al. (1956) indicate that vasodilation should appear only when the right ventricle begins to fail and *both* circulations are supported by the extracorporeal pump. During left heart bypass, a pressure of 80 to 100 mm. Hg. in the ascending aorta suffices to maintain a normal coronary flow, while pressures of 40 to 60 mm. Hg. in the carotid and femoral arteries allow the maintenance of a stable preparation for one hour (Vowles et al., 1958). The hemodynamic problems involved in left ventricular bypass in the case of aortic insufficiency have been ably discussed by Clauss, et al. (1959).

The main pitfalls of left heart bypass reside in the repair of thin-walled pulmonary vessels after cannulation, in the complete collection of arterial blood with a catheter introduced through the left atrium and, finally, in the occurrence of pulmonary edema if the lungs are not properly drained. A practical limitation to the application of unilateral bypass procedures in human surgery has been the hopeless situation the surgeon might face if an undiagnosed defect (shunt or abnormal vessel) should preclude the use of the circuit envisioned. From this point of view, total heart–lung bypass by means of a heart–lung machine offers a safer approach to the surgical treatment of congenital abnormalities. However, there may be a place for unilateral bypass procedures in the treatment of acquired diseases where diagnostic errors are less likely to occur.

Summarizing

In left heart bypass, arterialized blood drained from either pulmonary veins or the left atrium is mechanically pumped into a peripheral artery. Cannulation difficulties and the danger of unanticipated intra-cardiac shunts limit the applicability of this method in the surgical correction of congenital defects.

AUTOGENOUS LUNG OXYGENATION

Complete cardiac bypass with autogenous lung oxygenation is a natural development of right heart bypass and left heart bypass, since it is essentially a combination of these two procedures. Bilateral cardiac bypass is achieved by draining the blood from the caval veins and infusing it through a pump back into the pulmonary arterial bed. After arterialization in the lungs the blood is drained from the left atrium and infused by a second pump into the systemic arterial tree (fig. 12).

Complete cardiac bypass with lung oxygenation features both the advantages and disadvantages of the unilateral bypass procedures: the circuit is reasonably simple and short, the need for priming fluid limited and the oxygenating performance excellent. It was therefore proposed as one possible approach to open heart surgery in the pioneer years of extracorporeal circulation (Wesolowski and Welch, 1951, 1952; Dodrill, et al., 1952). The large bulk of the multiple cannulations and the unpredictability of pulmonary vasomotor reactions when the lungs are perfused under abnormal conditions seemed later to diminish the enthusiasm for this highly physiologic technique of oxygenation (Dennis, 1956). Difficulties in balancing precisely the output of the two pumps, although not fully recognized, contributed to the discouragement felt by many workers. At the period when low flow perfusions were in favor ("azygos principle"), Cohen, et al. (1953, 1954) simplified the cannulation technique by channeling all the blood drained from the central veins into one pulmonary lobe and collecting the oxygenated blood directly from the corresponding pulmonary vein. Since difficulties were experienced in pulmonary venous drainage by pump suction, Read, et al. (1956) separated the region of the mitral orifice from the area of the venous confluence in the left atrium by means of a non-crushing clamp, and drained this collecting chamber by simple gravity through soft latex tubing. Campbell, et al. (1955), carried the technique to its

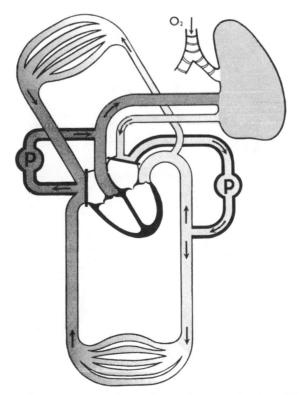

Fig. 12. Autogenous lung oxygenation. Through a combination of right and left heart bypass, the lungs of the patient are still able to provide regular gas exchange. Right and left heart cavities are clamped off at atrial or veno-atrial levels and are bloodless.

logical conclusion: they resected one pulmonary lobe of the patient, inserted it as oxygenator in an external circuit and collected the blood flowing freely out of the pulmonary veins into a reservoir, from which it could be infused into the arterial tree. Despite the success obtained by the Minneapolis school, autogenous lung oxygenation fell temporarily into oblivion.

More recently, however, some of the early investigators have come back to bilateral cardiac bypass with autogenous lung oxygenation (Mustard, et al., 1958; Blanco, et al., 1958, 1959; Létac and Létac, 1959). More refined cannulation techniques and increased knowledge of pulmonary circulation have permitted excellent results in animal experiments and have led to new clinical trials. Using perfusion flows which approximate the resting cardiac output, the best results are obtained using both lungs as oxygenators rather than one lung or one lobe (Blanco, et al., 1958). Gravity venous drainage has replaced pump suction. Open reservoirs, however, introduce the risk of air embolism when the amount of blood collected does not match the output of the pump.

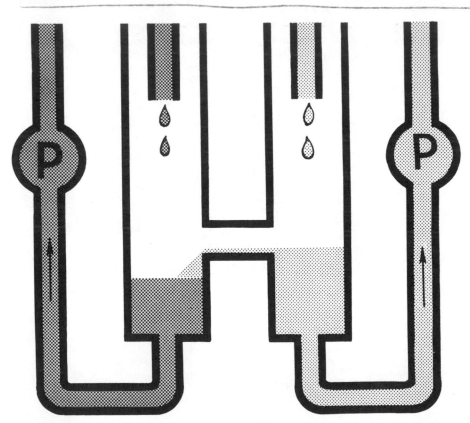

Fig. 13. Cross linked reservoir system used in connection with autogenous lung oxygenation. Venous blood (dark shading) drained by gravity from the caval veins is collected in a reservoir, from which it is infused by means of a pump (P) into the pulmonary artery to perfuse the patient's own lungs. Arterialized blood (light shading) drained by gravity from the left atrium is collected in a reservoir, from where it is infused by means of another pump into a peripheral artery to perfuse the patient's body. Any imbalance of the right and left circuit is counteracted by an overflow between the two reservoirs (modified after Cass and Ross, 1959).

An elegant solution to the problem of temporary imbalance is provided by the linked reservoir system proposed by Cass and Ross (1959). Having noted that in a bilateral bypass circuit, when one reservoir empties, the other tends to fill up, they fitted the reservoirs with a cross-link of plastic tubing (fig. 13). If either reservoir then fills above the level of the link, the excess blood automatically flows over to replenish the deficient chamber. The logical maneuver, to avoid an external "right to left shunt", is then to set the "right ventricle" pump at a slightly faster rate than the "left ventricle" pump. Another method for avoiding possible gas embolism consists of using closed plastic bags as drainage reservoirs (Holt, et al., 1960).

Autogenous lung oxygenation has been used recently as a means of gas exchange in the achievement of deep hypothermia (Ross, 1959, b; Shields and Lewis, 1959; Aletras, et al., 1960; Garcia Ortis, et al. 1960; Darbinian and Portnoy, 1961). Clinical application has been reported by Drew, et al. (1959), Gordon, et al. (1960) and Bjørk (1960). The method also seems particularly suited for prolonged bypass periods because it is definitely less traumatic to the blood than is the artificial heart–lung machine. Only time will tell whether these advantages outweigh the necessity for the extra cannulations involved in the autogenous lung oxygenation method.

Summarizing

When the patient's own lung serves for oxygenation, the entire heart can be bypassed by combining two separate circuits: one leading from the central veins to the pulmonary arterial bed (right heart bypass) and the other from the left atrium to the systemic arterial tree (left heart bypass). Since lungs are less traumatic oxygenators than mechanical gas exchange devices and require less priming volume, this method is sometimes preferred for prolonged cardiac surgery in man despite the technical difficulties of multiple cannulations.

III. Materials Used in Extracorporeal Circuits

It is almost impossible to handle blood without damaging its components to some extent. In fact, no man-made surface can closely approximate the natural environment provided for blood by the inner lining of the blood vessels. The continuously renewed contact between blood and a variety of foreign materials (pump, oxygenator parts and tubing) required for extracorporeal circulation creates a situation that is innately unphysiologic. Therefore the selection of construction materials is one of the major problems confronting designers of heart–lung machines.

Scattered information on testing of old and new substances is available in reports of a few studies dealing with the technology of perfusion. Unfortunately, however, very few scientists have devoted the necessary attention to the systemic investigation of construction materials. Even fewer have bothered to publish their observations. These problems are, therefore, approached empirically by most groups interested in development, resulting in a considerable duplication of work. This chapter constitutes an attempt to collect the information presently available—scant though it is—with the hope that it will stimulate other workers in the field to present their data.

EFFECT OF MATERIALS ON BLOOD

Bain (1903), working in T. G. Brodie's laboratory, seems to have been the first to undertake a systematic study of blood trauma by a perfusion apparatus. He established on experimental grounds that rubber and glass were the least traumatic materials available at the time. He also was able to trace some hemolysis to the fact that his pump was made of vulcanite and brass. His observations supported the common belief that smoothness and chemical inertness rank first among the desirable qualities of blood containers. In a review of perfusion techniques of 1920, F. Müller devotes only a few scattered lines to the construction materials for external blood circuits. The data collected by the early perfusionists substantiated the excellence of pure latex gum whenever resilient material was required. Tainter (1932) suggested aluminum and monel, a nickel alloy, as convenient metals for artificial heart–lung machines. In 1938, however, Beland, et al., pointed out the toxicity of aluminum in an extracorporeal circuit, thereby dimming the hopes which the advent of light metals had first elicited. More recently, stainless steel has emerged as the best metal, only to find itself competing with completely new organic materials such as polyethylenes, polyurethanes, methacrylates, nylons, epoxy resins, organosilicon and organofluorine compounds (Hirschboeck, 1941; Donovan, 1949; Blunt, 1959; Hufnagel, 1959; Perkins, et al., 1960).

Materials found empirically to be the least traumatic to blood have certain properties in common: a high degree of chemical inertness and resistance to corrosion; a naturally smooth surface, or polishable to a mirror-like finish; finally, a low surface energy, related to a physical quality loosely defined as "unwettability." It is not clear at present which of the features, viz., chemical inertness, smoothness of the walls or water repellency is primary in determining the most effective blood handling qualities of different materials. Obviously, a high degree of smoothness is a first requirement to avoid local turbulence and deposition of fibrin or red cell ghosts (Hufnagel, 1959). The development of plastic substances and of water repellent coatings for other materials has led to the view that the physical properties of the surfaces have a causative relationship to the improved preservation of blood. This belief is often referred to as Lampert's rule, after the German hematologist (Neubauer and Lampert, 1930; Lampert, 1931) who first established that the capacity of a surface in delaying coagulation is usually inversely proportional to the force of adhesion exerted between the surface and water (*Benetzbarkeit*). Attractive and widespread as this view may be, it should be pointed out that there is no general evidence to support it (Strumia, et al., 1959). It is only confirmed by the measurements of surface profiles in tubing materials reported by Stewart and Sturridge (1959). Direct studies of the wettability of different polymers (Kawasaki, 1960) demonstrate that they do not range in the order expected from their blood handling properties. Furthermore, the fact that only a few of the synthetic materials developed have been found usable for blood preservation, despite similar physical properties, points to the importance of the chemical nature of the surface. The harmful effect of numerous materials may then be due to chemical radicals present in the wall with which blood comes into contact, or more likely, to substances leaching out of the container walls into the blood. Finally, the fact that roughness, wettability and chemical changes in the surfaces are interrelated (Allan, 1957; Allan and Roberts, 1959; Portela, 1961) points to the difficulty of ascribing the blood handling properties of materials to only one of their physico-chemical properties.

There is a great deal of confusion in the medical literature regarding the effects of various substances on blood. In fact, one may promote any one of them by proper selection of references. There are several reasons for these controversies. First is the marked progress which has taken place in glass manufacturing and siliconizing techniques. The second element of confusion, and possibly the most important, is the constant introduction of new and different polymers which vary widely in their chemical reactivity. The biologic evaluation of the materials often has been unable to keep pace with technologic progress. Therefore, a situation has developed in which some substances have proven empirically commendable before the reasons for their success could be established. Even more confusing in publications is the lack of identification tags for many of the synthetic polymers tested. Without the code number provided by the manufacturer, giving full information on the plasticizers, stabilizers and other chemicals used in the manufacturing process, the precise nature of the material used cannot be recognized. As stressed by McGregor (1960), if the medical evaluation of polymers is to keep up with the rapid pace of industrial development, it is imperative that any statement about specific substances made today can be precisely interpreted by the reader of tomorrow. Failure to ensure this destroys the usefulness of conclusions reached after great expenditure of time, talent and money.

A major reason for much of the prevailing confusion is that there are no universally accepted criteria for establishing experimentally which materials are best. The methods proposed can be arranged in three classes, which all pertain to a different facet of biological inertness. *Hematological* methods are primarily intended to measure the extent of blood damage caused by exposure to standard surfaces of different materials (Guendel, 1955; Aepli, 1960; Frei, 1960; Perkins, et al., 1960). The delay of clotting of non-heparinized blood, the liberation of free hemoglobin into the plasma by hemolysis, the counting of surviving platelets and leucocytes and the studies of numerous plasma proteins and coagulation factors are the most convenient indices of hematologic changes. Despite their practical significance in blood preservation studies, these methods may fail to correlate with observations during perfusion of living organisms, because the blood is then submitted to a continuous clearance which tends to minimize the actual blood trauma. Among the *biologic* methods, implantation of the material in the body provides a good test of chemical inertia. Perfusion of an isolated heart in a circuit made of the substance to be tested permits recognition of the liberation of some constituents, thanks to the exquisite sensitivity of the cardiac contractile mechanism to minute amounts of toxic substances (Meyler, et al., 1960). The growth of bacterial or tissue cultures is impeded by substances leaching out of foreign materials immersed in the medium. The respiration of tissue cultures can also be modified under similar conditions (Cruickshank, et al., 1960) and thereby serve as an index of toxicity for the tested material. Using these methods, the biologic inertness of polyvinyl polymers, nylons, latex and silicone rubber has been related to the fact that under most conditions these materials will neither absorb the chemicals they are in contact with nor release any of their components into solution. Finally, *physical methods* permit correlation of properties of surfaces with the damaging action they exert on blood. Low surface tensions characterize most of the substances used in blood handling techniques (Lampert, 1931). Micrometric analysis of surface profiles of the best tubing materials reveals that the smoothness and polish of the internal wall may be an even more important a factor of kindness to blood than the material from which the tubing is actually made (Stewart and Sturridge, 1959). Surfaces which cause hemolysis display irregularities in size which may exceed considerably that of the red blood cells. Electron microscopic studies (shadow cast technique) and reflection interference microscopy studies of medical grade tubing obtained by extrusion or dipping show that the ripples on the inner surface are less than 2 microns in all cases (Portela, 1961) thereby providing a physical explanation for their recognized blood handling qualities. In conclusion, it appears that the concept of biologic inertness has many aspects which need to be considered when developmental work is attempted in the field of artificial blood circulation.

Summarizing

The materials found to be least traumatic to blood have in common a high degree of chemical inertness, smoothness of surface, and unwettability. These qualities are partially interrelated. Since deterioration of blood has mostly been evaluated on an empiric basis, more systematic studies as to the relative effects of mechanical and chemical factors are necessary for future development. In this respect precise identification of the materials tested is imperative in view of the variability of the compounds available on the market.

METALS

Where mechanical strength and stiffness are the primary requirements for parts of an extracorporeal circuit, metals are commonly used. Though cheap and easy to machine, copper and brass have long been recognized as inadequate in perfusion technology because they are easily oxidized and release toxic ions when exposed to watery media. Chromium-plated surfaces have proven disappointing, because pinholes subsist in the plating, through which contact with the basic material is still possible. Nickel and nickel alloys appreciated for their unusual toughness and corrosion resistance, were proposed by Tainter (1932) but never gained a wide acceptance, possibly because of the price. Reports of nickel sensitivity as a cause of infusion reaction (Stoddart, 1960) may also deter from their use. Despite a lack of hardness, silver has been used where its high thermal conductivity coefficient is of particular benefit (heat exchanger surfaces). Gold and gold-plated parts are acceptable, but their price is prohibitive. Aluminum and light metal alloys are still the subject of controversy. Beland, et al. (1938) experienced a considerable degree of toxicity, which could, however, be overcome by simple passage of the arterialized blood through an animal lung. They surmised that aluminum hydroxide is formed on the surface of the metal exposed to blood, leading to the precipitation of plasma proteins and capillary embolisms. The lung was thought to act as a filter for the small particles because it was of no help when inserted in the venous line. Diettert, et al. (1958a, b) have used disposable aluminum screens in their artificial lung, but did not observe any toxic effect during the course of perfusion. It may very well be that the presence of other metals in aluminum alloys and the kind of finishing of the surfaces determine their blood handling properties and that a suitable material from that class will be developed someday.

From the evidence presently available, stainless steel is the material of choice. Not too expensive, it can be machined into complicated shapes and, provided special welding techniques are used, connected to other pieces without creating dangerous recesses or joints. It readily transmits heat, can be easily cleansed by mechanical or chemical means and permits sterilization by autoclaving. The chromium–nickel type alloys are the most widely used. They are normally nonmagnetic and show the highest corrosion resistance of all types of stainless steel as well as unusually fine mechanical properties. The types standardized as 304 (18–20 per cent chromium, 8–-12 per cent nickel) and 316 (16–18 per cent chromium, 10–14 per cent nickel, 2–3 per cent molybdenum) are preferred because they combine the mechanical qualities of steel with a high degree of biochemical inertia. They can be electropolished to the point where their surface becomes almost atraumatic to blood (Rose and Broida, 1954; Adams, et al., 1958). Other alloys, such as 303 and 17-4PH, are considered for special applications (Watkins and Hering, 1959). As for other surgical metals, it is still not clear whether the biochemical inertia and tissue tolerance of stainless steel is primarily dependent on the alloy composition, the degree of annealing, the hardness, the polish, or more complex properties such as electrical surface potential (Fleisch and Stauffer, 1961) or thermal electromotive forces. Development of better alloys must, therefore, be promoted by trial and error, so as to approach more closely the standard of the ideal metal for biologic use.

In Fleisch's laboratory Aepli (1960) has carried out a comparative study of the blood handling qualities of copper, brass, nickel and stainless steel. Human blood was exposed to standard surfaces of these metals, and the changes in blood chemistry and the modification of the formed elements brought about by mere contact of the metals with blood were measured. The toxic effects of copper and brass were evidenced by considerable protein deposits, loss of fibrinogen, hemolysis and disappearance of platelets. Nickel and steel, though not completely inert, exhibit more favorable properties: blood proteins were denatured to a slighter extent, whereas the formed elements were not drastically reduced in number as with copper and brass.

Summarizing

The advantages of metals for use in extracorporeal circuits lie in their mechanical strength, machinability and ease of fabricating and finishing. Copper alloys and light weight metals have markedly toxic effects on perfused organisms, while stainless steel alloys are not quite free from such drawbacks. Nevertheless, stainless steel is presently the metal of choice for various components in extracorporeal circuits. It is resistant to most chemicals, easily machinable and can be polished to a high degree of smoothness.

GLASS, TRANSPARENT PLASTICS, FLUORINATED AND EPOXY COMPOUNDS

The remarkable chemical inertness of glass has long been recognized in blood handling procedures. In fact, glass constituted most of the reservoirs, tubing and stopcocks of a number of perfusion units, from those of the pioneers (von Frey and Gruber, 1885; Jacobj, 1890) to the most elaborate ones of recent investigators (Lindbergh, 1935). Although breakable, glass offered the distinct advantage of transparency, thereby permitting a visual control of blood and of the perfused organ. Hard glass and pyrex represented a definite improvement and they still remain among the most acceptable substances for the construction of modern heart–lung machines. In recent years, water repellent coating of glass surfaces with silicone films has improved their physiologic qualities. At the same time, translucent plastic substances have been developed for essentially the same applications as glass. The hard ones, like plexiglas, lucite and some epoxy resins, are more easy to machine than glass and considerably less breakable; the soft ones, polyvinyl chloride, polyethylene and others, are widely used for manufacturing blood containers and disposable oxygenators.

In studies concerned with blood preservation and storage in siliconized glass containers and various plastic containers, Strumia, et al. (1959) have been unable to find any significant difference in any parameter throughout the period of normal storage of blood. They attributed the improvement noted with siliconized containers to the fact that plain glass releases silicates which are responsible for the damage to blood. In their experience, even high grade polyvinyl chloride, plasticized with a distilled grade of dioctylsebacate, exerted a toxic effect on the red cells. This effect could be eliminated when the basic plastic was compounded by the addition of a proper stabilizer, such as one containing zinc. Nevertheless, many reliable investigators still maintain that plastic containers and siliconized systems are in some way "kinder" to blood.

Rose and Broida (1954) and Aepli (1960) have compared glass, pyrex, plexiglas and siliconized glass in studies of the biochemical changes in blood exposed to standard surfaces of these substances. All of them ranged among the less traumatic materials commonly used in extracorporeal circulation techniques and appeared better than polished steel. Siliconized glass ranked first among the substances tested in both studies. Up to now, one of the main limitations to the use of hard and soft transparent plastics instead of glass has been the thermolability of the materials and of the adhesives used in manufacturing them. Consequently, heat sterilization cannot be used, and one has to rely upon chemical sterilization. It appears, however, that by new compounding this drawback can be overcome (Catchpole and Nixon, 1959b).

Nylon is used in the manufacture of connectors and filters. Although most of the brands developed for medical use are relatively bland with respect to blood, it has been reported that the presence in nylon of free monomers, which contain highly reactive end-amino groups, may be the cause of a marked toxicity (Cruickshank, et al., 1960). Epoxy compounds become increasingly important in the technology of artificial blood circulation, because of their qualities as adhesives, their mechanical resistance and their ability to be molded in any desired shape. However, some caution is indicated in the choice of the resins and of their "hardeners", since the less complicated polyfunctional epoxides, and the monofunctional epoxides with auxiliary active groups are capable of producing deleterious effects on the hemopoietic system (Kodama, et al., 1961).

Teflon, DuPont's tetrafluoroethylene resin, and other polymers of the polytrifluorchlorethylene group known as Hostaflon and KelF, compete with metals and glass in many applications. Organofluorine compounds offer a unique combination of chemical, physical and electrical properties which cannot be found in any other material. Teflon, for instance, is completely inert to almost all known chemicals, non-flammable, heat resistant and unaffected by humidity. Physically it is tough, resilient and not brittle. Besides possessing excellent dielectric properties, Teflon's most outstanding characteristic is its extremely low coefficient of friction. Its surface is so waxy and slippery that smooth metal surfaces do not stick to it, thus making Teflon an ideal material for bearing, bushings and pump parts. Finally, the wettability of Teflon is close to that of paraffin, which has long been considered the prototype of materials for blood containers (Kawasaki, 1960). Despite its outstanding qualities, Teflon, because it is considerably more expensive than stainless steel, is seldom machined to form the essential parts of artificial lungs. However, techniques for applying a thin coat of Teflon over metal surfaces are available (Tullis and Rochow, 1952). Finely divided particles are suspended in an appropriate dispersion agent and then poured or sprayed over the metal surfaces. After drying and heating, the resultant surface can be polished and remains as a semi-permanent coating. Thin plastic membranes, mostly made of polyethylene and Teflon, are used to separate the blood from the gas phase in some types of oxygenators. Their properties will be reviewed in Chapter VII.

Summarizing

At the present time, glass is still one of the most acceptable substances for use in blood handling. Its chemical inertia has been enhanced by water repellent coatings. Transparent plastics have been developed which compete with glass in most of its applications. Continuous changes and improvements in manufacturing techniques make definitive assessments impossible. Nylon, organofluorine compounds and epoxy resins are hard plastic substances whose remarkable chemical inertia offers advantages in many applications.

TUBING MATERIALS

At the present time the tubing for extracorporeal circulation apparatus is usually made of a translucent, flexible and non-wettable plastic. Within the versatile group of the vinyl polymers, some compounds have been developed which combine the chemical inertness, physical toughness and dependability characteristic of this class with properties especially required in blood handling: smoothness of the internal wall, translucency, absence of toxicity, ability to withstand sterilization at high temperature, no tendency to kinking, enough hardness to prevent the collapse of the tubing when the flow is restricted and enough resilience for the tubing to regain its shape after clamping, or any other external compression, is released.

Just as steel can be alloyed to change its basic properties to fit a specific need, so the basic vinyl polymer can be modified to provide the chemical and physical properties required for any particular use. Most flexible vinyl tubings for medical purposes are made up of a very inert resin such as polyvinyl chloride, and about 30 to 40 per cent of the mass is a high boiling point plasticizer (often an ester of phtalic acid) that gives the tubing flexibility. A good plasticizer must be very inert and not leach out into the blood. A small proportion of a stabilizer, which could be any of certain organic barium, cadmium, zinc or tin compounds, is also added to the mixture. Some stabilizers resist water migration into the plastic so well that the tubing remains clear when immersed in water over long periods. However, some stabilizers may display cardiotoxic properties, particularly the organic tin compounds (Steele, 1959; Strumia, et al., 1959; Meyler, et al., 1959, 1960; Autian and Kapadia, 1960; Keith, et al., 1961). Therefore, particular care must be exercised by the manufacturers in their choice of tubing for biologic purposes. Finally, certain waxes or lubricants are sometimes added to the polymer to give it a low surface tension for making it unwettable.

Polyvinyl plastic tubings are produced by extrusion. It has been empirically established that certain temperatures of extrusion as well as the right rate of flow and accurately machined dies will give a uniform, highly polished internal wall. Successive lots of plastic tubing may vary in wall thickness from 0.05 to 0.07 mm. (Watkins, et al., 1960). Tygon (S 22-1 or B 44-3 formulation) and Mayon are almost universally recognized brand names for dependable blood conducting tubes. They are presently marketed at such a price that most users discard them after one use. However, in the experimental laboratory, one can use them over and over again, provided they are thoroughly rinsed and cleaned after each contact with blood. Polyvinyl plastic rubings can be glued to each other by dipping their extremities in a solvent such as cyclohexanone, thereby providing for versatile laboratory circuits. They are readily sterilized by heat or chemicals. Tygon S 22-1 may be safely autoclaved at 15 lbs. of steam for one hour. B 44-3 can withstand such autoclaving for 30 minutes. Some shrinkage (2 to 4 per cent) may be noted following the first autoclaving. However, no further shrinkage should occur following the first exposure to high temperature. Although the tubing appears somewhat fogged and soft immediately after heat sterilization, it regains its natural clearness and resiliency within 48 hours, as it cools and dries. Owing to their chemical inertness, plastic tubings also lend themselves ideally to sterilization by chemical means.

Besides polyvinyl tubing, natural rubber and silicone rubber are also used in extracorporeal circuits. It has long been appreciated that some types of natural or artificial rubber are extremely toxic. The same holds true for many brands of silicone rubber not specifically developed for biologic purposes (Wilkinson, et al., 1956; Frei, 1960). The amber latex tubing for blood handling is manufactured by multiple dipping of forms in natural latex, a colloid dispersion of natural rubber obtained from the Hevea trees. The dipping process seemingly provides a higher degree of smoothness of the internal wall than the extrusion of dry rubber compounds. Latex rubbers are lighter in weight than polyvinyl chloride and somewhat easier to handle, owing to their greater elasticity. The inconveniences of hardening and deterioration by aging are of little concern in the field of extracorporeal circulation, since tubing is usually discarded after one use. Silicone rubbers are discussed with other silicone compounds (see below). Although inferior to polyvinyl in translucency, rubber tubings offer the advantage of a greater resiliency. They are often preferred for pump circuits, where their unusual ability to regain their shape quickly after decompression permits higher flows than polyvinyl tubings of the same internal diameter. The durability of rubber, when subject to strain and rough usage, makes it superior to any other material in occlusive type pumps. However, when the tubing is used many times in the experimental laboratory, it must be checked and replaced frequently because repeated mechanical stresses eventually produce crevices and internal structural defects.

Summarizing

The combination of transparency, resilience and non-wettability makes some new plastics materials suitable for tubing in extracorporeal circuits. Through proper choice of basic vinyl polymer, plasticizer and stabilizer, a biologically nontoxic tubing may be made which tolerates heat and chemical sterilization. Amber latex tubing although only moderately transparent, is used whenever its superior resilience is advantageous, for instance in pump circuits. Since small discrepancies in composition and manufacturing can result in marked differences in physical and chemical properties of plastics and rubbers, a medical evaluation must always refer to the specific material tested.

SILICONES, SURFACE AGENTS, ANTIFOAMS AND SILICONE RUBBERS

Silicones are synthetic, semiorganic polymers characterized by two distinctive features. First, the basic structure of the molecule is not carbon (C—C—C), but a chain skeleton of alternating silicone and oxygen atoms (Si—O—Si—O—Si). Each silicon atom has one or more organic groups attached to it. Second, depending upon the number or type of organic groups attached to the silicon and the degree of polymerization and cross linking, the final material may be a liquid, a resin or a rubber.

Silicones owe an unusual combination of properties to their unique chemical structure. With a basic structure closely related to that of silicon dioxide or quartz, they display a high degree of chemical inertness, a great heat resistance and good dielectric properties. From the organic groups attached to the silicon atoms they acquire the flexibility characteristic of purely organic compounds, e.g., the ability to act like oily fluids, to be soluble in many organic solvents, to form a film on surfaces and to impregnate porous material. Thus, looked upon as a class, silicones are notable for the fact that they are chemically and physiologically inert, stable at high and low temperatures, and water repellent.

The organic groups attached to the silicon atom may be any one of a number of hydrocarbons or substituted hydrocarbons. However, the methyl group, giving rise to a whole series of methyl siloxane polymers, is the one which produces the most interesting compounds. The number of hydroxyls attached is also important, because the number of directions in which a polymer might grow by condensation determines the character, properties and behavior of the finished product. Commercial silicones are prepared from chlorosilane monomers and vary in type of substituting groups and molecular weights. The basic products are available in the form of liquids, pastes and rubber gums. After ultimate polymerization and cross-linking, many of the silicones used in blood handling technology acquire a resin, or lacquer-type quality (Rochow, 1951; McGregor, 1954).

The *silicone fluids* include first the class of linear polymers of dimethylsiloxane. These are clear, oily liquids that are odorless, tasteless, insoluble in water and highly resistant to changes by heat or oxidation. Their viscosity is dependent on the average polymer chain length and may vary from less than 1 to more than 10,000,000 centistrokes. Thus the consistency ranges from water-thin fluid to non-flowing gum-like substances. They are endowed with a very low surface tension (around 21 dynes/cm., as compared with water at 72 dynes/cm.) and therefore spread easily. They are exceedingly repellent to water and all watery solutions although they will transmit water vapor. The temperature of polymerization is relatively high.

Silicone rubber compounds are formulated by blending the very high viscosity polymer gums with suitable fillers and vulcanizing agents (McGregor, 1954). Among the most satisfactory compositions are the dimethylpolysiloxane gums filled with amorphous precipitated silica (Wilkinson et al., 1956). No plasticizers are needed to obtain the desired characteristics, and hence, there is no material that can be leached out. The physiologic properties of the finished compounds may, in a large measure, be determined by the nature of the non-silicone compounds. The development of silicone rubber for medical application must include not only the proper formulation (silicone polymer, inorganic filler and organic peroxide) but also particular attention to the next steps in manufacturing. The raw stock is vulcanized under pressure at about 150°C., so as to decompose the peroxides and bring about the chemical reaction that develops rubbery properties. Finally, the material should be cured at high temperature for several hours so as to complete the vulcanization and drive off the decomposition products of the peroxides and any low polymers, since the vulcanizing agents do not become part of the rubber. One characteristic feature of these silicone rubber compounds is that they appear completely inert physiologically and can come in prolonged contact with body tissues without eliciting any kind of reaction. Another family of silicone rubbers is the room-temperature-vulcanizing (RTV) type. These employ catalysts which, when stirred into the fluid base, cause vulcanization to occur at room temperature. Some of these are toxic because of the catalyst employed, but others utilize acceptable catalysts and have been implanted subdermally for periods up to several years. They are also used for gaskets and seals in extracorporeal circuits.

Dow-Corning *Antifoam A*, a material with a honey-like consistency, is made by mixing into a silicone fluid a few per cent of finely divided amorphous silica particles about 20 millimicrons in diameter (McGregor, 1954). Dow-Corning *Antifoam B* is a 30 per cent emulsion of Antifoam A and emulsifiers primarily suitable for industrial uses. *Antifoam C* is a 10 per cent emulsion of Antifoam A which is acceptable in human blood. All are widely used whenever it is necessary to quell foam produced by admixture of gas into liquids.

Silicone resins, obtained from both the methyl and phenyl types of polymers, can be blended to meet different specifications. The rigidity of the structure is determined by the chain length and the number of cross-links from one chain to another in the polymer. Silicone resins are used for water repulsion and for electrical insulation. In the field of extracorporeal circulation their main application concerns the coating of surfaces exposed to blood.

Monomeric chlorosilanes have found some application in biologic technique. They are highly volatile materals which readily react with moisture to form silicones and as a byproduct, hydrochloric acid. When applied by vaporization they deposit a tightly bonded, water repellent film of molecular thickness on the walls of the container. Since they are corrosive in the presence of moisture, the chlorosilane monomers must be handled with care. They are somewhat unpleasant to use because of the hydrochloric acid given off, and of course, corrosive to materials affected by the acid.

Sodium methyl siliconate is particularly interesting in view of the convenience of its use. It is water soluble; yet, when it is properly applied to a porous surface, the coated surface becomes water repellent.

There are four main lines of use for silicones in the field of extracorporeal circulation.

1. Coating of surfaces exposed to blood: Jaques, et al. (1946) introduced silicones as a protective internal coating for reservoirs and tubes used in handling blood. By proper application an extremely smooth and thin film can be developed which prevents the adhesion of blood to glass, metal, plastic or rubber surfaces.

Certain precautions must be taken to obtain the most satisfactory results. The surfaces must be scrupulously clean, for traces of grease, oil and electrolytes yield less durable coats. Effective cleaning can be obtained by heating glass to above 400°C. for at least one hour. Other surfaces may be degreased by the use of organic solvents. A particular problem arises when the surface to be treated has been siliconized before. The previous coat must be removed before a fresh one is applied. Dipping in a 10 per cent aqueous solution of sodium hydroxide (Tullis and Rochow, 1952) or 20 per cent sodium hydroxide in ethanol (Osborn, et al., 1960) for at least two hours, gives excellent results. Small metal pieces can be conveniently stripped in 5 minutes by immersion and/or brushing in an organic remover, identified as Ensign No. 803 Cold Stripper. Care must be taken to prevent the stripper from touching skin or plastic parts. Thorough rinsing with water, acetone and water again, followed by thorough drying, should precede recoating. Ensign No. 803 is inadequate for removing all traces of silicone from intricate stainless steel pieces. An effective remover for such application can be made by adding 1 part of sodium hydroxide to 99 parts of Dowanol EB, and heating the mixture to obtain a solution. The container should be kept tightly closed, when not in use, to keep water from being absorbed into the solution. The silicone resin is removed by immersing the stainless steel pieces in this solution for 15 minutes, at 75°C.

The silicone coating may be applied by dipping, spraying or painting, using either an emulsion or a solution. No attempts should be made to lay down a heavy film, for a thin coating is just as effective as a heavy one (Fisher and Jaques, 1958). The silicone compounds recommended may be either resins or stable or volatile liquids.

Among the resin types, the most commonly used are known as Dow-Corning 1107 and R-671. Dow-Corning 803 and 804 resins have also been used extensively. The first is applied by dipping in a 5 per cent acetone solution (Osborn, et al., 1960) and the latter by painting lightly with a brush (Gross, et al., 1960) or by dipping in an organic solution of the compound (Kay, et al., 1957). After drying, they require prolonged baking at high temperature in all cases. The silicone on stainless steel, for instance, should be cured for 2 to 8 hours at 150-170°C. The coating so applied has an excellent life.

The liquid type available from the Dow-Corning Corporation is identified as DC 200 Fluid, whereas the corresponding product from the General Electric Company belongs to the SF-06 series. Viscosities of 100 to 350 centristrokes are commonly used, although almost any viscosity can be utilized if desired. A dilute solution (2 to 5 per cent in ether, chloroform, carbon tetrachloride, trichloroethylene or similar solvent) is prepared and allowed to flow over the surfaces to be coated. The solvent is removed by draining and passing a current of air over the surface. Care must be taken not to blow any dust or dirt particles which would mar the smooth silicone film. There is always an advantage in baking the objects treated, if practicable, for this brings about longer life of the coating.

Monomeric chlorosilanes, such as General Electric Company SC-77 or Dow-Corning 1208 offer another convenient way of applying a water repellent film over solid surfaces. The vaporization of these volatile compounds deposits a thin film which cannot accumulate in excessive quantity in some areas and then solidify, as solutions may easily do. This greatly simplifies the treatment of intricate forms. After processing into a silicone polymer, the film becomes a bland and inert substance. SC-87 (General Electric Company) is a polymeric silicone fluid containing some unhydrolyzed chloride-silicone bonds. Much less volatile than SC-77, it has been designed particularly for treating glass (Fisher and Jaques, 1958). When used in the unmodified form, a few drops are applied with a cloth to a previously cleaned surface. An oily film is formed at first which must be removed with a clean cloth. Thereafter the desired surface is obtained. The surface develops a high degree of water repellency without further processing.

Water soluble silicones in 1 per cent solution such as Dow-Corning Z-4141, sold for medical uses as Siliclad (Clay-Adams), offer the most easy way of siliconizing glassware since nothing more than dipping, rinsing in water and drying is required. However, the quality of the coating, though sufficient for some applications, does not equal that of other silicones (Fisher and Jaques, 1958).

2. Defoaming agent: Since the original application by Clark, et al. (1950), silicones have been enthusiastically accepted for repressing the foam developed in the artificial oxygenation and circulation of blood. For this purpose the intricate mixture of blood and gas bubbles is passed over beads, shreds, ribbons, sponges, meshes or cloths that have been given a thin coating of Dow-Corning Antifoam A or similar products. The surface tension of the bubbles coming into contact with the silicone is suddenly decreased and the bubbles burst. Thereby the foam is eliminated or at least reduced to such an extent that the remaining gas bubbles can be disposed of by physical separation.

The techniques for applying the Antifoam coat over the defoaming surfaces are essentially the same as for the application of silicones as a water repellent film. According to the nature of the support, spraying, dipping or painting is preferred. The choice of the proper silicones and vehicles and the production of as thin a coat as possible are important. One must obviously avoid the use of such large amounts that free droplets are carried away by the blood stream. Dow-Corning Antifoam A is the most widely used compound. A more viscous, salve-like material known as Dow-Corning Antifoam SC-20033 is also available. When simply diluted 1 to 5 in ether, globules in the order of 40 to 100 μ are present in the antifoam solution and may easily pass into the blood stream (Cassie, et al., 1960). To remove silica and the larger colloidal particles, techniques of ether extraction and centrifugation have been developed (DeWall, 1959; Barnard, et al., 1960). The material obtained, though not as potent a defoamer as the original Antifoam A, is adequate for most debubbling purposes. In our experience, however, when defoaming of blood must be carried out for 10 hours, either in vitro or in animal experiments, Antifoam A is still preferable.

It is admitted that Antifoam is effective only when it passes into the blood, and that attempts to fix it to the walls of the debubbling chamber are trivial in their effects (Cassie, et al., 1960). Since products of relatively low viscosity and high dispersibility give the best results, it seems obvious that some of the antifoam must be picked up by the blood stream and transported to the perfused tissues. While it may well be so, it should be stressed that there is presently no direct evidence that the progressive loss of defoaming capacity observed after a certain duration of use of Antifoam coated materials is due to the washing away of the active substances. Coating of the material itself with blood proteins could offer an alternate explanation. Detailed physico-chemical studies of this problem are needed if techniques of defoaming are to be improved. It would be particularly useful to determine the amount of Antifoam required by measuring how much of it is actually removed from the support, instead of relying on empiric estimates based solely on satisfactory defoaming performance.

The organism tolerates well the minute amounts of Antifoam picked up by the blood, as indicated by the large number of successful operations performed with these silicone compounds properly applied. Nevertheless, there are some hazards associated with the use of the regular defoaming compounds, as suggested by recent toxicologic studies. Gianelli, et al. (1958) have shown that Antifoam A may produce severe neurologic changes. According to Reed and Kittle (1959) Antifoam A, when given intravenously in large doses, may cause death acutely through a pulmonary embolus, or may cause chronic pulmonary fibrosis. Intra-arterial injections cause embolic phenomena in much smaller doses than do intravenous injections. Penry, et al. (1959, 1960) have also demonstrated that Antifoam injected in sufficient amounts into the cerebral circulation will result in capillary obstruction and elicit the clinical and pathologic picture of cerebral fat embolism. Yates, et al. (1959), and Cassie, et al., (1960) recognized some Antifoam globules in microscopic preparations of brain tissue, even when the animals did not display any evidence of brain damage. Smith (1960) confirmed that focal cerebral lesions are much more frequent than simple clinical examination let one suppose, while Thomassen, et al. (1961) recognized the particulate matter present in Antifoam A as the foreign material which obstructs terminal vessels.

However, contrary to the above findings, when radioactive silicone was properly applied to the parts of a bubble oxygenator and cardiopulmonary bypass was carried out, no evidence for the presence of silicone in the brain or in the kidneys could be established (Close, et al., 1960). When large amounts of purified dimethylsiloxane (Antifoam A without silica filler) were injected into the left ventricle, no signs of coronary or cerebral infarction were noted (Fitzgerald and Malette, 1960). Partial perfusions with bubble oxygenators have been successfully carried out for 10 hours (Galletti, et al., 1960) without having recourse to the high doses of Antifoam quoted by Cassie, et al. (1960): 0.44 g. for a flow of 1000 ml./min. during 30 minutes. On the other hand, surface tension reducing substances mixed with blood minimize the toxicity of gas emboli resulting from prolonged cardiopulmonary bypass (Adams, et al., 1959). As summarized by McGregor (1960), in spite of the recognized difficulties and care required in the use of Antifoam, there is no good alternative as yet to the use of silicone defoamers in certain types of heart–lung machines. The hazard involved in their use appears to be appreciably less than the hazard entailed in failure to use them.

3. Blood carrying tubing: By the addition of the proper fillers and additives to basic silicone polymers, it has been possible to develop certain rubbery solids which lend themselves to many of the applications of organic rubber. However, many of the commercial products are not adequate for blood handling (Wilkinson, et al., 1956; Aepli, 1960; Frei, 1960). A review of the problems involved in the medical application of silicone rubber tubing has been given by McGregor (1961).

Several types of silicone rubber tubing (Silastic S-2000, S-9711, X-30146, etc.) are now available which are translucent and contain no toxic additives. Their surface characteristics are similar to those of silicone treated glass or plastic tubing. They can be sterilized by hot air or by steam without damage and used repeatedly. Since it is not affected by temperature, silicone rubber tubing does not become stiff in contact with cold blood. It is therefore the material of choice for pump and tubing in hypothermic perfusions. Silastic is remarkably atraumatic since it has been implanted in the brain and jugular veins of thousands of children with hydrocephales for periods up to 5 years. By appropriate molding it can be manufactured so as to form the gaskets and blood handling parts of a number of pump-oxygenators.

4. Lubricant for blood pumps: Silicones are often used with advantage as an external lubricant in blood pumps where a rubber or plastic to metal surface-to-surface contact occurs. Silicone fluids such as General Electric Company SF-96 or the Dow-Corning 200 fluids are also excellent lubricants for gears and bearings made of nylon and other plastics. Some of these fluids have an unusual resistance to breakdown by mechanical shearing. The high viscosity compounds (1000 centristrokes) seem to give the best results. Organic rubber is not affected by mere surface coating with silicone fluids, but silicone rubber will absorb them and swell. Vinyl plastics are generally unaffected but could possibly increase in hardness as a result of partial leaching of plasticizers by a prolonged contact. There is some evidence that silicone fluids contribute to stress—cracking of polyethylene. Caution is therefore indicated when applying lubricating silicones to polyvinyl and polyethylene materials.

Summarizing

Silicones are semiorganic synthetic materials with a basic structure related to that of quartz, endowing them with resistance to chemicals, heat and electricity. The organic groups that may be attached to the silicon atoms yield a wide variety of fluidity, elasticity and solubility properties. Some silicones are used in the preparation of water repellent coatings for blood reservoirs. Special compounds serve as antifoam because they can be dispersed over large surfaces in order to burst the gas bubbles present in foamy blood. Silicone rubbers prepared for medical purposes are physiologically inert, and combine the virtues of plastic and rubber tubing as regards to transparency, heat resistance, elasticity and unwettability. Some viscous silicone fluids are excellent lubricants for rubber and nylon parts in blood pumps.

IV. Principles of Extracorporeal Gas Exchange

The task of replacing adequately the heart and lungs of an average human adult by artificial devices presents a formidable challenge: within one minute, four to five liters of blood must be collected and spread in a thin film exposed to oxygen, the liquid phase must then be separated from the gas phase, pooled and infused under pressure back into the organism. This process has to be continuously repeated for half an hour or more without damaging the delicate blood elements. The maintenance of viable biochemical conditions for all tissues in the organism is required throughout the period of perfusion. Finally, one must be able to discontinue the procedure on short notice, so as to let the organism's heart and lungs resume their function.

The early perfusion machines were crude in design and could at best saturate a few hundred milliliters of venous blood up to 90 per cent. It took Gibbon and his group more than 15 years of perseverent laboratory work before they achieved the gas exchange capacity which permitted extracorporeal circulation in man. Refinements in oxygenating and pumping techniques have now minimized the blood trauma, once conspicuous, to a point where the organism itself can perform the necessary clearance and regeneration, after the perfusion period is over. Advances in mechanical engineering have made it possible to meet most of the hemodynamic and metabolic requirements of the totally perfused organism. Nevertheless, further refinements and simplifications are still needed. A more detailed understanding of the physicochemical laws of gas exchange may provide the necessary background for the successful collaboration of biologists and engineers in meeting these needs.

Oxygen, carbon dioxide—and in some cases—nitrogen, water vapor and anesthetic gases are exchanged between the blood and the adjacent atmosphere in artificial gas exchange devices. The major physical problem is no doubt the rapid introduction of oxygen into the blood. However, in some artificial lungs, the limiting factor of the gas exchanges is not the oxygen uptake, but the elimination of carbon dioxide. Another problem is related to equilibrium of the water vapor tensions between gaseous and liquid phases. At times so much heat of vaporization is required that it interferes with the thermoregulation of the artificial lung. The discussion below is devoted to some details of the mechanisms involved in the transport of respiratory gases in artificial lungs regardless of type. The effect of turbulence in blood films will be discussed in detail in Chapter VI. The passage of gases across artificial membranes will be considered in Chapter VII.

NATURAL LUNG

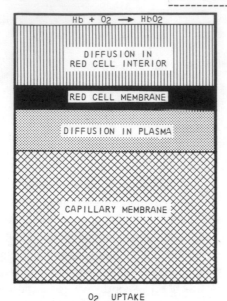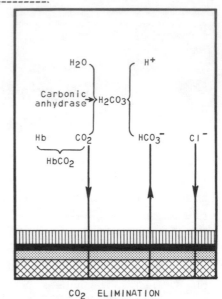

Fig. 14. Barriers to gas exchange in the natural lung. This scheme features the relative importance of various processes in the overall speed of O_2 uptake and CO_2 elimination. Heights of rectangles are proportional to the "resistance" of the consecutive processes: diffusion through capillary membrane (cross hatched); diffusion in plasma surrounding the red cells (stippled); passage through red cell membrane (black); diffusion in the red cell interior (hatched); chemical reaction within the red cell (white). In the case of oxygen uptake the chemical reaction $O_2 + Hb \rightarrow O_2Hb$ (narrow white bar) is so rapid that the time required is negligible in comparison to the time needed for diffusion within the red cell. In contrast, in the case of CO_2 elimination, the time needed for diffusion within the red cell (narrow hatched bar) is negligible in comparison to the time required for the chemical reactions involved (white). (Modified after Roughton and Rupp, 1958)

PROCESS OF OXYGEN UPTAKE

Three steps can be considered in the chain of processes involved in oxygen uptake by blood directly exposed to an oxygen atmosphere (figs. 14 and 15):

1. Diffusion of O_2 through the layer of plasma surrounding the red cells. In an artificial gas exchange device, this process is a composite one, consisting partly of diffusion and partly of mechanical mixing of the plasma. It differs from the corresponding stage in the natural lungs in many respects. In the natural lungs, a monocorpuscular film of blood is exposed to a partial pressure of oxygen of around 100 mm. Hg. for 0.1 (Vogel, 1947; Müller, 1948) to 0.75 seconds (Roughton, 1945). On the contrary, artificial oxygenators expose a relatively thick layer of blood (0.1 to 0.3 mm. according to Gibbon, 1939a, b; Taylor, 1957; Borst, 1959) comprising approximately 20 to 60 layers of erythrocytes, to a partial pressure of oxygen usually of about 700 mm. Hg. for many seconds. The thickness of the film is such that some degree of stirring is needed to permit oxygen to advance through the plasma within the time available. Then the surface of contact between blood and oxygen does not begin to approach the huge alveolar-capillary interface of the natural lung. For instance, the gas

ARTIFICIAL LUNG

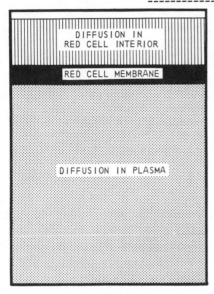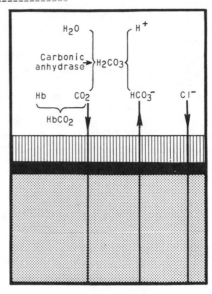

O₂ UPTAKE   CO₂ ELIMINATION

Fig. 15. Barriers to gas exchange in an artificial lung with free blood–gas interface. The additional resistance offered by artificial membranes (usually greater for CO_2 than for O_2, chap. VII) is not considered in this diagram. The main factor of resistance to gas exchange is the limited rate of diffusion of gases in a relatively thick blood film. (Chemical reactions of O_2 uptake not entered.)

blood interface in a stationary film oxygenator ranges from 2 to 10 m² as compared to 50 to 200 m² in the human lung.

The passage of oxygen through the plasma begins when the gaseous oxygen is dissolved in the watery phase and then by diffusion progresses towards the red cells. The diffusion of oxygen in plasma obeys Fick's law:

$$\dot{V}_{O_2} = \frac{D\alpha(P_1 - P_2)}{l} \text{ or } \frac{D'(P_1 - P_2)}{l}$$

where $\dot{V}_{O_2}$ is the volume of oxygen passing through a layer of plasma per unit of time, D the (physical) diffusion coefficient of O_2, α the coefficient of solubility of oxygen in plasma, P_1 and P_2 the pressures of oxygen on either side of the plasma layer, l the thickness of the layer and D' the permeation coefficient (or Krogh's diffusion coefficient). Expressed in the standard physico-chemical units of cm² sec⁻¹, the diffusion coefficient (D) of oxygen in plasma approximates 1.6×10^{-5} at 20°C. (*Handbook of Respiration*, 1958; Thews and Niesel, 1959). The corresponding value for D' (6.5×10^{-10} ml. O_2/cm./sec./mm.Hg.) is not far from that obtained by Hüfner (1897), recalculated by Krogh (1919) and since then quoted in many physiology textbooks. These permeation coefficient values indicate that the diffusion of oxygen in plasma is rapid, but by no means instantaneous. In fact, it accounts for at least 20 per cent of the overall "resistance" to the natural process of oxygenation in the lungs.

Mechanical mixing of the plasma is also a factor in the rate of passage of oxygen through the fluid surrounding the red cells (Roughton and Rupp, 1958), although its importance can hardly be estimated in the conditions of the natural lung. Vogel (1947) reported that plasma passes through the pulmonary capillary bed more slowly than red cells, an observation which suggests some sliding of the formed elements over the watery layer through which diffusion first occurs. Contrasting to the thin layer of blood exposed to gas exchange in the pulmonary capillaries, artificial oxygenators feature a thick blood film. The rate of diffusion of oxygen through plasma then becomes the major factor limiting the binding of oxygen on hemoglobin. Streamlined flow in the blood film leads to a poor performance in terms of gas exchange. As empirically discovered by Stokes and Flick in 1950, turbulence is the major factor of efficiency in artificial oxygenators because it enhances the admixture between the inner and outer layers of the blood film (See fig. 24, 1, B). The impediment to oxygenation as brought about by diffusion alone has been firmly established by Marx, et al. (1960). Until a practical way is found to expose a monocorpuscular blood layer to oxygen without undue denaturation, all artificial gas exchange devices will have to feature some degree of turbulent flow to overcome the resistance due to the limited rate of gas diffusion through a thick blood film.

2. Diffusion of O_2 through the red cell membrane. The resistance to passage of dissolved gas from the exterior to the interior of the red cell is possibly significant, since Hartridge and Roughton (1927) observed that the rate of increase of oxyhemoglobin is about 10 times smaller when the erythrocytes are intact than when they are hemolyzed. Recently, Forster, et al. (1957) have reinvestigated the additional resistance to gas diffusion into the erythrocytes imposed by the cell membrane. They found that the rate of oxygen uptake is about 3.6 times smaller when the erythrocyte membrane is intact. Roughton and Rupp (1958) estimated that the red cell membrane contributes about 25 per cent of the whole resistance in the natural process of lung oxygenation. As such, it should also be time consuming in artificial oxygenation. However, this view is not universally accepted. Thews (1959) denies any specific resistance effect of the red cell membrane. From recent observations Kreuzer and Yahr (1960) also conclude that the red cell membrane does not represent an essential impediment to the movement of oxygen

3. Diffusion of O_2 within the red cell and chemical combination of O_2 with hemoglobin. The reaction of hemoglobin with oxygen is an extremely rapid one (Gomez, 1961). However, the combined process of oxygen diffusion within the red cell and subsequent chemical reaction is only about one tenth as fast as the pure rate of chemical combination of oxygen with hemoglobin in a homogenous solution (Roughton and Rupp, 1958). According to Thews and Niesel (1959), the diffusion coefficient of O_2 in the red cells is 0.8×10^{-5} cm^2 sec^{-1} (permeation coefficient 3.3×10^{-10} ml O_2/cm./sec./mm. Hg.), or about one-half of that in plasma. Recently Scholander (1960) and Hemmingsen and Scholander (1960) have suggested a specific role of the hemoglobin molecules in the transport of oxygen which should enhance the effect of regular diffusion.

Owing to the finite permeability of the red cell interior to oxygen, the last step of oxygenation represents a notable part of resistance to the overall process of oxygen uptake. This part is estimated to be around 25 per cent of the total resistance in natural lung oxygenation (Roughton and Rupp, 1958) and reaches 66 per cent under conditions of artificial oxygenation where there is only one layer of erythrocytes in the blood film (Thews, 1959). The speed of all the processes involved in artificial oxygenation, with the exception of the final chemical reaction, may be significantly accelerated by increasing the oxygen pressure. Therefore, all modern oxygenators utilize a mixture containing from 95 to 100 per cent O_2 in their gas phase. Theoretically a gain in efficiency could be obtained by placing the oxygenator at a pressure higher than atmospheric. However, the disadvantage of more complicated construction still outweighs any gain in efficiency of gas exchange (Bjørk, 1959).

Summarizing

Oxygenation by exposure of a blood film to an oxygen atmosphere involves three steps: (1) diffusion through the layer of plasma surrounding the red cells; (2) diffusion across the red cell membrane; (3) diffusion within the red cell; and (4) the chemical combination of O_2 with hemoglobin. In artificial lungs, the blood film is much thicker than in the pulmonary capillaries. Consequently, the rate of diffusion of oxygen through the film represents an essential impediment to oxygen which can only be alleviated by mechanical stirring, prolongation of contact time or thinning of the film.

PROCESS OF CARBON DIOXIDE ELIMINATION

Little attention has been devoted to the process of carbon dioxide release in artificial gas exchange devices. Physiology textbooks state that CO_2 is 20 to 40 times more "diffusible" in aqueous fluids and body tissues than is O_2. Thus most builders and users of heart–lung machines implicitly admit that the CO_2 elimination is adequate as long as there is no defect in oxygenation. However, there are artificial lungs, particularly the "membrane", "small bubble", and "foam" type of gas exchange devices, which may favor CO_2 retention in the presence of perfect oxygenation. The mechanism of this anomaly of gas exchange will be discussed in the chapters devoted to each type of artificial lung (V, VI, VII). We shall consider here only the basic physico-chemical principles of CO_2 binding or elimination.

Little is known about the relative kinetic importance of the various factors involved in the rate of CO_2 uptake by the blood in the tissues and of CO_2 release from the blood in the lungs. Nevertheless, one can distinguish two main steps:

1. **Diffusion of CO_2 through the plasma and the red cell membrane.** The actual diffusion coefficient (D) of carbon dioxide through these media is probably 85 per cent of the corresponding diffusion coefficient of oxygen, since, in liquid media, dissolved gases tend to diffuse at rates inversely proportional to the square root of their molecular weight ($\sqrt{32/44}$ = 0.85). The actual partial pressure of dissolved CO_2 in venous blood is of the order of 50 mm. Hg., that is about two-thirds of the partial pressure of dissolved oxygen. Since, however, the solubility coefficient of CO_2 in plasma is 25 times the solubility of O_2 (*Handbook of Respiratory Data*, 1958), the actual concentration of dissolved CO_2 in venous blood will be of the order of $25 \times {}^2/_3$ of 17 times the concentration of dissolved oxygen. Therefore, the time taken for diffusion of a given quantity of CO_2 across biologic barriers should be only about one-fifteenth

to one-twentieth the time of that for O_2. The resistance to diffusion of CO_2 from the tissues to the inside surface of the red cell membrane is normally of the order of three to five per cent of the total resistance to CO_2 uptake. Such a fraction is barely significant as a limiting factor (Roughton and Rupp, 1958).

The conditions prevailing in an artificial lung differ somewhat from those in the body. Assuming that the incoming venous blood has a CO_2 partial pressure of 50 mm. Hg., and an O_2 pressure of 70 mm. Hg., and that pure oxygen is used in the gas phase, then the pressure gradient of oxygen from liquid to gas phase will be at least 12 times as large as the CO_2 pressure gradient. Due to its overwhelmingly greater solubility, the CO_2 will still diffuse faster than oxygen, but the difference is by no means so striking as in the natural lung: the time taken for diffusion of CO_2 across the plasma and the red cell membrane will be no less than one-half the time for diffusion of O_2.

2. Diffusion of the CO_2 within the red cell and chemical processes. Within the red cell, CO_2 like O_2 must diffuse as well as react chemically. In the case of oxygen, the speed of chemical reaction is extremely high, and consequently, the process is slowed down, and limited by diffusion. In the case of carbon dioxide a different situation prevails: diffusion is very fast and its effect is such as to reduce the chemical reaction rate by only a few per cent.

Once the CO_2 molecules have entered the interior of the red cell, three chemical processes occur, the first two of which are concurrent (Roughton and Rupp, 1958): (a) reversible combination of CO_2 with hemoglobin in the carbamino form; (b) reversible combination of CO_2 with H_2O to form the H_2CO_3 under the catalytic influence of carbonic anhydrase; (c) exchange of HCO_3^- ions formed within the red cell by ionic dissociation of H_2CO_3 with Cl^- ions from the plasma (the so-called "chloride shift"). Of these three processes, the first two account for about 30 percent each of the physiologic transport of CO_2, and the third for most or all of the remainder (Roughton and Rupp, 1958; Davenport, 1958).

Little is known about the kinetics of the different processes of CO_2 binding under physiologic conditions in mammalian blood. Up to now, orders of magnitude rather than accurate data have been determined (Roughton and Rupp, 1958; Dettli, et al., 1955; Bucher and Grun, 1958; Baltzer and Bucher, 1960). Even less can be said concerning CO_2 release in an artificial gas exchanger. Nevertheless, the possibility that biochemical reactions may be to some extent a rate limiting step of CO_2 elimination in an artificial lung should be kept in mind when new techniques of gas exchange are devised.

Summarizing

Since the permeation coefficient of CO_2 through watery media is markedly greater than that of O_2, an adequate CO_2 release can be assumed under the conditions of the normal lung, as long as oxygenation is unimpaired. Such an assumption cannot be made for some types of artificial lung in which CO_2 elimination may be the limiting factor of gas exchange. Two main steps in CO_2 release can be distinguished: (1) diffusion through the plasma and the red cell membrane; (2) diffusion within the red cell and chemical processes involved in CO_2 binding. In artificial lungs, the gradient of pressure available for oxygen diffusion is at least 12 times that for CO_2. Therefore the difference in the rate of movement of CO_2 and O_2 is never as conspicuous as in the normal lungs.

EXCHANGE OF NITROGEN

Nitrogen dissolves easily in blood and body fluids. It dissolves to an even greater extent in fatty tissues, because it is about five times as soluble in fat as it is in water. Normally, the nitrogen in the body tissues is very nearly in equilibrium with the nitrogen in the alveoli (Rahn, 1960). Hence, when air is breathed, the partial pressure of nitrogen throughout the body tissues is approximately 570 mm. Hg. In a 70 Kg. man, this pressure will cause around 930 ml. of nitrogen to be stored in the body (Noll and Bartels, 1960).

The gas mixture used in artificial lungs does not carry appreciable amounts of nitrogen. Therefore, denitrogenation of the body tissues usually occurs during heart–lung bypass. No experimental study has yet been devoted to this particular aspect of extracorporeal oxygenation. In fact, it is likely to be of little practical importance in ordinary bypass procedures. Usually the subject has undergone artificial ventilation with a mixture of high oxygen content for quite a long period prior to functional exclusion of the lungs. Therefore, the body nitrogen stores are partly depleted before the perfusion. Further, most *total* bypass procedures now performed are of too short duration (10 to 20 minutes) to result in complete denitrogenation. Thus no equilibrium is ever reached. Throughout the period preceding and following the heart–lung bypass, the body nitrogen content undergoes fluctuations to which no harmful effect has been ascribed as yet.

A different situation prevails during partial heart–lung bypass. First, far longer periods of perfusion are compatible with survival when this type of extracorporeal circulation is used; second, gas exchange (in this case, nitrogen) occurs at two sites, namely in the lungs and in the extracorporeal exchange device. When both the natural and the artificial lungs are ventilated with pure oxygen or oxygen–carbon dioxide mixtures, all nitrogen may be removed in the long run. When air is breathed while pure oxygen is introduced into the heart–lung machine, nitrogen will be continuously taken up by the pulmonary circulation and eliminated in the extracorporeal circuit. Since the subject has not been studied, it is still unknown whether variations of nitrogen content of blood and tissue fluids have physiologic consequences under the conditions of extracorporeal circulation.

Summarizing

The amount of nitrogen normally dissolved in the body tissues is reduced during heart–lung bypass, because the gas mixtures, to which blood is exposed in the artificial lung, do not contain nitrogen. This reduction is of no practical importance in the usual heart–lung bypass procedures. However, it could pose a problem in long term perfusions particularly when gas exchanges occur simultaneously at two different sites.

THE IDEAL OXYGENATOR

Since 1950, mechanical oxygenators have evolved from the stage of crude laboratory devices into dependable pieces of surgical equipment. From the wealth of information gained in empirical development and laboratory trials, a concept of the "ideal oxygenator" has emerged. Even now heart–lung machines still fall short of this ideal in many respects. However, the remarkable advances made in the last 10 years justify a reasonable optimism about future progress.

The qualities of an ideal oxygenator are usually described in terms of the efficient performance of the human lung as a gas exchanger and of the gentleness of the normal circulatory system in handling blood. Most authors (Templeton, 1958; Melrose, 1958; Bahnson, 1958a; Gibbon, 1959a, b; Clark, 1959; Griesser, 1960) agree on the following requirements:

1. The artificial lung must be able to oxygenate up to five liters of venous blood per minute to the range of 95-100 percent saturation.

2. Simultaneously, the gas exchange device must remove carbon dioxide in appropriate amounts so as to avoid either CO_2 retention (respiratory acidosis) or CO_2 depletion (respiratory alkalosis).

3. A suitably large gas exchange capacity must be provided while keeping the blood content of the artificial lung within reasonable limits.

4. The mechanical process of gas exchange must be gentle enough to avoid destruction of formed elements of the blood or denaturation of plasma proteins.

5. The artificial lung must be of simple and dependable construction so as to permit safe oxygenation over prolonged periods, easy cleaning and assembly, and reliable sterilization.

The lungs of an average human adult are able to introduce, according to the metabolic needs of the organism, from 250 to 5000 ml. of oxygen into the blood, and to remove about the same amounts of carbon dioxide. This performance requires a gas exchange surface of 80 to 100 m^2 and a relatively steady blood volume of 700 to 900 ml. in the lungs, which is continuously removed and replenished at a flow rate varying from 4 to 30 liters per minute. The various artificial lungs need only to equal the minimal performance of the human lung, because they are used for perfusion of the resting organism. They should be able to bind up to 300 ml. of oxygen per minute to the venous blood. If one admits that the arterio-venous oyxgen difference should not ideally exceed 6 vol. per cent, the blood flow requirement may be as large as 5 liters/min.

Most oxygenators are limited to an oxygen uptake of between 150 and 250 ml./min. Unlike the natural lung, they require an increasingly large surface for gas exchange as the demand for oxygenated blood is augmented. In other words, a maximum oxygen binding capacity is obtained only at the price of a larger blood content. In fact, the priming volume of pump oxygenators sufficient in capacity to carry on the perfusion of human adults varies from 1200 to 6000 ml. The largest volumes of blood are almost prohibitive in terms of cost and time required for preparation. On the other hand, there is probably little practical advantage in reducing the priming volume below 1000 ml. for human perfusions. Most surgeons find it comforting to have a 20 to 60 seconds supply of blood in the extracorporeal circuit, in case of massive bleeding or any other accident leading to temporary absence of venous return from the organism into the heart–lung machine. Seen in this light, satisfying the need for increasingly large priming volumes, as higher flows are required, tends to keep constant the ratio of oxygenator blood content to blood flow. This is a safety factor which cannot be neglected under practical conditions.

Since the efficiency of gas exchange in most oxygenators depends closely upon the volume of blood each contains, an easy method for determining the blood volume in the extracorporeal circuit is convenient for the operator of the respirator. The ability to control the blood content in the artificial lung also provides an important safety check, because the blood content of the oxygenator reflects the blood volume of the patient. Providing no blood loss occurs in the operative field, the organism and the heart–lung machine form a closed-circuit. Changes in the amount of blood of the circulatory system are reflected by the level of blood in the oxygenator. Thus the blood level in the oxygenator indirectly monitors the body blood volume and gives valuable indications as to the need of transfusion (see Chapter XVI).

Absence of mechanical or biochemic trauma to the blood is a requirement whose desirability hardly needs comment. All parts in the circuit should be smooth and have rounded edges not only to avoid recesses where clots or protein deposits may accumulate, but also to facilitate cleaning. Despite the many refinements introduced since the advent of human perfusion, denaturation of blood remains one of the factors which presently preclude the maintenance of heart–lung bypass beyond approximately two hours. The imperfections of blood handling in artificial oxygenators also necessitate blood filters and bubble traps in the circuit, in order to remove gas bubbles, cell clumps or fibrin strands for the arterial stream.

Finally, gas exchange devices must be of a simple design and have as few components as practicable. The simpler and less numerous the parts, the easier and less troublesome will be the assembly, functioning and sterilization. Despite the appeal which many designers feel for monitoring gadgets feeding automatic regulation devices, it must be stated that simple designs of inherent safety which avoid complicated mechanical or electrical systems are still to be preferred. At any rate, provisions for manual operation of the oxygenator must be made in case of power failure during bypass.

Summarizing

The ideal artificial lung should be simple and dependable. It should oxygenate up to five liters of venous blood, adequately remove carbon dioxide, have a reasonably small blood content and avoid damage to blood. Since there is no universally recognized criterion for defining performance of mechanical oxygenators, it is not possible to state definitely which device best approaches the ideal.

TESTING OF OXYGENATOR PERFORMANCE

Despite the early attempts of Gimbel and Engelberg (1954), there is still no generally accepted method for establishing the efficiency of gas exchange in mechanical oxygenators. Most authors simply state that their machine is able to saturate (above 95 percent) with oxygen a certain number of liters of blood per minute. Such a quantification may be misleading because the performance of the oxygenator will be related to the hemoglobin content and the degree of desaturation of the venous blood. The venous saturation in turn depends upon the oxygen consumption of the organism connected to the heart–lung machine. In other words, any statement as to the efficiency of an oxygenator expressed in terms of maximal blood flow per minute cannot be taken at face value without information as to the actual oxygen consumption of the perfused organism.

Determination of maximal gas exchange capacity of an oxygenator can hardly be obtained in the human operating room for obvious reasons. Further, the usual laboratory animals are too small in size to lend themselves to such determinations. Attempts at using very large mammals (cows, calves or horses) or two dogs in parallel have met with only partial success, because of the difficulties involved in maintaining steady perfusion conditions. Clearly, one of the reasons why most experimentators are reluctant to compare quantitatively the performances of different oxygenators is the lack of a convenient in vitro method.

The testing of an artificial lung requires an unlimited pool of venous blood with standardized hemoglobin content, oxygen saturation, carbon dioxide content, pH and temperature. These requirements are dictated by a few basic physiologic considerations: (1) in terms of overall gas transfer, it is not equivalent to saturate diluted blood or concentrated blood; (2) owing to the particular shape of the whole blood oxygen-dissociation curve depicting the affinity of hemoglobin for oxygen, it is much easier to raise oxygen saturation in the lower range (i.e., from 50 per cent to 75 per cent) than in the upper range (i.e., from 75 per cent to 100 per cent); (3) a drop in pH, an increase in CO_2 pressure or an increase in blood temperature, all decrease the affinity of hemoglobin for oxygen; (4) conversely, a rise in pH, a decrease in CO_2 pressure or a decrease in temperature all increase the affinity of hemoglobin for oxygen. Since it is not practical to collect the exceedingly large amounts of fresh blood needed for comparisons of gas exchange devices by "one-passage" techniques, closed circuit methods have to be devised. We have already stressed the difficulties involved in obtaining from perfused organisms a standard venous blood over any long period of testing. The most promising way therefore, is to couple to a regular oxygenator another gas exchange device used as a "desoxygenator," or source of venous blood. In such a circuit, the same venous blood is continuously arterialized in one artificial lung, then deprived of oxygen and loaded with CO_2 in a second artificial lung which is ventilated with a convenient CO_2-N_2 mixture (fig. 16).

The rates at which blood acquires or loses oxygen were first investigated and compared by Barcroft and Hill (1910) and later by Oinuma (1911). The feeling prevailed that the rate of in vitro reduction of blood is slow, out of all proportion to the rate of oxygenation. Barcroft (1928) discovered that, however important these observations were, they did not yield any information concerning the time required for the actual chemical process of oxygen binding to hemoglobin. They rather reflected the properties of the equilibrium curves of the reactions involved. Since Barcroft's interest was in the kinetics of the chemical reaction, rather than in the overall gas transport, he dropped the subject. Bjørk (1948) found empirically that the rate of desoxygenation in his artificial lung was too slow to permit simultaneous testing of another artificial lung. Jongbloed (1954) must be credited with the first successful design of a circuit for measuring the efficiency of gas

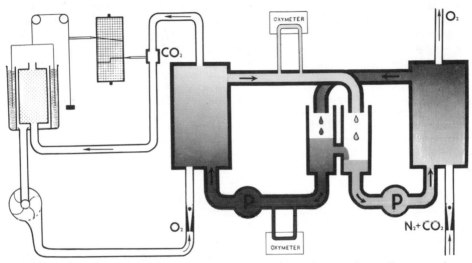

Fig. 16. Blood and gas circuits for in vitro testing of heart–lung machines. The gas exchange device under study (left) is provided with venous blood (dark shading) from one chamber of the central reservoir. The blood, once arterialized (light shading), returns to the other chamber of the central reservoir. A second gas exchange device (right) performs the opposite cycle of gas exchange: it is fed with arterial blood (light shading) by the pump P. In the desoxygenator, the arterial blood is exposed to a mixture of nitrogen and carbon dioxide. Thus oxyhemoglobin is reduced and venous blood is returned to the central reservoir. The oxygen and carbon dioxide contents of the venous blood are regulated by varying the blood and gas flow through the desoxygenator, as well as the internal stirring of the gas exchange device (a rotating disc oxygenator is usually preferred). The arrangement depicted for the central reservoir permits obtaining a constant quantity of venous blood by setting the pump which feeds the desoxygenator at a somewhat higher flow than that which feeds the oxygenator. The oxygen and carbon dioxide saturations, contents, or tensions are measured by suitable devices in the blood entering and leaving the gas exchange device under study. Whenever possible, the oxygen uptake and CO_2 elimination of the artificial lung under test are measured directly. For this purpose, oxygen is delivered by a centrifugal pump from a closed–circuit spirometer (upper left) though a precision ball flowmeter into the oxygenator. Gas leaving the oxygenator first passes through the "breathe-through" cell of a CO_2 analyzer, then is returned to the spirometer where CO_2 is chemically absorbed. A continuous recording of oxygen uptake and CO_2 tension in the "expired" gas is obtained (symbolized by rotating drum).

exchange devices under prolonged, steady conditions. Since desoxygenation was more difficult to achieve than oxygenation, the blood flow through each of the machines had to be regulated in order to maintain a constant venous saturation. Jongbloed was able to demonstrate that the efficiency of artificial oxygenation did not vary over a period of five hours.

Similar circuits have been used occasionally by different authors such as Head, et al. (1958), and Levin, et al. (1960). This technique has been extended in our laboratory so as to permit reliable testing of different types of oxygenators. An artificial lung of the rotating disc principle is at present the most convenient "desoxygenator" because the amount of gas exchange, and consequently, the characteristics of the venous blood, can be modified at any time by acting on one or many of the controlling parameters: blood flow, gas flow, or rate of rotation of the discs. If the oxygenator itself is gas-tight and a constant blood volume is maintained, its oxygen uptake can be monitored continuously by means of a closed spirometer circuit as originally suggested by Staub (1929). The CO_2 tension in the atmosphere of the oxygenator, which closely reflects the CO_2 tension in arterialized blood, is displayed by an infrared CO_2 analyzer. Since the gas flow through the oxygenator and the CO_2 fraction in the spirometer circuit are known, the CO_2 removal in the oxygenator can easily be calculated. The blood temperature is kept constant by adequate heat exchangers; blood flow and gas flow are established at all times by using pump calibration charts and/or flowmeters. Arterial and venous blood oxygen saturations are measured by a cuvette oximeter, fed by an auxilliary pump. Similar information can be obtained using polarographic electrodes for the measurement of oxygen tensions. Sampling for pH measurements or van Slyke analysis are carried out as required. Blood cell counts and biochemical determinations, such as free hemoglobin, serum potassium or coagulation factors, are performed to ascertain the traumatic effect of the heart–lung machine in the absence of any biological correction by the perfused organism. Antibiotics are usually added to the blood, as are small amounts of heparin and glucose.

Using the circuit depicted in fig. 16, testing of oxygenator performance has been carried out for periods exceeding 10 hours without alterations in gas exchange efficiency. It has proven a very reliable and, in the long run, economical way of investigating developmental items. It should, in our opinion, replace a number of poorly controlled animal experiments.

Summarizing

The peak performance of oxygenators cannot be determined satisfactorily by animal experiments because of hemodynamic and metabolic fluctuations in the organism which functions as a "desoxygenator". In vitro testing of oxygenators is best performed using a closed circuit method with two heart–lung machines in tandem. One of them is the oxygenator to be tested, whereas the other acts as a desoxygenator in which venous blood is continuously produced by addition of CO_2 and removal of O_2. Constant and reproducible conditions can be created by constant control of blood flow, gas flow, temperature, gas pressures, pH, oxygen uptake and removal, as well as carbon dioxide binding and elimination. The traumatic effect on blood caused by artificial lungs and pumps can be ascertained in the absence of any biologic correction by the perfused organism.

THE ACTUAL OXYGENATORS

In the flurry of publications on heart–lung machines which blossomed out during the pioneer years of extracorporeal circulation, it was sometimes difficult to distinguish between real advances and remodeling of past gadgets.

More recently, however, the situation has stabilized, and attempts can now be made to systematize the description of the characteristic features of the different types of oxygenator. Such a presentation must necessarily rely on data from the literature, where only a few unbiased comparative studies are available. Therefore, it would be rather presumptuous to attach any grade, or figure of merit to specific models. It remains the responsibility of the surgeon, or investigator, to weigh the advantages and inconveniences of each type of

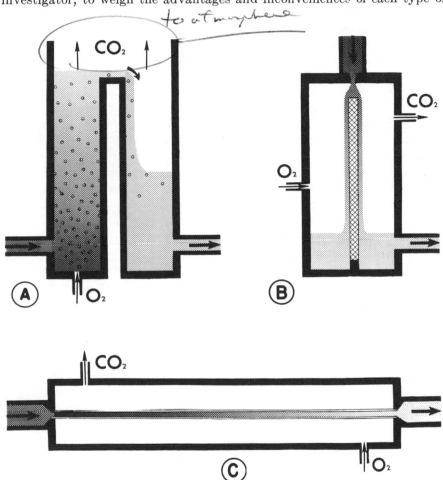

to atmosphere

Fig. 17. The three basic classes of artificial lung.

A. Bubble oxygenators comprise essentially two components: a bubble chimney (left) in which oxygen is admixed with venous blood and connected via an overflow weir to a debubbling or settling chamber (right) from which the arterialized blood is led off. Carbon dioxide escapes to the atmosphere.

B. Film oxygenators comprise essentially a solid support (center) over which venous blood (top) is spread for exposure to oxygen and removal of carbon dioxide. Arterialized blood is led off (right) from a settling chamber at the bottom of the oxygenator.

C. Membrane oxygenators comprise essentially two membranes between which venous blood (left) is conducted through a gas chamber. Oxygen and carbon dioxide are exchanged across the membranes and arterialized blood is led off (right).

machine and to decide which one is best fitted to his particular needs and circumstances.

Gas exchange in artificial lungs relies on the creation of a large surface of equilibration between blood and gas. Such a surface is obtained by the dispersion of gas in the blood, ("bubble oxygenator," "foam oxygenator"), or by dispersion of blood in the gas ("spray oxygenator," "film oxygenator"). The maintenance of a film of blood in a gaseous atmosphere necessitates a mechanical support, either a moving one (e.g., rotating disc oxygenator) or a fixed one (e.g., stationary screen oxygenator). Finally, a membrane permeable to respiratory gases can be interposed between the liquid and gaseous phases to avoid the trauma to blood associated with a large free blood–gas interface ("membrane oxygenator").

In some gas exchange devices, equilibrium of gas tensions between the blood and the respiratory mixture is satisfactorily achieved by a single exposure of the blood film (e.g., "spiral oxygenator," "rotating screen oxygenator"); in others a recirculation pump is required to protract the contact time between blood and gas in order to obtain steady conditions of gas transfer (many "stationary screen" and "stationary membrane oxygenators"). In several models an unpredictable amount of recirculation, or mechanical mixing, of the blood to be arterialized, is produced by the gas flow ("bubble oxygenator") or by the movement of the film support ("rotating disc" and "rotating cylinder oxygenator").

It is customary to categorize oxygenators into three classes: "bubblers," "filmers" and "membrane oxygenators" (fig. 17). We shall follow this convenient classification. However, it should be pointed out that the assigning of many machines in one or another class is arbitrary, because many gas exchange devices combine features of more than one.

Summarizing

The actual oxygenators are difficult to evaluate on a comparative basis, since unbiased studies attaching a figure of merit to specific models are largely missing. The customary classification of "bubblers," "filmers," and "membrane oxygenators," based upon the nature of the gas and blood distribution used for obtaining a large blood–gas interface, is somewhat arbitrary, but convenient. In fact, however, several gas exchange devices combine the features of more than one.

V. Bubble Oxygenators

The oxygenation of blood by gas dispersion is based upon the age-old knowledge that a huge gas–liquid interface can be created in a relatively small volume by bubbling the gas through the liquid. Gas exchange devices, in which this technique of exposing blood to oxygen is prepotent, are grouped under the class of "bubble oxygenators," or more familiarly, "bubblers."

PRINCIPLES OF BUBBLE OXYGENATORS

Continuous arterialization of blood by a stream of oxygen bubbles was devised some 80 years ago (Schröder, 1882). In the early days of total body perfusion, the potentialities of bubble oxygenators were explored by Bencini (1949) and Thomas and Beaudouin (1950). However, no consistent survival of experimental animals could be achieved, owing to the impossibility of removing the excess of gas bubbles from the blood stream. The decisive forward step was made in 1950, when Clark, Gollan and Gupta thought of using silicone compounds as defoaming agents. Once oxygenated, the blood was exposed to surfaces coated with suitable silicone polymers. The bubbles then burst and perfusion could be carried on without involving the risk of gas embolism.

In bubble oxygenators, the gas is dispersed into the venous blood through small holes in a distributing manifold usually located at the bottom, or along the longitudinal axis, of the bubble chimney. The foam, which is continuously generated, imparts a swirling motion to the blood stream and ascends to the surface, resulting in a cushion of mixed liquid–gas phase which floats over the blood. Gas exchange happens during the ascent of the foam at which time intimate mixing of blood and oxygen occurs. Once this is completed, coalescence of the foam and removal of the remaining bubbles are carried out by the action of surface active susbstances, by settling, trapping, filtration or centrifugation of the bubbles, or by a combination of these means. (*See* Chapter XI.)

The amount of oxygen that can be transferred into the blood depends primarily upon the total surface of exchange achieved by the bubbling process (Clark, 1958; 1959). Thus it first appears that the oxygen should be distributed in bubbles as small as possible, because the surface of each individual bubble decreases relatively less than its volume when the radius is diminished (fig. 18). If for instance, the arterio-venous oxygen difference is 5 vol. per cent, it may suffice to inject 5 ml. of O_2 for each 100 ml. of blood flow, provided only the bubbles are small enough to combine with hemoglobin within the time available. Such a device would be a pure "oxygenator," since obviously it could not eliminate carbon dioxide in any amount. Let us now consider the gas exchange from the point of view of carbon dioxide release: If the blood features a venoarterial CO_2 difference of 4 vol. per cent, and the arterial CO_2 tension does not exceed 40 mm. Hg., then 76 ml. of O_2 must be provided for each 100 ml. of blood flow, in order to make the CO_2 tension in the bubbles equal to that expected in arterial blood. Since the equilibration of gas tensions between blood phase and gas phase is never perfect, mainly because of

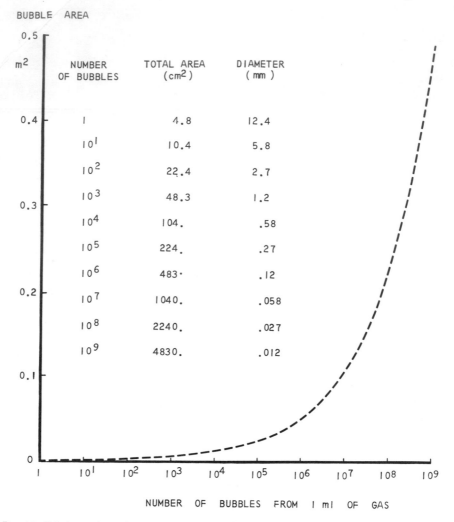

BUBBLE AREA

NUMBER OF BUBBLES	TOTAL AREA (cm²)	DIAMETER (mm)
1	4.8	12.4
10^1	10.4	5.8
10^2	22.4	2.7
10^3	48.3	1.2
10^4	104.	.58
10^5	224.	.27
10^6	483·	.12
10^7	1040.	.058
10^8	2240.	.027
10^9	4830.	.012

NUMBER OF BUBBLES FROM 1 ml OF GAS

Fig. 18. Tabular and graphic representation of the total surface area produced by 1 ml. of gas when it is divided into an increasingly larger number of bubbles of progressively smaller diameter. (Modified from Clark, 1959.)

incomplete mixing, bubble oxygenators usually require equal oxygen and blood flows in order to achieve adequate gas exchange. Actually the ratio of oxygen flow to blood flow is often far above 1, reaching 3, 5 and even 10 in some commercial gas exchange devices where the stirring action of large gas flows through the bubble chimney is needed to provide sufficient hematosis. However, this in turn is not without its disadvantages: large gas flows require large oxygenation chambers, tend to create a rather "dry" foam, to increase the damage to the blood and to remove too much CO_2 by a mechanism of "hyperventilation." This last inconvenience can be obviated by the admixture of 2 to 5 per cent carbon dioxide in the oxygen supplied, in order to set a minimal value below which the arterial CO_2 tension cannot fall, regardless of gas flow. Since the flow of oxygen gas must be at least 25 times larger than the oxygen uptake, there is actually no need to disperse the oxygen into the smallest possible bubbles. In fact, one must avoid this because the tiniest bubbles are the most difficult to eliminate from the blood stream owing to their low buoyancy. (*See* Chapter XI.)

From the above considerations, it is obvious that the amount of gas flow, the size of the bubbles and the composition of the gas mixture are all critical factors in bubble oxygenators. Small bubbles produce an excellent oxygenation, but they are not very efficient in terms of CO_2 removal. Furthermore, they may cause hemolysis by jet action at the site of emergence and may become exceedingly difficult to remove. Large bubbles are less efficient as far as oxygen transfer is concerned, but are essential for CO_2 elimination. The gas–liquid ratio of the foam they form is high, thereby increasing the tendency to plasma protein denaturation. However, large bubbles are easily removed by the action of antifoaming compounds, or simply by buoyancy. Compromises between these opposing specifications have been worked out empirically. Some theoretic basis for this can be found in studies dealing with the production of gas bubbles from orifices submerged in liquids.

Maier (1927) demonstrated that the radius of the bubble increases as a cube root of the radius of the tip at which it is formed. Guyer and Peterhans (1943 a) established the following relationship:

$$D = K_1\sigma + K_2 \log \eta + A \left(\sqrt[3]{d} \right),$$

where D is the diameter of the bubble, σ the surface tension and η the viscosity of the liquid; K_1, K_2 and A numerical constants and d the diameter of the orifice. In studies devoted to bubbling through filter plates, Guyer and Peterhans (1943 b) also demonstrated that the size of the bubbles increased with the flow of gas. The size of the bubbles decreased with decreasing superficial tension of the liquid, whereas the effect of viscosity was remarkably slight. A critical survey of the literature concerning gas bubble formation (Jackson 1952 a, b) revealed that most processes have an optimal bubble size. Where mass transfer is involved (as in oxygenation), an increase in the fineness of subdivision of the gas results in a higher surface area and longer contact time. However, it also decreases the mass transfer coefficient owing to increase in thickness of the liquid film and to changes in the internal circulation of the bubble. Jackson (1952 a) also pointed to the complexity of the relationship between pore size and bubble size when filter plates with somewhat irregular openings are used. As the applied gas pressure increases, the pore which first emits gas is that for which the narrowest cross-section is wider than that of any other pore. Successive pores, with decreasing values of the narrowest cross-section, are then brought into play, but their openings, and therefore the bubbles produced, are not necessarily in the same order of succession in regard to size. Another approach to a similar problem has been reported by Harrison and Leung (1961).

Clark (1958) has summarized the technologic knowledge as it relates to ways of regulating the relative numbers of small and large bubbles in oxygenators:

(1) A coarse and a fine porosity bubbler with separate oxygen feed lines can be used simultaneously.

(2) As oxygen flow through a porous material in contact with blood is increased, the amount of gas emerging as large bubbles increases, accompanied by a slight decrease in the amount of small bubbles.

(3) As the interfacial tension between the blood and the porous material is lowered, the size of the emerging bubbles at a given gas flow is greatly decreased. In this way, surface active agents such as detergents may function (by design or unexpectedly) as a means of enormously increasing the oxygen-liquid interface. But a porous surface rendered hydrophobic by siliconing, produces huge bubbles which are relatively ineffective in oxygenating.

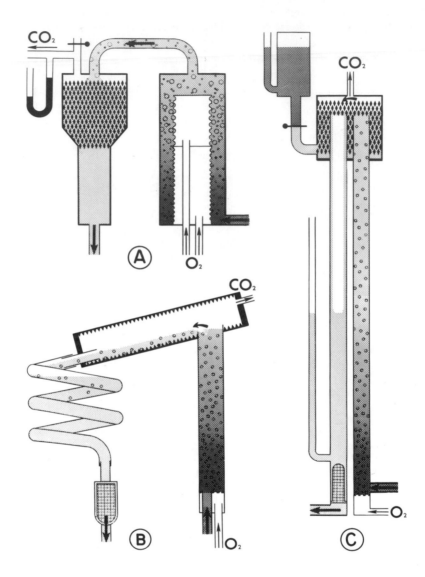

Fig. 19. Basic design of sequential bubble oxygenators. Venous blood (dark shading) and oxy-gen are injected simultaneously at the bottom of the oxygenating column. Oxygen bubbles ascend in the blood and progressively arterialize it. Antifoam coated surfaces (black, vertical rhombs) in the debubbling chamber serve to eliminate the excess oxygen and CO_2, which escape in the at-mosphere. The arterial blood (light shading) accumulates in a settling chamber and passes through a filter (cross-hatching) before entering the arterial infusion line.

    A. Oxygenator described by Clark, et al. (1950, 1952).

    B. Oxygenator designed by DeWall, et al. (1956b, 1957b).

    C. Oxygenator designed by Jordan, et al. (1958a). (See details in text.)

Ever since the introduction of defoaming agents by Clark and his associates in 1950, oxygenators of the bubbler type have consisted of three main chambers: a bubbler, a defoamer and a blood settling chamber, serving the three functions involved in blood oxygenation and separation from the gas phase. The three chambers can be arranged either in a row, or concentrically. The last two chambers are often combined. We shall distinguish the sequentially arranged oxygenators (simpler in design, but somewhat cumbersome) from the concentrically built oxygenators (more compact and also usually more expensive).

Summarizing

Bubble oxygenators take advantage of the fact that a large gas–blood contact surface can be created in a relatively small amount of blood by bubbling oxygen through the blood. The greater the number of small bubbles, the larger the gas exchange surface will be. On the other hand, the finer the subdivision of the gas, the less efficient is the carbon dioxide elimination and the more difficult the removal of the bubbles by defoaming agents. It is technically possible to vary the proportion of small and large bubbles to achieve the best compromise between oxygenation and carbon dioxide elimination.

SEQUENTIAL BUBBLE OXYGENATORS

The gas exchange device designed by Clark (fig. 19 A) may be considered as the prototype of this class. The bubbling chamber is a siliconized glass reservoir in which oxygen is bubbled through a combination of coarse and fine pores in two sintered glass cylinders placed on top of each other. The flow of oxygen to each of the distributing manifolds can be regulated independently. Thereby, it is possible to control both oxygen tension and pH of the blood. The defoaming occurs in the next chamber, held under 90 mm. Hg. suction, where blood is spilled over teflon shreds coated with antifoam. The blood then flows into a third chamber, (not represented in fig. 19 A), which serves simultaneously as an arterial reservoir and an arterial pump. The most interesting feature of the Clark oxygenator is that it combines the gas exchange unit and the pumps in one compact series of containers. The size of the different chambers can be easily modified according to the perfusion requirements. The small model for instance, with an oxygenating capacity of 1.2 L./min., requires only 450 ml. of blood for priming. It includes monitoring devices for blood pH, pO_2 and temperature, so that in the hands of a skilled operator, these parameters can be maintained within close limits. The machine has served since 1952 without undergoing any major modification, a tribute to the soundness of its design. The oxygenator described by Clark, et al. (1950, 1952) has been successful both in experimental and clinical perfusions. Therefore it has been widely imitated all over the world (Costantini, et al., 1953a; Dogliotti, et al., 1954; Battezatti and Taddei, 1954; Bucherl, 1956; Vanpeperstraete and Ardenne, 1958).

Clowes, et al. (1954) experienced difficulties in the removal of the small gas bubbles. Therefore, they incorporated into their artificial lung an oxygen distributing head which produced bubbles 2 to 7 mm. in diameter. Many of these large bubbles exploded in an ascending bubble breaking chamber. The remainder encountered a defoaming airjet, as originally proposed by Thomas and Beaudoin (1950). For further safety, a chamber filled with antifoam coated spheres was placed on top of the bubblebreaker. The oxygenating capacity of this machine amounted to 4.5 L./min., with a priming volume of 2.6 L.

The oxygenator designed by DeWall, et al. (1956b, 1957b, 1958) incorporates the defoaming principle initiated by Clark. It has been used with conspicuous success at the University of Minnesota and has firmly established the reliability of the bubbling technique combined with defoaming. In the DeWall oxygenator (fig. 19, B), large volumes of oxygen are bubbled through a column filled with venous blood from the perfused organism. Most of the resulting foam is destroyed in an oblique coalescence chamber which is coated with an antifoam compound. The blood then flows through a long helicoidal settling tube which has proven to be a most efficient bubble trap. Then it is filtered and passed into the arterial line. The DeWall equipment is relatively inexpensive; it may be turned out easily by the central supply service of most hospitals, is heat sterilizable and is easy to assemble and to check (Lillehei, et al., 1956a). Care must be taken to remove all gas bubbles on priming the blood circuit (Faggella, et al., 1958; McKenzie and Barnard, 1960). The usual design permits blood flows of at least 2 L./min. with a priming volume below 3 L. Higher flow rates (4 L./min. and more) can be achieved by doubling the oxygenating and defoaming chambers and increasing the size of the helix (Lenfant, 1956; Taber and Tomatis, 1959). The gas flow needed is about three times the blood flow. Two to three per cent CO_2 content in the gas mixture prevents a marked hyperventilation.

The success of the DeWall oxygenator, as compared with its many unsuccessful precursors, is due to its adequate defoaming capacity. A few minor improvements have been proposed, such as immersion of the helix in a water bath, the insertion of a steel debubbling canister at the top of the oxygenating column, or that of an antifoam coated mesh in the dependent part of the debubbling chamber. Although the design of the machine may look relatively crude at first sight, the critical size and shape of all parts of the circuit have been thoroughly worked out. Unfortunately, because this oxygenator looks so simple, and possibly because it is not available as one "ready to use" unit, but must be assembled for each perfusion, there has been an almost irresistible temptation to "improve" the original DeWall design. Most of the modifications (or actually deviations) devised by the followers of the Minneapolis group have resulted in disasters (see, for instance, Diesh, et al., 1957; Abrams, et al., 1958). Failures have been ascribed to gas, antifoam or fibrin embolization, although it is improbable that these complications ever occurred to any serious extent in the hands of the originators of the technique. In fact, the DeWall oxygenator has benefited from its extensive clinical application and has served for more human perfusions than any other machine. Its success has spread all over the world and the machine has been tested everywhere from France (Dubost, et al., 1956; Lenfant, et al., 1956b; Ducuing, et al., 1957; Devin, et al., 1959), England (Drew, et al., 1957; Cass, et al., 1958; Taylor, 1959), Holland (Eerland, et al. 1957, 1959), Norway (Semb, 1959a, b), Sweden (Swedberg and Nettleblad, 1959), to Czechoslovakia (Bednarik, et al., 1959), Argentina (Guastavino, et al., 1959 b), South Africa (McKensie and Barnard, 1958), and China (Koo, et al., 1958).

A permanent type of sequential bubble oxygenator has been proposed by Jordan, et al. (1958a, b), and Chevret and Besson (1960). Jordan, et al. have used two stainless steel tubes joined in a common debubbling chamber (fig. 19 C). The gas exchange tube is 100 cm. in length and 3.5 cm. in internal diameter. The oxygen distributing manifold is a stainless steel disc perforated with 250 minute holes, 0.06 mm. in diameter, through which gas is injected into the venous blood stream. The debubbling chamber is a 4 L.

stock gauze container, in which a fitted wire basket holding stainless steel sponges is inserted. No antifoaming substance is needed. The second tube, 2.5 cm. in diameter serves as an arterial reservoir. After passing through a stainless steel wire mesh filter, the arterialized blood is returned to the perfused organism. The level of blood in the arterial reservoir can be seen through a sight glass. A stainless steel blood reservoir of 3 L. capacity is connected by plastic tubing to the bottom of the defoaming chamber. This reservoir can be raised or lowered either to transfuse or to bleed the system. A particular feature of this oxygenator is that the two tubes, though having different inside diameters, are interchangeable in their seats in the debubbling chamber. The oxygen manifold chamber and the filter manifold chamber are also interchangeable. Thus blood can be arterialized in the small tube when low flows are needed and in the large one for higher flows.

A particular feature of the DeWall oxygenator was the use of disposable plastic material so as to eliminate the problems of scrubbing. This idea led to the development by the Minneapolis group (Gott, et al., 1957 a, b) of a compact, disposable oxygenator constructed of two sheets of polyvinyl plastic (fig. 20, A). The blood chambers and channels are delineated by a heat seal of the plastic material so as to obtain a two-dimensional version of the DeWall oxygenator. The gas exchange device is a complete, self-contained, ready-to-use, sterile unit which has become commercially available. Its performance, in the low flow range needed for infants and children, compares favorably with the three-dimensional prototype of that unit. A regional perfusion oxygenator of similar design, which features a capacity of 500 ml./min. and efficient debubbling for at least an hour, has been described by Ausman and Aust (1960).

A simple, disposable plastic lung has been devised by Hyman, et al. (1956). The oxygenating chamber and the defoaming chamber are placed on top of each other (fig. 20 B). A saran screen inserted between the trough and the arterial reservoir slows the blood entering the reservoir, minimizes the introduction of air bubbles and allows a variable drop to the blood level in the reservoir. The incorporation of this filter (Hyman, 1959a) has permitted a substantial increase in the blood flow rate. Presently, the oxygenator has a capacity above 1.5 L./min. with a priming volume of about 600 ml. The gas flow: blood flow ratio does not need to exceed 1:1 to insure proper gas exchange. In our own experience, the debubbling action becomes less efficient after 60 to 90 minutes of use and, in principle, the machine should not serve for longer perfusions. The Hyman oxygenator is commercially available in a sterile package. In clinical emergencies, it can be put into service on 30 minutes' notice (Halley, et al., 1959a).

Another interesting development along the same lines is the Rygg-Kyvsgaard (1956 a, b; 1958) plastic bag oxygenator (fig. 20 C). It is made of two polyethylene sheets, heat sealed so as to delineate an oxygenating chamber, a debubbling chamber, a settling chamber and an arterial reservoir. Oxygen is introduced through holes in a plastic tube. Debubbling and filtration occur over polyurethane sponges coated with antifoam. The width of these sponges (35 mm.) confers a three dimensional shape to the plastic bag, which therefore has a higher oxygenating capacity (above 3 L./min.) and a larger priming volume (1200 ml.) than the other plastic bag oxygenators. A somewhat smaller model with no settling chamber is also available. The defoaming action as

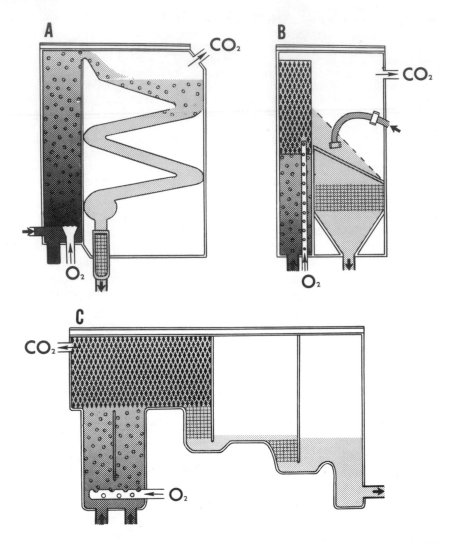

Fig. 20. Disposable plastic bag oxygenators featuring the principle of sequential bubble oxygenators. Symbols as in fig. 19.

A. Oxygenator described by Gott, et al. (1957a,b). The main features are the perforated plate for oxygen distribution, the winding settling chamber delineated in the plastic bag and the cylindrical stainless steel filter in the arterial line.

B. Oxygenator proposed by Hyman, et al. (1956). Oxygen enters through multiple holes in a vertical distributing tube. The gas exchange chamber is capped by a saran sleeve coated with antifoam. Blood traverses a vertically disposed nylon filter before entering the arterial line. Cardiotomy blood is returned to the top of the arterial reservoir.

C. Oxygenator described by Rygg and Kyvsgaard (1956a,b; 1958). Polyurethane sponges coated with antifoam serve for debubbling and filtration purposes. (See details in text.)

tested in our laboratory is extremely efficient for at least five hours and is usually satisfactory for 10-hour perfusions. Successful application of this device has been reported by Gammelgard, et al. (1957) and Saegesser, et al. (1960).

Summarizing

In the sequential bubble oxygenator the three chambers for respectively producing foam, defoaming and settling of the blood are arranged in series so blood passes from one chamber to the next. The last chamber serves simultaneously as an arterial reservoir. Permanent as well as disposable gas exchange devices have been developed on this principle. The oxygenating capacity of these devices is usually limited by the extent of their ability to remove the excess of gas bubbles.

CONCENTRIC BUBBLE OXYGENATORS

The idea of arranging the different elements of an artificial lung concentrically rather than sequentially was prompted by the desire for a compact gas exchange unit which would save on surface of contact between blood and foreign material, decrease the amount of priming blood and minimize the heat loss.

This design originated in the elegant small bubble oxygenator described by Gollan, et al. (1952a, 1955), for low flow perfusion under hypothermic conditions (fig. 21 A). Gollan's design embodies all the advantageous features of the concentric bubble oxygenator, namely compactness, simplicity and ease of assembly and control. It consists of a glass column through which venous blood mixed with oxygen ascends. Plastic fibers coated with antifoam are placed in the top cylinder for disposing of the bubbles, and oxygenated blood is withdrawn from the bottom of the arterial reservoir. The apparatus features an internal glass coil through which a temperature regulating fluid can be circulated. Thus the temperature of the blood can be altered simultaneously with its chemical composition. The use of a sintered glass filter as oxygen distributing head makes the size of the bubbles extremely small. The oxygenation is therefore very efficient, but the carbon dioxide removal lags behind somewhat. Owing to the protective effect of hypercapnia at low body temperatures, the retention of CO_2 is not a drawback for a gas exchange unit designed for hypothermic perfusions (see Chapter XIX).

The oxygenator proposed by Dodrill, et al. (1955) employed a stainless steel plate with holes, 10 micra in diameter, as the oxygen distributing manifold. The rate of arterialization could be regulated by the pressure beneath the metallic plate. Owing to the extremely small size of the bubbles obtained, and consequently, the huge surface of contact between gas and blood, the total amount of oxygen needed for complete saturation was merely 50 per cent in excess of the actual oxygen requirement of the perfused organism. On that basis one would expect a marked CO_2 retention, since a gas flow of a few hundred ml. can eliminate only negligible amounts of CO_2 when normal arterial tensions are maintained. Therefore, it is difficult to understand the authors' statement that, if pure oxygen was bubbled in sufficient quantities to fully arterialize the venous blood, any excessive amount of CO_2 was washed away.

An oxygenator consisting essentially of two bubble chimneys located in a large cylindrical reservoir was described by Shumway, et al. (1956). Porcelain filter discs served for oxygen distribution. The entire oxygenator was made of Plexiglas or Lucite and could be disassembled for cleaning. Around 1956-1957, the difficulties associated with the removal of small gas bubbles caused most designers to give up sintered glass and porcelain filters as oxygen distributing heads, and to turn to larger bubble-producing orifices. Nelson, et al. (1956), chose size 14 French oxygen catheters immersed vertically in the

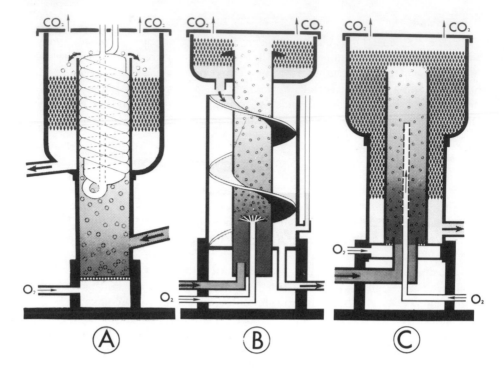

Fig. 21. Schematic representation of three models of concentric bubble oxygenators. All devices feature a central oxygenating column, at the bottom of which venous blood and oxygen are simultaneously injected. At the top of the oxygenating column, the foam overflows in a debubbling chamber where the excess of gas bubbles is removed by contact with antifoam coated surfaces. The arterialized blood, freed of bubbles, then settles in an arterial reservoir from where it is tapped for perfusion.

A. Small bubble oxygenator devised by Gollan, et al. (1952a). The coil wound in the oxygenating column serves to bring a thermoregulating fluid into contact with the blood.

B. Oxygenator utilized by Cooley, et al. (1957, 1958 a,b). Made completely of stainless steel, it is particularly sturdy and reliable.

C. Oxygenator described by Hufnagel, et al. (1959), built of transparent, plastic material. (See details in the text.)

oxygenating column. Milnes, et al. (1957 a, b) delivered the oxygen at the bottom of the bubble chimney through a vertical lucite tube which displayed 20 holes 0.8 mm. in diameter. Despite the use of antifoam in the debubbling chamber, and the interposition of a fine stainless steel filter, they found that a column of at least 8 cm. had to be maintained in the outer cylinder to provide a safety barrier against small bubbles and fibrin embolization. They stated that a gas flow about seven times that of venous blood was required for sufficient oxygenation. The specific aim of the oxygenator described by Merendino, et al. (1957) was to produce a large number of uniform sized bubbles, 3 mm. in diameter, which could readily be eliminated from the arterialized blood. A 1 mm. thick base plate containing 20 drilled holes 0.33 mm. in diameter produced a uniform stream of large sized bubbles when a gas flow of 10 L./min. was maintained. The priming volume of the machine was 1.5 L. and blood flows up to 4 L./min. could be achieved. Oxygenators of somewhat similar design have been described by Painter, et al. (1957), Keown, et al. (1957), Weiss and Bailey (1960), Trubetskoy (1960) and Malette, et al. (1960).

The oxygenator of Cooley, et al. (1957, 1958a, b) is made entirely of stainless steel and thus can be cleaned and sterilized as are surgical instruments. It consists of four principal parts (fig. 21 B): (a) a diffusion head for oxygen dispersal; (b) an oxygenating column; (c) a defoaming chamber; and (d) an inclined helicoidal trough. The diffusion head is perforated by approximately 150 small holes, 0.5 mm. in diameter, around which the venous blood enters. The oxygenating column is 75 cm. long and has an inside diameter of 3.75 cm. On top of the oxygenating column is the defoaming chamber, into which the blood gas mixture overflows. This chamber, which is approximately 15 cm. in diameter, contains disposable stainless steel scouring sponges sprayed with antifoam. From the defoaming chamber the liquid blood, purged of its gas bubbles, is drained through a spigot and passes into the inclined helicoidal trough that leads to an arterial reservoir. Attached to the reservoir is a side tube to indicate the blood level. The apparatus provides blood flows up to 3 L./min. with a priming requirement between 1 and 1.5 L. The rate of oxygen flow is set at 10 times the intended rate of blood flow. To avoid hypocapnia, a mixture of 97% O_2-3% CO_2 is recommended. Very similar in design is the oxygenator constructed by Taber and Tomatis (1959). To satisfy the demands of extended, high flow perfusions, the vertical oxygenating column has been enlarged to 5 cm. in internal diameter. Venous blood may be pumped into the oxygenating column or the oxygenator may be placed on the floor thereby allowing the venous blood to drain into it by gravity. Arterialized blood flows from the debubbling canister into the arterial reservoir through a polyvinyl plastic helix which serves to complete the defoaming and also to gauge the amount of blood in the reservoir. A filter of stainless steel mesh is provided at the bottom of the reservoir. All steel surfaces in contact with blood are coated with baked-on Teflon. Thermoregulation is accomplished by placing the lower two-thirds of the oxygenator in a water bath.

The oxygenator described by Hufnagel, et al. (1959) is also of the double concentric column bubbler type (fig. 21 C). The base plate and all the fittings are made of nylon. The columns and exterior shell consist of treated plexiglas which can be autoclaved. The entire unit is therefore transparent and sterilizable by heat. Blood is admitted into the inner oxygenating column (68 cm. in length) through a central opening. The base plate is perforated for the admission of oxygen. A central tube of nylon extending three-fourths of the distance up the inner column also supplies oxygen through small radial holes arranged in a spiral throughout the length of the tube. This central distribution is said to increase greatly the oxygenation of the blood over that obtainable by distribution through the base plate alone. The top portion of the outer chamber is enlarged and filled with siliconized steel mesh, thereby acting as a debubbling chamber. Siliconized steel mesh also fills the upper two-thirds of the outer column or arterial reservoir. Blood overflowing from the central oxygenating tube trickles downward through the steel mesh into the lowest portion of the outer chamber. The blood level in this reservoir is kept sufficiently high to include the lower portion of the siliconized steel mesh, so that there is no free fall of blood. The total priming volume necessary to fill this apparatus is 1.2 L. The oxygenating capacity approaches 5 L./min.

Summarizing

In concentric bubble oxygenators the components are so arranged as to surround one another. Thereby the surfaces of contact between blood and foreign material, the priming volume and the heat loss are minimized. Oxygen is finely dispersed in venous blood into an oxygenating column, thereby forcing the foaming mixture upward. At the top, defoaming agents coalesce the arterialized blood which is then collected in a suitable reservoir.

FOAM OXYGENATORS

Although foam oxygenators are classified for simplicity under the heading of bubble oxygenators, they utilize a different oxygenation principle: oxygen is bubbled into blood at the bottom of a container, and the resulting foam is permitted to accumulate upon the surface of the liquid. Venous blood is poured over the top of a densely packed column of this foam and cascades downwards, spreading over the surface of the bubbles. The resulting film is oxygenated while falling through the interspaces of the mass of oxygen bubbles. Eventually, it runs off into the blood pool upon which the foam column rests. Arterialized blood can then be tapped from the bottom of the container.

In such a gas exchange device, oxygen and carbon dioxide transfer depend mainly upon filming of the venous blood over an aggregation of oxygen bubbles, rather than upon the bubbling of oxygen through the arterialized blood. Thus foam oxygenators differ from bubble oxygenators in two main features: (a) by applying the counter-current principle, venous blood and oxygen are injected in opposite directions; (b) gas exchange occurs primarily in the foam phase and not in the liquid phase. In bubble oxygenators, the foam is a nuisance and must be disposed of as early as possible, whereas in the foam oxygenators, the foam is a necessity—but must be kept within limits. The ideal foam oxygenator depends upon the filming principle for its efficient gas exchange and, hence, can hardly be considered as an ordinary bubbler.

As new bubbles are continually blown into the blood at the bottom of the gas exchange device, the foam column is displaced upward, while the liquid blood is separated by gravity and collected at the dependent part of the container. The foam may overflow unless the bubbles are ruptured at the end of their course in order to let their gas content escape from the oxygenator and permit the liquid in their walls to trickle down into the column. The tendency of the bubbles to coalesce and to burst is enhanced by the mechanical action of rivulets of venous blood distributed by a kind of shower head over the foam cushion. Because continuous percolation makes the foam very thick, there is a tendency for blood to accumulate in the foam phase, and for the level of liquid at the bottom of the container to drop as times goes on.

The amount of foam formed depends upon the flow rate of the gas injected. Thus the maximum volume of bubbles that can be ruptured per unit of time sets the limits for the gas exchange capacity of a foam oxygenator. The smaller the bubbles, the larger is the surface area of the blood film coming in contact with the oxygen, and seemingly, the less is the necessary gas flow. In practice, it is found that foam oxygenators are extremely efficient as far as oxygen transfer is concerned. There is no special need for tiny bubbles to increase their oxygenating capability because the limit is set by carbon dioxide elimination. One can easily calculate that, if complete equilibrium is established between foam and venous blood by the time the bubbles have reached the top of the column, 70 ml. of CO_2 at best will be removed by a gas flow of 1 L./min. Therefore, 3 L./min. of oxygen bubbles must be ruptured if the metabolic needs of a normal adult are to be fully covered.

The desire to increase the oxygenating capacity by using small bubbles must be tempered by considerations of safety. Large bubbles climb more rapidly in the foam column than do small ones. If the velocity of ascent of gas bubbles is not greater than the downwards velocity of the blood, they will be carried away in the arterial blood stream. Therefore the smallest permissible bubbles are much larger in a foam oxygenator than in a regular bubble oxygenator. In fact, the historical development of foam oxygenators is characterized by a progressive increase in the diameter of the holes in the oxygen distributing manifold. It has also been found necessary to eliminate stray bubbles by including some kind of bubble trap in the arterial line.

The first design of a foam oxygenator originated in Brukhonenko's laboratory (Iankovskii, et al., 1939). Venous blood was converted into foam by the admixture of moist oxygen at the bottom of a container, whereas octyl alcohol vapors were injected on top of the foam in order to dispose of it after sufficient oxygenation. When large gas bubbles were produced, this artificial lung contained 500 ml. of blood in the liquid phase and 50 ml. in the foam phase, which was limited to 1.5 L. The oxygenating capacity was sufficient to maintain a 15 Kg. dog on total heart–lung bypass. The artificial lung described by Waud (1952) also used the counter-current motion of blood and foam for the continuous renewal of a gas exchange surface. It consisted mainly of a funnel-shaped glass percolator, the bottom hole of which was large enough to admit the oxygen inlet and the arterial blood outlet. The venous blood was distributed evenly over the cushion of oxygen bubbles in the percolator. Since no specific defoaming agent was provided, it was necessary at times to shut off the oxygen completely, to avoid overflow. The foam oxygenator of Gimbel and Engelberg (1953, 1954) designed to process 2.5 L./min. of blood, consisted of a 5 cm. diameter, 45 cm. high glass column surmounted by a short, wide glass bowl (fig. 22 A). Bubbles were produced at the foot of the column by forcing pure oxygen through a manifold of 100 segments of 25 gauge hypodermic needles (0.25 mm. internal diameter). The bubbles blown in such a manner were about 2 mm. in diameter and could ascend against a blood flow of 10 L./min. When the foam column rose above the shower head distributor of venous blood in the bowl, it encountered a baffle of high surface area smeared with an antifoam compound. This defoaming system was not very efficient, since it did not break up more than 0.8 L./min. of bubbles. As a consequence it severely limited the elimination of carbon dioxide. On the contrary, the oxygen transfer capacity was extremely high when compared to other types of lung built on the stationary screen or rotating disc principle (Gimbel and Engelberg, 1954). When 21 gauge needles (0.50 mm. inner diameter) were used, the efficiency of oxygenation decreased by 20 per cent only. Therefore, the authors suggested that the use of larger gas bubbles could result in a better overall performance because defoaming would be easier, the risk of gas embolism lessened and the hold-up of blood in the column diminished.

Foam oxygenators of somewhat similar design, but utilizing large bubbles, have been described by Clowes, et al. (1954), Wilkens (1955), Folga and Semerau-Siemianowski (1955) and Schimert (1956). The design developed by Sakakibara (1957b, 1959) features a particular oxygen distributing head located almost at the surface of the blood, in order to avoid gas bubbles being carried away with the arterial stream (fig. 22 B). A refined model described by Semerau-Siemianowski, et al. (1958) features rhythmical oscillations in the pressure of oxygen distributed. This property should help to maintain the foaming process within the desired limits.

The artificial lung devised by Salisbury (1956a) was the first percolating oxygenator model to achieve a really large gas exchange capacity. In this machine (fig. 22 D) a thick layer of foam is created by dispersing oxygen through blood at the bottom of a stainless steel funnel coated with teflon. Venous

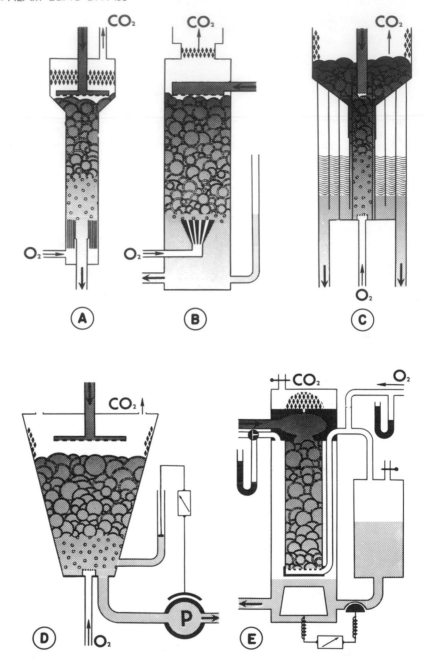

Fig. 22. Scheme of five different models of foam oxygenators. All feature counter-current injection of venous blood and oxygen.

A. Oxygenator described by Gimbel and Engelberg (1953, 1954).
B. Oxygenator of Sakakibara, et al. (1957b, 1959).
C. Oxygenator described by Neptune, et al. (1960) and Panico (1960).
D. Oxygenator of Salisbury (1956a).
E. Oxygenator described by Ananiev, et al. (1958). (See details in text.)

blood is trickled over the foam from a teflon head in which it is distributed in many small rivulets by a spiral gutter. The foam is killed at the top of the cone by the mechanical action of the blood shower as well as by an antifoam compound coated over the upper fifth of the container walls. The level of arterial blood at the bottom of the cone is maintained at a constant, safe level, by a sensing device which can modify the output of the arterial pump. The blood also passes in a shallow layer through a long, horizontal bubble trap, where a slow transit enables even small stray bubbles with little buoyancy to rise to the surface (*see* fig. 53). This oxygenator requires 2.5 L. of blood for priming purposes and has a capacity of up to 5 L./min. Its efficiency in debubbling makes it possible to use large oxygen flows, and consequently, to control the CO_2 content of the blood by regulating the gas admixture.

One of the most interesting developments in the field of foam oxygenators is the AIK artificial lung described by Ananiev, et al. (1958). In this unit (fig. 22 E) the venous blood is injected under pressure at the top of the foam column, and distributed centrifugally over the inner wall of a spheroidal chamber, in order to warrant a good dispersion. The amount of foam within the gas exchange unit is limited by a cylindrical filter of kapron (nylon) which prevents foam from escaping across its mesh into the glass container. Moist oxygen is forced through a porous membrane at the bottom of the foam column and distributed by 30 apertures in bubbles of uniform size. The overall gas pressure in the oxygenating chamber is monitored by a manometer and any excess is permitted to escape through a valve. The foam which is not destroyed by the mechanical action of blood distribution in the centrifugal chamber overflows into the defoaming chamber at the top of the oxygenator, where it condenses by contact with antifoam coated sponges. The arterialized blood settles at the bottom of the oxygenator in a kind of reservoir, which provides an additional defense against gas embolism. A float in the arterial reservoir monitors the level of blood. When it falls too close to an electro-magnet placed beneath the oxygenator, a clamp is released permitting blood to empty from a side reservoir into the main circuit.

The AIK machine comes closer than does any other to the ideal of a foam oxygenator, namely to achieve gas exchange by filming only and not by bubbling. The blood content of the foam is extremely small in comparison with other devices of the same type (3 per cent of the priming volume, instead of 25 per cent or more). Using a foam column twice as long as the one originally proposed, between 4 and 5 L./min. of blood can be fully oxygenated (Ananiev, et al., 1959; Kharnas, 1960). The flow of oxygen does not exceed 1.2 L./min. which makes occurrence of CO_2 retention likely when large organisms are perfused (Babskaga and Pogosova, 1960). On the other hand, a 3 per cent CO_2-97 per cent O_2 mixture is said to be used in certain circumstances, probably when the metabolic production of CO_2 is less than the amount blown out by the rigidly maintained volume of ventilation. There is no information available concerning one inherent weakness in the foaming principle, namely the difficulty of keeping the amount of foam within the preset limits for a period exceeding one or two hours. According to Ananiev, et al. (1959), a more viscous siloxane should perform better than does regular Antifoam A.

The latest design of foam oxygenator is that proposed by Neptune, et al. (1960). Venous blood falls by gravity on a stream of oxygen emanating from a diffusion disc at the base of a central bubble chimney (fig. 22 C). Oxygen transports the blood to an antifoam coated debubbling chamber situated on top of the oxygenator. From there the blood flows into a series of concentric chambers arranged as a labyrinth. These chambers serve a double purpose— they provide skimming of any stray bubble which may have entered the blood stream, and they function as arterial blood reservoirs. One of the most interesting features of this oxygenator is its extremely low priming volume. Owing to the extremely smooth conditions of flow which prevail between the inner and outer reservoir, it is possible to superpose saline over the blood and to keep the two fluids separated for rather long periods of time. If the oxygenator is primed from the arterial line in a retrograde fashion as for instance, by slow arterial bleeding from the organism to be perfused, simultaneously compensated by intravenous transfusion, one may actually operate the oxygenator with a minimal amount of blood in the extracorporeal circuit. A smaller model of oxygenator, working on the same principle, has been described by Panico (1960).

Summarizing

In foam oxygenators foam is produced by injecting oxygen at the bottom of a container filled with blood. Venous blood, poured on top of the foam, spreads in a thin film over the surface of the bubbles and becomes arterialized. Foam oxygenators differ from other bubble oxygenators in that venous blood and oxygen are injected in opposite directions. Therefore gas exchange occurs in the foam phase and not in the liquid phase. Foam oxygenators are extremely efficient as far as oxygen binding is concerned, but their capacity for CO_2 elimination is often limited. Some models feature an extremely small priming volume.

SPRAY OXYGENATORS

The technique of spreading blood out in fine drops by means of compressed oxygen, in order to achieve arterialization was first applied by von Euler and Cornelius Heymans (1932). In fact, the use of a spray for accelerating a chemical reaction between a liquid and a gas was suggested by J. F. Heymans (1921), who devised on that principle an apparatus for the continuous absorption of CO_2 in the expired air by an alkaline solution. An artificial lung was built on the same principle (fig. 23 A): blood and oxygen were injected under pressure through closely spaced openings of about 1.0-1.5 mm. in diameter. Blood was blown in fine droplets against the inside of a spherical glass bulb, then collected at the bottom of the container, whence it could be tapped for perfusion. At a blood flow up to 250 ml./min., as much as 20 ml. of oxygen could be transferred. No frothing occurred as long as defibrinated blood was employed. Von Euler and Heymans observed hemolysis only when the dispersion of the droplets was too fine, or when blood was more than 24 hours old. However, the investigators who have attempted to develop spray oxygenators for the purpose of total body perfusion have been impressed by the marked blood damage this technique entails (Bjørk, 1948a; Bencini, 1949; Kunlin, 1952; Fleisch, 1958). The fact that their reports are rather scanty seems to indicate that at high blood flows, this type of artificial lung produces too much hemolysis to become practicable, despite its efficiency in terms of gas transfer. Nobody has been able to achieve a consistently successful heart–lung substitution by means of a spray oxygenator, and today the method appears somewhat obsolete.

A different approach to the technique of dispersing blood droplets in an atmosphere of oxygen has been proposed by Smith, et al. (1957), and Vasli, et al. (1959). To avoid hemolysis and foaming, their "multiple stage droplet oxygenator" (fig. 23 C) features low blood flow velocities and relatively large

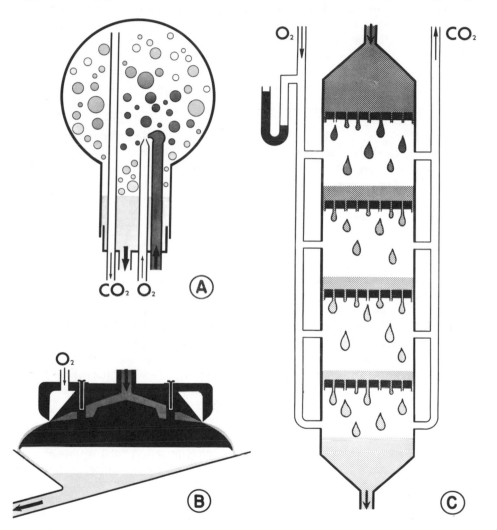

Fig. 23. Spray oxygenators. The three devices represented have in common that oxygen under pressure is used to force venous blood in small drops or a thin film. The drops or the film are then easily oxygenated thanks to their relatively large surface volume ratio.

A. Oxygenator proposed by von Euler and Heymans (1932).
B. Oxygenator devised by Marx, et al. (1959).
C. Oxygenator described by Smith, et al. (1957) and Vasli, et al. (1959). (See details in text.)

drops. Perforated stainles steel plates positioned horizontally are mounted into a vertical tower in a plastic cylinder. Venous blood enters at the top of the tower and cascades downwards through the holes in the plates. The droplets formed under each plate fall through an oxygen atmosphere into the pool on the plate beneath, where mixing occurs. The blood is finally arterialized when it accumulates at the bottom of the column. From pilot studies, it was found that coalescence of droplets on the undersurface of the plate could be prevented by spacing the holes, coating the metal surface with antifoam or using short tubes extending about 3 mm. below the plate. Oxygenation was better with higher cylinders and therefore with longer droplet fall, as well as with larger tubes (around 2 mm. I.D.). It was calculated that a tower made of 40 plates, each carrying about 50 tubes, would be needed for properly oxygenating a blood flow of 3 L./min., while requiring a priming volume in the order of 500 ml. However, no further studies on this artificial lung have been reported.

While searching for a simpler and safer way of accomplishing gas exchange in blood, Marx, et al. (1959) have proposed the "impingement oxygenator" (fig. 23, B). In this apparatus, a jet of oxygen emerging from a narrow nozzle orifice impinges on the venous blood flowing over the oxygenator base. The gas, which changes direction as it is reflected off the base, imparts a certain amount of its kinetic energy to the blood thereby forcing it into an ultrathin film and achieving a large surface per unit of volume. A circular knife-edge lip configuration is achieved by bolting together the basic parts of the oxygenator, so as to adjust the oxygen and blood nozzle openings exactly to 0.1 mm. width. When the oxygenator is assembled, two completely separate chambers are created, one distributing oxygen and the other blood. All parts are made of solid steel, precision lathed and gold plated. A lucite reservoir collects arterialized blood dropping at the periphery of the oxygenator. Laboratory experience with the impingement oxygenator has been disappointing. Tremendous oxygen flow rates are required to maintain a nozzle pressure of 100 mm. Hg. The oxygen transfer is limited to 50 ml./min. despite the high blood flow through the artificial lung provided by a recirculation pump. Carbon dioxide is not effectively eliminated. Finally, hemolysis is marked owing to the jet effect and high linear velocities of blood reached.

Summarizing

Spray oxygenators are devices in which compressed oxygen impinges upon blood at such high velocities that fine droplets instead of bubbles are formed. Although this technique of mixing blood with oxygen is efficient in terms of gas transfer, it entails considerable hemolysis. Several oxygenators based on the spray principle have been described but none has been found practicable for total body perfusion.

VI. Film Oxygenators

Film oxygenators bring about a large blood–gas interface by spreading out a swiftly moving stream of blood into a relatively thin film. Gas exchange is then facilitated by exposing the blood film to an atmosphere of oxygen. There are various ways in which such a film can be produced. Blood can be made to flow over a stationary support such as a hanging plate, a cloth curtain, a metal screen or a pile of beads. Blood can also be distributed over moving supports, such as spinning cylinders, discs or cones. Film oxygenators are conveniently classified according to the type of support used. We shall follow this convention and describe oxygenators with stationary film support and oxygenators with moving film support.

PRINCIPLES AND HISTORICAL BACKGROUND

The thickness of the film obtained by gentle spreading of blood over a solid surface is by necessity greater than the diameter of the pulmonary capillaries. Nevertheless, satisfactory oxygen uptake and carbon dioxide removal can be achieved in this type of artificial lung provided a few requirements are suitably met: marked gas tension differences between the blood film and the adjacent atmosphere; prolonged time of exposure of the film; turbulent flow to renew constantly the surfaces of exchange; finally, recirculation of blood through the artificial lung if one passage does not permit completion of the gas transfer.

Early application of the filming process involved stationary supports, usually glass beads, glass bulbs or glass plates. Foaming, frothing and hemolysis were among the problems encountered. Even when these difficulties with respect to blood handling were mastered, arterialization of blood remained rather inefficient, because the superficial layer of the blood film acted as a barrier to gas exchange between the atmosphere and the layer immediately adjacent to the support (fig. 24, A). Since gas diffusion was thus limited to a certain depth of film, some degree of stirring had to be provided in the liquid phase, or the same blood had to be exposed repeatedly to oxygen in order to achieve full arterialization. The fundamental contribution of Gibbon's group was the observation that an irregular support, such as a wire mesh screen, would cause a gentle turbulence in the blood film and thereby promote continuous admixture between the inner and outer layers of the film (fig. 24 B). The concept, that the superficial layer of blood acts as a barrier to the diffusion of oxygen in the depth of the film, was established on firm experimental ground by Marx (1960) with documentation by direct measurements of the diffusion barrier in moving blood films. The hydrodynamic theory of thin

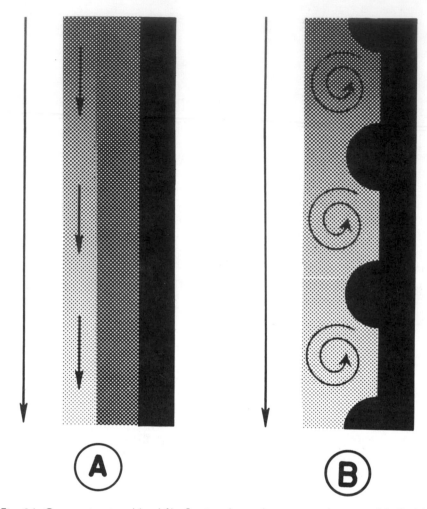

Fig. 24. Oxygenation in a blood film flowing down along a vertical support (black). Venous blood indicated by dark shading, arterialized blood by light shading.

A. Film on a smooth, flat support. The superficial layer of blood is properly oxygenated, but acts as a barrier to diffusion of oxygen into the depths of the film. Frictional resistance decreases the speed of descent of the blood layer immediately adjacent to the support, so that the arterialized blood flows as a sleeve over the blood which is not in direct contact with the oxygen atmosphere.

B. Film on an uneven corrugated support. Mild turbulence (spiral arrows) is induced by the irregularities in the supporting surface and causes continuous admixture of the deep blood layers with the superficial layers. Gas exchange is thereby enhanced.

films put forward by Kapitza and recently extended by Tailby and Portalski (1960) may serve as a base for future engineering developments in this field.

Early in the development of film oxygenators it became apparent that a thinner film could be achieved by forceful spreading of the blood over a rotating support. Since the exchange surface was built in such a way that venous blood could be continuously dispersed and arterialized blood continuously removed, the area of blood film exposed to gas increased in proportion to the rotational speed of the support. Consequently, the equilibration time could be reduced without detracting from the efficiency of gas transfer. By proper arrangement of the gas exchange surfaces, artificial lungs involving moving film supports have been brought to a high degree of practical utility. They occupy less space than do stationary film oxygenators, require a smaller priming volume, and can be conveniently autoclaved. These advantageous features compensate for the presence of moving parts in the blood phase and the inherent risk of blood trauma. They have brought about the ever increasing acceptance of rotating disc and cylinder oxygenators.

The physical operation of mass transfer across a surface involves many surface properties which are still poorly understood. For example, interfacial turbulence, rippling of liquid films flowing on a vertical support, traction of a moving monolayer on the underlying liquid are but a few phenomena about which fundamental information has just recently become available (Davies, 1960). Since biologists are largely unaware of the literature in chemical engineering, it is not surprising that in the past 80 years, film oxygenators have been developed on a purely empiric basis.

The first film oxygenator was designed by von Frey and Gruber (1885). It employed a slowly rotating, slanted cylinder on whose inner surface an equilibrium of gas tensions between blood and a controlled atmosphere was brought about (*see frontispiece*). This moving support was later abandoned because of irreducible blood foaming. One of the early artificial lungs which offers more than just historical interest is that described in 1928 by Bayliss, et al. (*see* fig. 31, A). A series of inversed truncated cones is held together on a vertical axle which is rotated by means of a worm gear. These movable cones are intersealed between a series of stationary plates which nest into one another accurately at their periphery. Blood entering at the top of the machine falls on the first revolving plate (the basis of the upper truncated cone) and is thrown in a thin film to the periphery. It collects on the upright wall of the first stationary plate, flows down the inclined surface and passes to the second revolving plate where the process is repeated. The Bayliss oxygenator, a small machine for organ perfusion, was able to transfer up to 19 ml. O_2 per minute at a flow of about 200 ml./min. and contained 54 ml. of blood. It served for years as a model of efficient gas exchange on a limited scale and was revived as late as 1954 by Osborn in attempts at total body perfusion.

Most of the early film oxygenators featured a stationary support. Of the many primitive devices described, one is worth mentioning since definitive advances in biologic knowledge resulted from its use: the oxygenator of Lindbergh (1935). Intended for organ perfusion under sterile conditions, it relied upon spreading the venous blood over the smooth surface of glass bulbs within an incubator. Its action was so gentle and efficient that isolated organs could be kept alive for many weeks.

When the feasibility of artificial maintenance of cardiorespiratory function in patients was seriously considered a decade ago, it seemed obvious that a larger oxygenating capacity could be obtained if the size of the early gas exchange devices were simply increased. Actual results at first did not meet this expectation, because the design characteristics of the blood films produced were inherently inefficient. The following devices illustrate the trend of developmental ideas in meeting the demand for the oxygenation of large blood volumes.

(*1*) Bailey, et al. (1951) attempted filming on the "Stedman packing," a stainless steel mesh used in chemical engineering when large surfaces of contact between gaseous and liquid reagents are needed. The Stedman packing consists of stacks of discs made of 60 x 40 mesh wire cloth, embossed and perforated so as to present a pattern of pyramids, valleys and holes. The device was critically studied by Gimbel and Engelberg (1954), who found its efficiency rather low as compared to other types of oxygenators. It was also imitated by Erickson and Hjørt (1956), who used saddle-shaped pieces of porcelain stacked in a plastic cylinder to produce a large filming surface (*see* fig. 28, A).

(2) Dubbelman (1951b) and Hayes, et al. (1955) employed gauze or nylon cloth as the filming support in artificial lungs, comparable to the original Richards and Drinker (1915) oxygenator. Venous blood spurted out of a perforated distributing tube to be caught immediately in the mesh of a heavy, but loosely woven cloth hanging in an oxygen atmosphere. Here again the gas exchange capacity was too low to permit total body perfusion in large-sized organisms and the development did not go beyond preliminary laboratory trials.

(3) Osborn, et al. (1956b), following an idea first successfully employed by Staub (1931), used a battery of fluted glass plates over which blood passed as a thin film. A recirculation pump maintained a constant flow over the slanted glass plates, thereby maintaining a blood film independently of variations in venous drainage or perfusion flow. This artificial lung was remarkable for its smooth performance and gentle blood handling.

(4) In the "smear oxygenator" of Poth (1958) the gas exchange chamber was a tygon tube filled with a rolled nylon mesh material. The mesh protruded from the end of the tube and dipped into the blood reservoir below, thus functioning as a wick to permit smooth flow without splashing or bubble formation. This artificial lung entrapped around 800 ml. of blood at a flow rate of 4 ml./min. However, the length of the nylon cloth used was such that it required a double decked operating room. Venous blood flowed directly into the oxygenator placed under the operating table and a pump on the floor of the lower deck returned the arterial blood to the organism. This arrangement was too inconvenient to find general acceptance.

Summarizing

In film oxygenators a swiftly moving stream of blood is spread out as a film and exposed to an oxygen atmosphere. The support for the film can be either a stationary or a moving surface. Large gas tension differences between blood and surrounding atmosphere, prolonged period of equilibration or repeated exposure of the blood film, and mechanical mixing of the liquid phase, are all factors to be considered in the design of an artificial lung based on the filming principle.

STATIONARY SCREEN OXYGENATORS

In their quest for a filming device capable of oxygenating large volumes of blood without undue trauma, Gibbon and his associates recognized the usefulness of mild turbulence avoiding a "sleevelike" flow in the blood film and promoting adequate gas exchange (see fig. 24). Stokes and Flick (1950) suggested the use of a wire screen as the support for the blood film. Blood flowing by gravity over a wire screen travels rapidly in a very thin film across the meshes, is first trapped on the upper surface of the horizontal wires and then descends again in a thin film across the mesh below. Thus there is a thorough mixing of all blood elements without foaming. The observation of an eightfold increase in efficiency of gas transfer when a wire screen was employed instead of a smooth plate led to the study of a large number of turbulence-producing surfaces. Screens made of stainless steel wire 0.7 mm. in diameter with rectangular mesh placed so as to have the greatest dimension of the mesh in the horizontal plane appeared the most efficient (Miller, et al., 1951). Larger wires produced an objectionable increase in hold-up and difficulties in maintaining the film without significant gain in oxygen transfer. Smaller wires held less blood, but produced inadequate turbulence. The historical sequence of achievements, which resulted in the design of the first machine to be successfully applied for total heart–lung bypass in man, has been reviewed by Kay and Anderson (1957, 1959), Dodd (1958), Griesser (1959 a, b) and Gibbon himself (1959 a, b).

The first screen oxygenator was constructed in the form of a vertical cylinder capped by a bullet shaped head of stainless steel. Blood was distributed by a revolving jet, passed down the screen in the form of a turbulent film and accumulated at the bottom in a collecting cup. It was necessary to brush the screen with blood in order to establish initially a complete film. From then on, the film was stable and gas exchange was performed steadily for periods of up to 4 hours. The device had an area of around 0.4 m² and an oxygenating capacity of 1 L./min. (Miller, et al., 1951).

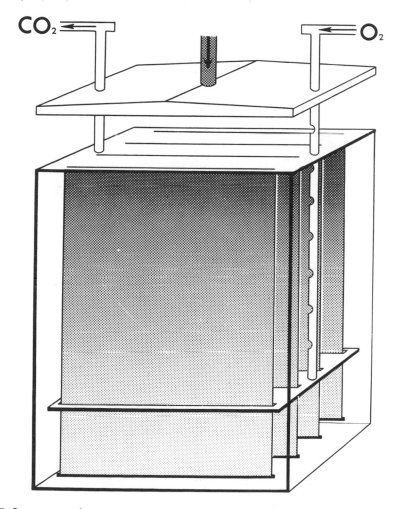

Fig. 25. Battery type of stationary screen oxygenator. Venous blood (dark shading) enters from the top into a distributing chamber under the roof of the oxygenator casing. Through narrow slits in the floor of the distributing chamber, blood is spread over wire mesh screens (shaded rectangular areas). At the end of its descent in an oxygen atmosphere, arterialized blood (light shading) collects in a reservoir (not shown) at the bottom of the oxygenator casing. The horizontal frame encircling the lower part of the screens is the filming device, or "comb." It is moved up and down to paint an even film of blood on the screens in order to start the gas exchange. The handles of the comb serve to carry gas in and out of the oxygenating chamber.

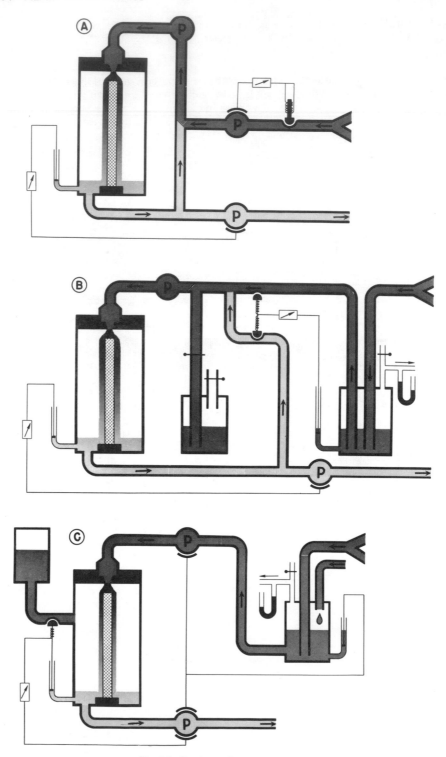

Fig. 26. See legend on opposite page.

In order to carry the entire circulation of an average adult, the geometric form was changed from the cumbersome vertical cylinder to a series of flat screens arranged in parallel and suspended in a clear plastic case. Through the cooperation of International Business Machine Corporation (I.B.M.), Gibbon, et al. (1953) constructed the battery type of screen oxygenator (fig. 25). The length of screen necessary to raise the oxygen saturation of the blood from 65 to 95 per cent at the optimum thickness of film was found to be 46 cm. Obviously the number of screens or their width had to be varied according to the blood flow in order to maintain the most efficient film thickness. A nomogram was constructed which related flow rate, screen width, volume of blood on the screens and oxygen saturation of the blood (Taylor, 1957). The original oxygenator consisted of six screens of stainless steel, each 45 cm. high and 30 cm. wide. The floor of the distributing chamber at the top of the oxygenator was made of seven bars of monel metal. Blood passed onto both faces of the screens through six narrow slits, or weirs, between the bars. The weirs extended the length of the chamber and were approximately 0.15 mm. in width and 16 mm. in depth. The lower extremity of each screen was inserted into a slot milled in a solid block of plastic, which served both to keep the screens in position and to reduce the volume of the collecting chamber. In order to establish the film, it was necessary to flood the whole oxygenator with saline immediately before blood was passed onto the screens. The saline was withdrawn by gravity at about the same rate that the blood would flow down the screens. When the solution was completely evacuated, blood was introduced and gas exchange began. Oxygen entered the plastic case through multiple perforations in a tube along a lateral wall and the excess escaped with the carbon dioxide through multiple outlets in the opposite wall. For reasons of convenience in engineering design, the flow of oxygen was set at such a high rate that excessive amounts of carbon dioxide were removed. A normal CO_2 tension of the arterialized blood was then maintained by the intermittent addition of small amounts of carbon dioxide into the gas entering the artificial lung. This type of control was achieved automatically by continuous measurement of the pH of the blood leaving the oxygenator. Condensation from the atmosphere within the oxygenator was prevented by heating elements imbedded within the lucite walls of the oxygenating chamber.

The original design of Gibbon's vertical screen oxygenator established one essential feature, namely the necessity of maintaining a constant volume of blood in the extracorporeal circuit and, thereby, a constant thickness of the blood film, independent of fluctuations in blood flow to or from the perfused organism. The problem was solved simply by incorporating in the circuit (fig. 26, A) a pump which constantly recirculated blood from the bottom to the

Fig. 26. Blood circuit schemes in various stationary screen oxygenators (screen symbolized by diagonal cross-hatching in the rectangular box on the left of each scheme).

A. Gibbon's original oxygenator (Miller, et al., 1951). The venous line includes a segment of soft resilient tubing provided with a diameter sensing device based on the principle of the differential transformer. If the venous pump generates too much suction, fluttering of the soft rubber tube actuates an electrical circuit which slows down the pump before actual caval collapse occurs. The recirculation pump (top P) is set at a constant flow rate which is always higher than that of the venous and arterial pumps. Consequently, there is always an upward flow of blood in the recirculating line (vertical connection between arterial and venous line). The rate of arterial pumping is automatically controlled by a level-sensing device in the collecting chamber, which tends to maintain a constant volume of blood in the extracorporeal circuit (electrical circuit acting on pump "P" on lower right side).

B. Gibbon-Mayo oxygenator: venous blood is transferred in a closed reservoir by the action of a controlled vacuum. The recirculation pump, set at a constant flow rate, aspirates, in varying proportions, blood from the venous line and from the arterial line in such a way that the levels in the venous reservoir and in the oxygenator remain constant.

C. Oxygenator described by Griesser (1958 a, b). Venous and coronary return are obtained by a controlled vacuum. The venous pump serves solely to transfer blood from the venous reservoir into the artificial lung. The output of both the venous and arterial pumps is under the control of level sensing devices in the venous reservoir and in the artificial lung. (Further details in text.)

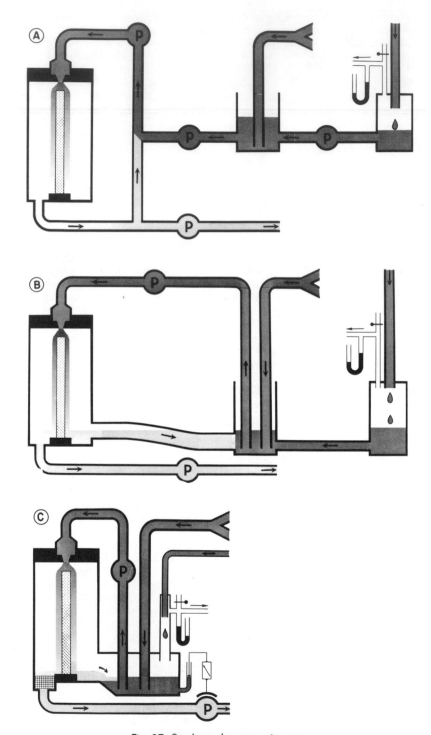

Fig. 27. See legend on opposite page.

top of the oxygenator. The first apparatus of the Gibbon type, built at the Mayo Clinic by Jones, et al. (1955), was essentially the original stationary screen oxygenator adapted to the needs of human surgery (Bernats, et al., 1956). It included 15 wire mesh screens, each 30 by 45 cm. Later the height of the screens was extended from 45 to 61 cm. (Kirklin, et al., 1958a). Blood gained access to the top of each screen through a series of carefully machined and polished slits in the stainless steel floor of the upper oxygenator reservoir. The weirs were 16 mm. deep and 0.20 or 0.25 mm. wide (instead of 0.15 mm.) in order to prevent the infrequent, but distressing, plugging during perfusion of polycythemic patients.

The most recent model of the Gibbon-Mayo pump-oxygenator retains the same essential features. Provision is made for reducing the number of screens to as few as four by replacing the distributing blocks, to which the screens are attached, by a solid block. The oxygenator provides adequate gas exchange at blood flows ranging between 220 and 280 ml./min. per screen (Lewin, et al., 1960), or up to 4.8 L./min. for the entire lung. The actual priming volume amounts to 2.2 to 3.5 L. The circuit used (fig. 26B) employs ingenious controls to maintain a constant volume of blood in the extracorporeal circuit. Both venous blood and cardiotomy return blood are aspirated in the same venous reservoir by a controlled vacuum. There is a single pump on the venous side of the oxygenator, which aspirates blood in varying proportions from the venous reservoir and from the recirculation lines. The volume control mechanism acts in the following way: should there be an increase in the amount of blood drained from the organism, then the level of blood in the venous reservoir will rise slightly. In response, a level-sensing device activates an occluder so as to open the venous line more fully and partly compress the recirculation line. Since the recirculation pump is set at constant rate (larger than the maximum anticipated blood flow), a greater fraction of the blood brought to the distributing head will then consist of venous blood. Simultaneously, the reduction in the amount of blood withdrawn from the collecting chamber at the bottom of the oxygenator via the recirculation line will cause a slight rise of the blood level in that chamber. The second level-sensing device is in turn activated and speeds up the arterial pump. A diminishing return from the veins causes the level in the venous reservoir, and secondarily in the oxygenator, to fall, which automatically results in a slower action of the arterial pump. In this way the variations in venous drainage lead to equal variations in arterial infusion. At the same time the maintenance of both a constant thickness of the blood film on the screens and a constant level of blood in the oxygenator makes it impossible unknowingly to increase or decrease the organism's blood volume during bypass.

The recirculation pump has been abandoned in the circuit described by Griesser (1958 a, b). The blood circuit is thereby simplified (fig. 26 C). However numerous controls are needed to achieve smooth performance of the oxygenator: the level sensing device in the venous reservoir acts on both the venous and arterial pumps, whereas the level sensing device in the artificial lung itself drives the arterial pump and an occluder on a feed line from a blood reservoir outside of the circuit.

Fig. 27. Blood circuit schemes in various stationary screen oxygenators (rectangular box toward the left with screen symbolized by diagonal cross-hatching).

A. First circuit used by Kay and Gaertner (1957). It requires four pumps: coronary suction pump (right), venous pump (center), recirculation pump (top), arterial pump (bottom).
B. Second circuit proposed by Kay and Gaertner (1957) provides a large recirculation shunt between the artificial lung and the venous reservoir (center).
C. Single-chambered oxygenator of Kay and Anderson (1957) in which a reservoir appended to the artificial lung collects the venous blood, the coronary sinus blood and the excess of arterial blood which are then mixed before circulating through the oxygenator. (Details in text.)

Kay and Gaertner (1957) have advocated the use of screens only 25 cm. in height, because the oxygen uptake by the blood occurs mainly on the upper portion of the screens. Their first apparatus included four pumps, i.e., for venous suction, coronary suction, recirculation and arterial infusion (fig. 27 A). The circuit was soon simplified and the number of pumps reduced to two by allowing venous blood to drain by gravity and by collecting cardiotomy blood under a slight vacuum (fig. 27, B). A single pump served for the transfer of venous blood into the oxygenator and for recirculation, because of the presence of a large internal shunt from the bottom of the oxygenator to the venous reservoir. Thereby the apparatus required less priming blood, produced less hemolysis and became easier to handle.

In 1959 Kay and Anderson described a single chambered screen oxygenator with only one container for the venous and arterialized blood (fig. 27, C). The foremost feature is the use of the recirculating pump to prevent the venous blood from reaching the arterial outlet without first going over the oxygenating screens. This eliminates separate storage containers for the venous reservoir, coronary sinus reservoir, arterial blood reservoir, arterial filter and bubble trap. Venous blood enters the unit on one side as does the blood from the coronary sinus suction tip. Mixed blood consisting of venous and recirculating arterialized blood reaches the screens via the internal circuit pump. Fully oxygenated blood collected at the other side of the unit is distributed to the organism via the arterial pump. In other words, the pump-oxygenator has a "ventricular septal defect with a left to right shunt." This offers the advantage of eliminating tubing dead space and of reducing the priming volume. The distributing chamber at the top of the artificial lung is emptied of air and filled completely with blood before starting the oxygenation. This provides equal pressure throughout the distributing chamber and causes similar flow through all the openings. The priming volume is as follows: oxygenator top 500 ml., screens 100 ml. each, oxygenator bottom 500 ml., tubing 500 ml.

Recent stationary screen oxygenators have a special device for establishing the film (Anderson, et al., 1957; Guastavino, et al., 1959 b). A sheet of teflon or stainless steel, with slots for the screens and two handles, (see fig. 25) can be raised just beneath the distribution chamber and then lowered to paint an even film of blood in a few seconds, or to reestablish it, should the film break and channeling occur. In addition the handles are utilized to introduce oxygen and to remove the excess gases from the oxygenator case. This "comb" permits replacement of the saline priming method and elimination of the waste of blood, dilution and delay inherent in the former technique.

Guastavino, et al. (1959 a) have demonstrated experimentally that the width of the slits in the blood distributing head should be at least 0.30 mm. wide (instead of 0.15 mm. as originally proposed) to permit the most efficient flow. Since blood viscosity is the main determinant of flow at a given head of pressure their results should be particularly borne in mind when the stationary screen oxygenator is used for hypothermic perfusion. Griesser (1958 a, b) has proposed to distribute the venous blood on the upper border of the screens by a row of tiny tubes under the floor of the upper reservoir. The drops formed at the lower extremity of the tubes are attracted by capillary action to the rim of the screens placed 1.0-1.5 mm. below. Since the mesh of the screens used is smaller than that of the Gibbon-type oxygenators, the film developed is also thinner and affords a faster gas exchange so that no recirculation pump is needed (see fig. 26, C). Similarly, Meyer-Wegener and Ney (1960) have employed a blood distributing manifold made of 1120 needles attached to holes in the base plate of the upper reservoir. They also used corrugated sheet-iron plates instead of a screen, in order to create a moderate amount of turbulence in the blood film.

Other stationary screen oxygenators have been described by Dietman (1955), Adams, et al. (1958), Kamm (1959), Margaglia, et al. (1959), and Guastavino, et al. (1959 a). Most authors agree that the main advantages of the stationary screen oxygenator are that it handles the blood gently and features reliable guards against hypercapnia, overoxygenation and gas embolism. Indeed this type of gas exchange device is, more than any other, susceptible to quantitative analysis, which in turn, leads to predictability of performance and optimal design. It often includes a wealth of controls which tend to run the machine almost automatically, a feature which may be explained historically by the attention devoted to it by large engineering companies such as International Business Machines (Taylor, 1957) and Convair (Kamm, 1959). Drawbacks of the stationary screen oxygenator are the relatively large priming volume and the necessity for relying on chemical sterilization for the oxygenator plastic case. Efforts have been made to minimize these inconveniences. In many commercial models the venous reservoir and the top as well as the bottom chamber of the oxygenator are designed to operate on a minimum blood volume, whereas a priming reservoir, capable of receiving large amounts of blood, is set for emergency requirements. As far as sterilization is concerned, two opposite solutions have been proposed. Some modern machines are made entirely of stainless steel (Kay and Anderson, 1959; Adams, et al., 1959; Griesser, 1960). Such apparatus can be sterilized repeatedly. Attempts are also made to develop disposable aluminum screens which can be discarded after use (Diettert, et al., 1958 a, b; Roe, et al., 1960).

Osborn, et al. (1959), have developed a disposable screen oxygenator where a blood film is spread on the inside of a series of partly inflated polyvinyl bags, each 76 cm. long and 40 cm. wide. The bags are inserted into a Lucite retaining frame and then inflated against the frame with an oxygen-carbon dioxide mixture. Blood is introduced into the top of each bag through a siliconed glass manifold. A Y-shaped distributing tube rocks back and forth inside the bags and spreads the blood into an even film on the inside of the bag at the top, as originally proposed by Long (1947). The bottom of each bag serves as a blood reservoir and drains into a common collecting manifold. Blood is continuously recirculated to maintain a constant film, using a circuit similar to that of fig. 26, A and B. The lack of efficiency in oxygen transfer due to filming over a smooth surface has been remedied in an ingenious way. Rapid changes in the thickness of the film are produced by the slowly moving oscillating jet. In this way blood runs down in rather thick waves, one following the other, and red cells at the surface can mix with those deeper in the falling film.

Summarizing

Stationary screen oxygenators take advantage of periodic changes in thickness of a blood film as it flows on a wire mesh. The turbulence needed for adequate gas exchange can also be provided by the use of a corrugated film support or by the pulsating distribution of blood at the top of the support. A recirculating pump is usually needed to maintain a constant volume of blood over the support despite changes in venous or arterial blood flow. Automatic devices which prevent any change in extracorporeal blood volume are also required for optimal performance.

STATIONARY SPONGE OXYGENATORS

The principle of sponge oxygenators is based on the fact that plasma appears to be the ideal surface for filming blood. Attempts have been made to

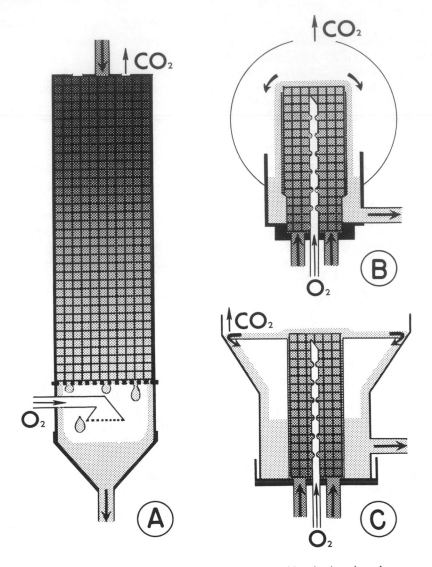

Fig. 28. Stationary sponge oxygenators (sponge represented by checkered area).

A. Artificial lung proposed by Erickson and Hjort (1956), which, like that of Bailey, et al. (1951), may be considered as a precursor of the sponge oxygenators. Venous blood enters at the top, cascades over intricate structures of porcelain or stainless steel and drips into an arterial reservoir at the bottom.

B. Oxygenator of Bencini and Parola (1956), featuring a polyurethane sponge enclosed in a plexiglas cylinder. Venous blood enters through the baseplate. Oxygen is distributed by a long, multiperforated needle standing in the center of the sponge. Arterialized blood overflows at the top of the cylinder and accumulates in the reservoir around the gas exchange column. The upper part of the oxygenator is protected by a plexiglas sphere with a hole at the top to permit the escape of gas.

C. Oxygenator devised by Gertz, et al. (1960). Arterialized blood spreads in a thin film on a horizontal plate to promote removal of the foam. At the periphery of this plate, the blood passes through a narrow slit and descends against the inner wall of a funnel shaped arterial reservoir. (Details in text.)

provide such a surface by filming blood over blood foam, as already mentioned. Another approach consists of using an absorbent surface saturated with plasma. Artificial sponges with large inter-connecting pores, saturated with water, provide in a small volume a large surface area on which blood will film naturally. If oxygen is simultaneously distributed in the sponge, gas exchange occurs in these artificial alveoli, and the blood is thereby arterialized. Such oxygenators are called "sponge oxygenators." Since oxygen must be injected into the sponge by some kind of dispersion manifold, sponge oxygenators are often confused with the usual bubble oxygenators. According to Bencini and Parola (1956), who pioneered the development of the sponge oxygenator, the efficiency of this type of artificial lung is extremely high, exceeding that of any other system, except the spray-oxygenator. The priming volume needed to establish the film in the sponge is limited to a few ml. and need scarcely be greater when the blood flow is increased (Bencini, et al., 1957, 1958 a; Parola and Bencini, 1957; Oselladore, et al., 1957).

One problem with the oxygenator developed by Bencini and Parola (fig. 28, B) is the formation of foam. By siliconizing the sponge it is possible to reduce considerably the number of bubbles emerging at the top of the gas exchange column. An annular nylon filter coated with antifoam, placed at the upper level of the arterial reservoir, provides a further defense against bubbles. Venous blood comes into contact with oxygen in the sponge for only 5 to 10 seconds. Nevertheless, even without recirculation, adequate oxygenation is provided for blood flows of up to 4.8 L./min. In a similar device proposed by Gertz, et al. (1960), a 1:5 ratio of gas flow to blood flow is sufficient to achieve complete oxygen saturation (fig. 28, C.). However, CO_2 retention is likely to occur with this degree of hypoventilation.

Another sponge oxygenator system was suggested by Heupel and Wild (1956). This artificial lung consists of a battery of polyvinyl formol (Ivalon) sponge leaves separated by inert wax plates. The assembly is placed vertically in a polyethylene support which is widely open at the bottom. Venous blood is distributed over the top of the frame and initially soaks down through the sponge leaves. The blood then films down and runs smoothly into an arterial reservoir below the tray. Oxygen is distributed from the side by a dispersion manifold fitted with a polyurethane sponge diffuser. It passes edgewise into the suspended sponge leaves and is exhausted to the outside through a hole on the opposite side of the container. An experimental unit based on this design was able to oxygenate 430 ml. of blood per minute with a priming volume no larger than 60 ml.

Sponge oxygenators are meant to simulate capillary flow through myriads of alveoli of different sizes. When flow is constant mild agitation will spread the film over a far larger surface than that provided by a smooth sheet. It remains to be proved whether a plasma absorbing sponge will be superior, as a film support, to a siliconized, unwettable surface which is less likely to create foam. The optimal gas flow in regard to blood flow also deserves further attention. The sponge oxygenator principle, unduly neglected in recent years, still offers a valuable approach to extracorporeal gas exchange.

Summarizing

Sponge oxygenators employ synthetic, spongy material as a mechanical support for filming blood. The surface is saturated with plasma and forms oxygen-filled spaces simulating the alveoli in the natural lung. These artificial lungs provide an extremely efficient oxygenation of blood and require only a small priming volume.

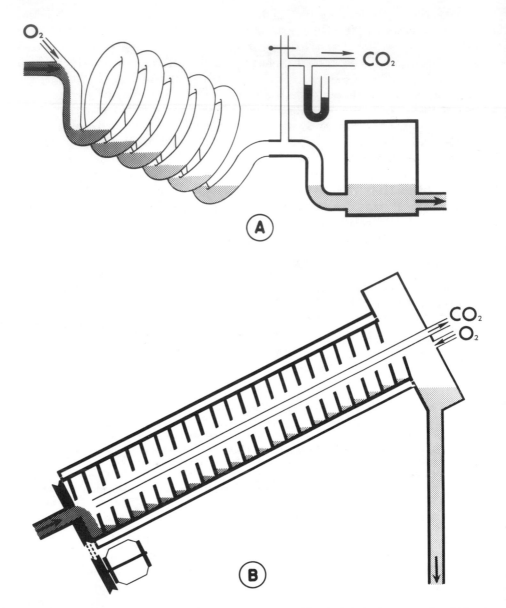

Fig. 29. Schemes of rotating spiral oxygenators (venous blood, dark shading; arterialized blood, light shading).

A. Basic unit of the oxygenator described by Jongbloed (1949). Venous blood enters a slanted helix of plastic tubing which revolves slowly around its axis. Oxygenation occurs during the downward course of the blood, and arterialized blood accumulates in a closed reservoir, from which it is infused into the organism.

B. Oxygenator devised by Westin, et al. (1958), for the perfusion of small organs or organisms. A plastic or steel band is bent into a spiral inserted within a rotating cylinder. Venous blood entering at left is filmed while ascending through an archimedean screw. (Details in text.)

ROTATING SPIRAL OXYGENATORS

In the pioneer years of extracorporeal circulation, two chief difficulties confronted the designers who attempted to support a blood film on moving surfaces. The first was related to the occurrence of frothing when the rate of venous blood distribution was suddenly varied. The second difficulty was that of preventing leaks around the rotating pulley-bearing spindle needed to spin the film support. Leaks were particularly annoying when a gas-tight oxygenator was required in order that direct measurements of gas exchanges in a closed gas circuit might be made.

To remedy these difficulties, Cruickshank (1934) devised the "magnetic blood oxygenator", which used magnetic power for rotation of a spiral plate supported upon a central axle enclosed within the gas chamber. Blood was evenly distributed from the center onto the spiral plate and forceful movements in the film were thereby avoided.

In the modern era of extracorporeal circulation, Jongbloed (1948, 1951) was the first to design a machine on the rotating spiral principle which was capable of equaling the basal cardiac output. The basic unit of his artificial lung (fig. 29, A) consisted of a plastic tube, 18 mm. in internal diameter and 10 m. long, bent into a spiral for compactness, with both ends of the tube lying in the central axis, around which the slanted helix revolved slowly. Venous blood entered the upper winding of the spiral, formed a thin film against the wall and was thus readily arterialized by oxygen which was simultaneously introduced. The rotation of the helix was synchronized with the ejection of the pulsatile venous pump. Thus each stroke of blood was filmed on one spire of tubing before the next stroke was distributed. The arterialized blood collected in a glass reservoir under a slight vacuum, was then taken by the arterial pump. The arterial reservoir hung from spiral springs. When its weight, which reflected the quantity of blood inside decreased below a given limit, the resulting upward movement of the reservoir pushed a mercury column and turned off the arterial pump. In a more recent model (Jongbloed, 1953), the weight of the arterial reservoir regulated the "leak" of compressed air in the gas chamber of a Dale-Schuster pump, and thereby modified the output of the arterial pump. In this way air embolism was prevented automatically. Jongbloed's artificial lung was made of six spiral tubes, each capable of accommodating a flow of 700 ml./min. Since 30 to 35 ml. O_2/min. could be transferred in each unit of the artificial lung when the venous saturation ranged around 60 per cent, this machine could carry the gaseous metabolism of a human adult under basal conditions. The priming volume of 2.5 L., however, was rather large.

A similar technique for oxygenation was proposed in 1955 by Miller. Gentle turbulence was induced in the bloodstream by causing the blood to tumble and ripple over irregularities in the wall of the artificial lung. The gas exchange chamber consisted of a tygon tube 6.6 m. long, 2.5 cm. internal diameter and 0.3 mm. wall thickness. A metal wire was tightly spiraled around the outside of the tube so as to cause 2 mm. indentation in the inner wall. The tube itself was wrapped, in eight evenly spaced windings, around a metal drum inclined 10° from the horizontal. Further distorsion of the tubing was achieved by 64 evenly spaced U-shaped clamps that constricted the lumen to an internal

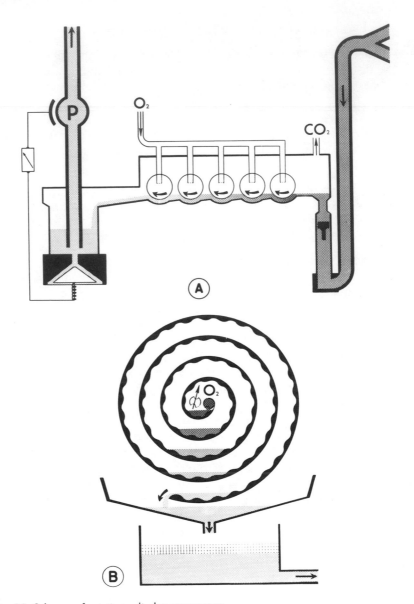

Fig. 30. Schemes of rotating cylinder oxygenators.

    A. Oxygenator of Crafoord, et al. (1957a): Venous blood flows by gravity into a large horizontal tray in which 6 cylinders are disposed horizontally (center). By spinning the cylinders a thin blood film is created over them and is exposed to an oxygen atmosphere. The arterialized blood is diverted into a reservoir (bottom, left), where a level sensing device controls the output of the arterial pump. The flow of venous blood is constantly displayed by a rotameter.

    B. Transverse section through the rotating drum oxygenator proposed by Schimert, et al. (1958): Venous blood is distributed along the axis of the drum and spreads over a corrugated plastic surface which revolves around the axis. Once blood reaches the periphery of the plastic sheet, it is arterialized and falls through a filter (cross-hatched horizontal band) into a receiving pan from which it can be tapped for perfusion. (Details in text.)

width of 1.5 cm. As the helix rotated, the blood was carried along and after eight revolutions emptied into the arterial reservoir. With a blood flow of 1 L./min. and with the drum rotating at the optimum rate of 72 rpm, the blood traversed the artificial lung in seven seconds. At any one time 110 ml. of blood would be in transit, while 20 ml. would cling to the wall. Five of the above mentioned helices, containing a total 650 ml. of blood, could handle a flow of 5 L./min.

At the other extreme of the volume rate of flow Westin, et al. (1958) described an apparatus for perfusing previable human fetus, which involves an original kind of spiral oxygenator. This artificial lung (fig. 29, B) consists of a plastic cylinder with a spiral band attached to its inner wall. The cylinder is placed at an angle of 30° to the horizontal plane and rotates at a variable rate between 10 and 50 rpm. The venous blood from the umbilical arteries is introduced at the lower end of the cylinder and transported in 30 to 70 seconds to the upper end of the cylinder by the archimedean screw mechanism. During this operation the blood is spread in a thin film over the inner wall of the cylinder and the spiral lucite band while moist oxygen is injected at the upper end of the cylinder. The arterialized blood accumulates in a chamber at the upper extremity of the archimedean screw. Part of it flows by gravity into the umbilical vein while the excess returns through a straight backflow tube to the lower end of the cylinder. Blood flow in the artificial lung can be regulated by changing the spread of rotation of the cylinder. According to in vitro experiments conducted in our laboratory with Westin's oxygenator, adequate gas exchange is achieved for blood flows up to 150 ml./min. when a priming volume of 300 ml. is used. Foaming does not occur. This artificial lung, as other spiral oxygenators, handles the blood very gently and hemolysis is barely noticeable.

Summarizing

In rotating spiral oxygenators the blood is suitably filmed over a moving helicoidal surface of metal or plastic and is moved spirally in the desired direction. Gentle turbulence and thinning out of the film are the main factors which enhance gas exchange.

ROTATING CYLINDER OXYGENATORS

The revolving cylinder of von Frey and Gruber (1885) may be considered as the ancestor of artificial lungs (*see frontispiece*). Venous blood was gently spread on the inner surface of a slowly rotating cylinder, and exposed to air or oxygen for arterialization. It was then collected in a chamber and served to perfuse isolated organs. That a swiftly moving stream of blood could be oxygenated without developing too much froth was first demonstrated with this device. Nonetheless, the surface area of the blood film exposed per unit of time was small and hence the scope of application limited.

Before designing screen oxygenators, Gibbon (1939 a) first experimented with spinning cylinders. Blood was filmed on the inner surface of a vertical cylinder. Fast revolution of the cylinder was necessary to maintain the blood film by centrifugal force. Otherwise, the blood descended in rivulets. At the top of the cylinder the blood was introduced tangentially in the direction of revolution by a fan-shaped horizontal jet. It was collected in a stationary cup which closely surrounded the knifelike edge of the bottom of the cylinder. This device was limited to an oxygen uptake of 18 ml./min. A larger artificial lung, capable of introducing 30 ml./min. of oxygen into blood, was described in 1941 by Gibbon and Kraul. Somewhat similar in performance was the oxygenator described by

Thomas (1948) and Ambrus (1955). In vitro studies by Karlson, et al. (1949 b), with a vertical revolving cylinder 28 cm. high and 18 cm. in diameter demonstrated that 80 per cent of oxygen uptake occurred in the upper half of the cylinder. Consequently, it served little purpose to increase the height of the cylinder. Karlson and his associates (1949 c) described the performance of an oxygenator made of eight spinning cylinders: 53 to 82 ml./min. of oxygen could be introduced into the blood.

Horizontal cylinder oxygenators were also investigated by Karlson, et al. (1949 a). They found that the rate of spinning could not be increased without causing undue foaming and hemolysis. Attempts at using concentric cylinders to increase the surface of contact failed to increase the oxygenating capacity. However, Kunlin (1952), using 11 coaxial stainless cylinders, with a total surface of 7 m.^{2}, was able to perform total body perfusion in dogs at flow rates of around 1.5 L./min.

The first oxygenator which featured spinning cylinders to achieve successful human perfusion was that of Craafoord, et al. (1957 a). Their first artificial lung (fig. 30, A) consisted of a basin containing six cylinders of perforated plastic foil. The outer surface of the cylinders lay 1 mm. from the bottom of the basin. The inflowing venous blood was filmed over the cylinders and so conveyed to the other extremity of the basin, where it collected in an arterial reservoir. The oxygenator could arterialize up to 1.5 L./min. of blood. To meet higher flow requirements, a second tray with six more rollers was added. This doubled the oxygenating capacity, but the priming requirement then lay between 2.1 (Craafoord and Senning, 1957 a; Lukac and Prcic, 1959) and 3.2 L (Spohn, et al., 1958). Since still higher flows were occasionally needed, the Swedish authors first resorted to a "preoxygenator." This was a bubbling device in which 50 to 100 ml./min. of oxygen were allowed to pass through a filter with pores of three to four microns in diameter directly into the venous blood before it entered the filming unit. More recently, the first tray has been equipped with six special rollers, made of two layers of perforated plastic foil concentrically arranged 3 mm. apart, in order to double the surface. Owing to the danger of foaming, the double rollers are used only in the first tray entered by the venous blood (Norlander, et al., 1958). With this arrangement, the maximal flow rate which can be arterialized reaches 5.5 to 6.0 L./min. with a priming volume of 3 L. The idea of using multiple, concentric cylinders has been recently revived by Wilson and Vowles (1960) and Barsamian, et al., (1960). It remains to be seen whether the advantage of compactness will outweigh the risk of foaming and splashing and the inherently limited performance of the cylinder oxygenators.

A design which combines features of the spiral and the cylinder oxygenator is represented by the rotating drum film oxygenator of Schimert, et al. (1958). It consists of a disposable drum, the surface of which is made of a corrugated polyethylene sheet wound into a spiral, resulting in a continuous concentric surface which rotates slowly within an oxygen atmosphere (fig. 30, B). Venous blood and oxygen are delivered into the center of the drum and arterialization occurs as the slow rotation carries a thin film of blood steadily towards the periphery. The blood which leaves the peripheral edge of the plastic sheet falls into a receiving pan placed below. Then it is filtered by gravity through a large surface of fine mesh nylon cloth. No part of this artificial lung needs to be siliconized. Polyethylene is used because it is less water repellent than most of the other plastics and, therefore, permits the maintenance of an excellent blood film. The corrugations in the polyethylene sheet are 4 mm. apart and 1 mm. deep. This particular shape increases the surface by about one-third. It also introduces a moderate amount of turbulence in the blood film, since the ridges contribute to the even distribution of the blood. The plastic sheet measures 7 m. in length and 76 cm. in width. Each successive turn is separated by a distance of 6 mm. The plastic sheet is held in place by two grooved end plates of stainless steel. As might be expected there is a definite relationship between surface area of the drum, speed of revolution, blood flow rate and oxygen transfer. The performance of this artificial lung has not been reported beyond the stage of the experimental evaluation. Nevertheless, it appears promising because it provides a large surface of blood–gas equilibration and a smooth circular motion combined with space saving qualities.

Summarizing

In rotating cylinder oxygenators, venous blood is spread over the wall of horizontal, slanted or vertical cylinders. Cylinder oxygenators are relatively inefficient when smooth surfaces are used for blood filming. Wire screen mesh or corrugated surfaces, which introduce gentle turbulence, greatly increase the oxygen transfer. Concentric cylinders can achieve optimal performance without the need of overly cumbersome devices.

ROTATING DISC OXYGENATORS

Rotating disc contactors are widely used in chemical engineering practice whenever mass transfer is enhanced by repeated break-up of droplets of a dispersed phase with exposure of fresh interface followed by coalescence and further break-up (Davies, et al., 1960). Their obvious drawback in the field of blood oxygenation is in the high degree of trauma inflicted upon blood by rapidly moving parts. Hooker (1915), Bayliss, et al. (1928), and Shen, et al. (1931), are often mentioned among the originators of the disc oxygenator. Actually these authors used flat revolving discs merely for the purpose of spreading blood centrifugally onto the walls of a container (fig. 31, A). Most of the gas exchange occurred in the film developed on the stationary support provided by the walls of the container.

The first artificial lung in which rotating discs provided the support for the blood film was that built by Bjørk (1948 b) in Crafoord's laboratory. Since the oxygenation of the hemoglobin molecule is a very rapid reaction, the Swedish authors thought it advisable to expose the blood film to oxygen for only a short time. In compensation, rapid renewal of the film would yield a large surface of gas exchange per unit of time in a comparatively small apparatus. Their first lung consisted of a horizontal cylinder containing a number of vertical plates, or discs, mounted on a central axle (fig. 31, B). Blood filled the bottom of the cylinder so that only the outer edge of each disc was immersed. Rotation caused a thin film of blood to form on the periphery of the plates. After a short exposure to the oxygen atmosphere (0.4 second at 120 rpm) the blood was wiped off and returned to the bottom pool of yet unoxygenated blood while a new film of mixed blood was exposed. This was an ingenious method of continuously and rapidly renewing the film and of transferring the blood from plate to plate. In a segmented trough at the bottom of the cylinder, the blood flowed alternately above and below partitions, in order to achieve a better mixing. The discs were made of rhodium-plated stainless steel, 0.5 mm. thick and were kept 4 mm. apart to avoid foaming at high rotational speed. Each group of 4 discs revolved in one segment of the

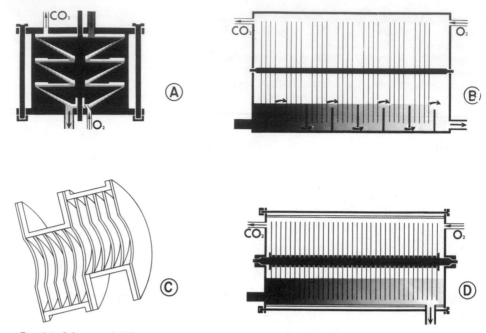

Fig. 31. Schemes of different types of rotating disc oxygenators.

A. Oxygenator of Bayliss, et al. (1928), consisting of inverted truncated cones revolving about a vertical axle. Venous blood is distributed centrifugally over the top plate of each cone and collects on the slanted inner wall of the casing to be filmed again on the next disc. Arterial blood is collected at the bottom of the gas exchange device.

B. Disc oxygenator of Bjørk (1948a). The main feature is the segmentation of the bottom part of the oxygenator casing, in order to improve mixing of the blood during the course of arterialization.

C. Sagittal section across the Melrose oxygenator (1953) demonstrates the inner arrangement of plates and washers.

D. Disc oxygenator proposed by Kay and Cross (1957). Immersion of the discs up to two-thirds of their radius in blood and moderate clearance between disc edges and oxygenator casing are among the paramount features of this design. (Details in text.)

trough. A stream of oxygen moved in the direction opposite to that of the blood flow. Since less than 100 ml. of O_2 were taken up by the blood from a chamber containing 5 L. of gas, variations of gas flow from 0.1 to 10 L./min. had no effect upon oxygenation.

Bjørk's basic idea was improved upon by Melrose and Aird (1953) in a design which combined features of the rotating disc and rotating cylinder oxygenators. Melrose's artificial lung consisted essentially of a rotating cylinder set at a slight angle to the horizontal. Blood traveled under the influence of gravity from one end to the other and was spread over a multitude of surfaces formed by blades projecting into the lumen of the cylinder. Originally, 76 perforated plates and 75 separating washers were mounted in the cylinder. The holes in the plates were all concentric and thus formed a cylindrical cavity coaxial with the enclosing cylinder. The holes in the washers were larger and cut excentrically, so that the plates projected as crescents within the cavity formed by the holes in the washers. Each group of five washers was arranged at 180° relative to the next group, in order to place the crescentic protrusions of the plates at opposite poles. This resulted in an arrangement of the cavities somewhat in the form of a helix. In sagittal section, the cylinder presented as a series of alternating platforms and troughs, each trough being subdivided into five compartments by the five plates (fig. 31, C).

Since the holes in the washers are eccentric with respect to the holes in the plates, the passage of blood down the slanted cylinder depends upon where the holes are tangent. When the point of contact is at the upper pole, a pool of blood is formed in the trough. During revolution of the assembly, as the point of contact approaches the lower pole, the pool will be emptied by the action of the washers which rise to the level of the holes in the plates. An alternation of phase between adjacent groups ensures that as a pool in one group empties, it is recreated in the next group. Simultaneously, the crescentic projections of the plates are alternately immersed in the pool of blood and exposed to the gas atmosphere with the resulting adherent film of blood. The stream of blood passing down the oxygenator is thus alternately raised and lowered by the action of the washers. This action avoids the need for the edges of the plates to cut across the streamline in order that they may become covered with blood. In fact, blood is poured over the plates and into the pool formed between them, then raised up and carried down the oxygenator before being poured over the succeeding group of plates. This arrangement permits a thorough mixing of the blood with a rapid passage along the machine. It also ensures that all the available surface area is utilized without reference to the volume of blood contained in the machine.

The first artificial lung model described by Melrose (1953) was made of a perspex cylinder 76 cm. in length and 20.3 cm. in diameter. The plates were 1 mm. thick and the washers were 8 mm. thick. Later it was found that the distance between the plates could be reduced to 5 mm. without increasing the danger of foaming, thereby allowing a reduction in the length of the cylinder. Moulding of prespex, nylon or teflon could combine both washer and plate and thus enable the number of parts to be halved (Catchpole and Nixon, 1959 b). The most recent model of Melrose's artificial lung features considerable simplification. The cylinder is made of six stainless steel chambers with stainless steel discs forming a complex of baffles on which the blood is filmed as the oxygenator rotates. The chambers retain the crenated arrangement visible on the sectional sketch (fig. 31, C). They are separated by silicone rubber washers and bolted together by external tie rods. There are 21 perforated discs in each chamber. The size and the excentricity of the holes in the discs is constant within any one chamber. However, there are three different patterns of perforation distributed between the six chambers, so as to keep a helicoidal arrangement of the space within the cylinder. A technique of electropolishing is used to renew periodically the metal surfaces and ensure a clean finish. The form of construction makes for easy assembly and is particularly suited to the use of disposable internal discs.

In the Melrose oxygenator, the inlet and outlet port for the blood, together with the inlet for oxygen, enter at one extremity of the cylinder. The tubes are carried by a stainless steel rod which passes through a simple seal in one end plate, along the axis of the cylinder to a stainless steel bearing on the other end plate. No reservoir is required.

Systemic and coronary venous blood are returned directly to the oxygenator. Arterial blood is pumped from the arterial outlet to a filter block utilizing a stainless steel gauze of 150 mesh to form a large area filter. The design of the filter enables it to function also as a bubble trap. A mechanical weighing device provides a sensitive indication of the blood volume within the machine at all times. The apparatus also includes an alarm system which, after operating a warning buzzer, brings the pump to a standstill in the event of sudden emptying of the artificial lung. The filling volume of the machine is around 1 L., though priming of 1.5 to 2 L. is used for high flow perfusion (Nixon, et al., 1960). The apparatus can fully oxygenate 4 L./min. of blood (Barratt-Boyes, et al., 1960). while the pumping system is designed to handle volumes considerably in excess of that amount.

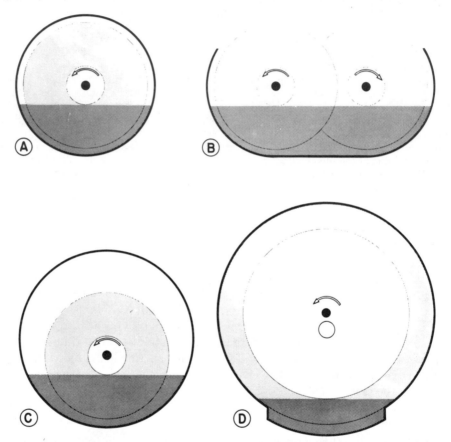

Fig. 32. Face view of various disc arrangements in oxygenators (dark shading: blood pool; light shading: film of blood spread over the disc to undergo arterialization).

A. Kay-Cross oxygenator (1956, 1957) features discs of 12 cm. diameter, immersed 4 cm. deep with 0.5 cm. clearance at the edge.

B. Twin-oxygenator of Kay, et al. (1958a), designed to make the casing more compact when numerous discs are needed.

C. Eccentric arrangement suggested by Milnes and Vanderwoode (1957) to provide a 2 cm. clearance at the level where the discs enter and leave the blood pool.

D. Oxygenator of Osborn, et al. (1960), utilizes 21 cm. discs with minimal clearance between disc edge and casing and with filming limited to the periphery of the disc. Note blood channel at the bottom of the oxygenator and hole for circulation of oxygen near the center of the disc. (Details in text.)

A rotating disc oxygenator which more closely resembles Bjørk's design than that of Melrose was put forward by Kay, Cross and their associates in 1956. Through the effort of these initiators and of their followers, the rotating disc oxygenator has gained widespread recognition. It is now produced commercially by several leading firms. Its engineering features are well understood and the machine has become one of the most commonly used. The original oxygenator of Kay and Cross (1957) consists of 59 stainless steel discs 0.4 mm. thick and 12.2 cm. in diameter, mounted 0.5 mm. apart by means of stainless steel spacers on a central shaft (fig. 31, D). The disc assembly is held horizontally within a pyrex cylinder 33 cm. long and 13.3 cm. in diameter by gasketed endplates of stainless steel. Venous blood is introduced at one end of the cylinder and is removed from the bottom of the opposite end. The rotation of the discs effectively prevents channeling of the blood along the bottom of the oxygenator. The cylinder is filled to a higher level than that recommended by Bjørk. This practice results in a larger surface of oxygenation because a wider area of the disc is covered with blood for the same diameter of the disc (fig. 32, A). There is also less tendency for the blood to splash against the inner wall of the cylinder and consequently foaming is no problem up to 120 rpm. When the oxygenator is primed with 1.4 L of blood, the static area of the film is 0.84 m.^{2} Dynamically it reaches 110 m.^{2} per minute at the usual rate of revolution of 120 rpm. This is enough to arterialize fully a blood flow of 2 L./min. with an oxygen uptake in the order of 120 ml./min.

The rotating disc oxygenator proved to be such an effective and safe means of oxygenating blood that numerous improvements were soon proposed to adapt it to any local oxygen requirements likely to be encountered:

(1) The first suggestion was to increase the oxygenating surface area by increasing the revolutions of the discs from 120 to 140 per minute. Kay, et al. (1958a) and Bjørk (1961) noted that when 5 mm. spacers were used between discs, no significant "columning" of blood occurred at the greater speeds, nor did foaming become a problem, even at low temperature. Although the oxygenating surface increased by one-sixth, it is dubious, in view of the experimental results of Bjørk (1948), that the oxygenating capacity increased to that extent. Data from Paton, et al. (1961), and from our own laboratory trials confirm that the oxygen transfer does not vary significantly between 110 and 150 rpm.

(2) Another method of enlarging the oxygenating capacity consisted in increasing the length of the cylinder and the number of discs employed. This method has been found efficient and practical. Cylinders are now available in sizes ranging from 10 cm., (e.g., Cartwright and Palich, 1960b), to 63 cm. (e.g., Waldhausen, et al., 1959b) with conversion assemblies allowing any adaptation of oxygenating capacity to the expected requirements. Table I gives data concerning the average priming volume, oxygen transfer and oxygenating capacity of rotating disc assemblies of different sizes.

(3) Instead of increasing the number of discs in one cylinder, the use of many oxygenators in parallel has been suggested (Senning, 1952; Kolff, et al., 1937). A twin unit, in which two series of discs interdigitate in a common container (fig. 32, B), was proposed by Kay, et al. (1958). Each series of discs revolves upward at the center. This machine is very effective, but requires a complicated casing and does not allow easy visual control of the oxygenator in operation. At the present time, its increased mechanical complexity still outweighs the advantages of compactness and efficiency.

(4) Convoluted discs have been developed as a way of increasing the oxygenating area without increasing the priming volume (Kay, et al., 1958; Micozzi, et al., 1960a). These convoluted discs are stamped with 90 degree impressions of corrugations in a

Table 1. Relationship between cylinder length, priming requirement and oxygenating capacity in the conventional rotating disc oxygenator.

LENGTH OF CYLINDER		PRIMING VOLUME	MAXIMUM BLOOD FLOW	OXYGEN TRANSFER
Inches	*cm.*	*ml.*	*L./min.*	*ml./min.*
3	10	400	0.4	25
6	15	600	0.7	45
9	23	900	1.2	80
12	30	1300	1.7	110
15	38	1700	2.6	150
18	46	2100	3.2	180
21	53	2500	4.5	210
25	63	3000	6.0	250

concentric manner, thus increasing the oxygenating capacity by 30 per cent over that of the flat discs. However, convoluted discs require more space between them (4.7 mm. instead of 3.6 mm. in one commercial model) to avoid "bridging" of blood from one disc to the next, and the increased space requirement for the entire assembly diminishes the advantage of increased filming area.

(5) Theoretically, one should enhance gas transfer by exposing the blood to oxygen pressures in excess of atmospheric pressures. Bjørk and Rodriquez (1959) demonstrated the feasibility of such a solution. In their opinion, however, the technical complexity involved in making the apparatus leak proof at the pressures studied (up to 10 Kg./ cm.²) has not justified itself by a sufficient increase in performance. One may also wonder whether very high partial pressures of oxygen in the arterial blood could not have deleterious effects upon the organism perfused.

(6) Finally, the oxygenating capacity might be enhanced by increasing the diameter of the discs. As Osborn, et al. (1960) pointed out, relative efficiency is related to the area of the disc submerged in the blood trough as compared with the filmed area which is exposed to oxygen. Therefore, a disc oxygenator is most efficient (as measured by the ratio of oxygenating surface to contained volume) if the disc is very large and dips only slightly into the blood trough. The 12 cm. diameter discs are limited in their oxygenating efficiency largely by the occurrence of foaming when the linear speed of the disc rim exceeds an empirically established limit. However, a higher rim speed can be achieved without foam formation if the clearance between disc edges and casing is very small, so that a continuous seal of blood bridges disc and casing all around its periphery. Based on these considerations, Osborn, et al. (1960) used discs 21 cm. in diameter (fig. 32, D). The enclosing cylinder is thus far wider than that of the Kay-Cross models, but the priming volume is smaller, because the discs are immersed to only 25 per cent of their radius, instead of 65 to 70 per cent as recommended for the 12 cm. disc. The centrifugal force acting on blood at the periphery of a 12 cm. disc revolving at 120 rpm is around 1 g., whereas it is 1.7 g for a 21 cm. disc. Thereby the tendency of droplets to be flung off the discs and splash against the inner wall of the cylinder is increased. Osborn and his associates have reduced the danger of foam formation by reducing the clearance between the discs and the cylinder wall to 0.4 mm., which is small enough to be easily and consistently spanned by the centrifugally formed blood seal. Obviously, though, this arrangement does not leave room for blood and oxygen to flow along the axis of the oxygenator as in the Kay-Cross design. Blood flows in a longitudinal canal at the bottom of the cylinder, the cross-section of which is a concentric annular segment 6.3 mm. deep, subtending an angle of about 64 degrees, and permits a 4 L./min. gravity flow under a 5 cm. H_2O head of pressure. The gaseous oxygen flows through a hole 9.5 mm. in diameter located in each disc near the shaft.

On assembly, each hole is oriented at 180 degrees to those in adjacent discs, so as to encourage mild gas turbulence.

To prevent excessive blood turbulence and foaming along the line where the rotating discs enter or leave the blood, Milnes and Vanderwoude (1957) and Sloan, et al. (1959), adopted a solution opposed to that of Osborn, et al. They proposed that clearance between discs and inner wall should be enlarged beyond the usual 5 mm. To achieve this goal without disproportionately increasing the priming volume, they devised an oxygenator in which the usual 12 cm. discs line eccentrically in a cylinder 16 cm. in diameter so that the lateral walls of the cylinder are well separated from the edges of the discs (fig. 32, C).

Most authors reporting modifications of the rotating disc oxygenator (Felipozzi, et al., 1958; De Rabago, et al., 1958; Loeschke, et al., 1959; Goldberg, et al., 1959; Lawrence, et al., 1960; Simkovic, et al., 1960; Servelle, et al., 1960) have followed a pattern of construction similar to that of Cross, et al. (1956). A scaled down version, utilizing discs 7.8 cm. in diameter, was constructed by Ross (1960) for low-flow perfusions. An even smaller model for hypothermic perfusions was proposed by Benichoux (1960).

The discs of the Kay-Cross oxygenator were made of stainless steel coated with teflon. Further experience has shown that simple silicone coating of the stainless steel discs is enough to prevent fibrin deposits and blood denaturation. According to the siliconizing technique used and the demand of any particular team, the silicone coating may be renewed for every perfusion (Osborn, et al., 1960), after 20 to 25 runs (Kay and Cross, 1956 b) or only once a year (Gross, et al., 1960). Plastic discs, such as phonograph discs, were first used by Kolff, et al. (1957), because of low cost and easy disposability. This idea has been extended by Esmond and Cowley (1958, 1959) in their single use, disposable disc oxygenator. Their apparatus consists of a 12.7 cm. diameter, interlocked plastic disc assembly mounted on a stainless steel shaft. The discs are injection molded from methylmetacrylate. Two identical draw formed methylmetacrylate half shells fit together to form a cylinder surrounding the discs and support the two nylon bearings for the shaft. Removable plastic tube fittings are installed in the top and bottom shells to serve as admittance and discharge ports for blood and gas. The oxygenator is provided ready for use in sterile boxes with all tubing in place. Thus, a perfusion can be initiated in a matter of minutes. A 33 and a 56 cm. long model have been developed. Their priming volume and flow performance compare with those of permanent disc oxygenators.

Among the recently studied technical problems connected with the use of disc oxygenators, those related to thermoregulation, control of blood volume within the oxygenator and control of the gas exchange are worth mentioning.

Difficulty in thermoregulation is undoubtedly one drawback of the rotating disc oxygenator because discontinuity between blood and cylinder over most of the surface prevents direct heat conduction. The use of a heating wire wrapped around the cylinder is rather inefficient; this also promotes clotting at the blood–gas boundary, because oscillations of the blood level result in a thin film which can be dried by contact with the overheated wall. The same criticism applies to the primitive technique of heating by external lamps. Attempts at circulating thermostabilized water through the central shaft supporting the discs have proven inadequate. A water bath in which the belly of the oxygenator rests suffices for maintaining the circulating blood at its normal temperature

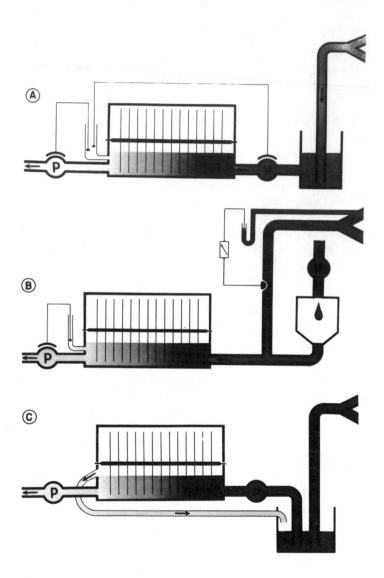

Fig. 33. Circuits proposed for maintaining constant blood volume in rotating disc oxygenators.

A. System devised by Olmsted, et al. (1958), in which level-sensing devices in the oxygenator regulate both the venous and the arterial pumps.

B. Circuit used by Kantrowitz, et al. (1959). On the venous side, a motor driven clamp compresses or releases the syphonage line so as to maintain a constant venous pressure. On the arterial side, a device which monitors the blood level in the oxygenator controls the output of the arterial pump so as to maintain constant volume.

C. Blood circuit designed by Cartwright and Palich (1960 a, b), which precludes any change of blood level in the oxygenator by the use of an overflow line from the arterial endplate. The venous pump is set at a rate which exceeds at all times that of the arterial pump, so that a small amount of arterial blood is constantly recirculated through the oxygenator.

(Gross, et al., 1960), but does not allow for rapid heat exchange in either direction. There-fore, many groups prefer to insert a special heat exchange device (*see* Chapter XI) in the arterial blood line, at the price of a higher priming volume of the complete circuit. Owing to the continuous blood seal between disc edges and the enclosing cylinder, the oxygenator described by Osborn, et al (1960) can be equilibrated rapidly with water circulating in a concentric steel cylinder. Since visual control of blood arterialization is thereby lost, Osborn has resorted to the use of transparent end plates for safety of oper-ation.

Early in 1958 a number of important contributions to the design of a good circuit were made by Gross. He included a collecting reservoir, the height of which could be regulated for gravity–venous drainage; a settling chamber, interposed between the collecting res-ervoir and the artificial lung, to provide smooth flow towards the oxygenator and to re-move the residual bubbles which become a problem when blood flow exceeds 2.5 L./min. (*see* fig. 72, C and D); finally, an arterial filter and bubble trap interposed between the arterial pump and the site of the arterial cannula (*see* fig. 54, C).

To control the blood volume in the extracorporeal circuit, Olmsted, et al. (1958), de-scribed a level sensing electrode which increases or decreases the speed of the venous and arterial pump as the blood level rises or falls (fig. 33, A). Their circuit can detect and correct volume changes in the oxygenator of less than 125 ml. Osborn, et al. (1960) rely on continuous measurement of the oxygenator weight for assessing the blood content of the oxygenator and thereby regulating the arterial blood flow so as to maintain a safe level in the oxygenator. Kantrowitz, et al. (1959) mounted a photoelectric sensing de-vice on the outside of the oxygenator chamber in such a way that changes in blood level modify the amount of light falling on the photocell. The electrical output of the cell is used to control the speed of the arterial pump. Venous return occurs by gravity. Its amount is automatically regulated by a motor driven clamp on the venous line, so as to maintain the venous pressure constant. Thus the arterial blood flow necessarily equals the amount of venous blood drained and the blood level in the oxygenator is effectively locked within ± 50 ml. An even more refined system was proposed by Waldhausen et al. (1959) in order to maintain constant blood volume in the oxygenator while obviating the decrease in perfusion flow brought about by a decrease in venous return (*see* fig. 84). Level sensing electrodes located in a small side arm of the arterial end plate activate a bidirectional blood pump connecting the oxygenator with a calibrated reservoir. If the level in the artificial lung rises, this pump withdraws blood into the reservoir. Conversely, if the level falls, owing to a decreased amount of venous drainage (in case of sudden hemorrhage for instance), the pump transfers blood into the oxygenator.

The simplest system for maintaining a constant blood level is that described by Cart-wright and Palich (1960 a, b). They simply added, at the arterial endplate of the oxy-genator, an overflow tap which connects the cylinder with a gravity drainage venous reservoir (fig. 33, C). Venous blood is pumped from this reservoir into the oxygenator at a flow rate exceeding somewhat that of the arterial pump. Thus, a small amount of ar-terialized blood continuously runs back into the venous reservoir. The blood level in the oxygenator is maintained constant as long as the recirculating shunt can accommodate the difference in flow between the venous and the arterial pumps. The changes in blood volume of the extracorporeal circuit can be read accurately by the level of the venous reservoir, and volume fluctuations due to transfer of fluid occur only in a noncritical area. Surface bubbles are also continuously removed by way of the overflow tap. In our own laboratory a similar overflow arrangement permits us to maintain a constant volume of gas in the oxygenator and thereby to obtain a continuous reading of the oxygen up-take in the extracorporeal circuit (*see* fig. 16). This technique requires the cylinder to be made airtight which is achieved by using precision bearings for supporting the central shaft.

Summarizing

In rotating disc oxygenators, the rapid renewal of the blood film yields a large surface of gas exchange per unit of time in a comparatively small appa-ratus. The speed of rotation of the discs, the distance between discs and the depth of immersion of the discs into the blood, are critical in achieving optimal oxygenation in the shortest time with the smallest priming volume. Through the introduction of numerous technical refinements the rotating disc oxygenator has become an effective and safe means of oxygenating large volumes of blood and is now widely used in clinical heart–lung bypass.

ROTATING SCREEN OXYGENATOR

The rotating screen oxygenator of Dennis, et al. (1951 a, b) combines the principle of filming blood over revolving discs introduced by Bjørk (1948) with the increased efficiency of a screen-type support, as demonstrated by Stokes and Flick (1950). In the usual disc oxygenator design, formation of the film is accomplished by immersion of the dependent portion of each revolving disc in a stream of blood. Recirculation is provided by the rotatory movement of the discs on a horizontal shaft and is limited only by the rate of blood flow through the oxygenator. To the contrary in Dennis' design (fig. 34), blood is laid centrifugally over a revolving screen disc by a low-speed jet in the center of the disc, and spreads but once in the oxygen atmosphere before collecting in the arterial reservoir. To achieve full arterialization, a disc of large diameter and a low speed of revolution are necessary. Empirically, Dennis (1956) found that a screen disc 50 cm. in diameter, rotating at 23 rpm, introduces 36.5 ml. of oxygen per minute at a blood flow rate of 500 ml./min. The blood retained over the disc at this flow rate is 97 ml. The disc is cut in a stainless steel screen, 18 by 10 mesh, made of wire 0.22 mm. in diameter. The central part of the disc, over which the blood is first distributed, consists of a solid sheet of stainless steel. A solid disc margin of carefully smoothed metal has been found to reduce hemolysis. Arterialized blood drops a few millimeters from the dependent margin of the disc to collect in the central chamber of a bubble trap (*see* fig. 53, A) filled with a stainless steel scouring sponge coated with antifoam. Blood overflows from the top of this column into an outer jacket, which serves as arterial reservoir.

Several discs can be mounted on a horizontal shaft. A four disc assembly in a closed chamber contains around 1000 ml. of blood, of which 600 ml. are in the arterial reservoir at the bottom of the unit. Oxygen is run into the tank at the rate of 10 L./min. through four jets adjacent to the blood jets. The film, initiated by laying blood on the central portion of the disc and spread by centrifugation and gravity, is remarkably stable. Dry discs film spontaneously in a matter of seconds and can be easily called into service, if more oxygenating capacity is desired while the apparatus is in use. This feature is almost unique among mechanical lungs. The rotating screen oxygenator has proven its clinical usefulness in total heart–lung bypass. It is efficient, easily cleaned and sterilized, and air embolism is not a problem, according to Dennis (1956) and Dennis and Karlson (1958).

Summarizing

The rotating screen oxygenator combines centrifugal distribution of blood with the advantages of a wire mesh screen support. To achieve arterialization of the blood film in a single passage over the rotating screen disc, a large disc diameter and a slow rate of revolution are necessary. Dry discs film within seconds and can be easily put into service if the oxygenating capacity of the apparatus must be increased.

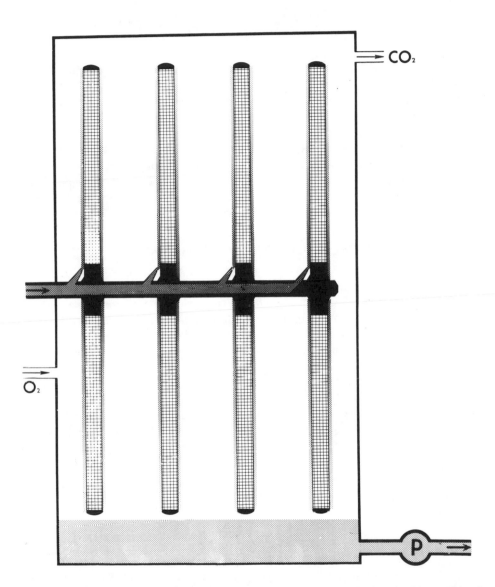

Fig. 34. Rotating screen oxygenator proposed by Dennis, et al. (1951 a, b). Venous blood enters through the shaft and is distributed centrifugally by a low speed jet at the center of the disc. It spreads over discs made of wire mesh (cross-hatched areas) and collects at the bottom of the oxygenator casing. For simplicity, the oxygen distributing manifold has been represented off center, and the arterial bubble trap has been omitted. (Details in text.)

VII. Membrane Oxygenators

$\mathbf{D}$uring the natural process of oxygenation, as occurs in lungs or gills, there is no direct contact between blood and the ambient gas. A semipermeable membrane separates the blood from the oxygen present in the alveolar gas or in the surrounding water. The gas transfer is then evoked by a process of molecular diffusion. Since many of the early difficulties encountered in using artificial lungs were associated with froth formation or fibrin deposits at the "raw" blood-gas interface, artificial membranes were proposed as a means of protecting the blood from direct exposure to the atmosphere. The concept that respiratory gas transfer is compatible with physical separation of blood and oxygen has evolved into a number of designs for artificial lungs during the last ten years.

PRINCIPLES AND EARLY DEVELOPMENTS

Fundamental studies by Barrer (1948) and van Amerongen (1950) indicated that natural or synthetic elastomers are permeable to gases. According to Barrer, the process of permeation of gas through a plastic or rubber membrane may be regarded as a sequence of three phenomena: (a) absorption and solution of the gas into the membrane at one surface; (b) diffusion of the gas through the body of the membrane; (c) dissolution and freeing of the gas from the membrane at the other surface. Physical chemists have demonstrated that permeation of gases and vapors through polymer films is primarily diffusion controlled (Waack, et al., 1955; Bell and Grosberg, 1961). Therefore, when a stationary state is attained, the flux or amount of gas passing through the film per unit area and time must satisfy Fick's first law, as expressed in Chapter IV.

In 1954, Brubaker and Kammermeyer compared the permeability of different membranes and found that polyethylene permitted more diffusion of oxygen and carbon dioxide than any other polymer available at the time. Stannet and Szwarc (1955) showed that for any pair of gases, the ratio of the permeability constants remains approximately constant for a wide variety of polymer films, even though the actual values of the permeability constants vary from polymer to polymer by as much as several thousand times. In the cases of respiratory gases, the ratio D'_{CO_2}/D'_{O_2} is in the order of five for most of the membranes tested (Stannet and Szwarc, 1955; Othmer and Frohlich, 1955; Kammermeyer, 1957; Michels and Parker, 1959), as compared to approximately 20 for the alveolar membranes. A large number of polymers have been tested for their permeatiliby to gases by chemical engineers as well as by biologists (Clowes, et al., 1955, 1956; Clowes and Neville, 1958; Peirce, 1958 b; McCaughan, et al., 1960). The permeability constants so obtained, when corrected to standard physical units, do not always agree. The methodologic difficulties involved in the measurements may account in part for the discrepancies. However, Michaels and Parker (1959) have recently demonstrated that, depending upon the polymerization and fabrication process, the gas permeability of polyethylene varies by a factor of 10, and is closely related to the crystallinity and density of the product.

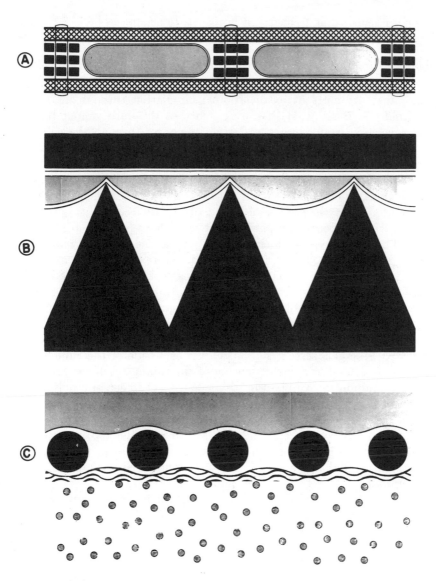

Fig. 35. Gas exchange principles in the three main types of membrane oxygenators.

A. Membrane oxygenator of Kolff, et al. (1956a). Blood (shaded area) flows through thin gas permeable polyethylene tubing which serves as a membrane. The expansion of the tubing is limited by spacers (black squares) and fiber glass screens (cross-hatched areas) which are held together with wires (vertical loops).

B. Membrane oxygenator of Clowes, et al. (1956). Only a single unit of the multilayered apparatus is represented. Blood (shaded area) flows as a thin film between two plastic membrane layers. Oxygen flows through grooves (white) in the solid supports (black) which separate each pair of membranes.

C. Membrane oxygenator of Thomas (1958a, b). A thin silicone film (white) is formed by evaporating silicone solution over a supporting nylon mesh (black). Blood (shaded area on top) is spread in a thin layer over the upper side of the membrane. Oxygen is carried by a saline mist (small circles at bottom) which condenses to form a moist coat on the lower side of the membrane.

Using special manufacturing technique, it is possible to obtain pores of a given size in polyethylene (McCaughan, et al., 1960) and cellophane sheets (Craig and Konigsberg, 1961). Therefore in this era of transition in the plastics field, the values collected in table 2 should be considered as dependent upon the particular brand tested, and open to revision.

In their first attempts at extracorporeal circulation through an artificial kidney, Kolff and Berk (1944) had observed that the dark venous blood entering the machine would brighten during its course through the cellophane dialyzing tube. Later Karlson, et al. (1949 a, 1951) compared this mechanism of arterialization to others and found it rather inefficient. Dubbelman (1951 b) also concluded that the process of oxygenation through cellophane is impractical when high rates of blood flow are needed, an opinion which has recently been substantiated by the studies of Firme, et al. (1960).

However, when it became apparent that total body perfusion at low flow rates, based on the "azygos principle," was compatible with survival, the old idea of oxygenating blood across membranes was revived. Kolff and Balzer (1955) demonstrated that the circulation of dogs could be supported with an artificial lung built of coils of thin polyethylene tubing. After trying out different arrangements, they described the following apparatus (Kolff, et al. 1956 a; Hale, et al. 1957): Two polyethylene tubes with a lay-flat diameter of 5 cm. and a wall thickness of 0.025 mm. are enveloped in long strips of plastic coated Fiberglas screen (fig. 35 A). On each side of the tube arrangement are spacers to allow some distension of the tubing when the blood flows through it. To minimize wrinkles the stitched strips of screen and polyethylene tubing are rolled around a can, and then provided with inlet and outlet tubes. The completed coil is placed in a transparent plastic bag. Oxygen is blown into the bottom part of the bag and escapes through the top, together with the CO_2 removed. Such a lung had an effective surface area of 1.4 sq. m. It was capable of arterializing about 75 ml. of venous blood per minute, and required a priming volume between 270 and 500 ml.

Clowes, et al. (1955) devised an artificial lung which depended upon grooved surfaces to hold two sheets of ethylcellulose together (fig. 35 B). Blood flowed between the membranes while oxygen flowed in the grooves outside. All four edges of the plastic sheets were supported by rubber gaskets to prevent leakage from one phase to the other. This arrangement was developed into a multilayered apparatus (Clowes, et al., 1956 a) with 6 sq. m. of membrane area. The oxygen pressure outside the membrane was maintained at a lower level than that of the blood inside, because ethylcellulose, being brittle and easily

---

Table 2. Permeation coefficients of the different materials used to manufacture semipermeable membranes. The data reported are subject to considerable variation because the experimental conditions of the measurements and the exact chemical nature of the polymers are not standardized. Therefore, the figures calculated here from the original data should be considered only as a first approximation. The values indicated for blood plasma are merely intended to serve as a yardstick for comparison.

Sources: 1. Stannet and Szwarc (1955), 2. Dow-Corning data sheet (1960), 3. McCaughan, et al. 1960), 4. Kammermeyer (1957), 5. Michaels and Parker (1959), 6. Handbook of Respiration (1958).

TABLE 2

MATERIAL	D'_{O_2}	D'_{H_2O}	$\dfrac{D'_{CO_2}}{D'_{O_2}}$
	$ml\ cm/cm^2/sec/cm\ Hg \times 10^{-11}$		
Polyvinylidene chloride (*Saran*)	0.05[1] 0.06[2]	0.01[2]	0.8[2]
Monochlorotrifluoroethylene (*Trithene A*)	0.09[2]	0.02[2]	10.7[2]
Polyester (*Mylar*)	0.22[1] 0.67[2]	0.09[2]	1.8[2]
Nylon 6	0.38[1]	—	—
Cellulose acetate	6.6[2] 6.0[3] 7.8[1]	5.4[2]	5.1[2]
Polypropylene	11.2[2]	0.04[2]	3.4[2]
Butyl rubber	13.0[1]	—	—
Polystyrene	18.6[2]	0.43[2]	4.9[2]
Polyethylene	35[4] 41[3] 55[1] 3.8–31.0[5] 8.5–34.4[2]	0.01–0.07[2]	4–5[5] 2.6–4.6[2]
Tetrafluoroethylene (*Teflon*)	66[2] 105[3]	0.02[2]	2.7[2] 2.6–4.0
Ethylcellulose (*Ethocel*)	96[2] 100[3] 265[1 4]	4.5[2]	4.1[2] 4.3[3]
Natural rubber	230[1 4] 327[3]	—	5[3] 5.6[5]
Silicone rubber (*Silastic 50*) (*Silastic S–2000*)	2600[4] 5890[2] 6500[3]	10.2[2]	4–5[4]
Microporous polyethylene (*Permax*)	130,000– 400,000[3]		
Blood plasma	6.5–10.1[6]	—	32–15

Legend on facing page.

torn, could otherwise admit bubbles through pinholes in the membrane. This apparatus trapped around 140 ml. of blood per sq. m. of membrane and could support the circulation of a dog. Later, teflon was substituted for ethylcellulose and polyethylene because it had more strength than the other membranes and displayed a somewhat higher permeability to oxygen and carbon dioxide.

Another method of blood oxygenation across membranes, pioneered by Thomas (1958 a, b), employs a film of silicone coated over a nylon cloth. The nylon fibers lend structural solidity to the thin and delicate membrane, which otherwise would not withstand the mechanical conditions to which it is subjected. Blood is spread on one side of the membrane while on the other side, a mist of oxygenated, buffered saline provides a thin layer of liquid saturated with oxygen (fig. 35 C).

The basic problems in the design of membrane lungs are logistic in nature. Some are associated with the membrane itself, others with the manifolding and distributing system for the blood.

When artificial membranes were first proposed, it was not immediately recognized that carbon dioxide transfer might be more difficult to carry out than oxygen transfer under the particular pressure conditions which prevail in an artificial lung. One manufacturer even recommended the use of an O_2-CO_2 mixture in the gas phase—a confusion probably resulting from misleading analogies among the mechanisms of gas exchange in the different types of lungs. Actually, one of the factors which limits the performance of the membrane lung is the resistance imposed by the membrane to the diffusion of carbon dioxide (Peirce 1958 b, 1960 a; Melrose, et al., 1958; Hassler, 1959). The basic physiologic concepts involved in the transfer of gases across membranes can be summarized as follows: Three factors are involved in the passage of gas across a membrane: the nature of the gas, the degree of hydration of the membrane, or wettability, which strongly influences the degree of solubility of the gas in the membrane, and the gas tension difference between the two sides of the membrane. In the case of an artificial lung, since pure oxygen is used in the gas phase and since the partial pressure of CO_2 in blood should not exceed 50 mm. Hg., a ratio of at least 12:1 exists in favor of oxygen in terms of pressure gradient. To counteract the partial pressure ratio and insure an equal transmission of CO_2 and O_2, the membrane should be 12 times more permeable to CO_2 than to O_2. Only then can a gas exchange ratio of 1 be maintained when the artificial lung is ventilated with pure oxygen. Unfortunately most synthetic membranes are only four to five times more permeable to CO_2 than to O_2 (table 2), and this is insufficient for the transfer of equal volumes of oxygen and carbon dioxide. Membrane lungs have to be designed in terms of CO_2 release, and will therefore feature a considerable reserve in oxygen transfer capacity. In other words, the rate of permeation of CO_2 is the bottleneck and dictates the area of membrane required.

In the liquid and in the gaseous phase on either side of the membrane, CO_2 diffuses very rapidly, so that these steps in gas transfer hardly influence the overall rate of exchange. On the contrary, for the oxygen factors such as blood film thickness or transit time are critical. Peirce (1958 a) established experimentally that the oxygenating capacity of a membrane lung depends much more upon the blood distribution pattern than upon the membrane actually employed. This view is supported by a theoretic analysis of gas diffusion in a membrane lung (Prados and Peirce, 1960). Recently, Marx, et al. (1960) have demonstrated both theoretically and experimentally that when highly permeable membranes are used in a blood oxygenator, the relative permeabilities of the blood film and of the membrane are such that the resistance of the blood film is the controlling factor. As in the case of film oxygenators which do not feature turbulent flow or continuous refilming, the length of the oxygen diffusion path is the rate limiting factor as soon as the thickness of the film exceeds a certain degree as compared to the size of an erythrocyte. One can thus summarize the logistic problems of the membrane lung by stating that CO_2 elimination depends upon the membrane area available, whereas O_2 uptake depends upon the design of the blood distributing system.

Melrose, et al. (1958) suggested that in place of nonwettable membranes, atraumatic to blood as they may be, marked solubility of CO_2 in aqueous media should be exploited. Possibly two types of membrane in combination, one favoring oxygen transfer (teflon, polyethylene, or silicone rubber), the other markedly permeable to CO_2 (such as wettable cellophane) might result in the greatest overall efficiency of O_2 and CO_2 exchange. In the future, physicochemists may be able to rearrange "upon order" the molecular structure of plastic films by irradiation or by new techniques of polymerization. "Microporous" membranes, which feature extremely high gas permeation coefficients, are already available (McCaughan, et al., 1960). Unfortunately, oozing of blood results when pressure in the liquid phase reaches the levels required for blood distribution. Alternately improvements may depend upon more satisfactory designs of the manifolding and blood distributing system, and upon the production of thinner blood films than now obtained. For the time being, the best indication for use of the membrane oxygenator is in the field of hypothermic perfusion, because advantage can be taken of the decreased metabolism, the increased solubility of CO_2 and the desirability of moderate CO_2 retention in hypothermia. Another possible application is to partial heart–lung bypass. The CO_2 retained, when the membrane area is chosen in relationship to oxygen transfer alone, is then eliminated through the lungs, which are normally endowed with a considerable reserve capacity for CO_2 transfer: The different permeability characteristics of the natural and the artificial lung complement each other in partial heart–lung bypass.

Summarizing

In membrane oxygenators, a blood film and gaseous oxygen are separated by a semipermeable membrane. Gas transfer across the membrane depends upon the nature, thickness, surface and degree of hydration of the membrane, and also upon the partial pressure difference of the diffusing gases on opposite sides of the membrane. Theoretic and experimental studies indicate that CO_2 transfer is primarily limited by the membrane barrier, while oxygen transfer is controlled by the thickness of the blood film, or in other words by the characteristics of the blood distributing system.

STATIONARY MEMBRANE OXYGENATORS

The first membrane oxygenator practical for human perfusion resulted from a development of the multilayered lung originally described by Clowes, et al., (1956 a). This improved oxygenator (Clowes and Neville 1957, 1958) again consisted of a number of units, placed one on top of another, in which blood flowed between double membrane layers. The solid plates separating each unit featured a grooved surface on the upper surface in order to support the membranes and a saran screen mesh serving for oxygen distribution on the lower membrane.

Details of construction of the Clowes oxygenator are depicted in fig. 35, B and 36, A. Blood channels are created by distending the membranes into the grooves in the outside supporting plate. Obviously, the longer the blood path, the higher the resistance to flow, the higher the injection pressure necessary to overcome such resistance, and thus, the

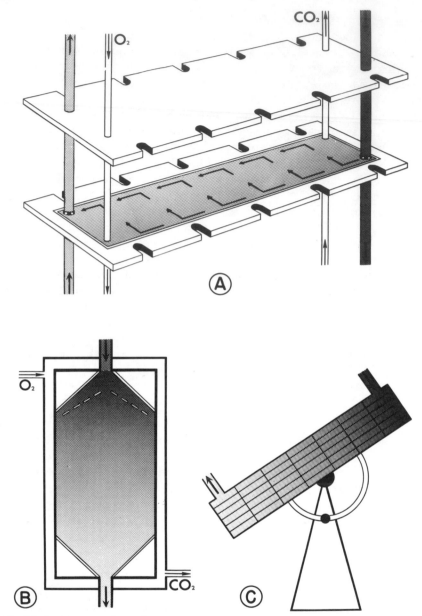

Fig. 36. Stationary membrane lungs.

A. Oxygenator proposed by Clowes, et al. (1956). Venous blood is carried by a vertical column and distributed between each pair of membranes by a radially pierced ring. Arterialized blood is collected in a similar column at the opposite angle of the assembly. Oxygen is circulated through grooves in the supporting plates or through interspaces of woven spacers between consecutive blood layers.

B. Stretched plastic bag proposed as a membrane oxygenator by Lewis, et al. (1958). Blood flows in a thin film in the bag which is encased in an oxygen-filled box (rectangle).

C. Multilayered membrane oxygenator mounted on a tilt table to take advantage of the most favorable angle, since blood transit time depends upon gravity (Benvenuto and Lewis, 1959).

more marked the bulging of the membranes into the grooves. To avoid trapping large volumes of blood in the oxygenator, the expansion of the membranes must be limited. The best oxygenating performance is achieved when the distance the blood travels along the membranes is reduced to a minimum. The blood enters at one corner of the stacked assembly, distends the membrane into a large channel (6.3 mm.) at the edge of each supporting plate and flows along the long side of each oxygenating surface. As the pressure is increased, the blood then distends the membranes into the little grooves (3 mm. from ridge to ridge) which run across each supporting plate. Finally, the oxygenated blood collects in a channel on the opposite side and leaves each unit by the corner diagonally opposite to that at which it entered. Blood is distributed by a series of rings placed one above another between the sheets of teflon when the apparatus is assembled. When the requisite number of units is attained, the membranes are pierced by passing a heated rod down through the column of rings. From the lumen of that column, blood flows between the membranes through small horizontal side holes pierced radially in the width of each ring. Thus blood can be fed to all units simultaneously through a single inlet at the top of the apparatus. It is removed in a similar fashion after arterialization.

Oxygen flows in the grooves and screens on the outside of the membranes. It reaches these spaces through little channels cut into the back of the grooved surface so as to communicate with each groove. A small tube communicates with the main oxygen distributing channel, which is formed by the superposition of cylindrical perforations at one corner of each supporting unit. Assembly is facilitated by alignment posts set in the steel or aluminum base plate and which protrudes through the top plate. Each supporting plate has a pair of holes which fit over the alignment posts. Clamps above the top plate firmly hold the complete assembly together.

Since the membranes stretch to a different extent with different pressures, one must keep a constant pressure within the artificial lung to obtain a regular performance. The pressure at the outflow end is usually maintained between 20 and 30 mm. Hg., which in turn asks for an injection pressure into the oxygenator ranging from 100 to 200 mm. Hg., depending upon the resilience of the membrane and the exact design of the blood channels. Two commonly used circuits are portrayed in fig. 37. A small amount of arterialized blood is continuously being recirculated and the flow through the artificial lung is independent of fluctuations in venous return. The apparatus contains a constant volume of blood, so that the arterial blood flow to the organism must equal the amount of venous blood drained from the organism. The priming requirement of the Clowes oxygenator amounts to 120 ml. per sq. m. of surface area. Since a teflon membrane of 0.5 mil. thickness transmits around 20 ml. O_2 sq./m./min., the surface area of the membrane and the priming volume needed for sufficient oxygenation may be easily calculated.

Peirce (1960) has described in great detail a modification of the Clowes artificial lung which is somewhat simpler, easier to assemble, much less expensive and which has approximately half the bulk of the Clowes model. The key to simple construction of each supporting unit is the preparation of an accurate gasket made of one-sixteenth inch rubber matting. The holes for the guide posts, blood distribution columns and gas distribution columns are pierced at the periphery of the rubber gasket. Fiberglas woven spacers separate consecutive pairs of membrane and act as an oxygenating bed. The priming volume is approximately the same as that of the original Clowes lung. A nomogram relating the area of membrane needed to body weight and oxygen requirement has been worked out by Peirce, et al. (1959). This chart is based on the ability of the membrane to transfer carbon dioxide and thus provides a large reserve of oxygenation. Recently, the fiberglas spacers have been replaced by grooved polyvinyl mats designed by Bluemle (1960) for enhancing mass transfer in an artificial kidney. The gas transfer capacity is more than doubled, owing to a more favorable distribution of the blood film. The priming volume is decreased, because the system is more rigid. The blood content of the lung is hardly affected by changes in flow. Nevertheless, the resistance to flow is not significantly increased, provided the proper gaskets are used.

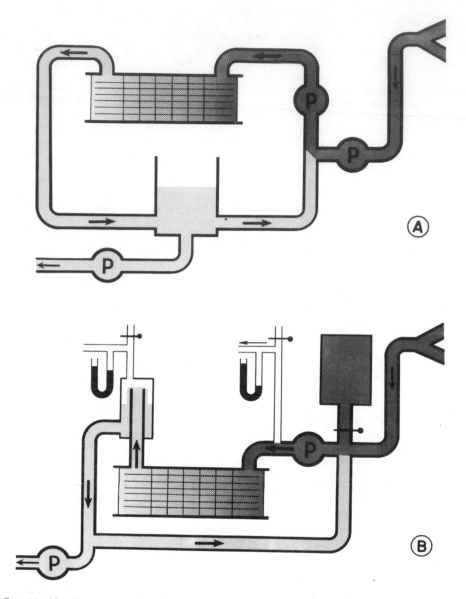

Fig. 37. Blood circuits employed with membrane oxygenators. Since the membranes are distensible, it is mandatory that a constant injection pressure and a constant blood flow through the artificial lung be maintained to keep blood content constant.

A. Circuit arrangement used by Kolff, et al. (1956a). A recirculation pump (upper right) is used in addition to the venous (right) and arterial pumps (lower left). Volume changes in the extracorporeal circuit are then limited to a noncritical reservoir between arterial and venous lines.

B. Circuit used by Peirce (1960a). The venous pump (right) is set at a somewhat higher flow than the arterial pump (lower left) and thus maintains a small amount of recirculation through the artificial lung. The pressure at the arterial outlet of the lung is maintained constant by the level of a bubble trap (upper left). The blood content of the extracorporeal circuit is fixed. A plastic bag (rectangle at upper right) filled with blood and located on the suction side of the venous pump may be opened to dampen the effects of possible fluctuations in venous return.

Gentle handling of the blood, disposability of the parts in contact with blood, freedom from formation of gas bubbles or fibrin emboli and simplicity of volume control are the outstanding virtues of the membrane lung. Blood leakage through pinholes in the membrane, which have not been recognized at the time of assembly present the greatest hazard, because dangerously large volumes of blood can be lost in a short time. Therefore, careful attention to details of assembly is an absolute prerequisite to successful perfusion. The time spent in preparation and the relatively high cost of the materials involved have been considered by some users as almost prohibitive (Gentsch, et al., 1960). Sterilization of the artificial lung may also present some problems. The original Clowes oxygenator is too large to fit into a standard autoclave. Gas sterilization has been suggested. Prior to use, a sterile saline or dextran solution must be recirculated through the apparatus in order to remove all trapped air bubbles. The priming blood is then admitted and must replace all the fluid between the membranes; otherwise hemodilution occurs. The membrane lung does not lend itself to any practical method of thermostabilization. Since much heat can be lost in the stacked assembly, a heat exchanger is often inserted in the arterial line.

In the Clowes type of artificial lung, the design of the supporting mats and plates and the pattern of blood distribution between the horizontally disposed membranes are critical in obtaining a good oxygen transfer. Flow difficulties leading to the formation of rivulets, instead of a thin capillary film, were quite common in the early experience with this type of lung. Lewis, et al. (1958) have tried to overcome these difficulties by using a different blood and oxygen distribution system. Each unit of their lung consists of a large tube of polyethylene held flat by means of a pair of aluminum stretching bars (fig. 36, B). These bars are provided with holes which fit over pins in a basic frame placed at 30 degrees to the horizontal. In the first model a blood distribution and collection pattern was heat sealed in each bag, which thus was an independent lung. In a more recent design, an unmodified tube cut directly from the foil is used. The pattern which directs the blood flow is impressed on the membrane by an aluminum and rubber divider plate placed over the membrane and slipped down on the pins of the basic frame. One face of the divider has the design in rubber and this, when pressed against the membrane, occludes it at the necessary points. The back of the divider then forms the base for the next membrane unit. Each membrane unit has a surface area of 0.9 sq. m. The number of these units in the final assembly is in accordance with the anticipated gas exchange requirement. The last dividers added, both in front and in back, are solid plates, and all membranes are encased without the need for a large oxygenating box. Perforated lucite discs, inserted at the top and bottom of each polyethylene tube and stacked on each other, form the blood distributing and collecting columns. Oxygen flows into the assembly through tubes in each divider. Each unit can oxygenate approximately 200 ml./min. of venous blood. Since the CO_2/O_2 permeability ratio for polyethylene is between four and five, the same limitation of CO_2 elimination prevails as in the Clowes' artificial lung.

Other attempts to modify the stationary membrane lung were reported by Crescenzi, et al. (1959, 1960) and Hofstra, et al. (1960). They designed a vertical lung made of one-quarter mil heat-sealed teflon bags separated by plastic aerated spacers. Such a thin teflon membrane may transmit as much as 65 ml./sq. m./min. of oxygen, but teflon's inherent weakness of low CO_2 permeability still remains. The plastic woven spacers, designed as oxygenating beds, are thinner than the grooved rubber mats and saran mesh originally proposed by Clowes, present more grooves and are made of a less compressible material. The principle of short distance flow is further applied by the use of a double blood collecting system. All these modifications result in minimal stretching of the membrane, thin film flow and a decrease in the amount of blood trapped in the artificial lung. Crescenzi's design has successfully passed the trial of human perfusion.

It is obvious that no improvement in the balance of oxygen and carbon dioxide transfer can be brought about by the use of oxygen pressures higher than atmospheric since this leaves completely unaffected the carbon dioxide diffusion gradient across the membrane (Benvenuto and Lewis, 1959). Although trials by Dagher (1959) indicate that oxygen transfer is increased by a factor of seven when a pressure of 1 Kg./sq.cm. is used in the gaseous phase, little can be expected from this technique. In most circumstances, carbon dioxide retention and the development of oxygen microbubbles and high oxygen tensions, should the blood not be circulated fast enough, will deter from its use.

The membrane lung is usually regarded as the lung of the future. Most authors are of the opinion that its blood handling properties are superior to those of other types of oxygenators, although there are in fact very few unbiased comparisons available. It is implicitly accepted by many that no toxic effect can occur without direct contact of blood with gas, or direct chemical reaction between blood and the walls of a container. However, as pointed out by Hassler (1959) this may be an error, because adsorption occurs on any kind of surface. It should also not be forgotten that presently available pumps cause more blood trauma than do currently existing oxygenators. For the time being, the bulk, large priming requirement and cost of preparation of the membrane lung are drawbacks to be considered in the case of high flow, normothermic perfusions. However, it appears likely that the limitations in oxygen transfer can be overcome by engineering skills. Plastic membranes of more suitable properties will probably be developed in the years to come. As suggested by Melrose, it may become possible to incorporate the blood pumps within the membrane oxygenator by using the supporting plates as pulsating diaphragms. Continued improvements in the membrane lung bring it ever closer to being the ideal device for extracorporeal gas exchange.

Summarizing

In stationary membrane oxygenators, alternating layers of blood and gas are arranged in sandwich form to create a large exchange surface. In order to maintain a constant blood volume within the oxygenator, overstretching of the membranes must be avoided. This is done by keeping pressure and flow in the apparatus constant. Gentle handling of the blood, disposability of parts in contact with blood, freedom from gas bubbles or fibrin emboli and simplicity of volume control are the outstanding virtues of the membrane lung. Difficulty of assembly and high cost of the disposable membranes are among the drawbacks.

ROTATING MEMBRANE OXYGENATORS

A completely different technique of gas exchange across a membrane has been developed by Thomas (1958 a, b). In this artificial lung, the membrane is made of a nylon woven support coated with a microporous silicone film (fig. 35 C) and forms the wall of a slanted rotating cylinder. Oxygen is introduced within the cylinder as a pressurized mist. A thin film of oxygenated saline is formed on the inner side of the membrane, while blood is filmed on the outer side. The respiratory gases diffuse through the membrane and adequate arterialization is achieved by adapting the rate of revolution of the cylinder to the blood flow.

Thomas' artificial lung (fig. 38) combines features of both the film and membrane oxygenator. The venous blood is spread over the revolving surface and thereby is exposed to the gas phase as in the classic rotating cylinder oxygenators. However, the exposure of the blood to the atmosphere surrounding the cylinder is too brief to achieve any significant gas exchange. Arterialization is mediated by the porous silicone membrane. If dry oxygen were injected into the cylinder, microbubbles would appear in the blood film. If, however, oxygen is dissolved in saline, gas exchange occurs by a process of molecular diffusion from the water film through the wetted silicone into the blood. In practice, oxygen and saline are nebulized as an aerosol. The excess liquid condenses at the bottom of the interior chamber and is automatically ejected, as is the excess gas. The arterialized blood accumulates in a thermostabilized reservoir below the cylinder before being returned to the perfused organism.

Experience with this oxygenator (Thomas, 1959) has shown the need for a disposable membrane of regular and constant thickness (0.08 to 0.10 mm.). The membrane is renewed prior to each use by coating a nylon cloth, stretched over the cylindrical frame, with a solution of silicone in an organic solvent. The cylinder is then spun briefly as the silicone dries. A light coating of the hard dry silicone film with an antifoam compound

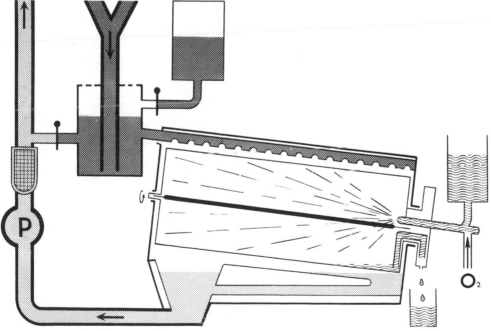

Fig. 38. Scheme of the rotating membrane oxygenator described by Thomas (1958 a, b). Venous blood is collected by syphonage and is spread over the outer face of a silicone membrane stretched over a cylindrical frame. Oxygen and saline (wavy shading) are nebulized under pressure inside the rotating cylinder. Blood is arterialized during a single exposure to the permeable membrane. It is collected in an arterial reservoir (bottom) enclosed in a water bath, before returning via pump and filter to the organism.

added is required for high flow rates over a prolonged period. A phosphate solution buffered at pH. 7.4 has also been found preferable to saline in producing the oxygen-carrying aerosol. Gas sterilization (ethylene oxyde and ozone) is recommended.

As is true of the rotating disc oxygenator, the capacity of the rotating membrane oxygenator can be adapted to changing requirements during the course of a perfusion and this is done by varying the rate of revolution of the membrane covered cylinder. However, when compared to stationary membrane oxygenators, the rotating type does not have the advantages of constant blood content and suppression of all blood–gas interfaces. With a functional surface of exchange of 60 sq.m./min., up to 6 L./min. of blood can be arterialized. Although no specific data have been published concerning the permeation rate of O_2 and CO_2 through the silicone membrane, one can calculate from the above data that it should be at least 4 ml. O_2/sq.m./min. Since the silicone film is wettable, there should be no problem with respect to CO_2 elimination. The oxygenator of Thomas has been extensively used for cardiac surgery in man (Thomas, et al., 1958; Vaysse, 1959). An excellent moving picture (Thomas, 1959) illustrates the simplicity of the assembly and the clinical usefulness of this unique oxygenator.

Summarizing

In the rotating membrane oxygenator, gas transfer occurs through a silicone membrane stretched over a cylindrical frame. The blood is spread as a film on the outer side of the membrane, while oxygen is introduced as a pressurized mist on the inside. The rate of revolution of the cylinder can be adjusted to the rate of blood flow.

VIII. Theory of Blood Pumps

Ernest Starling allegedly stated that an artificial lung capable of eq̲ ̲ing the performance of the natural lung would never be devised. It is not reported if Starling also believed that no mechanical pump could ever perform as well as the heart, although such an opinion is to some extent tenable nowadays. For one century, physiologists have been developing pumping mechanisms capable of displacing limited volumes of blood in perfusion experiments. However, as late as 1952, Folkow was forced to conclude that the trauma inflicted to blood by mechanical pumps was such that the perfused vascular beds soon lost their normal reactivity. It was the application of such blood pumping techniques to therapeutic procedures in man which promoted further research. Empirically, data were collected which now permit defining the requirements for a pump intended to replace temporarily the human heart (Bahnson, 1958 a; Melrose, 1959; Kolff, 1959; Bucherl, 1960).

THE IDEAL BLOOD PUMP

The ideal blood pump should have the following desirable features:

(1) It should be able to move blood volumes up to 5 L./min. against pressure up to 180 mm. Hg.

(2) The handling of blood by the pump should be at low velocities of flow.

(3) All parts in contact with blood should have smooth surfaces; their design should be simple and devoid of dead spaces and recesses; it should offer no opportunity for stagnation or turbulence, for the formation of gas bubbles, foam or clots.

(4) It should be possible to dismantle, clean and sterilize the pump with ease, and its blood handling components should be disposable.

(5) Calibration of the pump should be easy, reliable and always reproducible.

(6) The pump should be automatically controlled and operated for routine use, but designed for possible manual operation in case of power failure.

(7) The pump should have an adjustable stroke volume and a controllable pulse rate.

(8) The output should be linearly proportional to the pulse rate and independent of the resistance in the circuit.

The heart of an average human adult can pump up to 30 L./min. of blood. However, at the present time there is no need for the pump to reach this level of myocardial performance, which only occurs under the most extreme conditions of muscular activity. Since blood pumping systems are used exclusively for the perfusion of organisms under resting conditions, the desired volume flow corresponds to the minimal, or basal, performance of the human heart. Even so, the output of the pump must cover all ranges from that required for partial perfusion in small infants to that required for total perfusion of large adults. This range is conservatively estimated to extend from 200 to 5000 ml./min. The same pump components can seldom be used over the entire range. Therefore most of the pumps are designed for the approximate flow at which they are expected to operate: small units deliver precisely known outputs for the perfusion of isolated vascular beds, whereas large pumps are employed for complete heart–lung bypass in adults. Pump outputs approximating the blood flow under normal conditions usually produce mean pressures in the order of 100 mm. Hg. To provide a sufficient margin of safety, should the resistance of the vascular bed be particularly high, pressures up to 180 mm. Hg. must be overcome without any loss in efficiency of the pumping action.

Perhaps no other factor in the operation of a pump is so detrimental to blood as high flow velocity, and none has been so much disregarded. Pumps are the site of energy transfer from moving mechanical parts to the blood. For this reason the pump itself ranks first among the factors contributing to blood denaturation in any extracorporeal circuit. As we shall discern later, vasodilation and lack of responsiveness in perfused vascular beds can be partly ascribed to the release of depressor agents by mechanical destruction of erythrocytes when the kinetic energy imparted to blood exceeds a critical value. Since the kinetic energy of a given mass of blood increases with the square of the linear velocity, one can easily conceive why stenoses, tight valves or small bore outlets must be avoided. Squeezing of the blood between collapsible structures, heating by friction or shear during the pumping cycle, excessive turbulence or stagnation, and finally high positive or negative pressure waves also count among the most deleterious factors in blood handling (*see* chapter III, XII and XVII).

Experience has shown that the compressible or movable elements of the pump in direct contact with blood are among the most difficult parts to clean in any heart–lung machine. The designers therefore have tended to make the pumps easy to dismantle for thorough cleaning and sterilization. In human application it is in general most desirable to discard the pump tubing or diaphragm after use in order to prevent the disastrous consequences of improper cleaning.

Regulation of the ideal pump should be automatic. Its control should integrate hemodynamic data (perfusion flow, arterial and venous pressures) and metabolic data (arteriovenous oxygen difference) so as to maintain all these parameters within physiologic limits. At the same time the pump should be designed to take into account the peculiarities of an extracorporeal circuit, for instance: it should stop when the arterial reservoir is empty or the arterial line inadvertently clamped; it should adjust the volume of arterial infusion to that of venous return, and should stop suction when the caval veins start to collapse. At the present time, it is not practicable to include all the feedback systems necessary for such a wealth of controls. Fortunately, most of the needed features are interrelated, so that under most circumstances, one or two checking elements are sufficient. Despite the attractiveness of "gadgeteering," the best design for a pumping mechanism remains that which incorporates the largest number of inherent controls and therefore requires a minimum of compensatory safety devices.

Because pumps with their controls and power supply can fail during a perfusion, they must be equipped for manual operation, or manual override. Since a few instances of mechanical failure during human operations have been reported (e.g., Zaroff, et al., 1959), it is mandatory that the pump can be actuated at short notice with a crank, or be replaced instantaneously by another pump inserted in the same extracorporeal circuit.

Summarizing

The ideal blood pump should have a minute volume ranging from 200 to 5000 ml. against pressures up to 180 mm. Hg., an adjustable stroke volume and pulse rate, and a linear relationship between pulse rate and output. Design should be aimed at ease of maintenance and gentle blood handling; the operation should be manual as well as automatic. High flow velocities should be avoided. The automatic controls which adapt the output of the pump to the prevailing hemodynamic conditions should be simple and reliable.

PULSATILE VERSUS CONTINUOUS FLOW

Certainly the most controversial point concerning blood pumps is whether or not a pulsatile flow is necessary or desirable. Classic physiology from the time of Ludwig and Schmidt (1868) to that of Carell and Lindbergh (1938) has assigned to pulse pressure a specific role in maintaining normal functions in perfused organs. Most of the experimental work on which this opinion is based has dealt with kidneys. Hooker (1910) reported that reduction in pulse pressure during the course of perfusion of isolated kidneys lowered blood flow and urine volume. Gesell (1913) was not able to establish significant effects of pulse pressure changes on renal blood flow in vivo. Nevertheless, he believed that reduction in pulse pressure caused a diminution in urine flow and in chloride excretion. In recent years, such claims have been consistently refuted. Goodyear and Glenn (1951), Selkurt (1951) and Ritter (1952) did not observe any significant change in renal blood flow and renal function when the kidneys were perfused at normal *mean* pressures, using flows of greatly reduced amplitude. There was also surprisingly little difference between pulsatile and steady perfusion of the dog's hind leg in the experiments related by Randall and Stacy (1956).

In the field of total body perfusion, claims for the necessity of pulsatile flow have been made by Jongbloed (1951) and by Thomas and Beaudoin (1951). However, the maintenance of normal gas exchange function in the lungs during nonpulsatile perfusion was demonstrated by Wesolowski, et al. (1953 b). A parallel conclusion, as far as the central nervous system and the entire cardiovascular system are concerned, was later reached by the same authors (1955): Total body perfusion experiments were conducted using either a pulsatile pump or gravity for arterial infusion. No difference in the reactivity of the cardiovascular system could be demonstrated; organic function remained unaltered and the fate of the perfused animals, once the heart–lung bypass procedure was discontinued, was essentially the same. A different conclusion was reached in a recent series of comparative studies by Ogata, et al. (1960), Nonoyama (1960) and Takeda (1960). In the absence of pulsatile flow dogs exhibited a lower mean arterial pressure, a more marked tendency towards acidosis, a larger increase in weight (probably from edema) and more obvious signs of blood pooling in the splanchnic area than when they were perfused at the same flow with a pulsatile pump. All these signs of deterioration were associated with a primary disturbance of the peripheral circulation: capillary stasis and opening of arterio-venous shunts, when nonpulsatile flows were used. Edema was thought to result from the relative hypertension prevailing in the precapillary region because the dampening effect of the arterioles on rhythmic pressure oscillations was not called into action. Hemolysis was similar in the two parallel series of experiments, and the fact that the heart was arrested only in the nonpulsatile perfusions was considered as irrelevant.

There is no irreducible contradiction between the results of Wesolowski and those of the Japanese authors. As pointed out by Ogata, the discrepancies between the effects of pulsatile and nonpulsatile flow were impressive at low and medium flow rates but disappeared when the perfusion flow reached 100 ml./Kg./min. Since Wesolowski used flow rates in the order of 130 ml./Kg./min. adverse effects of nonpulsatile flow could not develop in his experiments. However, the problem may require further consideration in low flow rate and hypothermic perfusions, where sludging of blood in capillaries is most likely to occur.

There is a belief that a perfusion pump should mimic the physiologic action of the heart and thus, be pulsatile, with a stroke volume, a frequency and a pulse contour adjustable over the whole range of variation encountered in man. Such designs have a particular appeal to those who feel that natural structures present the ideal type of adaptation to function, and that artificial organs should closely simulate their natural counterparts. However, most of today's equipment is designed to perform organic functions under physical conditions which differ widely from those of the intact organism. As far as the circulation is concerned, there is little rational for claiming that the normal pulse contour should be aimed at when blood is injected from a peripheral artery towards vessels of *larger* diameter, since under natural conditions it flows from the root of the aorta in a distributing system progressively *decreasing* in size. Pulsatile action appears to be the solution reached by nature for attaining maximal pumping efficiency by a hollow muscle. There is at present no conclusive evidence that a mechanical system need be likewise. Many of the structures within the circulatory system act to convert pulsatile flow in the arteries into continuous flow in the capillaries (compression chamber or windkessel effect). As demonstrated by Peterson, et al. (1960), the usual consequence of the work performed by smooth muscle in the vessel walls is an increased absorption of mechanical energy generated by the heart. The concept that the arteries function as a "peripheral heart", i.e., rhythmically contracting in synchrony with the heart, is no longer justified. However, reflex mechanisms which depend not upon changes in vascular pressures, but upon the rate of these changes, can possibly be jeopardized by continuous perfusion. Electrical signals are elicited in the wall of arteries by the pulsatile nature of the blood flow (Rijlant, 1932), but nothing is known about the effects of rhythmical stimulation of baroreceptors by pulsatile flow at the level of the small vessels. Their inhibition could conceivably affect the balance of hemeostatic mechanisms in the cardiovascular system, although such an effect is, for the time being, purely hypothetic. Nevertheless, considerable ingenuity has been applied to design a pump capable of reproducing the arterial (or venous) pulse contour. Hooker (1915) empirically developed a cam by which the aortic pulse could be simulated with his piston pump. In Russia, groups led by Vainrib and Ananiev (1956) developed a mathematical model of the genesis and propagation of the pulse contour by means of which they could duplicate the normal arterial flow pattern by the use of a ventricle pump. Recently, McCabe (1959) has designed a multichambered pump which closely approximates all features of the venous and arterial circulation. Only the future will decide whether the approach of these investigators will be successful.

The above considerations do not apply under conditions of partial heart–lung bypass or of "assisted circulation," where synchronization with the heart action becomes of crucial importance. Then the pattern of flow (constant, dephased or synchronized) may be just as important as the flow itself. Therefore, stroke volume and frequency should ideally be variable over the entire range of human heart action (*see* chapter XX).

Summarizing:

From a biologic and philosophic viewpoint it is difficult to conceive that nature has endowed the circulatory system with pulsatile pressures and flow without deriving from this some benefit towards the function of the organism. Nonetheless, there is at present no conclusive evidence available to support the view that, at the organ level, pulsatile flow issuing from a blood pump is superior to constant flow at the same mean pressure.

OCCLUSIVE VERSUS NONOCCLUSIVE PUMPS

Whereas the controversy over the use of pulsatile or continuous flow is largely based on theory or prejudice, the debate concerning the use of occlusive or nonocclusive blood pumps is basically a matter of technical efficiency. The pump itself is usually the only flowmeter available in an extracorporeal circuit, so that any estimation of perfusion rate is dependent upon its calibration chart. The calibration of the pump must therefore be stable, easy to check immediately before initiating the perfusion, and must remain reliable throughout the period of use, regardless of temperature variations in the reduction gear or speed variator. In this respect, attention must be directed not only to the pump itself, but also to the elastic properties of the tubing and to the size and shape of the cannulae. Under conditions of total heart–lung bypass, the volume of arterialized blood distributed to the tissues must be independent of random fluctuations in vascular pressures. The pump must therefore be "load insensitive," meaning that within predetermined limits of pressure, the output is independent of the resistance in the circuit. If the pump is "load sensitive," then the effects of various filling or ejection pressures must be quantitatively established, and the pump setting modified accordingly.

The simplest approach to accurate control of perfusion rate consists in making the pump occlusive. The walls of the pumping chamber are rhythmically brought against each other so as to occlude the blood path. Unidirectional flow is provided by a system of valves. A constant stroke volume is obtained if the pumping chamber is thoroughly squeezed during the occlusion phase, or if the action of the pumping mechanism is restricted between two stops. Then the flow can be directly determined from the frequency of motion of the activator. Within the range of outflow pressures encountered in human perfusions a completely occlusive pump will deliver the same output regardless of resistance. When the pump is not occlusive, or when backflow occurs on the input or output side of the pump owing to valvular regurgitation, the flow is essentially pressure-dependent, and can only be estimated from the rate of motion of the activator. Provided the same size of pumping chamber is always used and the same degree of regurgitation always achieved, a graph can be constructed relating the outflow to the rate of actuation of the pump at various levels of peripheral resistance (D. P. Hall, et al. 1958; Griesser and Parson, 1960). Such a method of flow control is, to say the least, cumbersome. For total body perfusion, some authors adopt a compromise proposed by Griesser (1958 a, b): the venous pump, which works against a constant, low resistance, is set as nonocculsive, whereas the arterial pump is made occlusive to achieve regular flow calibration.

Occlusive action is associated with a marked degree of hemolysis in some of the commercially available pumps. The trauma is thought to occur because the forces developed in squeezing the blood between the walls of the pumping chamber exceed the mechanical resistance of the erythrocyte membrane. If, however, the forces exerted during occlusion are minimized by proper adjustment, the blood trauma can be reduced to acceptable levels. One possible improvement consists in using for the pumping chamber and valves a material which is softer than the erythrocytes such as some of the polyvinyl alcohols. Then the blood cells caught in the pump during the occlusive phase are merely imbedded in the neighboring walls (Majer, 1958). The most commonly adopted solution is that of "minimal occlusion," meaning that micrometric adjustment of the degree of occlusion prevents crushing of red cells by undue compression. The simplest means of reaching the proper degree of minimal occlusion consists of filling the outflow tube of the pump with a liquid (fig. 39): the pump is arrested and the adjustment of the occlusion mechanism is modified by small increments until no fall in level of the liquid column is observed (Shimomura, et al., 1958). One can also test the occlusivity by means of feeler gauges (Watkins, et al., 1960). Some authors believe that trauma is reduced by keeping the pump slightly insufficient. It should be observed, however, that under these conditions there will be a leakage which may be just as detrimental to the blood as is complete occlusion if high backflow velocities are reached. When the pump is adjusted for a given tubing size, it is mandatory to check the occlusivity with each new batch received from the factory, since the commercial tolerances on wall thickness exceed the desired adjustment.

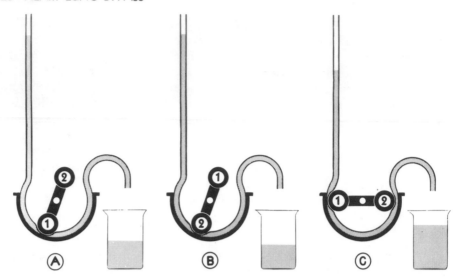

Fig. 39. Technique of adjusting blood pumps for minimal occlusion. The outflow line of the pump is filled with saline to the level corresponding to anticipated outflow pressure. The occlusion of the blood path by that part of the pump which acts as a valve (finger, roller, knife edge, compression cuff, etc.) is gradually released until saline starts to leak back through the occluded blood path. As illustrated in A and B, each external valve (e.g., roller 1 and 2) must be tested independently. Failure to do so (C), can lead to the erroneous conclusion that the pump is occlusive, where actually leakage under 2 is prevented by a particular position of roller 1.

Vadot (1960) has calculated that an occlusive pressure of 2 Kg./sq.cm. is the limit at which hemolysis begins to appear, because the mechanical resistance of the erythrocyte membrane is then surpassed. It is possible to prevent blood trauma if the occluder is spring loaded at a pressure below 2 Kg./sq.cm. Irregularities in the thickness of the tubing do not result in crushing of red cells, since the occluder "gives" before excessive pressures are attained. Vadot has also indicated another factor favoring blood trauma in those occlusive pumps which use a cylindrical tube as compression chamber. The deformation of the tube by the occluder (fig. 40 A) is such that with increasing compression the section first takes on the shape of an ellipse, then that of a "figure 8" before flattening completely. High pressure must be exerted in order to achieve complete occlusion. When a tubing which is diamond-shaped in cross-section is used (fig. 40 B), complete occlusion requires less pressure which is then more evenly distributed, the strain upon the lateral parts of the tubing being markedly diminished.

Summarizing

Occlusive pumps are useful for accurate control of perfusion rate because their output does not depend upon the resistance in the circuit. However, they can produce prohibitive degrees of blood trauma unless they are carefully adjusted.

THE ACTUAL BLOOD PUMPS

The most common classification of pumping equipment is based on the mechanism of moving, or adding energy to the fluid. Engineers (Serven and Rhodes, 1960) distinguish two main classes: kinetic pumps and positive displacement pumps (table 3). In *kinetic pumps*, the pumping action is performed by the addition of kinetic energy to the fluid through the forced rotation of

Table 3. Types of pumps used for extracorporeal circulation. Letters in parentheses refer to illustrations in fig. 41.

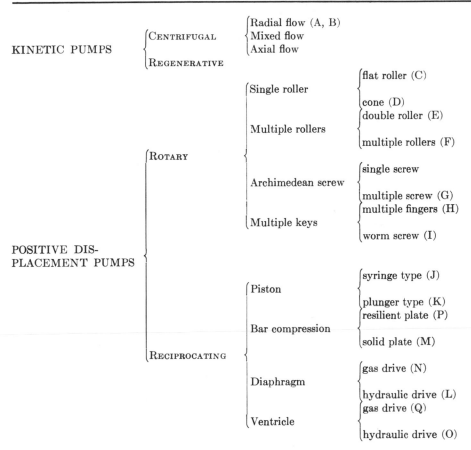

an impeller or other similar mechanism. Fluid velocity is then slowed down at the exit by passage through a diffuser which increases the pressure, or level of potential energy. Kinetic pumps are commonly used to move large volume flows against a minimal pressure difference between their input and output sides. From the engineering point of view, they involve a minimum of transmission and moving parts, and are very compact and efficient. However, they create high velocities of flow and thereby are likely to produce a marked hemolysis.

The output of a centrifugal pump is directly related to the input pressure, and inversely related to the pressure head against which it works. In other words, a centrifugal pump has the tendency to deliver a higher output as more blood is fed at the inlet; reciprocally, it will provide a lower flow when the resistance in the circuit increases. The extreme "load sensitivity" of centrifugal pumps appears to render them ideal for intracorporeal cardiac substitution (Saxton and Andrews, 1960). As pointed out by Melrose (1959), the different types of centrifugal pumps have in common an absence of valves to direct the flow, and they depend for pumping action on the rotation of a system of

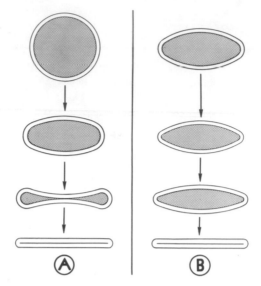

Fig. 40. Cross-sectional shape of a resilient tube at successive stages of compression against a solid flat surface. Lumen of tube is indicated by shading.

A. Conventional blood tubing of circular cross-section. When complete occlusion is achieved the axial part is submitted to higher external pressure than are the lateral parts.
B. Blood tubing diamond shaped in cross-section as proposed by Vadot (1960). Progressive compression leads to simultaneous occlusion over the entire cross-section with relatively minimal force applied (redrawn after Vadot, 1960).

blades set at an angle about the axis of rotation. While producing an inherently smooth flow, a certain amount of "slip" occurs—the rotating blade sliding inefficiently through the fluid pumped across its direction of flow. "Slip" may be associated with "cavitation," that is, areas of very low pressure developing along the leading edge of the blade and drawing from the fluid a quantity of dissolved gas. Both "slip" and "cavitation" contribute to hemolysis. In a comparative study by P. E. Hall, et al. (1958), centrifugal pumps were found to be far more traumatic than other models and consequently, no pump of this type has yet been developed for blood perfusion purposes.

Positive displacement pumps accomplish this purpose by displacing the liquid progressively from the suction to the discharge opening of the unit. They are divided into two classes: rotary pumps and reciprocating pumps. In rotary pumps, the displacement of fluid is managed by rotating members which trap a portion of the liquid and conduct it toward the outlet. No valves are needed. In reciprocating pumps, suction and discharge valves bind a cavity which is subjected to the reciprocating action of a piston, plunger, compression bar, or diaphragm. As the reciprocating member moves back and forth, liquid is drawn in through a suction valve and forced out through a discharge valve. In all positive displacement pumps, the capacity depends upon the displacement and the number of displacements per unit of time.

All pumps which have been found practicable for handling blood belong to the positive displacement class. The basic features of the various systems proposed in the last hundred years are illustrated in fig. 41. The blood pumps in actual use are described in Chapters IX and X.

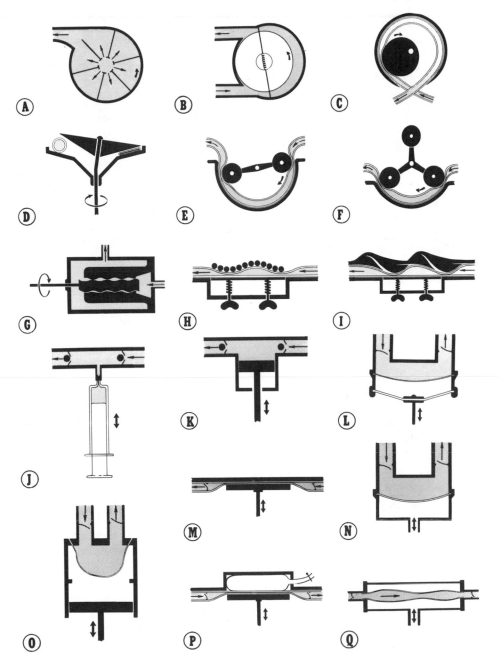

Fig. 41. Blood pump mechanisms. Blood represented by shaded areas. Solid parts in black.

A and B centrifugal pumps; C single flat roller pump; D single cone roller pump, E double roller pump. F triple roller pump; G archimedean screw pump. H multiple finger pump; I worm screw pump; J syringe piston pump; K plunger pump; L diaphragm pump with hydraulic drive; M bar compression pump with solid plate; N diaphragm pump with gas drive; O ventricle pump with hydraulic drive; P bar compression pump with resilient plate; Q ventricle pump with gas drive.

Before methods for reliable control of blood clotting were available, the pumping of large volumes of blood without undue denaturation was an impossible task. In the early era of extracorporeal circulation, two main designs were utilized: the diaphragm pump of Dale and Schuster (1928) was developed to high output capacity by DeBurgh Daly (1933) and Jongbloed (1949), mainly by multiplying the number of pumping units. On the other hand, the old roller principle was applied to perfusion equipment by International Business Machines for the Gibbon stationary screen oxygenator. Around 1954 the cooperation of pump engineers with cardiac surgeons at the University of Minnesota produced the Sigmamotor pump, a multiple finger pump which soon became extremely popular. For years these two basic types, multiple finger pump and roller pump, have dominated the market and they still occupy this position of prominence.

Design factors affecting the performance of the different models of pumps have been investigated and discussed in detail (Khayutin, 1958; Hall, et al., 1959). The engineering factors are still not as well defined as they are in pumps for chemical service (Hoffman and Calkin's, 1960; Flindle, 1961; Middeldorf, 1961). Nevertheless, they can be divided into the same three groups:
(1) Materials of construction;
(2) Specific factors (capacity, head of pressure, specific gravity of fluid pumped, suction conditions, partial pressures of dissolved gas, shape of pulse contour);
(3) General factors (cost, spare parts, space limitations, standardization).

From the biologic standpoint, the quality of a blood pump is usually estimated from measurements of the release of hemoglobin in the plasma following red cell destruction. Most comparative studies are quite deceptive because the experimental conditions are not standardized. Data obtained while conducting actual perfusions are not directly relevant, because of the clearing action exerted by the living organism which is part of the blood circuit. Measurable blood trauma will also be dependent upon the size of the priming volume and the cumulative amount of flow, since damage to blood elements is obviously proportional to the number of times they pass through the pump. Cahill and Kolff (1959) and Taylor, et al. (1959) have described a mock circuit for the testing of pumps under reproducible conditions. Their technique is dependable for comparative studies provided that the pitfalls of plasma hemoglobin determination are recognized (see chapter XVII). However, this technique is limited to testing periods of one to two hours since blood recirculated without undergoing gas exchange later shows unpredictable biochemic alterations which markedly increase the fragility of the formed elements. It is conceivable that the testing of pumps over long periods will require devices such as dialysers, in order to maintain viable conditions in the blood under study.

Summarizing:

Pumps are divided into two main classes: the kinetic type and the positive displacement type. In the former, kinetic energy is added to the fluid through the forced rotation of an impeller. These pumps are very traumatic to blood and are therefore unsuitable for extracorporeal circulation. Positive displacement pumps are divided into two main groups: rotary pumps and reciprocating pumps. In the former, liquid is progressively displaced toward the outlet by a rotating member with no valves required. In the latter, suction and discharge valves form the entrance and exit respectively of a cavity which is subjected to the reciprocating action of a piston or diaphragm.

IX. Rotary Pumps

$\mathbf{F}$luid is displaced in rotary pumps by moving members which trap a portion of the fluid and conduct it towards the outlet (*see* fig. 41, C to I). The blood is usually contained in a segment of flexible tubing introduced into the pump casing. The movement of the actuator, which compresses the tubing against a solid base plate, is circular. According to the type of pump, the axis of rotation may be parallel, perpendicular or at some other angle to the axis of propagation of blood flow.

ROLLER PUMPS

This type utilizes a roller which progresses along a resilient tube in order to squeeze blood out of it. The basic design is so old (list of U.S. patents in Shaw and Grove-Rasmussen, 1953) that it is difficult to decide to whom credit should be given for its first application to blood handling. Beck (1924), von Issekutz (1927), Bayliss and Muller (1928), Van Allen (1932), DeBakey (1934), Jouvelet and Henry (1934) and Thalimer, et al. (1938), all used roller pumps for human blood transfusion. In a review of perfusion equipment available at the time, Fleisch (1935) described a model of roller pump suitable for laboratory experiments. To avoid the use of anticoagulants, Brull (1950 a, b) even devised a roller pump in which the tubing could be replaced by a segment of aorta.

Since the beginning of the extracorporeal circulation era, the obvious advantages of simplicity and ease of cleaning and sterilization have favored the use of roller pumps. However, blood trauma inherent in the severe shearing forces developed during the squeezing process first appeared prohibitive. Difficulties were encountered in attempts to achieve radial compression of the blood tube without tangential displacement of its walls and grinding of the blood between them. Controversy arose over the degree of occlusion required to make the pump effective, and over the desirability of a nonpulsatile flow. Moreover, experimental studies are still needed to define the ideal pump speed and stroke volume and to assess the advantages and inconveniences of multiple roller systems versus single rollers.

Since roller pumps require tubing with a high degree of elastic rebound, rubber is usually preferred to plastic material. Nevertheless some type of polyvinyl tubing, such as Tygon R-3603, perform satisfactorily. Osborn (1953) suggested placing the tubing in a vacuum chamber in order to accelerate its elastic recoil. This scheme has not been followed further on account of the technical complexities involved. Rubber is also the material of choice when resistance to prolonged mechanical stress is a primary consideration because plastic tubing may split under conditions of total occlusion (McCaughan, et al., 1958b). Silicone rubber is ideal for hypothermic perfusions, since its resilience is not affected by temperature variations.

Highly accurate engineering of the pump housing, use of the proper material for both housing and roller, and adequate external lubrication of the tubing, are all factors to be considered in the design of a roller pump. A simple parallel arrangement between roller and backplate often fails to provide trouble-free pumping. Rubber tubes have the tendency to move forward as the roller passes over them. Bushings may be used to fix the tubing at the inlet and outlet of the pump and to keep constant the length of the segment acted upon by the roller. Thereby the stroke volume is constant and the pump remains true to its calibration curve. When not acted upon by a constant longitudinal tension, blood tubes tend to "float" laterally in their casing. In one popular model (Head, et al., 1960), a guide rod mounted on the central axle of the pump precedes each roller in order to keep the path of tubing straight (fig. 42, A). To avoid "creeping," DeBakey (1934) used rubber tubes with a flat projecting flange which could be clamped between two semicircular metal bars, thereby holding the tubing firmly in position during the passage of the roller (fig. 42, B). A more advanced design is that pioneered by Melrose (1959): the backplate is grooved to accept the tube, along which runs a roller, shaped to invaginate one wall of the tube into the other (fig. 42, C). If the radii of the roller and groove are arranged to match one another, an efficient occlusion is produced with a minimum of trauma.

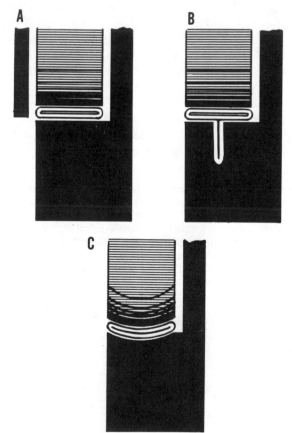

Fig. 42. The different systems employed in roller pumps to keep the tube in place. Pump housing black; roller marked by horizontal stripes; tubing shown compressed between roller and back plate.

A. Guide rod on the left of the tube prevents lateral movement.
B. Flange inserted into a slot of the backplate keeps the tube straight.
C. Tube compressed between convex roller and grooved backplate.

The blood trauma induced by modern roller pumps is well within acceptable limits. There is evidence that hemolysis is quantitatively related to the number of passages of the roller over the blood tube (Head, et al., 1960). Therefore it is advantageous to use tubing of the largest possible bore (Leonards and Ankeney, 1958) despite claims to the contrary (Hodges, et al., 1958). Recent reports of in vitro testing experiments (Cappeletti, et al. 1961; Brown, et al. 1961) demonstrate that roller pumps compare favorably to almost any other type of pump. Most commercial roller pumps were originally intended for nonocclusive action. Recently, there has been a swing in opinion back to occlusive setting which can be achieved with negligible levels of hemolysis, at least at low velocity and large stroke volume (Leonards and Ankeney, 1958). As pointed out by Melrose (1959), nonocclusive operation does not only deprive the operator of accurate flow control (*see* Chapter VIII), but it may also lead him astray, e.g., when all forward flow is canceled by an equal backflow, because of an increase in peripheral resistance, a nonocclusive roller pump still appears to be functioning satisfactorily. With the extremely regular and smooth latex and plastic tubings available nowadays, the degree of compression of the blood tube needs to be exactly adjusted if roller pumps are to be employed under occlusive conditions. One group (Kay and Anderson, 1958) prefers a permanently adjusted pump in order to eliminate unwanted changes during operation. This pump is accurately machined to be barely insufficient and limited to only one width of tubing wall. Another design (Head, et al., 1960) incorporates individual micrometric adjustment of each roller by worm screws which displace the center of the roller along the radial axis of the pump (fig. 43, A). Griesser (1958) relies on modifying the angles of a parallelogram at one top of which the roller is mounted (fig. 43, B). The use of spring tension (Melrose, 1959; Vadot, 1960; Esmond, et al., 1961) is probably the most sensible approach to occlusion because it prevents regurgitation while avoiding the development of exceedingly high pressure on the blood trapped in the pump (fig. 43, C). To minimize the friction of the rollers upon the tubing, which may result in slippage and bending of the boot, the manufacturer of the Mayo pump has chosen to spin the rollers actively with an auxiliary power transmission rather than letting them revolve by friction as the pump turns. Mechanically, roller pumps are simple and robust. However, they require very careful machining in order to avoid small irregularities in the shape of the pump casing, which may render a roller occlusive in one position and not in another one. Ideally, all pump backing and rollers should be concentric within one thousandth of an inch. Many manufacturers mount the roller pumps on a vertical support to facilitate elimination of gas bubbles and the check on minimal occlusion.

Roller pumps are conveniently described under the headings of single roller, twin roller and multiple roller pumps:

(1) Single roller pump: This type consists of a circular housing in which a complete 360 degree loop of tubing is inserted (*see* fig. 41, C). Within the loop is a large single, eccentric roller free to rotate on ball bearings mounted on a compound driving shaft. A cam can be adjusted so that the roller carried in the shaft just closes the lumen of the blood tube, or the roller can be spring loaded. A steadily progressive compression is produced as the ring of the roller rotates about the axis of the race bearing and "milks" the blood out of the tube. Adjustment is simple and rapid, and a pulsatile flow is ob-

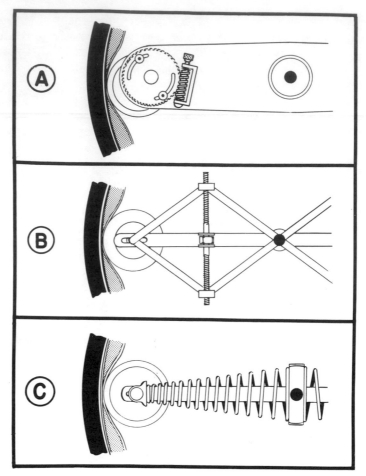

Fig. 43. Methods for adjusting the occlusion of the tube in a roller pump. Backplate black; blood tube shaded.

A. Micrometric adjustment used by Head et al. (1960).
B. Parallelogram arrangement proposed by Griesser (1958a, b).
C. Permanent adjustment by calibrated spring. Details in text.

tained. The stroke volume depends only upon the nature and bore of the tube, while the rate of pumping is controlled by a variable speed gearbox. Occlusive pumps of this type maintain a constant delivery in the face of sharp fluctuations in pressure at the outlet. When, however, marked changes in the inlet pressure are produced, the output may vary by six to eight per cent as a result of change in the diameter of the compressible tube (Khayutin, 1958). According to the same author, the degree of hemolysis produced by a single roller pump is considerably less than that produced by a three-roller pump enclosed in a similar housing.

Single eccentric roller pumps have been used in heart–lung machines by Shaw and Grove-Rasmussen (1953), Osborn (1953), Melrose (1954), Rygg, et al. (1956), and Esmond, et al. (1961). Recently, the artificial lung developed at the National Institutes of Health by Waldhausen, et al. (1959b), and the Mayo stationary screen oxygenator have been equipped with single roller pumps. Micropumps for laboratory studies and organ perfusion are also available.

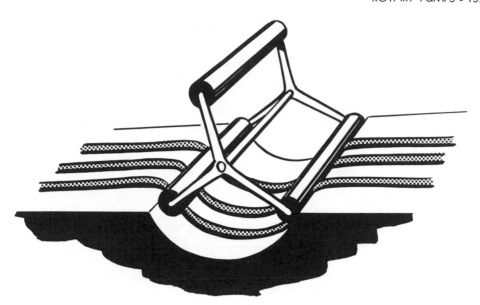

Fig. 44. A roller pump with three long rollers which can compress several tubes simultaneously.

(2) Twin roller pump: The twin roller blood pump is the most widely used at the present time. In this type (*see* fig. 41, E), a loop of tubing is fitted between a horseshoe-shaped housing and two rollers revolving at the same distance from a central axis. The rollers are 180 degrees out of phase and the pump casing subtends an angle of 210 degrees or more, so that at least one of the rollers is acting as a valve at all times. When one roller finishes its stroke, the other has already begun. If the setting is occlusive, the changeover from one roller to the other is accompanied by a momentary fall in forward flow and hence the output is pulsatile (Griesser and Parson, 1960). The pressure curve shows a sustained mean pressure interrupted by a dip at the changeover point (Melrose, 1959). If the setting is not occlusive, the output is more continuous (Gibbon, et al., 1953; Servelle, et al., 1958; Felipozzi, et al., 1958) although there may be a pronounced backflow past the roller if the resistance in the circuit is too high. A solution to the dampening of the pulsatile flow pattern generated by twin roller pumps has been proposed by Yasargil (1960). Two similar tubes are arranged in parallel in the housing of the pump and joined to the circuit by Y connectors. Two pairs of rollers are arranged at 180 degrees to each other, each compressing one of the blood tubes.

(3) Multiple roller pumps: Pumps using three or more rollers have been proposed for extracorporeal blood handling (Lenfant, 1956; Raderecht, 1958). The loop of tubing may then be reduced to 120 degrees or less (*see* fig. 41, F). Since the degree of hemolysis increases with the number of rollers (Khayutin, 1958; Head, et al., 1960), there is no obvious advantage to this design for a single pump. However, such pumps are often built so that the rollers compress the arterial and the venous line within the same housing (Battezatti and Taddei, 1954; Falor, et al., 1958). A recent model (fig. 44) consists of two rotating wheels supporting three long rollers. Latex rubber is stretched across the rollers and as the wheels rotate, the tubing is partially occluded and the blood propelled in a unidirectional fashion. Tooled metal part rings slip over the tubing and fit snugly into the holes at the base of the pump, preventing any tendency for the tubing and adaptors to be pulled into the pumping area.

Summarizing:

Roller pumps use a progression of rollers along a flexible tube filled with blood to provide the pumping stroke and to give direction to the flow. Occlusive setting makes the pump load-insensitive, but requires an exactly adjusted compression of the resilient tubing to prevent undue blood trauma. In general, the more rollers to a pump, the greater is the hemolysis. Single roller pumps have a circular housing in which a complete loop of tubing is inserted and compressed by an eccentrically revolving roller. In twin roller pumps a loop of tubing lies in a horseshoe-shaped housing and is compressed by two rollers 180 degrees out of phase. Pumps with three or more rollers are also available. Roller pumps are relatively simple in design and remarkably sturdy.

ARCHIMEDEAN SCREW PUMPS

The roller of a roller pump, by compressing the loop of tubing while moving along it, fulfills simultaneously the functions of a piston and of an external valve. A similar action can be obtained using a worm screw which revolves along a straight piece of resilient tubing (*see* fig. 41, I). Progressive compression of the tube against a solid plate results in unidirectional flow. Because of the "progressive cavity" principle embodied in this design, the flow delivered at the outlet of the pump is practically continuous. The worm screw pump does not present any obvious advantages over other types of equipment (Khayutin, et al., 1958). Indeed the mechanical action of the worm screw upon the blood tube involves a danger of rupture which cannot be neglected in perfusion experiments.

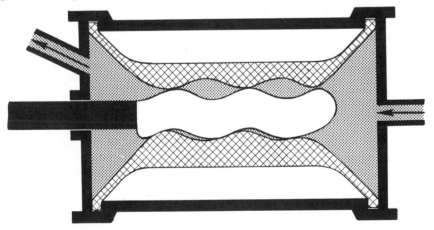

Fig. 45. Archimedean screw pump. Axis and casing: black; rotor: white in center; resilient stator: diagonally cross hatched; blood: shaded. Details in text.

A more advanced design, which does not feature a resilient tube, but incorporates the blood path into the moving organs of the pump, has been adapted from industrial pumping equipment. It consists of two helical shaped parts: a rotor and a stator (fig. 45). The rotor is a true helical screw and revolves within a stator of resilient material, which has a double internal helical thread. The stator thread pitch is, therefore, twice the pitch of the rotor. When the rotor is inserted into the stator, cavities, or pockets, are formed. Pumping starts as soon as the rotor begins to revolve, exerting a positive action comparable to that of a piston moving through a cylinder of infinite length. Rotary motion is used to move a seal through the stator at uniform velocity. The seal is continuously recreating itself at the inlet, or suction end, of the pump by the cooperative engagement of the helical rotor within the stator. During revolution, the fluid pockets between the stator and the rotor steadily progress along the thread toward the outlet, or delivery end, of the pump. The spiral sealing lines bring about perfect closure of the pockets; the pump is thus self-priming. The velocity of flow through the pump is a function of the rotor speed. The liquid trapped in the pockets is almost stationary with respect to itself. Therefore, no turbulence or foaming is likely to occur. The head of pressure developed is independent of speed, but the capacity is proportional to speed. Slippage is a function of viscosity and pressure, and thus easily predictable. Because the total entrance area and discharge area remain constant, the volume of fluid entering and leaving the pump remains at all times constant, the pump is thus an excellent metering device as well. It is also apparent that such a pump may work in either direction with equal efficiency.

The minimum length stator takes a rotor with a twist of slightly more than 720 degrees, thus having two seal lines (one seal line for each complete revolution). This is known as a single stage unit. Multiple stage units, featuring rotors and stators with many complete seals, can be devised to divide the outflow pressure equally among them all. Each revolution of the rotor, regardless of the number of stages, provides continuous displacement of a volume equal to 4 LDE, where L is the stator pitch length, D the diameter of the rotor and E the eccentricity of the axis of the rotor as related to the axis of the stator.

The English *Ormond-Mono* pump (Hall, et al., 1958) represents the first application of the archimedean screw principle to a blood pump of large capacity. The manufacturers have developed a pumping chamber which is easy to dismantle and to clean and which can be autoclaved while fully assembled. Junction of the cartridge and the pump driving head is achieved without affecting the sterility of the surfaces in contact with blood. The entrance to the stator is designed so as to present only smooth surfaces to the incoming blood, and to prevent trapping of air within the elements of the pump. Sharp edges, corners and recesses in the path of blood flow have been avoided. The pumping chamber is made of 316 stainless steel, while the pump stator is made of a synthetic rubber material. A range of output from 0.7 to 5 liters per minute can be delivered, using a variable speed drive in conjunction with a suitable motor. Attempts have been made to develop a "half-pitch" rotor-stator unit, interchangeable with the regular one, which would enable the pump to deliver, at the same speed, the above-mentioned range of outputs divided by half. In laboratory trials (Hal', et al., 1958, 1959), the Ormond-Mono was found to compare favorably with other types in terms of gentleness of blood handling. Clinically it has been used with satisfactory results by Cass, et al. (1958), Taylor (1959), and Shaw, et al. (1960).

The *Donaldson* heart pump, developed in the United States with the collaboration of a surgical group in Philadelphia, is essentially similar to the Ormond-Mono pump. It is mounted in cradles and the shaft-bearing assembly can be taken apart from the pump for sterilization. The unit is so designed that all of its parts, with the exception of the bearings, which can be readily disassembled, can be autoclaved without damage. The output can be adjusted from about 0.3 to 10 liters per minute by regulating the speed of the pump. The speed is controlled by operating a DC motor on an AC power supply, using a selenium rectifier with a variable transformer, which make the unit compact and easy to handle.

Summarizing:

The Archimedean screw pump operates on the principle of a solid helical rotor revolving within a resilient helical stator of different pitch so that blood is drawn along the thread. The fluid pockets trapped between the stator and the rotor progress steadily toward the outlet end of the pump and provide for a continuous flow. The pump is easily calibrated since there is no possible backflow. Pumps based on the Archimedean flow principle handle blood gently and are capable of a wide range of outputs.

MULTIPLE FINGER PUMPS

Like roller pumps, multiple finger pumps incorporate a blood tube which is physically separated from the moving organs of the pump. However, the blood tube is straight, and sequential compression along its axis provides an advancing seal line which resembles that of Archimedean screw pumps.

Finger pumps (fig. 46), utilize a series of keys operated by cams in a crankshaft, which press in a sine wave-like fashion against a flexible tube in order to impart a unidirectional movement to the fluid in the tube. The cycles of the operating fingers are timed so that the tube is always compressed against a solid plate at some position, thereby eliminating the need for external check valves. The attainable pressure head or suction depends to a large extent upon whether or not an occlusive setting is reached. These depend also upon the nature of the tubing used, and the strength of the springs used for plate adjustment. The cardinal advantage of this system resides in the fact that regular blood tubing, such as is used in all extracorporeal circuits, can be inserted

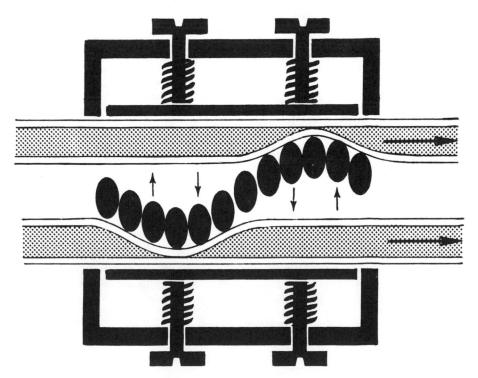

Fig. 46. Multiple finger pump. Casing, backplates and fingers: black; blood tubes: shaded. The occlusion of the blood tubes on either side of the moving keys is adjusted by spring tension.

into the pumping head with a minimum of manipulation. Maintenance of sterile conditions while connecting the pump to the rest of the circuit presents no problem. Cleaning and maintenance of the whole apparatus can also be carried out with ease.

This pumping principle was first applied to extracorporeal blood circulation by Saltzman and Rosenak (1949). Their pump consisted of a plastic tube of suitable wall thickness and diameter which was compressed in wave-like motion by a series of 12 keys that pushed the fluid column ahead. Behind the crest of the wave, the plastic tubing expanded by its own elastic recoil to fill up again. The baffle plate, against which the tubing was compressed, could be adjusted to nonocclusive conditions: pumping then ceased at a predetermined level of pressure if the outflow resistance increased above desirable limits. Since a key rather than a flat surface acted as a valve, the compression of the tubing was largely performed by one elevated edge at a time thereby reducing the area over which mechanical trauma could occur.

The Sigmamotor pump, which was adapted for blood handling by a surgical group in Minneapolis (Cohen, et al., 1954), embodies the same pumping principle. It was modified from a prototype first designed to handle liquids, slurries or gases in such a way that no contact could occur between the fluid pumped and the pump organs. Owing to its simplicity and highly dependable mechanical performance, this pump was of inestimable service in the pioneer years of extracorporeal circulation. Nevertheless, it was soon observed that the moving fingers principle entailed some degree of hemolysis, particularly when used at high speeds. The trauma to blood was ascribed to the very small stroke volume used and to the shock wave induced by rapid oscillation of the compressing fingers (Melrose, 1959). Flow adjustment for pumping under conditions of minimal occlusion was rather inaccurate (Shimomura, et al., 1958; Taber and Tomatis, 1959). The pump was found to be moderately load sensitive (Cross, 1957) and therefore accurate flow calibrations were not possible. Finally, the pumping unit was cumbersome and noisy.

Over the years, many improvements have been made. The most recent model Sigmamotor pump (fig. 47) is fairly compact and easy to clean. Two pumping heads, each driven by its own speed changer, have been incorporated into a single unit. The direction of flow in the two pump components is opposed, so that a unidirectional loop flow system results. The tubes are held in interchangeable split inserts contained in the head. The springs used in the older models have been eliminated. Instead, pressure plate adjustment is made by means of vernier knobs on the back of the pump head with lock nuts to secure the back plate. The noise level has been reduced by activating all moving parts with ball and roller bearings.

The performance characteristics of a finger pump are mainly dependent upon the nature and size of the tubing used. Most pumping heads can accommodate two or more blood tubes of widely different cross-section area and, therefore, cover a wide range of flows. The tubing used must be resilient enough to recover quickly its shape after compression. In general, surgical gum latex tubing produces the largest output. However, tygon tubes below a critical size (one inch inside diameter) often provide longer service. Certain types of silicone tubing operate very satisfactorily. External lubrication with

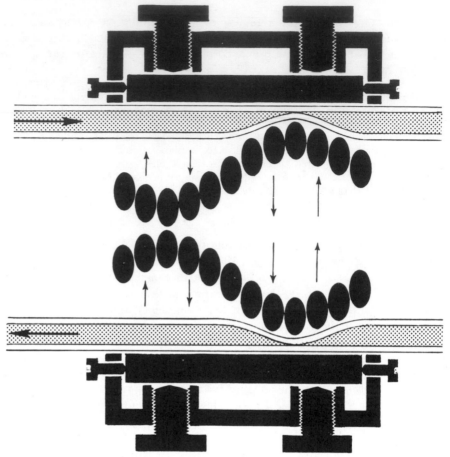

Fig. 47. Multiple finger pump with a double series of keys to permit flow in opposite directions (Symbols as in fig. 46. Details in text.)

a suitable silicone grease may considerably extend the life of the tubing. Besides the large finger pumps for heart–lung bypass, small units for organ perfusion are also available.

Summarizing:

In multiple finger pumps, unidirectional flow is produced by series of keys which press in sequence against a resilient tube. The cycles of the operating fingers are timed so that some part of the tubing is always occluded by pressure against a solid plate. Any convenient segment of an extracorporeal circuit can easily be inserted into the pumping head. In the pioneer years of extracorporeal circulation, the development of this principle in a practical blood pump (Sigmamotor) was one of the cardinal steps which made open heart surgery possible.

X. Reciprocating Pumps

All pumping systems in which a chamber is alternatingly filled and emptied by the back and forth displacement of a moving member are of the reciprocating type (see fig. 41, J to Q). They have in common some kind of eccentric transmission to transform the circular movement of a motor shaft into the longitudinal movement of the actuator, and valves are required in the flow line in order to obtain a unidirectional propagation of the fluid. The actuator may be either in direct contact with the blood, as in some piston pumps, or separated from it by a fluid transmission or a flexible diaphragm. The valves may be located within the blood stream, or some external mechanism may fulfill the same function. In all cases the type of flow is pulsatile and its characteristics depend upon the design of the actuator, transmission and valves.

PISTON PUMPS

Since Claude Bernard (1848) and Brown-Séquard (1858) used syringes for discontinuous manual perfusion of isolated organs, many pumps based on the motor-driven syringe principle have been devised. Pistons or plungers deliver a pulsatile flow, the character of which can be modified by the insertion of a damping chamber, or more subtly, by cams specially designed to permit variations in pulse pressure without essential changes in mean pressure. The perfusion pumps described by Bock (1907), Hooker (1910), Richards and Drinker (1915), von Skramlik (1920) and Binet and Mayer (1929) represent milestones along that path of development.

Motor-driven syringes are limited to a low output capacity sufficient only for isolated organs or small animals. Pistons often stick in their cylinder so that the pumps require constant attention. There are also surfaces of foreign material, considerable areas of which are in continuous or intermittent contact with blood, resulting in a progressive denaturation of the perfusion medium. It seems unlikely that regular piston pumps will ever be able to cope successfully with the high outputs required for cardiac substitution in man. Nevertheless, they will remain a useful laboratory tool owing mainly to easy visual control of the blood, ease in changing pumping rate and stroke volume, and their accuracy as flow metering devices (Waud, 1952; Spataru and Nicodium, 1959).

Much better adapted to extracorporeal blood circulation is the type of piston pumps in which there is no direct contact between blood and the piston or cylinder. A prototype is the small, compact unit used by Bluemle (1958), in which blood is pumped by two syringes via an air cushion (fig. 48). The valves are of the knife-edge type and operate against rubber tubing through which

141

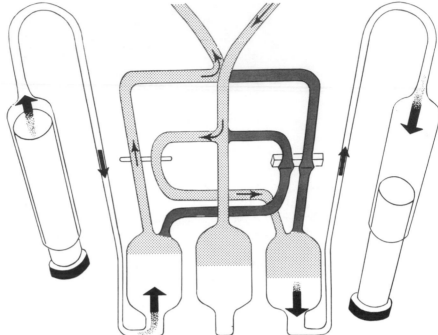

Fig. 48. Double piston pump devised by Bluemle (1958). Two motor driven syringes, 180 degrees out of phase, alternatively suck and compress air in the upper part of blood filled containers. Knife-edge valves synchronized with the movements of the pistons in the syringes regulate the flow so that one blood container fills while the other empties. Therefore, at any moment the blood moves in one half of the circuit (light shading), while it stays still in the other half of the circuit (dark shading). The central blood reservoir serves as a dampening and sampling chamber. (Courtesy of Dr. L. Bluemle and General Instrument Co., Inc., Philadelphia, Pa.)

the blood flows. Their timing is adjustable by means of graduated controls which can vary the open and closed time for each cylinder, and also the phase relationship between valve and cylinders. The flow capacity extends from 0 to 500 ml./min., and is essentially independent of intake and discharge pressures ("load insensitive"). All parts which handle blood directly are removable as a single assembly for sterilization.

By extension, one can also classify among piston pumps the air-driven pulsatile pumps in which intermittent gas pressure is applied directly to the blood in the pumping chamber. In this design, pioneered by Clark, et al. (1952), electrodes are in contact with the blood surface in a vertical pumping chamber. These electrodes actuate solenoid valves, which in turn control the alternation of positive and negative pressure within the chamber. The valves are controlled by the same mechanism. Clark's pump has been successfully employed in both experimental and clinical perfusions.

Summarizing:

Piston pumps utilize motor-driven syringes equipped with suitable valves to deliver a pulsatile flow. Regular piston pumps are limited to a low output capacity, sufficient only for the perfusion of isolated organs or small animals.

Pumps in which intermittent gas pressure is applied directly to the blood surface have a larger capacity and have been applied successfully in human perfusions.

BELLOW PUMPS

Thirty years ago, the pump originally proposed by Gibbs (1930, 1933) and later improved by Tainter (1932) was one of the first to make possible complete replacement of the heart while maintaining the experimental animal in responsive condition. Essentially, the device consisted of two rubber bellows functioning as the right and left chamber of the heart. When filled with blood by the venous inflow, the bellows could be squeezed empty into the arterial system by water pressure. Rubber flap valves retained by elastic "chordae tendineae" were used to maintain unidirectional flow. The beginning and the end of systole were signalled by an electric switch mechanism which in turn activated a two-way valve through which alternate positive and negative water pressure acted on the bellow.

The modifications in this apparatus as suggested by Tainter aimed mainly at obtaining a smoother action. Tainter's pump could maintain artificial circulation for a few hours in the heparinized animal. However, fluid loss into the tissues and a shock-like condition eventually resulted, a sign that blood was being denaturated during the procedure. More recently, Khayutin (1958) used a pump featuring a metal bellow, the base plate of which is actuated up and down to impart pulsatile motion to an elastic membrane at the other end of the bellow. This system was not found suitable for blood handling.

Summarizing:

Bellow pumps produce a pulsatile flow and there is no contact of blood with shearing components such as pistons. However, no model satisfactory for clinical heart–lung bypass has as yet been developed.

BAR COMPRESSION PUMPS

Compression of an elastic tube by a metal plate is a time-honored mechanism of blood pumping: Jacobj (1890) employed a rubber bulb for this purpose in his first primitive oxygenator. His design was later improved by Embly and Martin (1905), who used an eccentric on a motor-driven shaft alternately to squeeze and expand a rubber tube between two boards hinged at the back. Blum, et al. (1955) enclosed a silastic bladder in a partially evacuated chamber, and compressed it rhythmically by raising a platform towards the cover of the chamber. Houston, et al. (1960) used a somewhat similar principle in their pendulum type of artificial heart designed for implantation within the chest.

Although bar compression pumps are usually equipped with directional valves, it should be noted that fluid displacement can actually be achieved without valves. A difference in diameter of the conduits on either side of the compressed segment provides some degree of pulsatile flow (Liebau, 1954). This pumping principle was explored by Liebau (1955), yet it seems doubtful that it will find an application in extracorporeal blood circulation because so much backflow occurs that the net forward fluid displacement is limited.

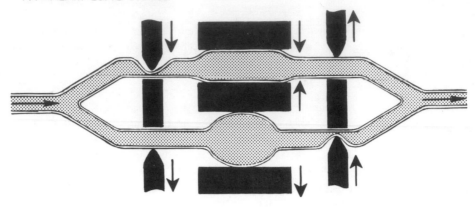

Fig. 49. Bar compression pump devised by Cowan (1952). Thrust plate and valves: black; blood: light shading. (Details in text.)

Recurrent compression of rubber tubing against a thrust plate was used in perfusion pumps by Benard and Henry (1941). Long (1947) described a blood pump in which a resilient tube was rhythmically compressed by the plate of an electromagnet. The first elaborate blood pumping system of large capacity was devised by Cowan (1952) and was used in heart–lung bypass procedures by Mustard, et al. (1952). The Cowan pump (fig. 49) consists of rubber bulbs alternately compressed and expanded by the sliding action of thrust plates over guide rods. The peripheral thrust plates are coupled together and slide back and forth in a direction opposite to that of the central plates, thus maintaining the bulbs in position. There is no tendency for the connecting rubber tubes to creep under the valves. The valves are of the knife-edge type and are actuated by the same crank shaft as are the plates. One bulb fills while the other empties. The frequency remains constant at 60 rpm but the stroke volume may be adjusted independently in each circuit to provide any flow rate between 0 and 3.75 L./min.

Pumps of basically similar design have been proposed by Cleland and Melrose (1955), Miller (1955), Nixon (1959), Breckler, et al. (1959), and Ogata, et al. (1959). The system used by Thomas differs in that it incorporates internal multicuspid valves. It consists of two elastic tubes alternately compressed by the lateral displacement of a crossbar. The pump is not occlusive and produces little hemolysis. There is a flowmeter for direct reading of instantaneous and mean flow. In the arrangement proposed by Nixon (1959), two parallel segments of plastic tubing lying on rigid platforms are alternately compressed by the movement of steel bars. The distance between the bars and the platform is such that the bars never lose contact with the tubing in diastole, and never completely occlude the lumen in systole. Changes in output are brought about by altering the rate of action of the bars by means of a variator.

Instead of compressing a resilient tube against solid plates as above, Bjørk (1948b) proposed insertion of the tube into an annular, inflatable cuff, a mechanism adapted from teat holder pumps in mechanical milkers. The gentleness

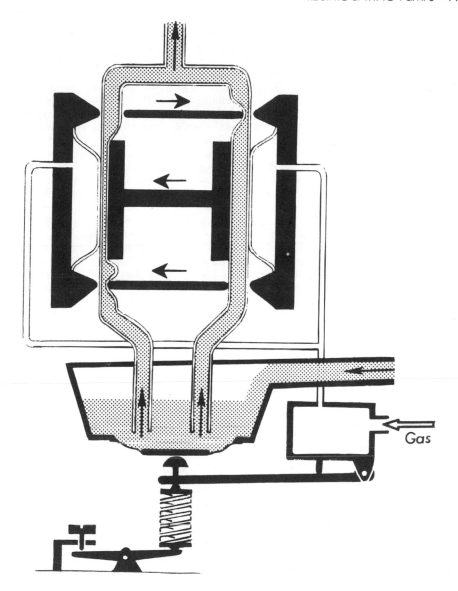

Fig. 50. Crafoord-Senning pump. Metal pieces: black; blood: light shading; gas filled space: white. The stroke volume of the pump is regulated by the gas pressure in inflatable cushions against which the blood tubes are alternately compressed. The gas pressure is regulated by a valve linked to a mechanism which senses the blood level in the arterial reservoir.

of blood handling and the flow control potentialities inherent in this design have been exploited with conspicuous success in the pumping-regulating unit of the Crafoord-Senning heart–lung machine (1957a).

The Crafoord-Senning pump (fig. 50) consists basically of two tubes alternately compressed by a crossbar which is driven to and fro by a crank mechanism. External valves operated by cam discs squeeze the bottom ends of the tubes during the compression phase, and the top ends when the tubes subsequently expand. The capacity of the pump is regulated by means of a "holding-on" unit consisting of two rubber cushions between the pump tubes and the rigid walls. The cushions are fed from an oxygen cylinder through a regulating valve, actuated by a lever and a diaphragm installed at the lowest part of the arterial reservoir in the bottom of the pumping unit. The regulating valve is so constructed that when the diaphragm is pressed downwards by the blood accumulated in the reservoir, the regulating valve opens to admit oxygen into the cushions. Once under pressure, the cushions offer a certain resistance to the lateral movement of the pump tubes, which are squeezed between the crossbar and the cushions, and thereby blood is expelled upwards. As long as the cushions are not under pressure, no pumping action occurs since the blood tubes follow the movements of the crossbar without being compressed. On the other hand, the greater the oxygen pressure within the cushions, the more the tubes are compressed and the larger is the capacity of the pump. Therefore, when the blood level in the arterial reservoir increases, more blood is expelled into the arterial line. However, should the level fall below a certain limit, the oxygen pressure within the cushion will drop to zero and the pumping action will stop entirely. The pump regulating system tends to maintain a constant volume blood in the arterial reservoir, but the blood level can be modified if desired by altering the pressure exerted on the diaphragm by the blood in the reservoir. The diaphragm is backed by a spring, the tension of which can be altered by means of a lever system adjusted by a screw. It is thus possible to change the blood level in the reservoir simply by turning the screw. Recently, Aletras, et al. (1960) have described a double pump based upon the same control principle. Their system balances exactly "right heart bypass" flow and "left heart bypass" flow during perfusion procedures employing autogenous lung oxygenation.

Summarizing:

Bar compression pumps move blood contained in a resilient tube or bulb by alternate compression and expansion of the tube or bulb between a moving bar and a solid backplate. Valves make the flow unidirectional. These pumps provide a large output with little blood trauma and can be adequately regulated for a variety of artificial circulation procedures.

DIAPHRAGM PUMPS

Valved pumps using a flat diaphragm or a finger-shaped membrane for imparting a movement to the blood have a well established position in the physiologic laboratory. The resilient part may be made of a thin sheet of rubber, plastic or metal. It may be actuated by any of hydraulic, pneumatic, mechanical or electromagnetic (Dietman, 1955) transmissions. The popularity of these pumps is due to their low cost and the ease with which they can be assembled from conventional laboratory equipment. In fact, most of the classic experiments on isolated organ perfusion in the first half of this century made use of diaphragm or membrane pumps.

Although there were precursors (for instance, Bornstein, 1926), Dale and Schuster (1928) are usually given credit for one of the earliest practical designs. The original Dale-Schuster pump (fig. 51, A) consists of a water chamber which is periodically compressed and decompressed by the movement of a plunger. Through a thin, finger-shaped, pliable rubber membrane, enough pressure is transmitted to propel the blood in its circuit. Internal inflow and outflow valves are necessary for proper performance. With minor modifications, this mechanism has been used for cardiac substitution by Lovat-Evans, et al. (1934), Sirak, et al. (1950), Dodrill, et al. (1952), Kunlin (1952), Tyrer

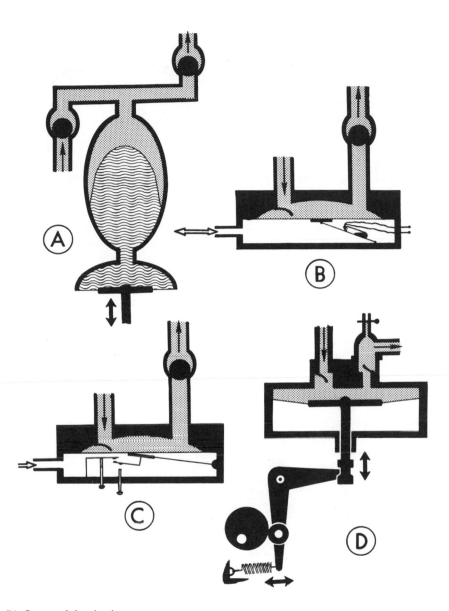

Fig. 51. Pumps of the diaphragm type.

A. Dale-Schuster pump in which a water-chamber (wavy horizontal pattern) is separated from a blood-chamber (light shading) by a thin elastic membrane. The movements of a piston (depicted by black double ended arrow) are transmitted to the water, then to the blood, causing internal valves (black circles) to open and close alternately.

B. Diaphragm pump described by Dennis (1956). The inflow and exhaust of compressed gas (depicted by white double-ended arrow) is regulated by a tilting mercury switch causing passage of blood alternately into and out of a chamber.

C. Pump devised by Newman (1958) on a principle similar to the preceeding one.

D. Tyson-Bowman pump in which blood is propelled by the movement of a diaphragm activated by a piston. (Details in text.)

(1952) and Ambrus (1955). Though ingenious, the Dale-Schuster pump does not cover a wide range of flow. To achieve higher outputs, DeBurgh Daly (1934) proposed using a seven horsepower Austin engine to drive a large model of this pump. A more practical arrangement was that of Jongbloed (1949) who used six Dale-Schuster pumps driven by a central sixfold crankshaft to obtain the high flows needed for total body perfusion.

Incompressible fluids, such as water (Dubbelman, 1951; Ananiev, et al., 1958; Vainrib, et al., 1959) or glycerol (Bucherl, 1956; Field, et al., 1958), faithfully transmit the displacement of the plunger to the membrane, but are apt to generate in the blood circuit peaks of positive or negative pressure which must be damped by an air cushion or elastic chamber unless reliable pressure sensing devices act to cut off the pump as required. Thomas and Baudoin (1951) were among the first to turn to pneumatic transmission. In their pump, compressed air and vacuum are alternately admitted under the membrane. A system of loaded valves permits regulating the head of pressure attainable by the pump so as to achieve a constant infusion pressure. However, according to the authors themselves (1959), this system proved dangerous in actual perfusions, owing probably to the large shifts in blood volume it entailed.

In the absence of special automatic tracking regulators, the stroke volume of a diaphragm pump decreases as the outflow resistance increases, and conversely. One solution for maintaining a constant stroke volume is that described by Dennis (1955): The inflow and exhaust of compressed air below the diaphragm is regulated by the tilting of a mercury switch (fig. 51 B). In a more refined model, devised by Newman (1958), the upper and lower limits of diaphragm excursion were made adjustable (fig. 51 C). As blood enters the pumping chamber, the rubber diaphragm is forced down. When a platinum contact on the moving paddle meets the bottom contact, a relay is actuated and locked. This switches on a solenoid valve and permits compressed air to enter the chamber below the diaphragm. The rubber diaphragm is forced upward and consequently, the fluid is ejected from the pump. The moving paddle makes contact with the upper platinum contact, and actuates another relay. Thereupon the solenoid is deactivated and returns to the exhaust position. A new cycle can then begin. In the blood circuit, a polyethylene flap valve is used on the inflow side and a ball valve on the outflow. The advantages of this system include simplicity of construction, since there are only two moving parts (diaphragm and follower). It is easy to clean and to maintain, and the blood can be continuously inspected. It always operates above atmospheric pressure and thus cannot suck in air. A drawback is that the pump head is made of mothacrylate plastic and therefore cannot be autoclaved. Furthermore, the system cannot be preset to deliver a constant output because the flow is dependent upon the pressure conditions prevailing at the outlet.

There has been a long search for a means of making a membrane pump load-insensitive, and yet to avoid the risks associated with excessive pressure or vacuum in the blood lines. Brukhonenko (1929) devised the first large capacity membrane pump which delivered a constant output regardless of the resistance in the circuit. In his pump, the vibrating metal diaphragm which causes the blood to move is directly actuated by an eccentric system connected to the shaft of an electric motor. Shunt lines controlled by Starling resistances serve as safety valves in case of sudden occlusion of a blood line (*see* fig. 9). In the pump employed by Blum and Megibow (1950), the floor of the pumping chamber is a solid sheet of tygon, to the undersurface of which is centrally attached a brass disc actuated by a lever system. The Tyson-Bowman pump described by Southworth and Peirce (1953) is somewhat similar. It consists of a chamber, the floor of which is made of a flexible diaphragm attached to the chamber at its periphery and to a piston centrally (fig. 51 D). Blood enters the pump chamber in response to a downward movement of the diaphragm and leaves it through an upwards motion. The diaphragm and its piston are driven by a linkage, consisting of a pump rod, bell crank, follower roller, actuating cam and return spring. In operation, the cam, acting through the bell crank, forces the diaphragm upwards to discharge the pump chamber. The return of the diaphragm, which refills the pump chamber, is dependent on the return spring, also acting through the bell crank. An increase in spring tension increases the interval during which the diaphragm is drawn downwards. This action may thus be used consequently as a means of regulating the quantity of blood drawn into the chamber during each cycle of the pump. Maximum output for any pulse rate is reached when the spring tension is sufficient to hold the follower roller against the cam throughout the cycle. If desired, the contour of the cam can be modified to obtain different pulse pressure contours.

Summarizing:

Diaphragm pumps are devices in whch a flat diaphragm or a finger-shaped membrane serves to impart movement to the blood. The diaphragm can be made of rubber, plastic or metal and can be actuated by hydraulic, pneumatic, mechanical or electromagnetic transmissions. The advantages of these pumps are their low cost, compactness and their fairly gentle handling of blood. They have the disadvantages of covering a relatively narrow range of flow. The output of pneumatically driven diaphragm pumps varies with the resistance to flow. Hydraulically or mechanically driven diaphragm pumps require control devices to dampen possible peaks of positive or negative pressure in the blood lines.

VENTRICLE PUMPS

Ventricle pumps consist of a compressible chamber mounted in a rigid casing and actuated by displacement of fluid in the surrounding space. When pressure is increased within the outer rigid chamber by injection of gas or liquid, the inner chamber is compressed and blood is expelled. When the outer chamber is vented, the inner chamber returns to its original shape and refills. The output of the chamber depends on its size, the resiliency of its walls, the characteristics of the valves, the rate of pumping action, and the pressure at which it operates. Ventricle pumps differ from diaphragm pumps only in the fact that pressure changes are not localized to any one face of the chamber through which blood flows, but rather surround a flexible organ inserted in a housing. Both systems use the same types of valves: knife-edge arm acting externally, intraluminal flap or flutter valves, or segments of tubing intermittently compressed by gas pressure.

The history of ventricle pumps is marked by the same difficulties as were encountered in the use of diaphragm pumps. The ventricle pump described in 1950 by Sewell and Glenn for temporary replacement of the right heart cavities consisted of a rubber tube with flap valves at each end and was driven by repeated cycles of alternating positive-negative pressures from a compressed air and vacuum line. The pumps used by Wesolowski and Welch (1950), Butterworth (1951), Guendel (1954), Illing (1958) and Demetrakopoulos, et al. (1959), were essentially the same. In 1954, Clowes, et al. found that among all pumps, ventricle pumps were the least traumatic to red cells. A similar opinion was expressed by Khayutin (1958) and Cahill and Kolff (1959) in their reviews of different types of perfusion equipment.

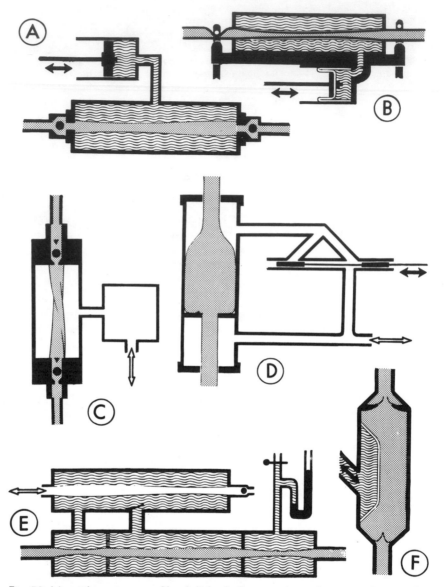

Fig. 52. Ventricle pump types. Blood: light shading; water or saline: wavy horizontal pattern; compressed gas: white; piston movement: black double ended arrows; admission and exhaust of compressed gas: white double ended arrows.

A. Water driven ventricle pump with internal valves.

B. Water driven ventricle pump with external valves, as proposed by Breckler, et al. (1959).

C. Gas driven ventricle pump with internal valves (Hufnagel, et al., 1958).

D. Gas driven ventricle pump with an external valve mechanism regulated by the movement of a piston (Röckeman, 1958).

E. McNeil-Collins pump in which air pressure fluctuations are transmitted to the blood chamber through a saline medium.

F. Davol pump, a pneumatically operated, hydraulically actuated ventricle pump with internal valves. (Details in text.)

Flow regulation of ventricle pumps has been a major problem. Pneumatic transmission not only involves the remote risk of rupture of the blood tube with passage of gas into the blood, but it also limits the force which can be applied at any given time. In other words, it renders the pump load-sensitive. By using water actuated by motor-driven syringes (fig. 52, A) as have Salisbury (1956), Khayutin (1958) and Sørensen (1960), a constant stroke volume can be maintained. However, the maximal negative pressure during "diastole" of the pump must then be closely regulated because no single factor causes as much blood trauma as does excessive suction. Hydraulic drive is highly satisfactory as long as the blood circuit is operating satisfactorily. But inadvertent occlusion of the arterial line or lack of blood in the venous line (as for instance in case of sudden hemorrhage) may lead to disaster.

One way of absorbing the peaks of pressure and of dampening the discontinuous flow from the compression chamber is illustrated in the pump of Rotellar (1958). Below and above the silicone rubber tube used as a pumping chamber are two similar tubes of equal diameter, but three times as long. These chambers tend to expand during systole and to contract during diastole of the pumping chamber, thereby providing an almost continuous flow. Kamm (1959) and Carmichael (1959) described a complex hydraulic drive system using a sterile saline compartment actuated by the pressure of the city water supply. Another solution to the problem of flow control is embodied in the hydraulic UPI pump described by Breckler, et al. (1959). A tygon ventricle with a mechanically actuated guillotine-type valve at inlet and outlet is surrounded by a fluid filled, annular chamber that has a slightly larger diameter tygon tube as its central wall (fig. 52 B). The outside diameter of the ventricle and the inside diameter of the actuating chamber are the same, so that there is close contact between the two concentric plastic tubes. Fluid is delivered to and taken from the annular chamber by mechanical displacement of a rubber diaphragm located in a side chamber linked hydraulically to the annular chamber. The mechanism is arranged so that at no time do the tygon walls of the ventricle actually touch each other. The valves are actuated through lever arms connected to cams located on the main drive shaft. The eccenter which operates the piston and the rubber diaphragm is on the same shaft. Synchronization is such that the outlet valve opens as the ventricle is compressed and the inlet valve opens as the ventricle returns to its normal shape. The flow rate can be varied from 0 to 5.8 L./min. by changing the pulse rate and the stroke volume.

The type of valve employed in a ventricle pump is quite critical in terms of flow turbulence. Elliot and Callaghan (1958) constructed plastic tricuspid valves that offer a satisfactory service. Hufnagel, et al. (1958) devised a pump including ventricles, valve seats and ball valves all in one disposable unit (fig. 52, C). The tube, made of silicone rubber, is so resilient that the balls can be squeezed out and removed when the pump is to be cleaned for repeated use in animal experiments. The wall of the ventricle thins out towards the inflow region so that when compression occurs it starts at the inflow region and progresses towards the outflow. A driving unit for this pump was described by Hufnagel, et al. (1959).

An ingenious system which does not require internal valves was described by Röckemann (1958). The compressible tubing is upright and housed in two separate chambers, one on top of the other (fig. 52 D). The lower segment of tubing is constantly exposed to the same external pressure as that which acts on the upper segment during systole only. During diastole, the upper chamber is vented and the blood tubing fills by gravity. At the beginning of systole, the external air pressures closes first the upper part of the blood tubing since the hydrostatic pressure there is the lowest in the pumping chamber. When the gas pressures in both outer chambers are equal, the hydrostatic pressure is added to the external pressure in the upper segment of the blood tubing and therefore pressure is higher than in the lower one. Blood then flows downwards until pressure in the lower external compartment again exceeds that in the upper one. This ingenious valve design is activated by the movement of a shaft which alternately admits compressed air around the pumping chamber and then vents it.

Another ventricle pump with external valves is that described by Doyle, et al. (1956) and MacNeill, et al. (1959). The pump is operated by a small piston whose displacement generates air pressures oscillating between $+90$ and -100 mm. Hg. These pressure variations are transferred to the pumping chamber through a sterile physiologic fluid medium (fig. 52 E). The blood conduit is a simple, seamless, thin walled vinyl tube divided into three segments: inlet valve area, pumping chamber and exit valve area. The pressure is first applied to the inlet valve area, occluding it. A delay mechanism then allows transfer of this pressure to the pumping chamber which is next compressed. The blood within the tube is propelled forward, opening the constantly pressurized exit valve area. The constant pressure on the exit valve prevents backflow between systoles. During the negative pressure phase of the piston, the air tube collapses; the saline rushes from the pumping chamber back into the pressure transfer box through a unidirectional flap valve. The blood tube then distends before the next pressure stroke. The pump runs at 180 strokes per minute. The stroke volume can be adjusted between 0 and 5 ml., resulting in an output between 0 and 900 ml./min. Some kind of flowmeter must be inserted into the line for accurate control of the output.

The Davol pump described by Harken (1958) is an electronically controlled, pneumatically operated, hydraulically activated ventricle pump with passive internal valves. It includes two pumping chambers and there is direct control over the volume of blood displaced. The design is quite refined. The ventricles are immersed in a leakproof housing filled with water and are provided with flutter valves at their inlet and outlet. The stroke volume is varied by altering the amount of water which compresses the wall and displaces the blood. Since diastole is brought about by removal of the liquid, any material which is flexible can be used for ventricles, regardless of its tensile strength and resilience. The amount of water displaced is regulated by the stroke volume of the actuators on a single shaft. The actuators, situated on either side of the power supply, are pneumatically operated from a compressor or a tank of gas. Their piston is spring-returned to a housing which affords accurate stroke measurement by means of a screw control. To make the operation of the pump proportionate between the two ventricles, the pneumatic operation of the actuators is restricted between two stops. By means of electronic timing circuits the pulse rate can be set arbitrarily anywhere between 10 and 120 strokes per minute, or the pump can be driven by the output from the oscillograph jack on electrocardiographic equipment. The two ventricles can be operated independently, in phase or out of phase, so that any type of pulsatile or nonpulsatile flow can be produced. With the Davol pump one can control the stroke volume (by altering the piston stroke), the pumping frequency (through the timing circuit) and the pulse contour (by varying the amount of gas pressure operating on the piston, and/or by synchronization of two ventricles). Double-ended ventricles are used for pumping blood in the usual circuits. Single-ended "ectopic ventricles" can be used for "synchronized circulatory assistance" (Harken, 1958, Clauss, et al., 1961).

The pump developed by McCabe (1959) is probably one of the most sophisticated ever invented. A replica of the heart, it has four inner chambers for blood handling and four semilunar and tricuspid valves. There is a common outer chamber for the two ventricles and one for the atria. Thus, if the stroke volume of homologous blood chambers is similar, the pressure produced will differ in relation to the peripheral resistance. There are controls for altering independently the stroke volume of the atria and of the ventricles, for altering the shape of the pulse contour with each individual chamber, for driving the pump at any rate and for regulating the interval between atrial and ventricular contractions. The McCabe pump runs by pneumatic operation and hydraulic transmission as do most modern ventricle pumps. It is primarily intended for cardiac substitution within the chest. However, it can be connected to an artificial lung.

Summarizing:

Ventricle pumps consist of a compressible chamber mounted in a rigid casing and are activated by displacement of liquid or gas in the casing. Unidirectional blood flow is maintained by the insertion of valves at the entrance and exit of the pumping chamber. The disadvantages of ventricle pumps—mechanical complexity, limitations in the range of output, load sensitivity or extreme peaks of pressure and suction—can be alleviated by modern sensing and regulating devices. Therefore, ventricle pumps appear most promising, because they potentially combine inherent gentleness in blood handling with safety of operation and the reliability of positive displacement pumps.

XI. Elements of Extracorporeal Circulation

Apart from the basic essential components, such as oxygenator, pump and tubing, modern heart–lung bypass equipment comprises various auxiliary elements which, depending upon the type of procedure planned, may or may not be dispensable. Pump oxygenators causing little trauma to blood and creating no bubbles can, under favorable circumstances, be used without blood filters or bubble traps in the extracorporeal circuit. Flowmeters can be dispensed with when adequately calibrated pumps provide the same information at less cost. Temperature regulating devices and heat exchangers are often unnecessary in short perfusions because a moderate decrease in body temperature is tolerated without detrimental effects.

The elimination of all of these components greatly simplifies the extracorporeal circulation procedure since each one of them adds to the inherent complexity of even the simplest bypass arrangement. It is therefore a good policy to reexamine critically from time to time the possibility of eliminating some elements in an extracorporeal circuit. On the other hand, when it is found that additional components contribute to the safety of perfusion, their inclusion in the extracorporeal circuit must be considered.

BLOOD FILTERS

In the pioneer years of extracorporeal circulation, the usefulness of blood filters was often debated. Some of the models available at the time offered considerable resistance to flow (Lenfant, et al., 1956a). They were difficult to free completely of air bubbles (Salisbury, 1956b) and apparently produced more emboli than they strained out. Osborne (1955) actually observed that in a series of filters of equal mesh, more debris was recovered from the last filter in the blood circuit than from the first.

At the present time most heart–lung machines incorporate some kind of blood filter in their circuit. The blood used for priming the oxygenator and the blood recovered from the operative field during open-heart surgery absolutely require filtration. Even the blood passing from the patient's veins into the extracorporeal circuit may need it because during any extended perfusion, some fibrin is almost inevitably deposited in the circuit, and may be subsequently embolized.

The characteristics of a good filter include: (1) the ability to remove all particles from the blood stream; (2) a negligible resistance to blood flow; (3)

minimal trauma to blood; (*4*) a large enough surface to permit the operation of the circuit despite the occurrence of partial plugging; (*5*) a design which allows the filter to be easily cleaned, sterilized, inserted at the proper place, and cleared of gas bubbles.

A suitable compromise among these different requirements is reached by using stainless steel, nylon or halofluorocarbon plastic filters of 70 to 100 mesh. The open area varies between 34 per cent (Gilman, et al., 1957) and 66 per cent (Lenfant, et al., 1956a). A filtering surface of 50 sq. cm. per liter of minute flow provides a wide safety margin should deposition of fibrin, red cells or platelets result in reduction of the effective filtering surface (Taylor, 1959). Blood trauma is minimized if excessive velocities and turbulence are avoided. The inlet and outlet of the filter must be designed accordingly. There is some discussion as to where in the circuit the filter should be located. To take advantage of the low velocity of flow, it may be placed immediately at the arterial end of the oxygenator itself (Milnes, et al., 1957b; Schimert, et al., 1958) or in the low pressure line between the oxygenator and the arterial pump (Taylor, 1959). In the experience of Hyman (1959) a saran sleeve which reduces the speed of blood flow before it enters the filter has been found beneficial. Others prefer to have the filter between the arterial pump and the arterial cannula, as the last element which the blood traverses before entering the vascular system (Senning, 1952; McKensie and Barnard, 1958; Gross, et al., 1960).

There are two main types of blood filters which can be inserted at appropriate locations in the circuit:

(*1*) Cylindrical filters have been modeled after those used in transfusion equipment. They consist of a roll of screen, about 10 times longer than wide, closed at one end and inserted into a casing. The blood enters by the open end and passes through the mesh openings to be collected in the casing made of transparent resins or polyvinyl tubing. Two filters are often mounted in parallel to increase the available surface and to reduce the resistance to flow. Disposable units including stainless steel or nylon mesh filters, plastic housing and Y connectors, to which the arterial line can be cemented or connected, are commercially available.

(*2*) Flat filters are used in a filtering chamber. Such a unit, as described by Gilman, et al. (1957), consists of a disc of stainless steel mesh sealed by a rubber gasket within a body composed of two assembled half shells. An inlet pierces one of the side walls and an outlet the other. This basic design has been improved in the filter-bubble trap described by Gross, et al. (1960), which is now widely used (*see* fig. 54, C). The housing consists of siliconized stainless steel and glass, and the gasket is made of silicone rubber. Blood enters the chamber on one side of a screen mesh disc and leaves it on the other side. Two escape vents, provided with stopcocks, are inserted at the top of the casing on either side of the filter. They permit elimination of gas bubbles, removal of the saline used for washing the circuit and monitoring of the pressure in the arterial line. The unit is heat sterilizable and the stainless steel filter can be replaced after each perfusion. A similar filter, but completely disposable, is available for use with disposable lungs (Esmond, et al., 1959).

Summarizing:

Blood filters serve to strain fibrin strands and debris from the extracorporeal blood before it is reinfused into the organism. Good filters are atraumatic, offer negligible resistance to flow, have enough free surface for blood to pass despite partial plugging, and are easy to clean, assemble and free of gas bubbles. Opinions vary as to the sites where filters are most effective in an extracorporeal circuit.

BUBBLE TRAPS

Gas bubbles in the blood stream of an extracorporeal circuit are caused in various ways: insufficient removal in the defoaming section of bubble oxygenators; admixture of air in the venous line or coronary suction line; foaming at the blood-gas interface in the oxygenator itself; wandering of gas bubbles inadvertently trapped in the circuit during the priming operation; release of gas dissolved in plasma owing to temperature variations, cavitation or extreme degrees of suction and finally, any leakage whenever negative pressure exists in the circuit. From this enumeration it is clear that the problem of gas bubble removal, of cardinal importance in bubble oxygenators, must be considered in every type of heart–lung machine.

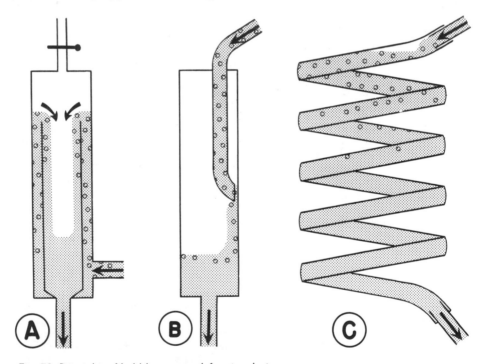

Fig. 53. Principles of bubble traps or defoaming devices:

A. Upflow-defoaming: The blood carrying gas bubbles enters at the lower part of a glass or plastic cylinder, rises through a relatively narrow path, then cascades into another cylinder located within the first one. An outlet at the top of the device permits removal of the excess gas.

B. Downflow-defoaming: The blood carrying gas bubbles is led against the wall and runs into a pool at the bottom of the chamber. Antifoam-coated baffles are often inserted to help in the coalescence of bubbles.

C. Helix blood settling column proposed by DeWall (1956b) for the separation of gas bubbles from blood.

As pointed out by Clark (1959), there are two main systems for defoaming blood. The first, upflow defoaming (fig. 53, A), is very efficient in coalescing and eliminating very small bubbles, because it gives them a "push" upwards. However, there is a definite limitation to the amount of gas which can be removed from the blood stream by this system. The second technique, downflow defoaming (fig. 53, B), is very efficient in breaking and removing large bubbles, and can dispose of virtually unlimited amounts of gas mixed with the blood phase. For this reason, it is chiefly employed with bubble oxygenators and coronary suction devices where large volumes of foam must be eliminated. Most of the systems proposed belong to one or the other of these categories. Many take advantage of the defoaming properties of certain silicone compounds (see Chapter III), smeared on the walls of the bubble trap or on some kind of baffle inserted in the blood stream.

Bubble traps have evolved mainly by a process of trial and error. Nevertheless a few theoretic considerations of the motion due to buoyancy of a gas bubble in a liquid (Epstein and Plesset, 1950) have been of help in the planning of adequate devices. The terminal velocity of ascent of a gas bubble is attained when the buoyant force (proportional to its volume and to the difference in density between liquid and gas) is balanced by the force of resistance to ascent (proportional to the radius of the bubble and to the viscosity of the liquid). The velocity of the vertical ascent of a spherical bubble in a liquid is expressed (Gertz, et al., 1960) by:

$$v = \frac{2}{9} \cdot \frac{\rho}{\eta} \cdot R^2 ,$$

where v is the velocity (in cm./sec.), ρ the specific gravity of the liquid (in g./cu. cm.), η the viscosity of the liquid (in poises) and R the radius of the bubble (in cm.). Replacing ρ and η by their actual values for blood ($\rho = 1.05$ g./cu. cm., $\eta = 2.7$ centipoise), one obtains $V = 8.5\ R^2$. From this equation, it can be calculated that only bubbles with a radius above 0.5 mm. will attain a velocity of 0.2 mm./sec., which can be considered as the minimum speed for removal in view of the circulation time and depth of the blood reservoir in most actual bubble traps.

Small bubbles do not have sufficient buoyancy to rise spontaneously to the surface of a flowing stream. In attempts to eliminate them, DeWall, et al. (1956b) recognized the de-bubbling property of a large bore tubing wound into a helix, the coils of which slope slightly downwards (fig. 53, C). The blood containing free gas bubbles is less dense and consequently tends to laminate on the upper layer within the tube. As the blood flows down the inclined plane of the helix, the heavier, gas-free blood descends beneath the lighter gas containing blood, forcing it continuously upward. In principle, a prolonged transit through a relatively shallow layer of blood gives the bubbles the best opportunity to coalesce and disappear. This can be achieved practically by circulating the blood through the lower half of a large tube placed horizontally (Salisbury, 1956a; fig. 54, A), spilling it radially over a horizontal disc (Gertz, et al., 1960; see fig. 28, C), or spreading it over the sloping surface of a series of consecutive glass bulbs disposed at a 30 degree angle with the horizontal (Chevret and Besson, 1960). The efficacy of a large, relatively stationary pool of blood open to atmospheric pressure (Gianelli, et al., 1957) is explained by the same considerations of buoyancy and transit time. The tendency of the bubbles to aggregate and burst at the surface of the blood is greatly enhanced by the presence of antifoam compounds.

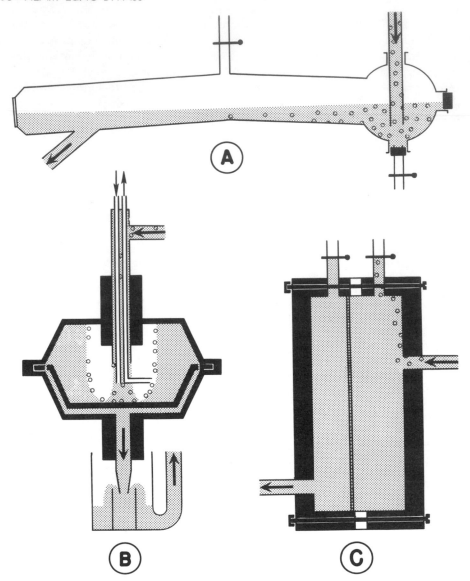

Fig. 54. Bubble traps of particular design:

A. Bubble trap-settling chamber of Salisbury (1956a) featuring a slow transit of the arterial blood stream through a long and wide glass tube.
B. Debubbling device proposed by Kusserow (1955). The foaming blood is distributed at the center of a rotating cup. Centrifugal force separates the blood which escapes through a narrow slit at the periphery and collects in a reservoir below. The aggregate of gas bubbles is continuously aspirated from the paraboloid surface of the blood pool by a suction device.
C. Filter-bubble trap described by Gross, et al. (1960). Blood enters on one face of the chamber, passes through a disc of stainless screen mesh, and leaves at the bottom on the other face of the chamber. The filter helps retain gas bubbles which accumulate at the top of the chamber and can be removed through a vent.

There are a few relatively simple de-bubbling devices which aid bubble clearing in particular situations. Fine mesh filters slow down the transit of bubbles and give them a chance to ascend, especially if the velocity of blood flow is low (Hyman, 1959; Gross, et al., 1960; fig. 54, C). Stainless steel sponges and polyethylene or teflon shavings immersed in the gas-trapping chamber (Dennis, 1956; Bucherl, 1956) help more by the antifoam coat they are given than by their mere physical presence. Pneumatic devices (air jets) have been long abandoned owing to their drying and defibrinating action (Thomas and Baudoin, 1950; Clowes, et al., 1954). Centrifugal skimming, as proposed by Kusserow (1955), involves complex mechanical devices (fig. 54, B). It is extremely efficient, but potentially traumatic because blood is in contact with rapidly moving parts of the device. The use of ultrasonic vibration (Dorsey, 1959) has not progressed beyond the experimental stage (Battezatti and Taddei, 1959).

Measures, such as priming of the heart–lung circuit with saline at 90°C., which is then allowed to cool down and thereby to take gas into solution (Faggella, et al., 1958), are useful for removing those small bubbles which so easily cling to new plastic tubing. Otherwise conscientious tapping with a patellar hammer is required. Such a procedure may take 20 to 30 minutes to get rid of all bubbles adherent to the walls in the helix-reservoir bubble oxygenator (McKensie and Barnard, 1960). Surface skimming by an overflow outlet on the arterial end place has been suggested recently, as an additional safety measure in rotating disc oxygenators, by Cartwright and Palich (1960 a, c); otherwise a Gross filter-bubble trap is ordinarily used with this type of equipment. Even in membrane lungs, a reservoir-bubble trap is useful to maintain a positive pressure at the arterial end and to collect minute bubbles which may be shaved off if some gas remains trapped during the priming operation (see fig. 37, B). In all circuits, careful attention to the tightness of connectors and stopcocks, and prevention of wide temperature fluctuations, minimize the risk of stray bubbles.

Useful in developmental studies are bubble monitors, or thin transparent chambers inserted in the arterial line to permit microscopic examination of a blood film for gas bubbles and other particles (Tepper, et al., 1958, 1959). Additional techniques for identifying microbubbles in the arterial stream have been suggested by Diesh, et al., (1957). The subject of microbubble embolization and "oxygen toxicity" is extensively discussed in Chapter XIV.

Summarizing:

Bubble traps are necessary safety devices in most extracorporeal blood circuits. Their design is based on theoretic considerations relating the velocity of vertical ascent of the bubbles to the duration of transit of the blood through the bubble trap. A prolonged transit through a relatively shallow layer of blood gives the bubbles the best chance to rise and dissipate. Auxiliary factors such as skimming, centrifugal separation or antifoam compounds are used to supplement bubble elimination by buoyancy.

FLOWMETERS

During heart–lung bypass, knowledge of the perfusion rate of flow is mandatory. If occlusive pumps are used, sufficient information is obtained from their calibration curves. It should also be possible to utilize, in the case of nonocclusive pumps, a family of curves relating mean arterial pressure, number of strokes per minute and flow rate. However, this latter method is cumbersome and fails to give information quickly at the time it is most urgently needed, for instance, in case of acute hypotension due to hemorrhage (see Chapter VIII).

Blood flowmeters for use in extracorporeal circulation must meet the following requirements (McMillan, 1958; Robiscek, et al., 1959; Griesser and Passon, 1960):

(*1*) continuous indication of the flow over the entire range expected in the procedure, with the possibility of recognizing the smallest significant deviation;

(*2*) accurate, easy and stable calibration, including absence of baseline drift and equal precision in the measurement of pulsatile or continuous flow;

(*3*) independence from variations in viscosity, specific gravity, temperature or other physical properties of the circulating blood;

(*4*) measurements in the main extracorporeal blood stream without interference from the pump or from alteration of blood flow;

(*5*) design which prevents hemolysis or fibrin deposits, and permits easy cleaning and sterilization.

Methods of flow measurement based upon the filling or emptying time of a reservoir somewhere in the extracorporeal circuit are known as *cumulative*, or *slope* recording of flow (Green, 1948; Bruner, 1960). By these means, flow determinations during heart–lung bypass can only be obtained by temporarily interrupting the continuity of the circulation. In view of the limited volume of blood available in an extracorporeal circuit, and of the high flow rates actually used, the measurement period cannot exceed 5 to 10 seconds. The error involved in timing and in reading the difference of two blood levels is usually so great that only the order of magnitude is determined. The ingenious flowmeter described by Hufnagel, et al. (1959), which takes advantage of an inclined spillway, graduated in width from bottom to top, partially escapes these criticisms. Though not highly accurate, it permits a continuous estimation of the venous flow rate during the period of bypass, and represents a transition towards more sophisticated equipment.

The instruments suitable for instantaneous reading of volume flow are the so-called flow *rate* recorders. Fortunately, the rate of blood flow is far easier to measure in extracorporeal circuits than in the vascular system because the blood line can readily be approached or even entered by the measuring device. Among the numerous types of flowmeters available, three have been incorporated most often in heart–lung machine circuits.

1. Differential pressure flowmeters: these meters use the difference in pressure between two points along the longitudinal axis of the blood stream to infer the rate of flow. To make the pressure differential measurable between two close sites, a stricture has to be produced in the line (resistance meter, Venturi meter and orifice meter) or a special pick-up device must be introduced in the blood stream to read the difference between total pressure and hydrostatic pressure (Pitot tube) (fig. 55).

A simple differential pressure flowmeter was first used in the heart–lung machine of Tosatti (1951). Cleland, et al., (1958) and Nixon (1959) pointed to the possibility of using the constriction already present at the site of arterial infusion for gauging the rate of flow: by subtracting the arterial pressure from the pressure in the infusion line, the drop in pressure across a previously calibrated cannula can be used as an index of flow (resistance meter). The venous flowmeter suggested by Robiscek, et al. (1961) is even simpler in design: It consists of two vertical glass cylinders communicating at their bottom through a contracted nozzle. Blood enters at the top of the first, or metering cylinder. Because of the impeded passage into the second cylinder, it reaches a level in the first cylinder which is proportional to the rate of flow. Empiric calibration permits ex-

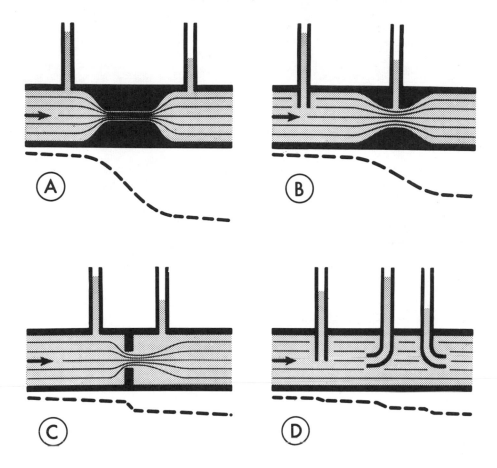

Fig. 55. Differential pressure flowmeters schemes, illustrating different ways of creating a pressure difference in a streaming fluid for the purpose of measuring the velocity of flow. Energy loss by friction is plotted as a broken line below each type of flowmeter:

A. Resistance meter: Narrowing of the lumen causes friction and loss of potential energy. The lateral pressure is therefore greatly decreased downstream to the stenosis as compared to upstream.

B. Venturi meter: In the narrowed segment, blood flows faster and potential energy is converted into kinetic energy. Therefore the downstream manometer records a much lower pressure than the upstream one without the need for a marked stenosis.

C. Orifice meter: When a tube is narrowed at one point, the stream lines continue to converge beyond the orifice. Consequently, lateral pressure is maximally reduced downstream from the orifice at a distance corresponding to half of the tube's internal diameter. This design features the advantages of both the resistance and the Venturi meter. However, the range of flow rates which can be covered without inducing turbulence is relatively narrow.

D. Pitot meter: In the opening facing upstream, the kinetic energy of the fluid is added to the potential energy indicated by purely lateral pressure. In the opening facing downstream, the kinetic energy is subtracted from the potential energy. The Pitot effect thereby results in a larger pressure difference than would be obtained if purely lateral pressure were measured upstream and downstream. The sensitivity is greater than in other types of differential pressure flowmeters but the pressure pickups must be placed rigorously in the same plane so as to avoid recording artifacts with pulsatile flows. (Redrawn from Brecher, 1956.)

pressing the height of the blood column, or pressure head, in terms of actual flow rate. Any suitable pressure monitoring device can be used for the recording of flow.

A Venturi meter mounted in the venous line has been described by Dow (1958). The instrument is bored from a lucite cylinder. The included angle of the entrance cone is 20 degrees and that of the diffusion cone 7 degrees. The system is stable, reliable and can be produced at low cost. The orifice plate flowmeter of Robiscek, et al. (1959 a, b, 1961) is the most elaborate instrument available in that class. It is made of stainless steel, provided with connectors for insertion into the arterial line and has Luer Lock pressure tape on either side of the orifice plate. The plate itself is made of Tygon and is disposable. The gauge is simple, robust and easy to clean. It produces more turbulence than a Venturi meter, but the differential pressure produced is also more easily measured. By using a sensitive differential manometer and proper amplification, a relatively large orifice is made to provide a sufficient signal and the resistance of the circuit is increased by only 3 per cent. The variations in blood viscosity and specific gravity encountered during heart–lung bypass procedures have a negligible effect on the reading.

All differential pressure flowmeters suffer from serious recording artifacts when highly pulsatile flow conditions prevail. Distortion caused by the acceleration and deceleration of the fluid column in the manometer were first described as "kinetic energy factor" and "acceleration factor" by Frank (1929, 1930, 1959) and extensively discussed by Müller, et al. (1954 a, b). Since the distortion is not the same during acceleration and deceleration, an error arises when pulsatile flow signals from differential flowmeters are averaged for the purpose of easy readability as "mean flow."

2. Rotameters: In rotameters, the blood flowing upward in a vertical tapered tube lifts a float to different levels according to the rate of flow (fig. 56). The float carries with it an iron rod, the extremity of which acts as the core of an induction coil wound in the housing of the flowmeter. The movements of the float thus result in changes in current which are recorded by a suitable galvanometer (Shipley and Wilson, 1951, 1960). The usual rotameters have a hat-shaped float which offers some resistance to blood transit and covers only a limited range of flow, with less accuracy for the low values than the high ones. In his heart–lung machine, Senning (1952) used two rotameters, one in the venous and one in the arterial line. A rotameter is still incorporated on the venous side of the Crafoord-

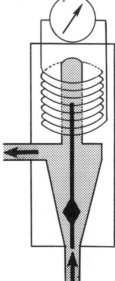

Fig. 56. Rotameter: The blood flowing up a tapered tube raises a float which carries with it an iron rod. One extremity of the rod moves in a recess surrounded by an induction coil embedded in the casing of the instrument. The current generated by the movement of the core in the induction coil is detected by a suitable galvanometer.

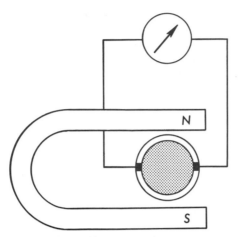

Fig. 57. Electromagnetic flowmeter: According to Faraday's principle, an electrolyte solution passing through a magnetic field generates at right angle to that field a voltage which is proportional to the velocity of flow. In this class of flowmeter, there is no restriction of the lumen because the sensing electrodes (black dots) are mounted flush with the inner wall of the blood tube.

Senning oxygenator (1956). Dennis (1956) also used a venous rotameter. Recently, Griesser and Passon (1960) described an arterial rotameter with a rhomboid-shaped float of the type previously described by Hilger and Brechtelsbauer (1957). This instrument features a linear calibration between 1 and 5 L./min.; causes a pressure drop in the line of only 2 to 3 mm. Hg. and is practically unaffected by changes in blood viscosity. Hemolysis and protein deposits are minimized by the favorable shape of the float.

Rotameters are suited only to record average flow, although the float can follow pulsatile changes to some extent. The flow signal to noise ratio is greater than that of most differential pressure flowmeters. The reliability of rotameters is therefore excellent. Their disadvantages are the extra tubing needed, the cumbersome mounting, and the inconvenience of a moving part and recesses in the blood stream.

3. Electromagnetic flowmeters: A conductive liquid flowing through a magnetic field generates a voltage which is proportional to the velocity. On that principle, instruments have been built which consist primarily of an electromagnet in the field of which blood passes through a tube of fixed diameter (fig. 57). Electrodes are mounted flush with the interior of the tube, in a plane perpendicular to the lines of force of the magnetic field and to the axis of the tube. The voltage sensed, which is linearly proportional to the average velocity of flow, is suitably amplified for recording. The frequency response of the system is limited only by the electrical characteristics of the amplifying circuit. Therefore electromagnetic flowmeters lend themselves to the monitoring of both phasic and mean flow. The considerable progress which has recently taken place in the development of electromagnetic flowmeters makes them most suitable for extracorporeal circuits. Their main advantage is that there is no need to enter the blood stream or to interfere with it in any way. The system is accurate and dependable, measures phasic as well as mean flow over a wide enough range and can be cleaned easily. It is not affected by changes in viscosity, specific gravity, temperature pressure or conductivity of the blood. Electromagnetic flowmeters have been used by Thomas, et al. (1958), Cordell and Spencer (1959, 1960), Spencer and Denison (1960), Waldhausen, et al. (1959 b), Albertal, et al. (1959, 1961), and Cannon, et al. (1960). The main disadvantage of electromagnetic flowmeters is their poor signal to noise ratio. Intricate electronic circuits are required to insure proper amplification and stability. The price of these flowmeters is therefore considerable.

Summarizing:

Since knowledge of the perfusion flow rate is mandatory in heart–lung bypass procedures, some means of measuring flow must be incorporated into the extracorporeal circuit. Occlusive pumps can serve as flowmeters. In the case of nonocclusive pumps, too many variables must be computed to obtain a flow reading which is of practical value. Cumulative recording of flow by temporarily interrupting the circulation is inaccurate. Most frequently used in extracorporeal circuits are differential pressure flowmeters, rotameters and electromagnetic flowmeters.

TEMPERATURE REGULATING DEVICES

In the early stages of clinical heart–lung machine development, temperature regulating devices were incorporated into the extracorporeal circuit to maintain the blood temperature within the normal physiological range. More recently, the success of hypothermic perfusions (*see* chap. XIX) has led to the development of special heat exchangers of large caloric capacity, which are capable of modifying the temperature of the blood in both directions at a very rapid rate. Obviously, the latter type of heat exchangers is also capable of stabilizing the temperature within the physiological range. For the sake of clarity, however, we shall discuss these two types separately. First we will take up the simpler devices proposed for temperature maintenance.

Heating systems are required in perfusion equipment because the large metal, glass or plastic parts of heart–lung machines present tremendous radiating surfaces and are responsible for most of the heat loss from the circulating blood. Operating rooms are usually thermostabilized at 12 to 15°C. below the normal body temperature. Some means of preventing or balancing the heat loss from the pump-oxygenator must therefore be utilized. The temperature of the patient during perfusion has been controlled by immersing all or part of the artificial lung in a water bath (e.g., Miller and Gibbon, 1951; DeWall, et al., 1956 a; Gross, et al., 1960) or by circulating thermostatically controlled warm air around the oxygenator (e.g., Rygg, et al., 1956; Westin, et al., 1958; Esmond, et al., 1959). Radiant heat, usually produced by infrared lamps (e.g., Gott, et al., 1957 a, b; Watkins, et al., 1960) or short wave radiation (Battezzatti and Taddei, 1954; Dietman, 1955) has also been suggested. Finally, thermostatically controlled heating wires have been either incorporated into the wall of the gas exchange unit (e.g., Jones, et al., 1955) or wrapped around it (Salisbury, 1956; Kay, et al., 1956; Kantrowitz, et al., 1959).

To fulfill their function, temperature regulating devices should maintain the blood temperature within ±0.5°C. The local temperature of surfaces in contact with moving blood must *never* be permitted to rise above 45°C., and preferably not above 43°C. because of the marked increase in mechanical and osmotic fragility of the red cells caused by thermal injury (Ham, et al., 1948; Gollan, et al., 1955). This requirement is even more stringent for surfaces in contact with foam where the temperature should not exceed 39°C. Since the risk of overheating is greatly enhanced when the blood circulation is arrested, many thermostabilizing circuits feature a safety switch which turns the heater off when the pumps are stopped (e.g., Gross, et al., 1960). The most difficult practical problem to solve in the design of such circuits is the location of the sensing device. If this is not carefully considered, local overheating may go undetected until denaturation of blood occurs.

Temperature stabilization at the physiological level is mandatory for those experimental perfusions in which a temperature variation may obscure the particular problem under investigation. Under clinical conditions, however, recent experience demonstrates that there is no inconvenience from, and probably some advantage in permitting the blood temperature to drift downward a few degrees. These considerations should be weighed when one examines the specifications of the different heating devices proposed.

Summarizing:

Since there is considerable heat loss in all extracorporeal circuits, devices have been introduced for the purpose of maintaining the temperature of the perfused organism within the normal physiologic range. Water baths, warm air, infrared radiant energy and heating wires have been used with varying success. Because of possible thermal injury to the red blood cells, the local temperature of surfaces in contact with blood should never be permitted to exceed 45°C.

HEAT EXCHANGERS

Bidirectional heat exchangers for heart–lung machines have been developed recently. Because they present a relatively well defined engineering problem, quantification has been easily introduced into their design. Performance, in terms of blood cooling or rewarming, can be measured and adequate comparison of different devices can be established (fig. 58). The biologic requirements,

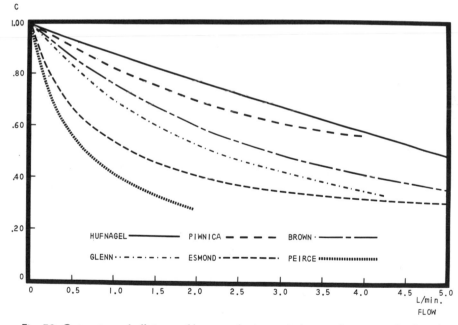

Fig. 58. Comparison of efficiency of heat transfer in certain heat exchangers used in hypothermic perfusion. Abscissa, blood flow in L./min. Ordinate heat transfer coefficient (C), defined as the blood temperature change across the heat exchanger—from inlet (T_{Bi}) to outlet (T_{Bo}) per degree centigarde of temperature difference between the inlet blood temperature and the inlet water temperature (T_{Wo}).

$$C = \frac{T_{Bi} - T_{Bo}}{T_{Bi} - T_{Wo}}$$

(Modified from Peirce, 1961.)

however, are still not fully known, particularly as far as the optimal rate of temperature variation is concerned. The criteria presented are, therefore, open to revision.

Heat exchangers must first meet the requirements for all elements in an extracorporeal blood circuit. Namely, they must be made of nontoxic material, easy to clean and sterilize, or else they should be disposable. Safety also requires that internal leakage should never occur to avoid contamination of the blood by the cooling or heating solution. Once inserted into the extracorporeal circuit, heat exchangers must neither materially increase the resistance to flow, nor inflict any trauma on blood. Efficiency of heat transfer calls for a minimum of foreign surface area in contact with blood, a low priming volume, and a design which permits adapting the size of the device to the caloric exchange required in different perfusions. Finally, the heat exchange unit must be assembled or produced at a reasonable cost.

Most exchangers in use are able to decrease the esophageal temperature of organisms perfused at flow rates from 1 to 4 L./min. by 1 to 3°C. per minute. Since the specific heat of blood is of the order of 0.86, depending upon the hematocrit (Mendlowitz, 1948), between 3 and 12 Kg. Cal./min. can be exchanged during a cooling procedure. The rate of rewarming is somewhat slower (0.5 to 1°C. per minute), owing not only to the narrower temperature gradient available (the temperature in the heat exchanger cannot exceed 45°C.), but also to the lower flow rates which are initially used because of the increased blood viscosity at low temperature. The necessity for overcoming the cooling effect of the ambient room temperature may also play a minor role in the sluggishness of the rewarming process. One of the advantages claimed for blood stream (or core) cooling over immersion (or external) hypothermia is the minimal caloric loss required for achieving low temperatures in such vital organs as the heart, brain, liver and kidney (*see* Chapter XIX). In view of this, the faster the rate of blood cooling, the less damaging the perfusion procedure will be. Presently, it is not yet apparent whether harmful effects resulting from local temperature differences within an organ or between organs limit the permissible rates of temperature variation. Because of the limitations in our knowledge, the way is still open for the development of more efficient heat exchangers.

Some heat-exchanger problems pertain to the safety measures required. The heat transferring surfaces can safely bear temperatures between 1 and 45°C. without damaging the blood. Simple thermostatic control of the cooling or heating fluid will easily prevent excessive temperature changes in either direction. More concern has been elicited by the possibility of bubble formation during rewarming because the oxygen solubility in plasma decreases as the temperature goes up. A bubble trap has been included in one of the most widely used heat exchangers (Brown, et al., 1958 a), although theoretic (Ross, 1959; Donald and Fellows, 1960) and practical (Young, et al., 1959; Urschell, et al., 1959 c) considerations indicate that the actual danger is rather limited. Another hazard resides in the possibility of blood contamination, should a leak develop between the blood conduits and the passageways for the heat-transferring water. Because of the large flows of water needed for efficient operation, the problem cannot be solved by maintaining the blood phase under a higher pressure, as is done in membrane oxygenators, for instance. One solution (Esmond, et al., 1959) consists of having joints only on the external surface of the unit, so that leaks can occur only to the outside where they will easily be observed.

Another method (Oselladore, et al., 1957) utilizes the rapid decompression of CO_2 instead of cold water circulation for the cooling process.

The ideal location of the heat-exchanger in the extracorporeal circuit is still not agreed upon. Heat transfer in the artificial lung itself using internal (e.g., Gollan, et al., 1952 a, b; Urschell, et al., 1960 c; Zuhdi, et al., 1960); or external (e.g., Osborne, et al., 1960) manifolds, is the most attractive method because wide surfaces of contact are available without increase in priming requirements. Location of the gas exchanger in the venous line (Esmond, et al., 1959; Aletras, et al., 1960) minimizes concern about gas bubbles because the artificial lung itself then acts as a bubble trap. Insertion of the heat exchanger into the arterial line (e.g., Brown, et al., 1958 a; Glenn, et al., 1960 a; Bjørk, 1960) presents the advantage of simplicity, because the heat exchanger can readily be joined to any existing circuit, and the additional resistance to blood flow is easily overcome by the arterial pump.

Of the three methods for transferring heat, namely radiation, convection and conduction, only conduction in combination with convection is useful for transferring significant quantities of heat in a small volume. Use has been made of this with different geometrical configurations: coils, cylinders or plates. Each of these three types feature advantages and drawbacks.

1. A simple silver *coil* immersed in the pump oxygenator has served successfully for cooling and warming of the entire circulation of dogs by Gollan, et al., (1952) (*see* fig. 21, A). Peirce and Polley (1953, 1956), Dietman (1955) and Oselladore, et al. (1957) found the same type of heat exchanger reliable. For autogenous lung oxygenation, Shields and Lewis (1959) inserted a stainless steel coil in both right heart bypass and left heart bypass circuits. A double lumen coil, with the blood circulating inside and the water outside, was proposed by Ross (1954 a). Zuhdi, et al. (1960 b, 1961) astutely thought of a long stainless steel spiral wound in the helix settling chamber of the DeWall-Lillehei bubble oxygenator (fig. 59 C). Their system is inexpensive and instead of requiring any priming blood, it actually diminishes the blood content of the helix without altering its efficiency as a bubble trap. Urschell, et al. (1960 c) devised an efficient system of coils which adapt to the inside of a rotating disc oxygenator. This system is made of a series of one-eighth inch outside diameter stainless steel tubes semicircularly molded, and connected in parallel (fig. 59 A). The inflow and outflow conduits perforate the end plates of the disc oxygenator near the top and are connected to a thermoregulation unit. The glass cylinder of the oxygenator must be one-half inch larger in diameter than the standard size in order to accommodate the coils and maintain the same priming volume. All coiled heat exchangers are efficient; the main objection is that cleaning is difficult, and that inspection of the inner surfaces is not possible before assembling the circuit.

2. Straight, *cylinder-shaped* heat exchangers escape the above criticism. They can be as simple as a concentric tube around a blood conduit (Bücherl, 1956) or around the oxygenator itself (Osborne, et al., 1960) or as complicated as the integral fin-type proposed by Glenn, et al. (1960a). This latter unit (fig. 59, D) is made of stainless steel and consists of three parts, an inner tube of 8 mm. (inner diameter) with the outer surface deeply grooved to form eight longitudinal integral fins; an outer tube of 1.6 cm. i.d.; and connecting tubes for inflow and outflow of blood and of the heat-transferring solution. Haglund and Lundberg (1960) reported favorably upon a heat-exchanger made of two silver-plated copper cylinders enclosing a blood path with water on each side. Because the space between the cylinders is only 1 mm. wide, a surface of 1400 cm.² can be developed without requiring more than 70 ml. as priming volume. The annular type of heat exchanger currently used by Drew (1961) also features concentric cylinders. The blood path is divided into four helical streams with entry ports designed to maintain even distribution over the heat exchange area. Somewhat similar designs have been advocated by Hufnagel, et al., (1961) and Anderson (1961).

A system of multiple parallel cylinders enclosed in a common chamber was described by Brown, et al. (1958a) and Zaconto (1958). The Brown-Harrison heat-exchanger (fig.

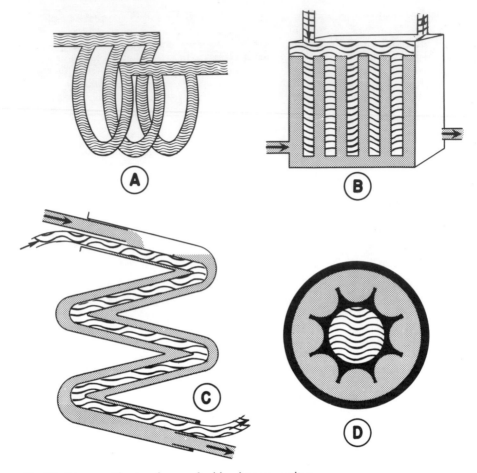

Fig. 59. Schemes of heat exchangers for blood stream cooling.

A. System of coils described by Urschell, et al. (1960c), for a rotating disc oxygenator. Since the refrigerated coils are largely immersed in the blood pool at the lower part of the glass cylinder, a very efficient heat transfer is achieved.

B. Disposable heat exchanger proposed by Esmond, et al. (1960). The device is made by folding a steel or silver sheet and enclosing it in a casing so that the streaming blood is on one side and the heat exchange fluid on the other side.

C. Cooling coil wound inside the helix settling chamber of the Lillehei-DeWall oxygenator, as proposed by Zuhdi, et al. (1960b, 1961).

D. Integral fin-type heat exchanger described by Glenn, et al. (1960a). Heat transfer between the liquid flowing in the inner cylinder and blood in the outer annular space is favored by the particular shape of the fins.

60, A) consists of a bundle of 24 thin-walled stainless steel tubes 38 cm. in length, heliarc welded into the drilled header plates of a 5.2 cm. diameter stainless steel outer jacket. The inlet and outlet water ports are near the ends of the jacket. The exchanger operates in a vertical position, the blood entering through a bottom cap, flowing upward through the tubes and out through the top cap. The priming volume is 175 ml. The Jehle's heat exchanger (Bailey and Lemmon, 1960), characterized by a rubber water jacket, has features essentially similar to the Brown-Harrison model. Other compact tubular heat exchangers made of parallel straight tubes welded at their end to blood distributing manifolds have been described by Bernhard, et al. (1960, 1961) and Drew (1961). Gebauer,

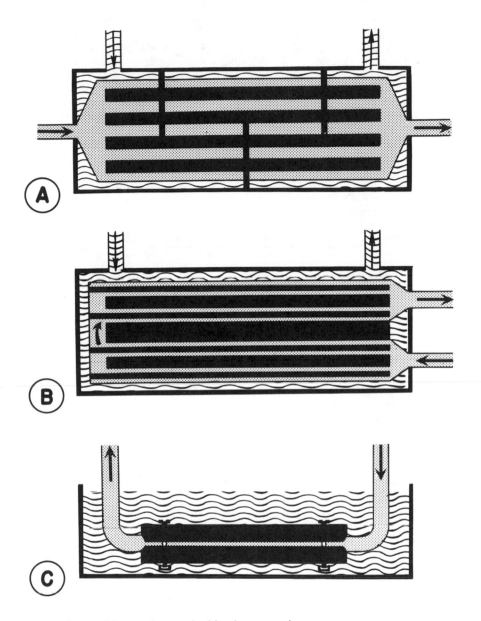

Fig. 60. Schemes of heat exchangers for blood stream cooling.

A. Principle of the Brown-Harrison (1958) heat exchanger. Blood flows through a number o parallel tubes immersed in a casing through which circulates the heat exchange fluid. Baffles in the water compartment help equalize the heat transfer in the different parts of the device.

B. Double-pipe heat exchanger as described by Bjørk (1960) and Piwnica, et al. (1960a, b). Rods (thick black bars) inserted axially within the blood tubes improve heat transfer because the blood path is reduced to an annular space in direct contact with the heat exchange fluid. In Bjork's design, blood enters and leaves on the same side of the exchanger.

C. Double-plate heat exchanger employed by Peirce (1961a). The blood flows in a thin layer between two opposing plates gasketed at their periphery, and immersed in a water bath.

et al. (1960) controlled temperature in a commercial rotating disc oxygenator by immersing a manifold of 18 parallel steel tubes at the bottom of the glass cylinder.

Double-pipe, or annular, heat exchangers are the most efficient (Sullivan and Holland, 1961; Volbrecht, et al., 1961). This well known engineering principle has been adopted in the devices described by Bjørk (1960) and Piwnica, et al. (1960 a, b). Their heat exchanger (fig. 60, B) consists of a bundle of straight parallel tubes with a steel or nylon rod introduced axially into each of them in order to expose a thin, annular layer of blood to heat exchange. The resistance to blood flow in the arterial line is said to be negligible, the priming volume is rather low and cleaning is easy upon withdrawal of the rods.

3. *Plate-shaped* heat exchangers also have their proponents. For laboratory use, the simple device described by Peirce (1961a) is undoubtedly the most practical. It consists (fig. 60, C) of two opposing plates of siliconed stainless steel, maintained 1.5 mm. apart by a teflon or silicone rubber gasket so as to form a thin blood path. The gasket is held tightly by a series of bolts and wing nuts placed about the periphery. The plates can be lined with teflon membrane if desired. The blood chamber, which is cooled or warmed by immersing the whole device in a water-filled bucket, can be easily and thoroughly cleaned. Aletras, et al. (1960), reported a similar system in which a thin-walled plastic bag (16 by 30 cm.) is placed between two metal plates maintained 1 to 4 mm. apart. The bag with its inlet and outlet are disposable. Also disposable is the stainless steel or silver heat exchanger proposed by Esmond, et al. (1960): a considerable flat area of heat transfer is provided by folding a thin sheet of stainless steel into a grid-like structure (fig. 59, B). A stainless steel rectangular casing surrounds the heat exchange elements and contains fittings for blood and water. The entire unit weighs only 230 gm. and requires but 60 ml. of blood for priming. Since it is produced at low cost, it can be discarded after use. A somewhat similar design is apparent in the heat exchanger employed by Benichoux (1960).

Summarizing:

Heat exchangers have been used to cool rapidly and rewarm the organism during surgical intervention in order to benefit from hypothermic conditions. These devices can decrease the esophageal temperature of the perfused organism by 1 to 3°C. per minute. The rate of rewarming is somewhat slower. In addition to their efficiency of heat transfer, heat exchangers must meet the same requirements as all other components of extracorporeal circuits, namely nontoxicity of construction materials, low priming volume, minimal resistance to flow, and ease of cleaning and sterilization.

XII. Connection of the Vascular System with an Extracorporeal Circuit

In connecting the vascular system of a living organism to an artificial heart–lung machine, the venous blood must be drained out of the central veins or right heart cavities in a continuous flow without inducing any marked change of the pressure within the large veins. Simultaneously, an equal amount of arterialized blood must be infused into the arterial tree under such conditions that each vascular bed receives its quota of blood under a normal head of pressure.

In dealing with the physical means of transferring blood from live vessels into inert tubes, and vice versa, one must integrate the basic physical laws which govern flow in the extracorporeal portion of the circuit, with the dynamics of pressure–flow–resistance relations on both the venous and arterial sides of the organism's circulatory system. In this chapter we shall, for convenience, consider venous drainage and arterial infusion separately. The dependence of each on the other will become apparent in chap. XIII.

PRESSURE-FLOW RELATIONS IN THE VENOUS LINE

The problem of venous drainage is essentially that of connecting wide, low–resistance, collapsible vessels to somewhat narrower, stiff, artificial conduits of known physical characteristics. A short analysis of the physical mechanisms involved is needed in order to understand how the blood can be made to flow out of the organism.

The pressure–flow relationships which exist in the veins do not differ materially from those established in vitro for collapsible tubes undergoing depletion upon suction (Holt, 1941; Brecher, 1956). When an increasing suction force is applied to collapsible tubing (fig. 61), the flow (*curve A*) first increases linearly with the pressure gradient, the resistance to flow (*curve C*) remaining nearly constant. However, when the suction is increased sufficiently to cause the tubing to collapse partially, the flow shows no further increase, and therefore the calculated resistance increases progressively. Actually, collapse does not occur instantaneously as pressure in the downstream portion of the line

171

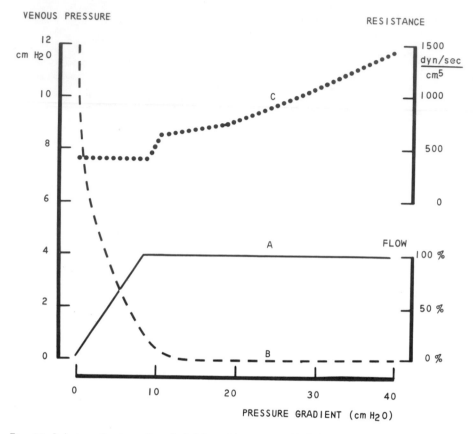

Fig. 61. Relation of volume flow (solid line **A**), pressure (dash line **B**) and resistance (dotted line **C**) in a vein subject to increasing degrees of suction (pressure gradient) on the venous outflow tube. At small degrees of suction (0 to about 10 cm. H_2O), the outflow **A** increases linearly (depleting stage). With greater degrees of suction (10 to 40 cm. H_2O), the outflow remains nearly constant because of a partial collapse of the vein (collapsed stage). Venous pressure **B** declines from a high value in the absence of outflow to zero when the vein is partially collapsed. It remains zero at higher degrees of suction. The resistance to flow in the vein **C** does not change at small degrees of suction (horizontal part of curve), but increases almost linearly with greater degrees of suction (incline of curve limb) when the collapsed stage is reached. The increase in resistance keeps the flow in partially collapsed veins nearly constant. (Modified from Brecher, 1956.)

is lowered (fig. 62, *curve A*). During a first stage, called the "depleting stage," the veins empty most of their content into the region of lower pressure, thereby further increasing the flow. Later, a "collapsed stage" is reached at which the vessel wall intermittently close the lumen, resulting in a decrease in the rate of volume flow through the suction line. From these considerations, it follows that there is little benefit in increasing the suction force beyond a critical level.

Since, however, the venous system is drained to the outside by tubes of relatively small caliber, an additional resistance to the outflow of blood must be taken into account. Assuming that the inner diameter of the venous catheter is at least 30 per cent less than that of the central veins, one can calculate that the resistance introduced by the catheters and tubing is at least four times larger than the low resistance of the intact venous system. Therefore

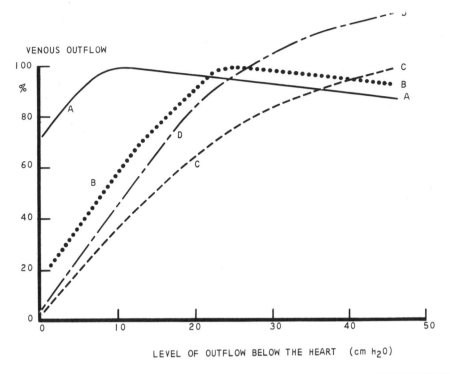

Fig. 62. Relation of venous outflow to the degree of suction applied (level of outflow tube below heart level).

A. Venous outflow through wide tubing offering negligible resistance. Flow increases from 75 per cent in the absence of suction to a maximum (100 per cent) at a suction of about 10 cm. (depleting stage), then diminishes slightly with greater degrees of suction (collapsed stage).

B. Curve calculated for a venous drainage line resistance 4 times that of the central veins. This value corresponds approximately to the resistance of the widest venous catheters used in extracorporeal circulation procedures. The maximal flow is reached at a suction of about 25 cm. H_2O.

C. Curve calculated for a venous drainage line resistance about 20 times larger than that of the central veins. This value corresponds approximately to the resistance offered by wide lumen catheters passed from a peripheral vein into the caval veins. The maximal flow is reached at a suction of about 50 cm. H_2O.

D. The resistance is taken to be the same as in curve **C,** but a blood reservoir is interposed in the venous outflow tract such as illustrated in fig. 82. By this means venous pressure always remains positive and partial venous collapse as a flow limiting factor is prevented. Flow reaches higher values because the gradient of pressure across the venous line is increased. (Modified from Brecher, 1956.)

more suction force than just a few centimeters of water will often be needed to bring about the largest possible outflow (fig. 62, *curves B and C*). In fact, according to the size of the tubing used, a negative pressure of 20 to 50 cm. H_2O can be developed at the downstream end of the venous line before venous collapse is induced.

Under practical conditions, it is hazardous to apply suction up to the point of collapse, or zero pressure, in the veins because the venous wall will then easily stick to—and even be drawn into—the openings of the cannulae, leading to irregular or intermittent flow. It is more advantageous to remain in the stage of venous depletion, which corresponds to a positive value of venous pressure at the cannula tip, and to the upward portion of the flow–pressure curve. By this means, one keeps some margin of suction pressure for flow regulation. Another practical approach to high flow venous drainage consists of preventing the decrease in venous pressure which normally accompanies the increase in suction force and venous flow (fig. 61, *curve B, left limb*) by some kind of regulating system such as a blood reservoir, under slight positive pressure, connected to the venous system. Under such conditions, the gradient of pressure from vein to the outflow site will be greater, and consequently the blood flow will be larger (fig. 62, *curve D*) than when the venous pressure is allowed to fall, as it would otherwise occur.

Summarizing:

The problem of venous drainage is essentially that of connecting wide, low-resistance, collapsible vessels to somewhat narrower, stiff, artificial conduits. The pressure-flow relationship in veins is similar to that in collapsible rubber tubing. When an increasing suction is applied, the flow increases, at first linearly (depleting stage), but later when the tubing begins to collapse, the flow does not increase further (collapsed stage). Increase in suction force beyond a critical level cannot increase the amount of venous drainage. High resistance in the drainage line necessitates higher degrees of suction than is needed with short, wide tubing. Maintenance of a positive pressure at the cannula tip broadens the margin of flow regulation because it prevents venous collapse.

SUCTION PUMP VERSUS GRAVITY SYPHONAGE FOR VENOUS DRAINAGE

There has been difference of opinion as to whether the venous blood should be made to flow from the central veins by syphon drainage into a "right atrium" collecting chamber placed underneath, or should be collected directly by the suction of a "right ventricle" pump. From the theoretic considerations developed above, one would conclude that both methods are equally effective, as long as venous collapse is avoided. Under practical conditions, however, the drawback of a suction pump is that it may accidentally develop too much negative pressure if there is not enough blood available. Syphons, on the other hand, are not self-priming and require adjustment to deliver a constant flow when the venous pressure fluctuates. Both systems can cause the walls of the great veins to collapse on the intake openings of the venous cannulae. This is not only liable to damage the formed blood elements and the venous walls, but also leads to a vicious cycle of lack of venous return calling for more and more suction, which actually decreases the amount of venous drainage.

Many techniques have been advocated for collecting the venous blood. In the early crude preparations, the perfused organ was simply placed on a funnel and the venous blood freely flowed out of the cut veins into a reservoir. Foaming and contamination were the main drawbacks of open air collection. Pumps were therefore proposed. The risk of excessive suction with venous flutter and collapse was soon recognized, and other procedures were developed to control negative pressure in the venous line. As clinical experience was gained in the management of total body perfusion, many surgeons felt that simple syphonage of the venous blood into the heart–lung machine, with or without an intermediate reservoir, was more satisfactory than the use of a suction pump.

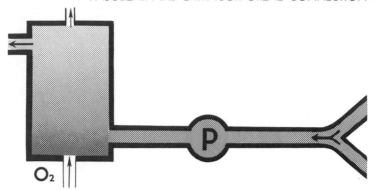

Fig. 63. Pump drainage of venous blood into an oxygenator. Venous blood (dark shading) is sucked by a pump (P) from the venous catheters (Y-shaped tubes at the right) into the artificial gas exchange device (upright rectangle with changing shade).

Others, disturbed by the necessity of placing a reservoir below the operating table, and of priming the syphon repeatedly, when it accidentally became empty, chose to apply the adjustable negative pressure of a vacuum line to a closed venous reservoir.

All these techniques have been successfully employed, and none is essentially superior to another. Yet controversies have arisen, because it is not always understood that the choice of the perfusion flow, the control exerted over the body blood volume and the fluctuations permitted or induced in the venous pressure, are all factors to consider in deciding for or against one or another technique of venous drainage. We shall review the advantages and limitations of each technique.

1. Pump drainage into the oxygenator: The blood from both caval veins is sucked by a pump directly into the artificial lung (fig. 63). The advantages of simplicity and flow metering by the pump are obvious. The oxygenator can be placed at any level above or below the heart. The hazard of excessive suction inducing venous collapse is minimal if relatively low perfusion flows are used (Cooley, et al., 1957, 1958b), if the body blood volume is increased for the bypass procedure (Yasargil, 1960) or if special care is taken to keep the venous pressure constant (Peirce, 1958a). Some circuits provide a shunt between the high-pressure arterial line and the negative pressure venous line, which can be transiently opened to unblock the venous cannulae if their openings are occluded (Salisbury, 1956). A more sophisticated safety system, already described in 1929 by Brukhonenko and perfected by Kantrowitz, et al. (1959), makes use of a venous manometer to actuate a relay and stop the venous pump when an excessive suction is developed (*see* figs. 9 and 26, A).

2. Direct gravity drainage into the oxygenator: The venous blood flows by direct syphon drainage into the artificial lung (fig. 64). This system is extremely simple, eliminates one pump in the circuit and reduces to a minimum the need for priming blood. However, it is necessary that the blood level in the oxygenator be considerably below heart level. The cannulae and tubing must be extra wide in order to minimize resistance, particularly when the oxygenator is at some distance from the organism. Priming of the venous line is cumbersome if the syphonage is lost during the procedure. Finally, each instance of blood loss in the perfused organism—as from hemorrhage, for instance—is reflected by a fall in the oxygenator blood level. For those gas exchange devices which work best at constant blood content—rotating disc oxygenator, for instance—direct gravity drainage is not recommended. At any rate, a continuous monitoring of the venous flow is often

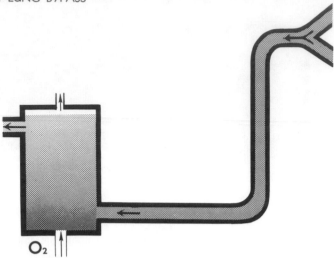

Fig. 64. Direct gravity drainage of venous blood into an oxygenator. The venous line connects the venous catheters directly to the artificial lung placed beneath.

found necessary (Dennis, 1956; Crafoord, et al., 1957a) to warrant a smooth functioning of the oxygenator.

3. Full gravity drainage with venous reservoir: The blood from the central veins first flows by syphon drainage into a collecting chamber, from which it then flows down into the oxygenator by simple gravity (fig. 65). This technique still requires that the oxygenator be at a level lower than the heart. The reservoir, however, gives it more flexibility. It can be moved along a vertical axis to vary the degree of suction, and it is built in such a way that the syphon can never be unprimed. At the beginning of the bypass procedure, when the blood content of the heart and of the lesser circulation empties into the extracorporeal circuit, the reservoir is often placed 50 cm. below heart level (Paneth, et al., 1957).

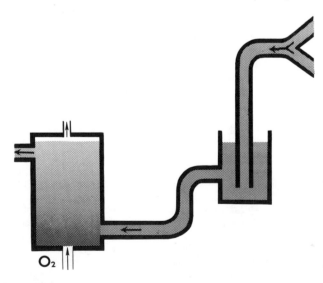

Fig. 65. Full gravity drainage with venous reservoir: Venous blood flows by syphon drainage into a reservoir, the height of which can be adjusted: From there it flows into the artificial lung by simple gravity.

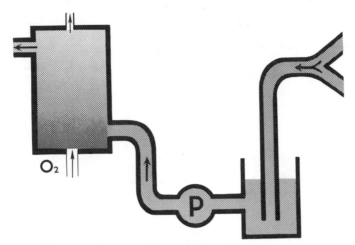

Fig. 66. Combined gravity and pump drainage: Blood flows from the venous catheters into a reservoir by syphon drainage. However, a pump (P) serves to transfer the blood into the artificial lung, which therefore can be placed at any level with respect to the perfused organism.

When an equilibrated perfusion is achieved, the level which brings about full drainage without unduly lowering venous pressure is usually of the order of 25 cm. (Olmsted, et al., 1958; Gross, et al., 1960). The reservoir also serves to damp the volume fluctuations in the oxygenator when blood is lost in the operative field.

4. Combined gravity and pump drainage: The blood from the central veins flows by syphon drainage into an open collecting chamber. A pump is then used for transferring the blood from this reservoir into the oxygenator (fig. 66). This arrangement combines the safety of gravity drainage with the advantages of a venous pump. The reservoir level is raised or lowered according to perfusion needs, yet the gas exchange device can be at or above the patient's level. A pump is also needed despite the use of gravity drainage when the venous blood must be distributed under pressure into the artificial lung, as is true, for instance, of most stationary membrane oxygenators (Clowes and Neville, 1958).

5. Vacuum suction drainage: The oxygenator, maintained under slightly subatmospheric pressure by a vacuum line, is connected directly to the central veins and blood is thereby drawn up continuously (fig. 67). This arrangement ideally combines all the conveniences

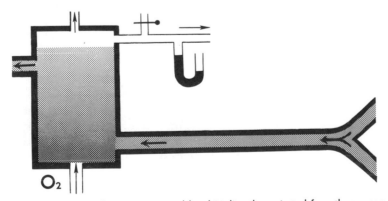

Fig. 67. Venous suction drainage: venous blood is directly aspirated from the venous catheters into the oxygenator by means of a vacuum suction system. The degree of suction exerted upon the oxygenator is indicated by a U-shaped manometer and regulated by a bleeder valve in the vacuum line.

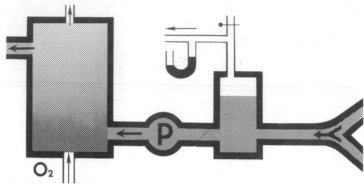

Fig. 68. Combined vacuum and pump drainage: venous blood is sucked into a closed venous reservoir by means of a regulated vacuum system. The reservoir can be placed at any level with respect to the heart and to the artificial lung, since a pump (P) is employed for transferring the blood from the reservoir into the oxygenator.

of syphon and pump drainage. The circuit is simple, no pump is required, the suction can be regulated and the artificial lung can be placed anywhere. Gas exchange occurs under a slightly subatmospheric pressure, which may be useful in preventing excessive oxygen tensions. The practical difficulty is that the whole system must be airtight to function correctly. Such a mechanism of venous drainage has been successfully used by Clark, et al. (1952).

6. Combined vacuum and pump drainage: Vacuum suction is used for transferring the blood from the central veins into a reservoir: thereafter a pump serves to feed the gas exchange device (fig. 68). The venous reservoir is a closed chamber with an outlet connected to a vacuum line. A bleeder valve is used to achieve the amount of suction required for adequate venous drainage without incurring venous collapse (Donald, et al., 1955; Kirklin, et al., 1957). The level of the venous reservoir can be anywhere with respect to that of the perfused organism. This system is often used with circuits which require a pump on the venous side of the oxygenator—as, for instance, the recirculation pump of stationary screen oxygenators. It can be refined by making the venous reservoir adjustable along a vertical axis below the heart. Then the venous reservoir can be opened to atmospheric pressure for conventional syphon drainage, or connected to the vacuum line either for priming or when more suction is required than is provided by the level of the chamber beneath the heart (Brecher, et al., 1955). This extra dimension in the regulating possibilities of syphon drainage has been found useful by Blanco, et al. (1959) in cases where syphonage is broken by malposition or displacement of the drainage catheters.

Summarizing:

Venous blood can be drained into an extracorporeal circuit, using either a suction pump or gravity syphonage. Theoretically, both methods are safe and efficient, provided venous collapse is avoided. A suction pump simplifies the circuit but may accidentally develop too much negative pressure and thereby lead abruptly to venous collapse. A syphon draining into an external venous reservoir must be primed and requires adjustment to venous pressure fluctuations. A number of different techniques have been proposed as practical solutions to the venous drainage problem: (1) direct suction of venous blood into the artificial lung by a pump; (2) direct syphonage by gravity into the artificial lung placed at a low level; (3) syphon drainage by gravity into an open venous reservoir, followed by gravity drainage into the oxygenator; (4) syphonage by gravity into an open venous reservoir from which the blood is transferred by a pump to the oxygenator; (5) vacuum suction drainage directly into the oxygenator which is maintained under a slight subatmospheric pressure; (6) vacuum suction drainage into a closed venous reservoir from which the blood is pumped into the oxygenator.

VENOUS DRAINAGE, CONDUITS AND RESERVOIRS

We shall now consider briefly the anatomical details of cannulation, the catheters and reservoirs actually used for transferring the venous blood from

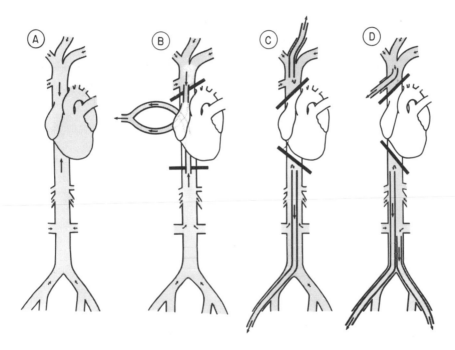

Fig. 69. Scheme of venous circulation and venous drainage towards an extracorporeal circuit for heart–lung bypass. Blood-filled vessels and conduits represented by gray shading; direction of blood stream indicated by arrows.

A. Normal venous return to the right heart cavities.

B. Drainage towards the extracorporeal circuit through catheters inserted in the right atrium and advanced into the caval veins. Tourniquets (heavy black bars) prevent blood from entering the right heart cavities. Normal direction of flow in the central veins is preserved, and wide, low resistance catheters can be used.

C. Drainage through peripherally advanced catheters. This technique can be used to perform partial heart–lung bypass in closed-chest conditions. For total heart–lung bypass, the chest must still be open to clamp or obstruct the caval veins close to the right atrium (heavy black bars). Centripetal flow in the caval veins is partially impaired by the presence of the catheters.

D. Mixed central and peripheral cannulation, using the azygos vein for draining the superior caval bed, and both femoral veins for draining the inferior caval bed. Systems with multiple cannulation are often deceptive and fail to provide the amount of venous drainage expected because the increased suction provided by multiple catheters is more than outweighed by the obstruction of numerous vessels.

the central veins or right heart cavities into an extracorporeal circuit. The problems encountered in drainage of the left heart cavities, although somewhat similar in nature, are beyond the scope of the present chapter (*see* Chapter II).

1. Cannulations: In open-chest surgery, the venous connections necessary for heart–lung bypass by a pump-oxygenator usually require the isolation of the superior and inferior caval veins and the insertion of catheters into each of these vessels. The caval catheters are introduced through purse-string controlled openings in the right atrium or right auricular appendage (fig. 69B). When the heart–lung bypass is to begin, their tips are positioned at the proper level in the veins, and tourniquets around the vessels are tightened to prevent the passage of blood into the right atrium. This arrangement brings the venous catheters close to the operative field where inadvertent manipulation may cause them to shift out of position. However, it offers the distinct advantage that wide cannulae of large flow capacity can be used without impairment of the venous circulation, if care is taken to advance the catheters into position only at the last minute to avoid interference with the cardiac output before bypass. A simplification was proposed recently by Blanco, et al. (1959), who use a single catheter introduced into the right atrium through the right auricular appendage or into the right ventricle through the right ventricular outflow tract. This technique is evidently limited to cases without shunts.

The venous catheters can also be introduced into peripherally located vessels such as the femoral, saphenous or jugular veins, and advanced into the caval veins close to the heart (fig. 69C). Bypass can then be initiated before, or without, opening the chest, and no suturing of the heart walls is required. The main limitation of this technique is that the size and length of the cannulae are dictated by the dimensions of the peripheral veins. The resistance offered to flow is considerably larger than is the case when catheters are inserted into the right heart cavities and this precludes high flow rates. Unless the organism is made hypervolemic, it is usually impossible to carry more than 60 to 70 ml./Kg./min. through such extrathoracic cannulation. Furthermore, insertion of the largest

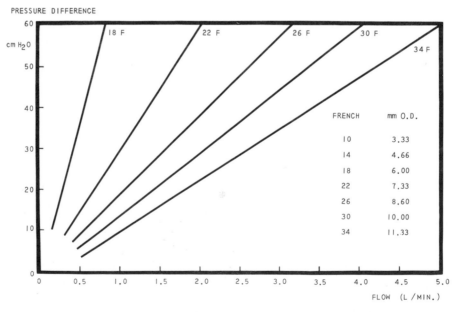

Fig. 70. Relationship between blood flow and the degree of suction needed with different sizes of plastic venous catheters (Redrawn from Borst, et al., 1959).

possible catheters from the periphery results in limitation of normal venous return owing to the space the catheters occupy in the caval vessels. This should therefore be reserved for hypothermic low flow perfusions, partial heart–lung bypass and emergency cases in which direct access to the chest is contraindicated.

In the pioneer years of extracorporeal circulation, rigid cannulae were used, as for instance that proposed by Leeds (1950) and modified by Helmsworth, et al. (1953c)—a right-angled cannula which was introduced through the azygos into the superior caval veins, and, in connection with an auxiliary catheter advanced from a femoral vessel, permitted complete venous drainage outside of the body (fig. 69 D). This type of multiple cannulation is now almost completely abandoned.

2. Catheters: The development of semiflexible tubing has made venous cannulation easier. Today's ideal catheter should be made of thin-walled plastic tubing, to offer the widest possible lumen, yet it should be rigid enough to avoid kinking and to resist flattening by an encircling tape (Bosher, 1959). Multiple side openings are desirable to avoid occlusion by collapse of the venous wall during strong suction. Translucency of the catheter facilitates the elimination of gas bubbles.

These specifications are not met entirely by commercially available catheters. The most commonly used catheters are made of transparent, disposable vinyl plastic. They are 42 cm. long, moderately rigid to facilitate insertion and prevent wall collapse, and feature a hole-in-tip and eight staggered perforations. The tapered end and the location of the openings makes them most suitable for insertion through the right auricular appendage, but causes some difficulties (resistance, bleeding) when introduction through peripheral vessels is attempted. A metal obturator can be employed at the point of in-

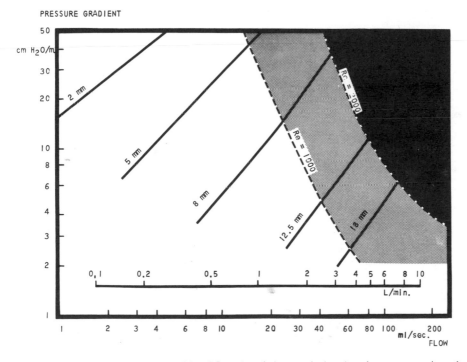

Fig. 71. Relationship between blood flow (in ml./sec. or L./min.) and pressure gradient (in cm. H_2O per meter) in plastic tubing of the type used for extracorporeal circulation procedures. The dark shaded area corresponds to turbulent flow (Reynolds number above 2000), whereas the light shaded area corresponds to the transition zone between laminal and turbulent flow (Reynolds number between 1000 and 2000). The figures along the oblique lines refer to the internal diameter of the tubing. (Modified from Vadot, 1959.)

sertion to prevent bleeding through the multiple perforations and to avoid kinking (Fitch and Bailey, 1959). One can also make a circumferential groove a short distance from the catheter tip to permit a firm anchorage in the caval veins (Heimbecker, 1960). Vinyl plastic catheters are fairly thick walled so that large sizes are necessary for high blood flow rates (fig. 70). Some authors (Bosher, 1959) prefer catheters made of polyvinyl tubing with attached perforated metal tips, largely because of the accuracy and dependability with which one can position and secure them. Moderately stiff, thin walled polyethylene or teflon tubing mounted on a nylon or stainless steel connector can be used in those procedures where no manipulation is required after insertion of the catheter. They offer much less resistance than vinyl catheters and are therefore advantageous for peripheral cannulation, although one has to be careful not to injure the vein walls.

3. Tubings and connectors: The catheters, the sizes of which are dictated by anatomical considerations, must remain the narrowest part of the venous line. Consequently, to keep resistance at a minimum, the cross section areas of the other elements of the venous line must always be wider (fig. 71), and no stenotic regions should be encountered by the blood once it leaves the catheters.

Most of the tapered nylon or stainless steel connectors in which the peripheral extremity of the venous catheters is inserted fit into plastic tubing three-eighths inch in internal diameter. The "Y" piece which is needed for uniting the two caval lines, must therefore present two three-eighths inch inner diameter inlets and one one-half inch or five-eighths inch i.d. outlet. This means that the main venous line will usually be made of one-half inch or five-eighths inch i.d. tubing. The Y-connector is often fitted with a lateral Luer-lock to which a syringe, or a vacuum line, can be attached for priming the line or removing gas bubbles (Guastavino, et al.. 1961). For the perfusion of small organisms, venous catheters with one-fourth inch connectors and three-eighths inch tubing for the venous line are permissible, particularly when the priming volume must be kept to a minimum.

4. Venous reservoirs: A reservoir in the venous line fulfills many purposes: it establishes and maintains the syphonage; it rapidly removes or adds blood to the oxygenator itself in case of fluid fluctuations; it mirrors the blood content of the extracorporeal circuit when the artificial lung is a constant volume device; and occasionally, it removes gas bubbles which may have entered the venous line before they reach the oxygenator.

The simplest venous reservoir is that advocated, with minor differences, by Paneth, et al. (1957); Olmsted, et al. (1958) and Blanco, et al. (1959). It is made of a cylindric segment of plastic tubing about 30 cm. long and 6 cm. in diameter (fig. 72). The drainage line enters at the top and blood flows out of the reservoir through an outlet at the bottom. The extra inlet at the top of the chamber is open to atmospheric pressure. It can be connected to a suction line if required.

The venous reservoir designed by Cartwright and Palich (1960a) is made of pyrex glass and stainless steel (fig. 72 B). The inlet and outlet for the venous blood are built into the base plate, as are special inlets for an overflow line from the oxygenator and for left atrial drainage. The main feature of this reservoir is a central obturator, which is immersed in the blood pool to decrease the priming requirement and provide for more accurate measurement of volume fluctuations. The whole assembly is mounted on a pulley system by which the height of syphonage can be readily varied. The system described by Gross, et al. (1960) is one of the most elaborate. It consists of two chambers (fig. 72 C and D). The upper one is a collecting chamber for blood from the caval veins and from the coronary sinus. The coronary blood enters at the top and passes through four stainless steel screens for removal of large bubbles and particles. The caval blood enters on the side. From the bottom of the reservoir, the blood cascades down into a settling chamber which rests at the level of the oxygenator. The purpose of this chamber is to smooth the venous inflow into the artificial lung and to permit volume fluctuations in the extracorporeal circuit to be detected. The double chamber system is particularly useful at very high blood flows because it acts as an efficient bubble trap for the small bubbles which must be prevented from going further.

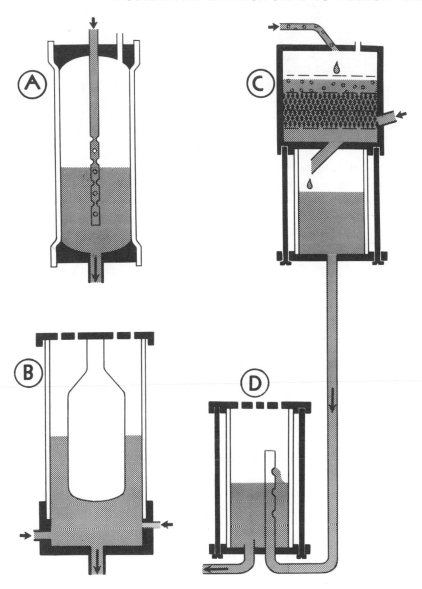

Fig. 72. Venous reservoirs used with heart–lung bypass equipment.

A. Simple gravity drainage reservoir made of a segment of plastic tubing and two stoppers (Paneth, et al., 1957).

B. Glass (double lines) and stainless steel (black) reservoir described by Cartwright and Palich (1960a). Venous blood enters through an inlet close to the lowest part of the reservoir (left) and leaves at the bottom of the base plate. One additional inlet (right) is provided for a recirculation line from the oxygenator (see also fig. 33, C). A hollow pyrex cylinder can be attached to the upper plate to diminish the blood content of the reservoir.

C. and **D.** System described by Gross, et al. (1960), for the collection of venous and coronary blood. The upper chamber **C** receives the foaming coronary blood at the top and the central venous blood on the right side. Filters (horizontal interrupted lines) and antifoam coated sponges (black diamonds) help in clearing the coronary blood. The lower chamber **D** is syphon connected to the upper one and permits settling of the blood before it enters the oxygenator.

Summarizing:

For open-chest surgery, low resistance catheters of large diameter are usually introduced through the right atrium into the superior and inferior vena
cava. In the closed-chest organism, one or more catheters are advanced from
a peripheral vein into the caval veins. The diameter of these latter catheters
is of necessity relatively small and flows corresponding to the cardiac output
are not attained. The catheters are best made of semiflexible, thin walled
plastic with multiple side openings to prevent occlusion by the venous walls
during suction. Tubing and connectors must always be wider than the cannulae so as to minimize resistance to flow. Venous reservoirs facilitate syphonage, can be used to remove or add blood to the oxygenator as required and
can mirror the blood volume of the extracorporeal circuit.

HEMODYNAMICS OF ARTERIAL RE-ENTRY

Just as the applied hemodynamics of venous drainage center on the problem of venous collapse, so the hemodynamics of arterial re-entry must be discussed primarily in terms of velocity of flow. The limit to arterial infusion is
not the volume of blood to be circulated—modern blood pumps can deliver
larger flow rates than the body ever requires. The limit is the stenosis at the
site of arterial re-entry, which results in high velocities of flow, turbulence,
and damage to the blood elements.

Turbulence appears in flowing blood (Coulter and Pappenheimer, 1949) when the
forces tending to drive the fluid particles apart (inertial) prevail over the forces tending
to hold them together (viscous). The inertial force per unit of volume is proportional to
$\dfrac{\rho \bar{v}^2}{r}$ (where ρ is the density, $\bar{v}$ the average velocity of flow and r the radius of the tube),
while the viscous force is proportional to $\dfrac{\eta \bar{v}}{r^2}$ (where η is the viscosity coefficient). The
ratio of inertial forces to the viscous forces can be stated for any specific flowing system
by a dimensionless expression called the Reynold's number R_e, which corresponds to
$\dfrac{\rho \bar{v} r}{\eta}$. When the viscous forces are dominant, laminar flow conditions prevail. As flow is
increased in a given system, the inertial force, proportional to the square of the flow velocity, increases faster than does the viscous force, which is proportional to the first
power of the flow velocity. The transition to turbulent flow occurs when the viscous
forces are no longer able to damp stray disturbances in the fluid. At that particular
point, the ratio between inertial and viscous force defines the critical Reynolds number.

The critical Reynolds number for blood has been found to be around 1,000 in vitro
(Coulter and Pappenheimer, 1949). It has been estimated to be about twice as high under
in vivo conditions by Reynolds, et al. (1952). The exact critical value depends upon a
variety of factors such as curvature of the tube, the smoothness of its walls and the flow
conditions at the inlet. For instance, a curvature in a pipe carrying water can raise the
threshold for the onset of turbulence from about 2,000 to over 7,000. It is therefore impossible to state a given Reynold's number above which turbulence will necessarily appear in the arterial infusion line. Nevertheless one can easily demonstrate that desirable
flow rates the use of relatively narrow arterial cannulae can indeed provoke turbulence
(see fig. 71). Andres, et al. (1954) measured the shearing stresses which rupture erythrocytes exposed to turbulent flow. Using a jet injection technique, they found that mechanical destruction of erythrocytes becomes detectable when the kinetic energy per second

of injection reaches 10,000 to 20,000 g. cm^2 sec^{-2}. If these data are directly applicable to the conditions of extracorporeal circulation, then the flow across an arterial cannula of 5 mm. i.d. should not exceed 1,200 to 2,400 ml./min.

Senning (1952) already noted that reduction by half in the cannula diameter would result in a twofold increase in hemolysis. The existence of a critical flow velocity at between 100 and 150 cm./sec. is also apparent in recent studies by Ruedi and Fleisch (1960), who furthermore observed that at velocities between 200 and 700 cm./sec., hemolysis is an exponential function of the blood flow velocity. As far as the tubing is concerned, the need for caution is suggested by the measurements of Stewart and Sturridge (1959). Using the best available material, these authors found that hemolysis could be completely prevented if very large bore tubing was employed. From their data, the maximum "safe" flow velocity is 6.5 cm./sec. for tubing 6 mm. i.d., 13.3 cm./sec. for tubing 12 mm. i.d. and 25.8 cm./sec. for tubing 24 mm. i.d. The problems associated with the linear speed of blood in the arterial line have been discussed by Baranov (1959).

There are other mechanical factors affecting arterial re-entry to consider besides the velocity of flow in the arterial line. One is the negative hydrostatic pressure generated at the emergence of the arterial cannula, either with laminar flow (Venturi effect) or with turbulent flow (vortices). Since the blood equilibrated with oxygen in the artificial lung is often supersaturated and contains gas nuclei, cavitation* at the cannula outlet may bring about the release of gas bubbles in the blood stream (Ross, 1959). Cavitation sites can be detected either audibly or by the appearance of gas bubbles using in vitro models. According to Ross, the volume of blood flow in relation to cannula size which is necessary for cavitation is considerably greater than that ordinarily encountered—with a cannula of 3 mm. diameter for instance, cavitation does not occur until the flow reaches 4.5 L./min. Nevertheless, the size and number of the gas particles present in the blood, as well as the addition of CO_2 to the gas equilibrating mixture in the artificial lung, are factors which could be critical in the development of cavitation under practical conditions.

The pressure in the arterial line as such could be a traumatic agent for certain blood elements, particularly for the platelets (Tullis, 1958; Chevret and Besson, 1958). The evidence for such a direct pressure effect is mainly inferential. Further studies under physically well controlled conditions are required.

The rate of pressure drop across the catheter itself or across the reducing connector must also be considered. The arterial line is usually three-eighths inch in diameter, or 50 to 100 per cent wider than the cannula. Thus a reduction is needed to connect the tubing to the relatively narrow arterial cannula. It has been established empirically that, for maximum security, the connecting piece should provide a gradual tapering of the inside diameter and present no shoulder to the blood stream (Guastavino, et al., 1959a). The curvature of the cannula itself may also help in preventing turbulence. However, as far as we know, no systematic study to determine the most favorable shape has been reported.

---

* Cavitation is a term used by physicists to indicate the formation of little gas-filled "caves" in a fluid passing at high velocity from a narrowed bed into a wide area. Owing to the subatmospheric pressure at the place of the tube widening, gas (oxygen, carbon dioxide or nitrogen) can be released from the flowing blood.

A final point to consider concerns the effects of infusion on the arterial wall. Watkins, et al. (1960), have noted that low amplitude pulsations produce less pulse recoil of small bore cannulae inserted in the arterial tree. With high amplitude pulsations, they have observed trauma to arteries inflicted by vigorous pulse recoil of the cannula. Dissecting aneurysms incident to cannulation for total body perfusion were reported by Jones, et al. (1960). Another subject which has been almost completely neglected concerns the effect of repeated arterial wall distension upon vasomotion. Vasoconstriction of the arterial wall following mechanical distension has been a subject of controversy among physiologists ever since Bayliss (1902) reported it. As pointed out recently by Thieblot, et al. (1959), this mechanism may play a role in every procedure involving countercurrent arterial infusion, and thus possibly in heart–lung bypass.

Summarizing:

The practical hemodynamics of arterial re-entry center primarily on damage to blood by high flow velocities through relatively narrow cannulae. Upon transition from laminar to turbulent flow, the formed blood elements are likely to be traumatized. The development of subatmospheric pressures at the site of emergence from the stenosed arterial cannula into the wider artery may result in gas bubble formation due to cavitation. It is not the flow capacity of the arterial pump, but the damage to blood by the extreme velocity of flow which limits the amount of blood which can safely be returned to the arterial system.

ARTERIAL INFUSION

With respect to arterial infusion, two factors can be singled out which have been subject to dispute in the past and are still controversial today. These are the best site for the arterial cannulation and the best material for the arterial cannulae.

1. Site of injection: In heart–lung bypass procedures the blood is returned to the organism through a peripheral artery with the catheter pointing towards the aorta (fig. 73). To accommodate the necessary flow, it must be infused into a large enough artery which then can be safely repaired or tied off after the cannulation. Since the area of ejection at the end of the cannula is smaller than the area of the aortic ostium, the blood flow velocity at the outlet must necessarily be larger than under normal circulatory conditions if the perfusion flow is to match the normal cardiac output. A jet-type of infusion must be expected, the characteristics of which depend upon the site of cannulation (Yasargil, 1960).

In experimental animals, the femoral, subclavian and carotid artery have been used for arterial infusion. In man, it was felt in the early days of cardiac surgery that the left subclavian artery (fig. 73 B) provided the best cannulation site for whole body perfusion. Some controversy arose about the biological advantage of returning the blood via a femoral artery (fig. 73 C) rather than via the subclavian. It may very well be that with the low perfusion rates used at the time, return of blood directly to the aortic arch provided better coronary and cerebral flow than could infusion through a smaller, more distant vessel. Some authors, however, felt that when femoral cannulation was used, the priming blood of the artificial circuit first perfused the lower part of the body, where it could be cleared and filtered in the kidneys before perfusing vital organs such as the brain or the heart (Salisbury, 1956b). With the perfection of gas exchange techniques and the advent of high perfusion rates, this controversy has lost some of its meaning. Simultaneously, the emergence of the median sternotomy incision as the incision of choice for most intracardiac operations (Julian, et al., 1957) has forced abandonment of the left subclavian artery. Lillehei and Cardozo (1959) recommended use of the femoral artery, while Kirklin and Lyons (1960) found it rather disadvantageous owing to its small size. They preferred the right external iliac artery or, if necessary, the common iliac artery, exposed extraperitoneally through a low abdominal incision. Simultaneous cannulation of two peripheral arteries has been advocated from time to time (Parola, et al., 1958b; Guastavino, et al., 1959a-d). The direct use of the aorta by means of special cannulae (Kunlin, 1952) or grafts implanted on the side (Dodrill, et al., 1957; Julian, et al., 1957) obviates the inconvenience of small bore vessels. This has been found to be useful for obtaining high perfusion flow rates in small infants (Nuñez and Bailey, 1959) Aortic cannulation provides the best approach to normal flow direction in the arterial system. Difficulties associated with reversed flow in the aorta were apparent in a clinical case, reported by Schmutzer (1959), in which it was impossible to prevent hypotension in the upper part of the body when arterial blood was perfused from a peripheral artery, although, normal direction of flow in the aortic arch resulted in normal circulatory conditions.

2. Arterial cannulae: Cannulae made of plastic material or metal are recommended. Thin-walled stainless steel cannulae offer a distinct advantage because almost their full cross-

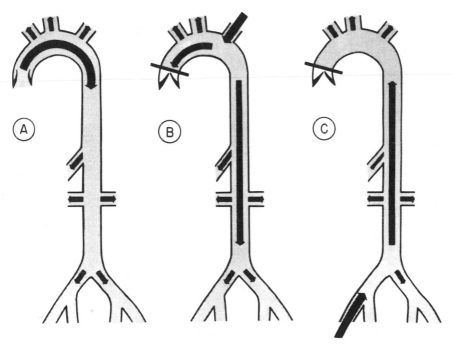

Fig. 73. Scheme of circulation in the arterial tree under normal conditions and during heart–lung bypass. The width of the arrows symbolizes the magnitude of the blood flow in the vessel.

A. Normal circulation: blood is ejected by the left ventricle, flows down the aorta and is distributed to the peripheral arteries.

B. Heart–lung bypass with arterial infusion through the left subclavian artery. The direction of blood flow is reversed only in the aortic arch.

C. Heart–lung bypass with arterial infusion through the right femoral artery. The direction of flow is reversed in the abdominal and thoracic aorta. (Modified from Yasargil, 1960.)

section can be used for blood flow. The usual plastic catheters on the other hand require a considerable wall thickness in order to be suitably rigid, and this cuts down the effective cross-section available for blood flow. The effect of such a lumen reduction upon the velocity of the blood stream is obvious. Furthermore, the narrow portion of a plastic arterial catheter is usually much longer than the narrow segment of the metal cannula, and thus offers more resistance to flow. On the other hand, a more careful catheterization technique is required when using a metal cannula and the repair of the vessel may be more difficult. Some are of the opinion that thin-walled teflon catheters mounted on metal connectors combine the advantages of both systems.

A tapered polyvinyl chloride arterial catheter has been proposed to improve over the relatively abrupt tapering in the metal connectors or cannulae (Elder, 1961). The decrease in diameter from the arterial line to the outlet is extended over the entire length of the catheter by this means. Once the perfused vessel is isolated, the tip of the catheter is cut at the place which matches the size of the artery.

The pressure difference across an arterial cannula should be kept to a minimum by selecting a size adapted to the perfusion flow expected (Bain and Mackey, 1959; McGoon, et al., 1960). With proper cannulation technique, it is possible to carry a flow of 2.4 to 2.8 L./sq. m./min. with a pressure difference along the arterial cannula of between 20 and 50 mm. Hg. (fig. 74). The resistance of the arterial line can be low enough to permit, under special circumstances, arterial infusion by gravity (Galletti, et al., 1960), as first suggested by Karlson (1952).

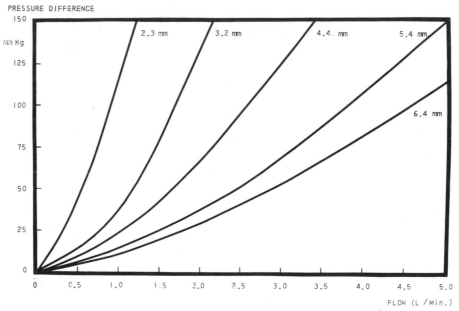

Fig. 74. Relationship between blood flow and gradient of pressure required with different sizes of short, stainless steel cannulae (Redrawn from Harshbarger, et al., 1958).

Summarizing:

The optimal site of blood infusion into the arterial system is not yet established. In the early days of open-heart surgery, the left subclavian artery was considered the best vessel because large bore cannulae could be inserted and better cerebral and coronary perfusion could be achieved. Smaller peripheral arteries such as the femoral or external iliac are now more convenient, but make high flow velocities the limiting factor for larger perfusion volumes.

With thin-walled stainless steel cannulae, almost the full cross-section can carry blood flow, whereas the usual plastic catheters require fairly thick walls to achieve the rigidity needed for cannulation—thus limiting the flow.

CARDIOTOMY BLOOD RETURN

When the caval veins are occluded for the purpose of diverting returning venous blood in the extracorporeal circuit, there is still a sizeable amount of venous blood returning directly to the right heart cavities via the coronary sinus, the anterior coronary veins, and the Thebesian vessels. If no cardiotomy is performed, this blood will fill the right ventricle, be ejected into the pulmonary vascular bed, return to the left heart, and then be ejected into the aorta. If the heart has been arrested, no ejection is possible and acute over dilatation will ensue, accompanied by flooding of the pulmonary vascular bed and pulmonary edema. Complete heart–lung bypass and a dry operative field for open heart surgery therefore require that the coronary sinus blood be removed to the outside. The same holds true for bronchial venous blood returning via the pulmonary veins to the left heart cavities. If the heart is arrested and if there is no defect in the cardiac septa to permit drainage towards the right heart cavities, some escape vent must be provided to prevent pulmonary and cardiac damage.

Under normal circulatory conditions, the coronary blood flow amounts to six to ten per cent, and the bronchial flow to one or two per cent of the cardiac output. Thus during heart–lung bypass, one may expect that about ten per cent of the blood infused into the arterial tree will pass to the heart instead of returning to the venous drainage line. While the blood accumulating in the heart can be discarded during perfusion of small organisms, in most cases the amount is so large that its loss would limit heart–lung bypass to no more than a few minutes. The recovery and utilization of this blood are therefore of major importance (Helmsworth, et al., 1953b; Miller, et al., 1953).

The venous blood which must be evacuated from the heart cavities is usually referred to as "cardiotomy return blood." Experience has demonstrated that the capacity of the system for removing the cardiotomy return blood must be far above the calculated ten per cent of the capacity of arterial infusion. To handle pathologic and emergency situations, the drainage capacity of the cardiotomy return system must reach at least 50 per cent of the perfusion flow. By simple comparison with the venous drainage system, one can deduce that a considerable degree of suction will at times be needed. However, this is primarily intermittent suction from an open well, so that much room air enters the cardiotomy return line, and must be eliminated before this blood is mixed with the regular venous blood. The technical aspects of cardiotomy return are therefore concerned with (a) large drainage capacity; (b) minimal degree of suction, to avoid blood trauma; (c) minimal admixture of air; and (d) reliable defoaming capacity (Miller and Allbritten, 1960).

Different systems have been proposed to handle the cardiotomy return blood. The simplest one (fig. 75 A) consists of a collection chamber into which the cardiotomy blood is aspirated by negative pressure. The blood then flows by gravity into the venous side of the extracorporeal circuit. The large gas bubbles collect and burst at the surface of

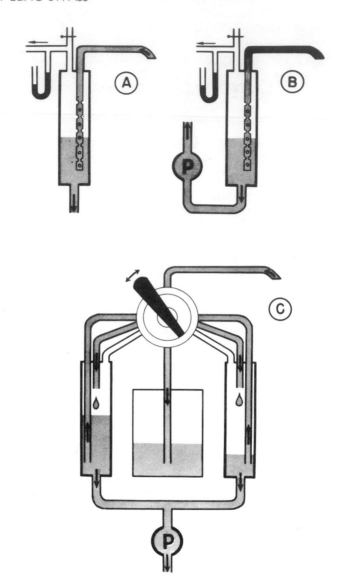

Fig. 75. Systems used for handling the cardiotomy return blood.

A. Suction tip connected to a reservoir maintained under a slight negative pressure. From the reservoir, blood flows by gravity into the main venous line or into the oxygenator.

B. Suction tip connected to a reservoir maintained under negative pressure, as in **A**. To prevent backflow from the oxygenator should considerable suction be exerted, a pump which acts simultaneously as a valve is used for transferring blood from the cardiotomy reservoir into the oxygenator.

C. Suction system devised by Watkins and Hering (1959). A valve manifold, or multiple stopcock (upper center) directs the blood aspirated at the suction tip into one or another graduated glass cylinder (left and right sides). The valve manifold also provides a negative pressure in the collecting reservoirs. When the graduated cylinders are full, blood can either be returned to the main circuit by means of a pump (P), or aspirated through the valve manifold into a storage reservoir (center), if the blood should not be returned to the organism. This system permits measurement of the blood volume aspirated from the cardiotomy.

the blood in the collecting chamber. When complete defoaming is needed (as is the case in all artificial lungs, except for bubble oxygenators), the walls of the reservoir may be smeared with antifoam, or an antifoam-coated baffle system may be interposed in the course of the blood stream. The negative pressure is maintained at the lowest effective value, by means of an adjustable control mechanism. Often this system does not provide enough suction to increase radically the flow when the need arises for rapid removal of large quantities of blood. It would then be necessary to increase the vacuum by occluding the air vent hose. The flow from aspirator tip to collection chamber will then increase, but the increased vacuum may also cause blood to flow back from the oxygenator into the collection chamber. As stressed by McCaughan, et al. (1958a), the maximum amount of blood which can be aspirated through a given size of aspirator and tubing equals the flow which would be obtained if gravity alone were used between the heart level and the oxygenator. Thus to increase capacity, the cardiac sucker and tubing should be as wide and short as practical usage will permit.

Owing to limitations of the combined vacuum-gravity system, many prefer to insert a pump of adjustable capacity between the cardiotomy collection chamber and the oxygenator (fig. 75 B). This pump can be accelerated to carry more flow when the vacuum suction is increased. In such situations the position of the oxygenator is also independent of the heart level.

A system incorporating a reservoir under negative pressure into which the blood is drawn from the sucker line, plus an occlusive pump which transports the blood from the reservoir to the oxygenator, and prevents backflow, has been described by Jones, et al. (1955) and Donald, et al. (1956). The main feature of the I.B.M.-Mayo system is that defoaming is achieved without the use of antifoam agents. Air bubbles are removed by a combination of several actions. As the blood enters the reservoir, it is spread on the surface of a stainless steel dispersion cone in order to achieve a thin, slow-moving film from which bubbles are easily released. Negative pressure contributes to the expansion of the bubbles and the pool at the bottom of the reservoir represents an additional safety against carrying away of foam.

The suction apparatus described by Watkins and Hering (1959) also features many refinements. Basically, it consists of a valve manifold by which blood can be directed from the suction tip into one or another narrow flask for accurate measurement of the blood volume collected (fig. 75 C). Blood can then either be returned to the extracorporeal circuit by means of a pump, or be sucked into a storage reservoir if its use is contraindicated.

Additional improvements in the cardiotomy return system include provisions for attaching other drainage lines for blood from the left atrium, and anomalous pulmonary vein, pulmonary artery or the pleural cavity. Suction tips which cannot be occluded by tissues drawn up into them have been designed for aspirating shallow pools of blood (Cross and Jones, 1961). Special sucker probes featuring a vacuum-regulating knob are also available. The flow of air can thus be cut down when little blood is to be removed, and thereby prevent the drying effect of large volumes of gas. Such a probe is used in the blood recovery system devised by Weiss and Sprovieri (1958), which includes a hand-controlled suction tip, an inclined spillway for debubbling, and a reservoir maintained under slight negative pressure, out of which the blood is intermittently returned to the main circuit (fig. 76 A).

In many circuits, the "coronary" pump is connected directly to the cardiotomy sucker (fig. 76 B). Although the negative pressure induced by such a device will at times undoubtedly exceed the values set by a controlled vacuum system, there are practical reasons for using a pump system when the cardiotomy venous return is expected to be high. In such situations, a relatively high suction can often be used without too much trauma to the blood since only minimal amounts of air are aspirated with the blood. It has now been proven that pump or negative pressure alone contribute little to hemolysis (McCaughan, et al., 1958b). The major cause of hemolysis is the turbulent mixing of air and blood (DeWall, et al., 1958; Gerbode, et al., 1960a) and this must be ascribed to the high flow velocities reached when small amounts of blood are mixed with considerable volumes

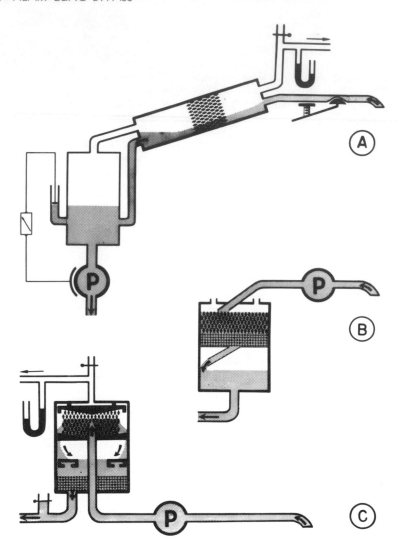

Fig. 76. Systems used for handling the cardiotomy return blood.

A. Circuit described by Weiss and Sprovieri (1958). Blood is aspirated by a hand-controlled suction tip into a sloping chamber filled with an antifoam-coated sponge (black diamonds). After defoaming, the blood settles in a reservoir (vertical rectangle), which is intermittently emptied by the pump (P). The pump is actuated by a level sensing device and its output is measured as a record of the volume of blood passing through the cardiotomy return system.

B. Suction system with a pump (P) for aspirating the cardiotomy blood into a reservoir. The blood mixed with air encounters an antifoam-coated sponge (black diamonds), then a filter (checked area), before accumulating in a pool at the bottom of the reservoir (Gross, et al., 1960).

C. Cardiotomy return system of Winterscheid, et al. (1960). The amount of suction generated at the suction tip depends upon the speed of the roller pump (P), which is regulated through a variac control by means of a foot switch (neither one represented). The blood entering the cardiotomy drainage reservoir, maintained under negative pressure, is defoamed on an antifoam-coated sponge (black diamonds). It spreads over the walls of the container and is prevented from splashing by means of floating baffles. The blood settles at the bottom of the reservoir and is still filtered (checkered area) before returning to the oxygenator.

of gas (Ruedi and Fleisch, 1960). The most sophisticated cardiotomy return system is that devised by Winterscheid, et al. (1960), which insures minimal air–blood mixing. This system also provides a reservoir where the velocity of blood approaches zero, a defoaming agent for removing the gas bubbles, a slight subatmospheric pressure to contribute to bubble expansion, and filters for removing any particles which may have entered the blood stream (fig. 76 C).

Summarizing:

"Cardiotomy return blood" comprises all blood from the coronary and bronchial circulation as well as from abnormal sources collecting in the right heart cavities. The capacity of the system for removing this blood must approach 50 per cent of the perfusion flow to handle pathologic and emergency situations. The cardiac sucker and tubing should be as wide and as short as is practical. Turbulent mixing of air and blood should be kept to a minimum, in order to prevent hemolysis, and the collected blood should be cleared of bubbles and debris before entering the oxygenator.

XIII. Hemodynamic Aspects of Total Heart-Lung Bypass

In the study of hemodynamic patterns associated with total heart–lung bypass, one usually takes the circulation in the normal intact organism as an ideal model of regulation. This attitude undoubtedly represents a safe approach to the problems of perfusion. Practically, however, normal and artificial circulation differ from each other in several important characteristics, which should be kept in mind in the following discussion. During total body perfusion, the organism is anesthetized, the heart and lungs are empty and the superior and inferior caval beds are usually separated. The distribution of blood among the organ systems is altered because of the exclusion of the heart and lungs and of abnomalous manner of drainage and infusion. Finally, owing to the geometric limitations imposed by the cannulations, the extracorporeal blood flow is often below the resting cardiac output.

Total body perfusion represents a most exciting hemodynamic experiment, since it offers the unique possibility of controlling blood flow, intravascular pressures and circulating blood volume at will. Because these parameters are interrelated in ways still not fully understood, total body perfusion also presents a difficult challenge to those who attempt it. Empirically one aims at performing bypass procedures with minimal deviations from normal physiologic function, which are followed by prompt and complete recovery of the patients. This chapter is an attempt to systematize the approach to this object.

PERFUSION FLOW, PRESSURE AND RESISTANCE

During total heart–lung bypass the perfusion flow rate in most instances is arbitrarily selected according to metabolic and hemodynamic criteria. The aim is a steady flow rate approximating the cardiac output of the lightly anesthetized patient prior to perfusion. In open-chest conditions, such flow rates can be reached, or at least approached, with maintenance of a normal blood volume, by proper positioning of large diameter venous cannulae and adequate operation of the pump-oxygenator. These flows initially result in a mean aortic pressure 10 to 30 mm. Hg. below that prior to cardiopulmonary bypass. The mean central venous pressure is ordinarily maintained between 5 and 15 mm. Hg., that is at a somewhat higher level than before surgery. As the perfusion continues, the arterial pressure gradually rises and tends to return to normal. When the pump oxygenator is discontinued and the heart and lungs are allowed to resume their function after a trouble-free perfusion, the arterial blood pressure often increases to a moderate extent (Dodrill, et al., 1957; Donald and Moffit, 1957; Mendelsohn, et al., 1957; Levowitz, et al., 1958; Andersen and Senning, 1958; Ivanova, 1958; Gianelli, et al., 1958; Moffit, et al., 1959; Melrose, 1959; McGoon, et al., 1960; Sanger, et al., 1960).

The pattern of pressure variation just described represents an ideal which is only approached when the perfusion flow rate is immediately adequate from both hemodynamic and metabolic points of view. It indicates that the total peripheral resistance is approximately normal, with possibly some degree of vasodilation at the beginning of bypass, followed by a vasoconstrictive phase. Actual determinations in man have not demonstrated any significant difference in total peripheral resistance between a perfusion period and a previous cardiac catheterization. In dogs, direct flow and pressure measurements immediately before and during perfusion at "normal" flow rates also did not indicate marked changes in peripheral resistance (Cordell, et al., 1960; Rowen, et al., 1960).

Much more care must be taken in the interpretation of such data than is often the case. First, a variation in arterio-venous pressure difference and in calculated peripheral resistance does not necessarily indicate active vasomotion unless the blood flow is kept constant throughout the period of comparison. In fact, resistance decreases with increased flow when one perfuses an inanimate model of the circulation. To establish that vasomotion has occurred between two periods of measurement, when there has been a change in flow, it must be demonstrated that the slope of the flow-pressure curve has

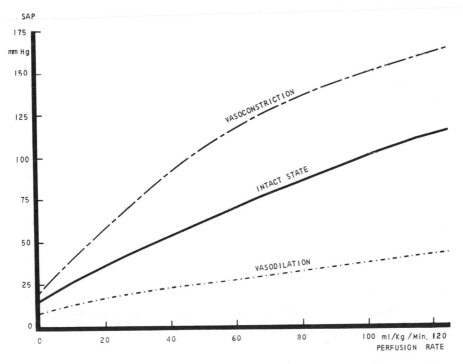

Fig. 77. Relationship of mean systemic arterial pressure (SAP) to perfusion flow rate in the normal vasomotor state and under the influence of vasoconstrictor or vasodilator agents. (Modified from Read, et al., 1957b.)

changed. This can hardly be ascertained in human perfusions. In dogs, transfusion reactions at the inception of bypass often result in vasodilation which must be ascribed to the blood mixing aspect of the procedure rather than to its hemodynamic features.

Within the range of flow encountered in total body perfusion, the arterial pressure is approximately a linear function of the perfusion rate (Read, et al., 1957b; Kirklin, et al., 1957; Birkeland, 1959; Grodins, et al., 1960). Extrapolation to zero flow intercepts the pressure axis at about 20 mm. Hg. (fig. 77). A convexity towards the pressure axis at flow rates below 20 ml./Kg./min. (about 0.5 L./sq. m./min.) and a leveling of pressure values when the perfusion exceeds the basal cardiac output are common findings. Increased vasomotor tone is not only associated with a steeper slope but also with a curvilinear pressure-flow function extending over the whole range of perfusion rates. On the other hand, vasodilation is characterized by a more linear plot (Read, et al., 1957b). These data indicate that under all conditions of vasomotion the total peripheral resistance is an inverse function of flow (fig. 78), as is the case in isolated vascular beds. In other words, increased peripheral resistance does not necessarily mean vasoconstriction, and decreased peripheral resistance is not synonymous of vasodilation. It is likely that, apart from passive changes in calculated resistance, which can be explained on purely mechanical considerations, there are reflex changes caused by active vasomotion. For instance, at very high flow rates, the aortic and carotid baroreceptor mechanism is ex-

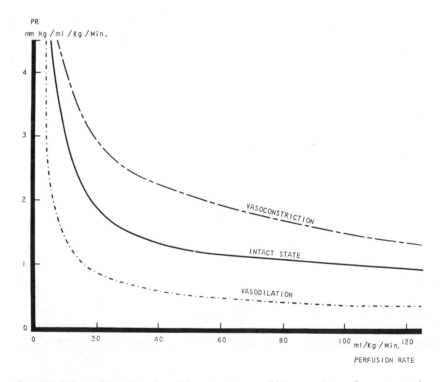

Fig. 78. Relationship of total peripheral resistance (PR) to perfusion flow rate in the normal vasomotor state and under the influence of vasoconstrictor or vasodilator agents. (Modified from Read, et al., 1957.)

pected to induce vasodilation, while at low flow rates hypoxia and release of catecholamines may contribute to the increase in resistance. As long as experiments under strictly controlled circulations have not been reported, it is impossible to decide whether changes in total peripheral resistance associated with flow variations are active or passive in nature or a combination of both.

Nevertheless, there is considerable evidence that vasomotor activity is maintained during total heart–lung bypass. By pharmacologic studies, Read, et al. (1957b) have been able to demonstrate that total peripheral resistance in the perfused state is made up of three elements, approximately equal in magnitude: Nervous influences account for one third, inherent myogenic tone of the blood vessel wall contributes another third, and the remainder results from viscous properties of the blood and dimensional factors in the completely relaxed vessels. The persistence of vasomotor activity, both intrinsic and neurogenic, during complete heart–lung bypass, is also demonstrated by the changes in resistance in response to stretching of the lungs (Salisbury, et al., 1959c), stretching of the ventricular walls (Salisbury, et al., 1960a; Ross, et al., 1961b), acute hypoxia (Sanger, et al., 1960), carotid sinus hypertension (Ross, et al., 1961a), and other similar stresses.

During successful perfusions, the total peripheral resistance tends to increase gradually (Moffit, et al., 1959; McGoon, et al., 1960; Cordell, et al., 1960). Thus, if there is some degree of vasodilation at the beginning of bypass, as is often the case, compensatory vasoconstriction soon occurs. When perfusion is prolonged for many hours, these initial reactions are often followed by a second, more pronounced, vasodilation (Sanger, et al., 1960). Upon termination of bypass, there is a sharp decrease in total peripheral resistance (Ankeney, et al., 1958; Cordell, et al., 1960; Rowen, et al., 1960), which may represent vasodilation, increase in flow or both.

The time course of these vasoreactive phases is not completely understood. It is a common observation during perfusions that the arterial pressure fluctuates despite unchanged flow rates. On the other hand, if efforts are made to keep the arterial pressure constant, the flow rate has to be adjusted repeatedly (Sanger, et al., 1960). Possible explanations for fluctuations in peripheral resistance during perfusion are numerous.

1. There could be a direct effect of circulating vasomotor substances liberated by destruction of formed blood elements, e.g., adenosine triphosphate and serotonin, as indicated by the early observations of Fleisch (1938), suggested again by Nyhus (1958), and recently substantiated by the investigations of Sarajas, et al. (1959, 1960). The formation of a vasopressor substance by incubation of plasma (Eichholtz and Verney, 1924; Khairallah and Page, 1960) could also be relevant to the conditions of extracorporeal circulation, although there is still no basis for deciding whether or not it plays a significant role.

2. Endogenous vasomotor substances could also be liberated by the stress of perfusion, the action being mediated either by local metabolic conditions (Freeburg and Hyman, 1960), or by the stimulation of local stretch receptors involved in the reflex control of hormonal secretion. Few actual data are available to support this hypothesis (Belisle, et al., 1960).

3. Fluctuations in the activity of the sympathetic nervous system related to fluctuations in the level of anesthesia play a role in partial perfusions of very long duration (Galletti, et al., 1960) and this may also occur in total perfusions (Read, et al., 1957b).

4. Local vascular changes at the periphery, such as arteriolar or venular occlusion, or opening of arteriovenous anastomoses, may affect peripheral resistance. Intravascular aggregation of red cells (sludging), leading to a marked decrease in the number of functional capillaries, has also been demonstrated by direct observations of the microcirculation (Takeda, 1960; Nonoyama, 1960).

5. The possibility of changes in viscosity of the perfusing blood due to loss of water from the vascular compartment, changes in temperature or other physical factors must be kept in mind.

In conclusion vasomotor reactions in the perfused state may have different origins. They are not necessarily the expressions of a pathologic mechanism. Moreover, it remains to be proved that in the course of a smooth, successful perfusion fluctuations in peripheral resistance exceed those encountered in the normal, intact organism.

Summarizing:

The pressure-flow-resistance relations as they prevail in a lightly anesthetized organism, are generally considered to be the most desirable during heart–lung bypass. That these can be achieved under ideal conditions suggests that there are only minor vasomotor changes during successful perfusions. The arterial pressure is approximately a linear function of the extracorporeal flow. Fluctuations in vasomotor activity are encountered in lengthy perfusions and may be caused by various hemodynamic or metabolic disturbances.

CONTROL OF THE CIRCULATING BLOOD VOLUME

It has long been recognized that maintenance of a constant systemic blood volume is one of the important factors in successful heart–lung bypass. In contrast with the intact circulatory system, which can readily compensate for moderate amounts of transfusion or blood loss, the mechanically supported circulation is extremely sensitive even to small variations in the blood content of the vascular system. Since the capillary and venous segments of the circulation contain about 80 per cent of the body blood volume, one would expect veins and capillaries to play a major role in the regulation of systemic blood volume and flow during perfusion. Indeed, Gibbs (1930) and Barcroft (1933) observed quite early that the body blood volume is the most important determinant of venous return to an artificial heart, and that transfusion markedly increases the systemic blood flow in a perfused animal. The details of the mechanism by which blood volume is associated with the regulation of flow are not fully understood, and there are only few reviews of the problem which take into account the mechanical aspects of artificial circulation as well as the reflex control of the peripheral circulation at the capillary and venous level (Galletti, et al., 1961). We shall attempt to delineate the question as it now stands.

Since there is no practical way of detecting changes in body blood volume directly and instantly during heart–lung bypass, the problem has first been approached by using indirect methods. The use of calibrated venous and arterial pumps, set to deliver exactly the same flow, makes the constancy of blood volume in the perfused organism dependent upon the accuracy of calibration. This also applies when equal venous and arterial flows are measured by rate recording flowmeters. Practically, the accuracy of such calibrations cannot exceed ±1 per cent. Therefore this type of blood volume control becomes grossly unreliable when the perfusion is maintained for longer than a few minutes. One can easily calculate that if the discrepancy between venous and arterial flow were as small as one per cent, and the total volume of blood available were exchanged every two minutes, the body blood volume could increase, or decrease, by as much as 25 per cent of its initial value within 30 minutes of perfusion without being detected.

Most techniques for controlling the body blood volume rely upon monitoring of the volume of blood in the extracorporeal circuit. The sum of body blood volume and extracorporeal blood volume is constant, so that an increase in one reflects a decrease in the other, and vice versa. Obviously, the recognition of alterations in the patient's blood volume then depends upon careful measurements of blood losses in the operative field (Klopstock, et al., 1959), and their immediate compensation. Assuming this condition is met, it suffices to monitor the blood level in the artificial lung and to alter the action of the pumps accordingly. Devices which perform such a control automatically are numerous. They usually include a level-sensing device: float (e.g., Crafoord, et al., 1957a), electrode (e.g., Olmsted, et al., 1958) or photo cell (e.g., Kantrowitz, et al., 1960), acting on the stroke (e.g., Crafoord, et al., 1957a) or rate setting of the arterial pump, or on a motor-actuated clamp on the gravity venous line (e.g., Kantrowitz, et al., 1960). One can also monitor the weight of the artificial lung using a scale, as suggested by Gott, et al. (1957a, b), or a mechanoelectrical transducer (Osborn, et al., 1960), and regulate the flow accordingly. Only recently has a simpler and more direct approach, following that originally proposed by Bazett and Quinby (1920) for regulating the body blood content in cross-circulation, been applied to partial (Galletti, et al., 1960) and total heart–lung bypass (Brecher, et al., 1955; Cordell, et al., 1960; Gianelli, et al., 1960). The operation board is mounted on a scale and equilibrated in the zero position just prior to perfusion. Thereafter changes in body weight should reflect changes in blood volume within the circulatory system. The drawback in this technique is that, for the time being, it is only applicable to experimental perfusions. One cannot distinguish between circulating blood and pooled blood (as often collects in the splanchnic circulation of the dog). Finally, in long term perfusions, fluid shifts between different body compartments mask or simulate blood volume changes. Despite these pitfalls, body weight measurements provide a simple direct approach to the control of blood volume. Clinically they are often used to check the compensation for blood losses after surgery. However, some doubt is cast on the reliability of weight measurements by the observations of Kaplan, et al. (1960) and of Redo and Arditi (1961), who usually found a moderately hypovolemic state after perfusion. It is likely that direct measurements of the circulating blood volume and of its elements, red blood cells and plasma, by radioactive isotopes dilution techniques, will soon be simplified to the extent that repeated measurements during and after bypass, procedures will be feasible (Rochlin, et al., 1957; Albert, et al., 1960, 1961; Swan, et al. 1960; Williams and Fine, 1961)

If there were no vasomotor reactions during total body perfusion, and no hemodynamic alterations due to connection of the vascular system to the extracorporeal circuit, blood flows approximating the basal cardiac output would result in normal blood pressures at the normal degree of filling of the vascular system. The ideal heart–lung bypass procedure would then require that the body blood volume be decreased at the beginning of the perfusion, because the heart and lungs are emptied by an amount equal to the central blood volume (that of the heart and lungs) that is approximately 20 per cent of the total blood volume. Conversely, at the end of the perfusion, this amount of blood would have to be returned to the circulation in order to refill the heart and lungs before disconnecting the pumps. Practically, there are many ways to deal with the blood content of the lesser circulation in heart–lung bypass procedures. Sometimes it is used to expand the blood content of the systemic circulation (fig. 79, 1). These workers who are careful to maintain a constant systemic blood volume add it to the extracorporeal circuit (fig. 79, 2) or store it in a reserve container if the artificial lung works best at constant blood volume (fig. 79, 3).

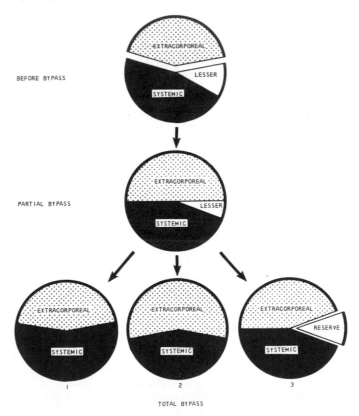

Fig. 79. Distribution of blood in the different compartments before and during heart–lung bypass. The blood in the extracorporeal circuit is represented by crosses, the blood volume of the systemic circulation (80 per cent of the total body blood content) is shown by black shading and the blood content of the lesser circulation, or central blood volume (about 20 per cent of the total blood volume) is unshaded. When the perfusion procedure is started, all three compartments are joined. The lesser circulation is progressively emptied during the period of partial heart–lung bypass. When total heart–lung bypass is achieved, the amount of blood corresponding to the central blood volume is either left in the systemic vascular bed (1), pooled in the extracorporeal circuit (2), or stored in a reserve compartment (3).

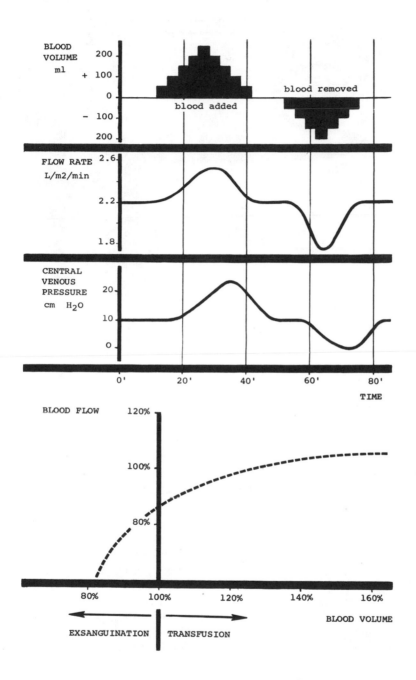

Fig. 80. Relationship between systemic blood volume and available venous return in dog (Modified after Bain and Mackey, 1959).

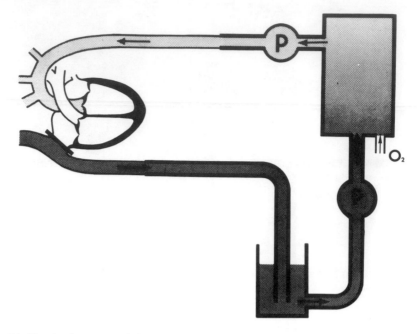

Fig. 81. Blood volume control during total body perfusion according to Gianelli, et al. (1958), and Kirby, et al. (1959, 1960). Provided wide, low resistance venous cannulae are used to permit low venous pressures, the systemic blood volume increases with increasing perfusion rates. The increment of blood needed is shifted from the extracorporeal circuit (venous reservoir or artificial lung) into the vascular system.

The expansion of the systemic blood volume by "transfusion" of the central blood volume or from the extracorporeal circuit is often necessary to achieve adequate blood flow. In fact, the relationship between body blood volume and attainable extracorporeal flow became apparent early in the development of perfusion techniques. Donald and Moffitt (1956) stated that in the dog, a 10 per cent reduction in blood volume causes a 50 per cent fall in venous return to the extracorporeal circuit, and consequently a 50 per cent fall in arterial infusion flow. Further quantitative investigation was pioneered by Herron, et al. (1958a, b), who demonstrated a direct, though widely scattered, relationship between body blood volume and available venous return. At control blood volume the spontaneous flow rate in dogs was usually in the range of 40 ml./Kg./min. To obtain flow approximating normal cardiac output, it was necessary to expand the blood volume to an average of 130 per cent of the control (fig. 80). These results have since been repeatedly confirmed. The data of Gianelli, et al. (1958) indicate a somewhat smaller expansion of blood volume at "normal" flow rates (5 to 25 per cent) than do those of Herron, et al. (1958a, b). Furthermore, the need for transfusion becomes relatively less as the flow is increased, and ceases altogether as the flow rate reaches 160 ml./Kg./min. On the other hand, Yarsagil (1960) had to transfuse an amount approximately 33 per cent of the body blood volume to achieve even subnormal flows. Observations by Levovitz, et al. (1958) and Lindberg (1959) fall in a similar range.

It should be pointed out that the results obtained in dogs are not directly transferable to man. It is a common experience, though not a widely published one, that dogs often undergo a mild transfusion reaction at the beginning of heart–lung bypass, with a fall in arterial pressure and a pooling of blood in the splanchnic circulation (*see* chap. XVI). The effects of this on venous return, perfusion flow and arterial pressure are minimized if one allows the animal to take up blood from the extracorporeal circuit (Dow, et al., 1960b), rather than losing to the artificial lung an amount corresponding to the central blood volume. The large transfusions sometimes needed at the beginning of heart–lung bypass in dogs do not necessarily mean a corresponding increase in circulating blood volume, since blood can simply be sequestered in the portal circulation. In lengthy perfusions, there is a tendency for moderate uptake of blood by the animal's vascular system. This trend has been documented in total (Gianelli, et al., 1960) as well as in partial heart–lung bypass (Galletti, et al., 1961).

In man, this tendency to blood pooling reaction is conspicuously absent and heart–lung bypass can be carried out without increase in systemic blood volume. However, a small transfusion (100 to 300 ml.) in the first minutes of bypass occasionally facilitates normal perfusion rates and thereby helps maintain acceptable pressure conditions. Gross, et al. (1960) state that if caval syphonage fails to drain more than 2 L./sq. m./min. and if the venous cannulae appear correctly placed, they transfuse to improve the venous return, though never more than five per cent of the calculated body blood volume. In general, experienced workers note a decrease in body blood volume at the beginning of perfusion at "normal" flow rates due to emptying of the heart and lungs (e.g., Waldhausen, et al., 1959b; McGoon, et al., 1960). This blood collects in the extracorporeal circuit, and must be returned to the organism during the perfusion only when the venous flow diminishes, as for example following surgical hemorrhage.

In view of the technical difficulties of maintaining a constant blood volume in the perfused organism, it is fortunate that the organism itself provides some degree of control. As demonstrated by Gianelli, et al. (1958) and Kirby, et al. (1959, 1960), there is a constant intravascular blood volume for each perfusion rate, as long as the venous pressure is maintained below 10 cm. H_2O by gravity venous suction (fig. 81). Under these conditions the amount of blood within the organism increases as the perfusion rate is increased. According to the data of Gianelli, et al. (1958) and Peirce (1958a), the body blood content increases by about 20 ml./Kg. when the perfusion flow changes from 30 ml./Kg./min. to 100 ml./Kg./min. This difference corresponds to about 20 per cent of the animal's blood volume prior to bypass. The essential condition for this train of events is the maintenance of a venous pressure within the normal range. This excludes distension of the great veins with increasing perfusion rates as a cause of blood uptake by the body, but does not permit further localization of that portion of the intracorporeal circuit which accommodates the larger volume of blood. The stability of the characteristic blood volume at each perfusion rate can be tested by transfusion or exsanguination. Following these maneuvers the body blood volume soon returns to control value, because the maneuver causes a decrease, or increase, in central venous pressure. The driving pressure along the venous catheter is then modified, resulting in a transient imbalance of venous drainage and arterial infusion until the central venous pressure comes back to normal. The adequacy of this compensatory

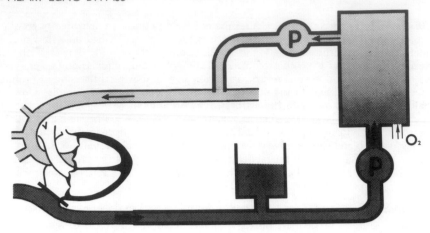

Fig. 82. Blood volume control during heart–lung bypass according to Peirce (1958a). A blood reservoir connected to the venous drainage line provides for constant venous pressure, transfuses the organism when the arterial perfusion flow is increased, stores blood when the perfusion flow is decreased.

shift depends upon the maintenance of central venous pressure in the "depleting" range, where small changes in pressure cause large changes in flow. It also requires the use of wide venous cannulae, capable of carrying the extra flow necessitated by transfusion with a minimal increase in pressure gradient. The same mechanism has been observed in our laboratory during *partial* heart–lung bypass with gravity venous drainage and gravity arterial infusion. The body blood content of a stable preparation cannot be radically modified by slow bleeding or transfusion because the organism automatically shifts a compensatory amount from or into the extracorporeal circuit. However, in both total and partial heart–lung bypass, the method does not work when a large, sudden hemorrhage occurs, or when vasoconstrictor drugs are injected. As pointed out by Herron, et al. (1958a, b), Kirby, et al. (1959), Ross, et al. (1961) and many others, adrenergic agents transiently increase the rate of venous return, and empty the venous system, thereby jeopardizing the basis for automatic control of the blood volume.

Essentially the same mechanisms operate when the blood volume is maintained constant as described by Peirce (1958a). Venous drainage and arterial infusion are performed by pumps set at a constant rate. The venous pressure is kept at the pre-perfusion level by raising or lowering a blood filled plastic bag, which acts as a venous pressure reservoir (fig. 82). If a transfusion is given to the organism during perfusion, the central venous pressure increases and more blood is lost to the extracorporeal circuit where it is stored in the bag. If there is hemorrhage which decreases the amount of venous blood available to the venous pump, blood is taken from the reservoir. Thus variations in reservoir weight accurately reflect changes in body blood volume. This system provides semi-automatic compensation for blood volume changes and is extremely stable.

The same physiological mechanisms also underlie control of body blood volume by regulation of the oxygenator blood content (fig. 83). Here the oxy-

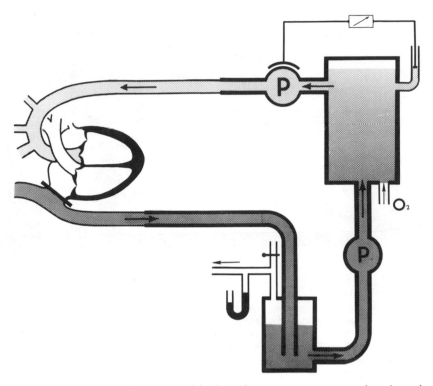

Fig. 83. Blood volume control during total body perfusion using a constant volume heart–lung machine. A level-sensing device in the artificial lung (upper right corner) controls the output of the arterial pump so as to maintain a constant volume of blood in the artificial lung. Variations in blood content of the vascular system are mirrored by variations in blood level in the venous reservoir (bottom). The amount of suction exerted on the reservoir can be varied to regulate the systemic blood content.

genator is a constant volume device, i.e., the volume of arterialized blood returned to the organism is exactly the same as the volume that the organism gives up to the machine. Should the patient bleed, the amount of venous blood drained into the extracorporeal circuit, for a given arrangement of cannulae and suction, will be decreased. Automatically the volume flow of the arterial infusion will slow down. Close observation of the arterial flow permits compensation for a decrease in perfusion rate by the addition of reserve blood to the oxygenator. The arterial perfusion rate then increases to the point when venous return is again able to match the desired output of the arterial pump. Thus the organism will be transfused and its initial blood volume restored by a transient imbalance of arterial infusion and venous drainage. Similarly, the system will react to an increased venous return, as caused, for example, by transfusion, by an increase in arterial perfusion rate.

In practical situations the flow regulating system should not react blindly to "physiologic" transfers of blood volumes, as for instance the emptying of the central compartment of the vascular system at the beginning of bypass. On the other hand, different types of artificial lungs require a relatively constant volume of blood to operate under the best conditions of efficiency and

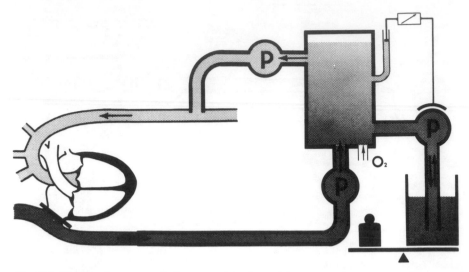

Fig. 84. Blood volume control during total body perfusion according to Waldhausen, et al. (1959b). The arterial pump is set at a constant flow rate. Any excess blood brought by the venous pump to the oxygenator causes a level-sensing device (upper right corner) to activate an auxiliary pump which transfers a corresponding amount to a reservoir. The reservoir can be placed on scales (lower right corner) or its volume measured in order to follow the changes in systemic blood volume. If the perfused organism requires a blood transfusion, the arterial pump is accelerated, while the auxiliary pump refills the oxygenator with blood from the reservoir.

safety. Some margin of operation can be provided by incorporating a storage compartment in the extracorporeal circuit. For instance Waldhausen, et al. (1959b), connected a blood reservoir to a rotating disc oxygenator by a reversible pump controlled through level sensing electrodes in the oxygenator (fig. 84). The arterial pump is set at constant flow rate and the reversible pump maintains a constant volume in the oxygenator by removing or adding appropriate amounts of blood from the reservoir. McGoon, et al. (1960) drain the venous blood by gentle suction into a reservoir. From there the blood is propelled to the top of the stationary screen oxygenator by a recirculation pump set to deliver at a constant flow rate (*see* fig. 26 B). The output of the arterial pump is regulated by level-sensing devices in the artificial lung so as to equal the rate of venous return from the organism, up to a maximum that equals the output of the recirculation pump. Venous return exceeding this minute volume is stored in the venous reservoir. This excess will be returned automatically to the circulation if venous return should diminish later as a result of surgical hemorrhage.

There is a recurrent tendency to explain the close relationship between systemic blood volume and available venous return in terms of "veno-venomotor," or "veno-vasomotor" reflexes. Although these mechanisms may exist, one should not forget that the pure hydro–hemodynamics in the open, mechanically supported circulation and in the closed, intact vascular system are not the same. There is no reason to believe that vasomotor mechanisms are "siderated" during artificial perfusion, since, for instance, the circulatory system continues to react to very small doses of vasoactive drugs. The absence of reservoir organs such as the heart and lungs does not prevent the marked increase in venous return when catecholamines are injected. Yet it is unlikely that venomotion plays an important role in the regulation of the flow–pressure relationship during heart–lung bypass (Read, et al., 1958). Recent studies by Ross, et al. (1961a, b) point to the control exerted by the carotid baroreceptor mechanism, and possibly by ventricular distension, over the tone of the venous bed. Their conclusions, associated with considerations of the mechanical particularities of the open circulation, give a satisfactory account of the role of blood volume in the regulation of perfusion flow (Galletti, et al., 1961).

Summarizing:

The maintenance of constant systemic blood volume is an essential condition for smooth perfusion. On the one hand, the perfused organism is extremely sensitive to variations in blood volume, and reacts to a small blood loss by marked reduction in venous return. On the other hand, the intravascular blood volume increases with the perfusion rate. Since the capillary and venous segments of the circulation contain 80 per cent of the body blood content, it is not surprising that venous pressure is closely related to systemic blood volume during perfusion. Mechanical factors characteristic of open circulation, together with reflex mechanisms which are best revealed when the heart and lungs are empty, account for the inability of the organism undergoing total perfusion to compensate for alterations in blood volume, and the observation of a characteristic blood volume for each steady perfusion rate.

DISTRIBUTION OF BLOOD FLOW AMONG VARIOUS VASCULAR BEDS

Under normal resting conditions, all tissues in the body do not receive an equal share of blood flow, nor is perfusion even proportional to the weight or apparent metabolic activity of an organ. Some organs or organ systems are profusely irrigated, while others receive a relatively small part of the cardiac output and extract proportionately more oxygen from their arterial blood quota. For instance the kidneys, which make up less than one per cent of body weight, receive about a quarter of the cardiac output. Since they use only about eight per cent of the total oxygen uptake, the renal arterio-venous oxygen difference is only one to three volumes per cent. The heart, with about the same weight as the kidneys, needs more oxygen, though its blood flow is less. Consequently, coronary venous blood is markedly desaturated.

The distribution of aortic blood flow among the various vascular beds in normal man is still not known in all details. Nevertheless, a tentative scheme can be formulated which is useful in considering what happens under conditions of artificial circulation. Furthermore, the mechanisms which regulate the distribution of blood flow, and maintain a balance in the face of changing hemodynamic conditions (Green and Kenchar, 1959) will also be involved when the organism is perfused by a mechanical device. Swan (1959) has given a lucid analysis of possible factors involved in control of the circulation when pressure and flow are artificially modified. Theoretically, two possibilities exist: "First the flow of blood to all organs may be reduced and all parts of the body share equally in the reduction of oxygen supply. Alternatively, and more probably, when the perfusion pressure is low, factors which control hindrance offered by the resistance vessels . . ., and which differ in different parts of the vascular system, may completely deprive certain organs of blood flow, while in other portions of the circulation flow may be normal."

The first determinant of regional flow is the vascular resistance of the organ system under consideration. This factor is best represented by the slope of the pressure-flow relationship which expresses how large an increase in flow is to be expected for an unitary increase in the head of pressure. The critical closing pressure, which is the transmural pressure at which collapse of the vessel walls occurs, is also an important factor in determining at what level of pressure the blood supply to an organ will cease. Geometric factors in the resistance vessels such as caliber, length, branching and taper must be considered. Finally the opening of new blood channels at capillary levels, such as arteriovenous anastomoses, may be involved under some conditions of perfusion. The curve relating pressure and flow for the whole body (see fig. 77) represents nothing but a weighted average of its regional components. Each individual organ has a different curve with a different slope and positive pressure intercept. It follows that when the perfusion pressure is decreased or increased, the variations in flow are *not* equal in all parts of the vascular bed on a purely hemodynamic basis.

Organs also have different mechanisms for coping with fluctuations in the gas tensions of the perfusing blood. The best protected organ, the brain, displays an exquisite sensitivity of vasomotor control to hypoxia and hypercapnia. It reacts by vasodilation to any decrease in the amount of oxygen distributed, thus providing for a relative constancy of cerebral blood flow despite fluctuations in cardiac output. The skin and the skeletal muscle, at the other extreme, do not enjoy the same degree of protection, and their blood supply is markedly reduced when the overall perfusion flow rate is inadequate.

Finally, the circulatory status of individual organs prior to bypass cannot be disregarded. The kidneys, because of their large blood supply and small arterio-venous oxygen difference, can most easily afford a decrease in perfusion flow without suffering unduly from hypoxia. On the other hand, the high oxygen extraction in the coronary vascular bed makes it impossible for the heart to function on a markedly reduced blood supply. In this respect, the pronounced coronary vasodilation induced by hypoxia or accumulated metabolic products represents a protective mechanism by which blood is shifted to the heart from more generously perfused organs (Gomori and Takacz, 1960).

The concept of "protective redistribution" of blood flow asserts that the more vital tissues in the body are selectively favored over less essential tissues when the volume of available blood is reduced. In the field of artificial perfusion this concept has evolved from cursory studies of the blood quota to individual vascular beds when the whole organism is perfused at different flow rates. Because of the surgical preparation it involves, complete heart–lung bypass easily allows separation of venous return from the inferior vena cava, superior vena cava and coronary sinus. Some insight into the distribution of blood flow can thus be gained by simple observation. From data of Paneth, et al., (1957), Levovitz, et al., (1958) and many others, one can estimate that in the most effective perfusion procedures, about two thirds of the blood flow is distributed to the lower part of the body (kidney, liver, gastrointestinal tract, lower extremities, etc.). The average superior caval flow is about one third of all flow rates in excess of 1.1 L./sq. m./min. (Kittle, et al., 1961). When total perfusion flow is experimentally increased over a wide range, the oxygen uptake in the regions drained by the superior vena cava (brain) and the coronary sinus (heart) seems to level off as soon as the flow rate reaches 0.5 to 0.8 L./sq. m./min. The oxygen needs of the tissues drained by the inferior vena cava are certainly not met before total flow exceeds 1.2 L./sq. m./min. In other words, at very low perfusion flows, one would expect proportionately more blood from the superior vena cava and the coronary sinus. Interestingly enough, adrenergic drugs, gangliopegic drugs and acute hypoxia, as induced by discontinuation of the oxygen supply to the artificial lung, all result in a relative increase of superior vena caval flow (Kittle, et al., 1961).

The problem of distribution of blood flow and oxygen uptake among different organs at various flow rates has been systematically studied by Creech's group in New Orleans (Halley, et al., 1958, 1959a, b; Reemstma, et al., 1959a), and more recently by other investigators (Brown, et al., 1958b; Schwartz, et al., 1958; Shumaker, 1960; Waldhausen, et al., 1960; Andersen, et al., 1961). It is beyond the scope of this chapter to discuss the many pitfalls involved in regional flow measurements. Despite some contradictory opinions among the above mentioned authors, the general picture supports the concept of selective redistribution. In the light of common physiologic knowledge (Bard, 1956; Brown, et al. 1958b; Feruglio, et al., 1960), we have attempted to delineate the changes in perfusion flow, arterio-venous oxygen difference and oxygen uptake in the more important organ systems (table 4). Using the fiction of the "average" human being (height 175 cm.; weight 70 Kg.; body surface area 1.84 sq. m., basal oxygen uptake 240 ml./min.; resting cardiac output 5 L./min.), the accepted standards for organ perfusion and metabolism in the resting state have been compared to the values obtained in normothermic artificial perfusion. The extracorporeal flow rates have been arbitrarily classified as high (2.4 L./sq. m./min.), medium (1.8 L./sq. m./min.), low (1.1 L./sq. m./min.) and "azygos" (0.5 L./sq. m./min.). Admitting that the representation given in fig. 85 is schematic, one can nevertheless visualize that brain and heart perfusion are the least affected by complete heart–lung bypass at any given flow rate. Compensatory mechanisms also insure that these vital organs will receive an almost unchanged share of oxygen. Kidney perfusion drops markedly with decreasing flow rates but the renal oxygen uptake is not seriously impaired at first. The gastrointestinal tract, liver and spleen follow a somewhat middle course. The splanchnic area is relatively well protected, and disproportionate deprivation of flow does not occur unless the perfusion rate is markedly decreased. Less information is available about the skin, musculature and other tissues than about the vital organs and there is less conclusive evidence for the mechanisms involved in adaptation. Despite the considerable difficulties encountered in measuring regional blood flow during heart–lung bypass and the reservations called for by some of the techniques used, much more information of this type is urgently needed for a better understanding of the reactions of the organism to total body perfusion.

Table 4. Distribution of blood flow and oxygen uptake among the main organ systems in the "average" human being. The resting cardiac output is taken as 5.0 L./min., and the basal oxygen consumption as 240 ml./min. The flow rates are arbitrarily classified as "normal" (intact organism), and "high," "medium," "low" and "azygos" (anesthetized, perfused organism). For each flow rate, an estimate is given of the quota of blood flow (F) and oxygen uptake ($\dot{V}_{O_2}$) of the individual organ systems, together with the arteriovenous oxygen difference usually observed (Δ_{O_2}). The lower line shows weighted means for the whole organism.

ORGAN	NORMAL FLOW			HIGH FLOW			MEDIUM FLOW			LOW FLOW			AZYGOS FLOW		
	F	Δ_{O_2}	$\dot{V}_{O_2}$	F	Δ_{O_2}	$\dot{V}_{O_2}$	F	Δ_{O_2}	$\dot{V}_{O_2}$	F	Δ_{O_2}	$\dot{V}_{O_2}$	F	Δ_{O_2}	$\dot{V}_{O_2}$
	L/min	Vol%	ml/min	L/min	Vol%	ml/min	L/min	Vol%	ml/min	L/min	Vol%	ml/min	L/min	Vol%	ml/min
Brain	.8	8.0	64	0.7	7.0	49	0.7	7.0	49	0.5	10.0	50	.3	15.0	45
Heart	.3	11.0	33	0.3	10.0	30	0.3	8.0	24	0.2	12.0	24	.15	15.0	22
Kidney	1.2	1.7	20	0.7	3.2	22	0.5	4.5	22	0.2	7.5	15	—	—	—
G.I. Tract, Liver, Spleen	1.3	2.7	48	1.3	3.0	39	0.8	5.0	40	0.5	8.0	40	.25	15.0	38
Muscle, Skin	1.4	5.3	75	1.5	4.0	60	1.0	5.5	55	0.6	8.5	51	.3	15.0	45
WHOLE BODY	5.0	4.8	240	4.5	4.4	200	3.3	5.8	190	2.0	9.0	180	1.0	15.0	150

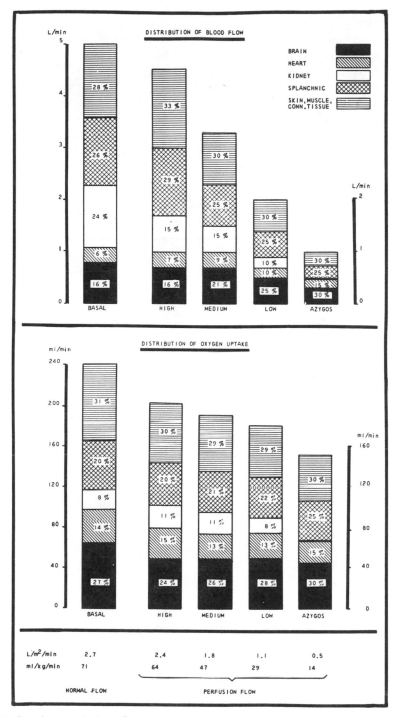

Fig. 85. Distribution of blood flow (upper graph) and oxygen uptake (lower graph) among the main organ systems in an "average" adult human (weight 70 Kg.; height 175 cm.; body surface area 1.84 sq. m.). The absolute values of flow or oxygen uptake in individual organ systems can be read from the scale; the relative values are inscribed in the appropriate blocks. Data from table 4.

Summarizing:

Under normal resting conditions, the distribution of blood flow to various organs is proportional neither to their weight nor to their metabolic activity. Under conditions of artificial perfusion, when the total perfusion rate is altered, the variations in flow are not the same in all vascular beds, because the pressure–flow relationship differs in each organ. Furthermore, organs react differently in their active vasomotion to changes in blood gasses. Owing to protective redistribution of blood flow, the heart and brain remain well perfused and are least affected by complete heart–lung bypass at low flow rates. Kidney perfusion drops markedly with decreasing flow rates. The splanchnic organs follow a somewhat middle course.

XIV. Metabolic Aspects of Total Heart-Lung Bypass

The end purpose of perfusion procedures is to provide all tissues in the body with the oxygen (and substrates) they need for survival, and to eliminate the carbon dioxide (and other wastes) which results from their metabolic activity (Clark, 1958). In terms of tissue gas exchange, artificial circulation must be considered from several aspects: perfusion rate, gas-carrying capacity of the blood, composition of the gas mixture used for equilibration with blood, temperature and metabolic demands. All developments brought forth in this chapter are concerned with perfusions at normal body temperature. Hypothermic perfusions are briefly discussed in chap. XIX. The data obtained in the most widely used experimental animal, the dog, will be distinguished from those directly applicable to man. For the sake of clarity, oxygen requirements will be considered first and carbon dioxide elimination subsequently.

OXYGEN NEED AND PERFUSION FLOW REQUIREMENTS

The metabolic conditions usually prevailing during total body perfusion correspond to those of light general anesthesia. General anesthesia as such does not reduce the oxygen requirement of the body tissues below that observed under strictly basal conditions (Brendel, et al., 1954). Frequent claims to the contrary stem from insufficiently controlled experiments where temperature is permitted to drop or a mild state of acidosis has developed. The fact that the classic metabolic standards of the normal subject are really seven to ten per cent too high (Fleisch, 1951) also contributes to the common belief in a "sommolent metabolic rate" lower than the "basal metabolic rate." It is therefore safe to base calculations of oxygen requirement of a perfused organism on the classic metabolic standards. The overestimation of values listed in the usual tables, plus the almost inescapable slight fall in temperature of the perfused organism, make the calculated oxygen requirement perhaps 20 per cent higher than that actually necessary (Engel, 1956). This margin of safety provides for most individual fluctuations around the average value of basal metabolic rate.

The oxygen requirements of the human body are usually based on parameters like weight, surface and age. Whereas standards based on surface are usually considered to be more significant from the biologic standpoint, weight standards are somewhat more convenient to use. In the field of artificial perfusion, it is also more practical to express basal metabolic rate in terms of ml. O_2/min. than in terms of Cal./hour or Cal./24 hours. Standard values for nor-

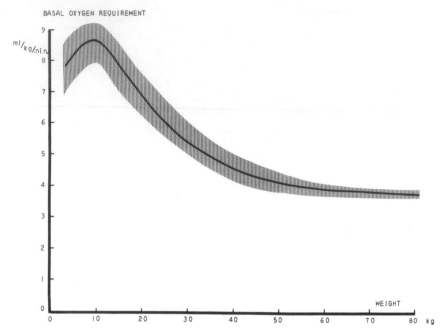

Fig. 86. Chart relating basal oxygen requirement (in ml./Kg./min.) to body weight (in Kg.) in man. The hatched area on either side of the curve includes 80 per cent of the normal population. The curve presents a maximum for a weight of about 12 Kg., which corresponds to an age of approximately two years. Younger infants have a lower metabolism per unit of weight. However, the actual values are rather uncertain and the scatter is probably large. The downward portion of the curve corresponds to the decrease of metabolism per unit of weight which occurs with growth. (Modified from Clark, 1958.)

mal man are given in figs. 86 and 87. It can be seen that the basal oxygen requirement per unit of weight is considerably larger during the period of growth than is true later. The difference is less conspicuous when the oxygen requirement is related to surface area. Both curves show a maximum for body dimensions corresponding to nine to twelve month old babies. The metabolic rate in the newborn and during early infancy is smaller than during the second year of life. The corresponding data for dogs are not as firmly established as they are in humans, and consequently, they cannot be presented in chart form. Estimates of the oxygen requirement at 37 to 38°C. range from 5.7 to 7.7 ml./Kg./min. (Levy and Blalock, 1937; Handbook of Respiration, 1958; Cheng et al., 1959; Galletti et al., 1960). The often accepted value of 130 ml./sq. m./min. corresponds to about 8 ml./Kg./min. in a 5 Kg. dog, and 5 ml./Kg./min. in a 25 Kg. animal. This compares with the values obtained in children of similar size.

On the basis of standard oxygen needs, theoretical equations relating the required perfusion rate to the parameters of body build can be derived from the Fick principle (Clark, 1958). The perfusion rate is indicated by the ratio of oxygen needed by the organism to the oxygen supply expected per unit of blood flow. The oxygen need is determined by the basal requirement per unit of weight (fig. 86) or surface (fig. 87) multiplied by the actual weight or surface. The oxygen which can be supplied per unit of time by a given volume of blood equals the hemoglobin content of the blood (as Gm. per 100 ml.), mul-

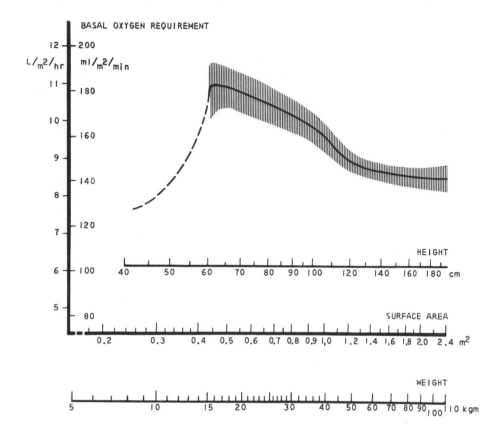

Fig. 87. Chart relating the basal oxygen requirement (in ml./sq. m./min. or L./sq. m./hour) to the body surface area (in sq. m.) in man. The horizontal scales for height (in cm.) and weight (in Kg.) are to be used as a nomogram. By joining the point on the upper scale, which corresponds to the height of an individual, to the point on the lower scale, which corresponds to his weight, one intercepts the axis of the abscissa at a point which indicates the body surface area. This point can then be used for estimating the basal oxygen requirement. (Other symbols as in fig. 86.)

tiplied by the oxygen capacity of one Gm. of hemoglobin (1.34 ml. O_2), multiplied in turn by the expected arteriovenous difference in oxygen saturation (in per cent). Clark has proposed the following formulas for calculating the "ideal" perfusion rate:

$$F = \frac{7.46\ W\ R}{H(A - V)} + C \quad \text{or} \quad F = \frac{25.8\ S\ R'}{H(A - V)} + C$$

where F is the perfusion rate (in L./min.); W the body weight (in Kg.); S the body area (in sq. m.); R the basal oxygen requirement (in ml./Kg./min.); R' the basal oxygen requirement (in Cal/sq. m./hour); H the blood hemoglobin content (in Gm. per cent); A the arterial blood saturation (in per cent); V the venous blood saturation (in per cent); C the cardiotomy blood return (in L./min.); 7.46 and 25.6 are numerical constants related to the units chosen. C is meant to indicate that, according to the volume of blood drained from the operative field, additional flow may be needed to compensate for this volume of blood which is no longer available to perfuse the peripheral tissues.

Assumptions must be made to transcribe these theoretic formulas into usable perfusion charts. Clark has admitted that the blood arterialized in an artificial lung is 100 per cent saturated (which is approximately true in most instances) and carries an extra amount of oxygen dissolved in plasma equiva-

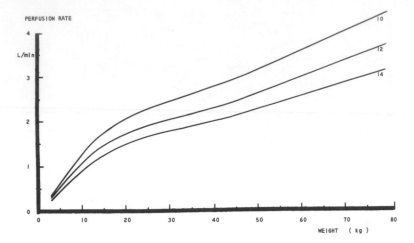

Fig. 88. Chart indicating the perfusion rate (in L./min.) as a function of the body weight (in Kg.) in man. The figures appended to each curve correspond to the hemoglobin content of the blood. (Modified from Clark, 1958.)

lent to the capacity of one gm of hemoglobin (at normal body temperature such a plasma oxygen content corresponds to a partial pressure of oxygen of around 600 mm. Hg., a value achieved only by a few bubble oxygenators). A venous saturation of 50 per cent has been chosen to represent a compromise between normal venous saturation and a favorable decline in tissue oxygen requirements during open-chest surgery. Because the hemoglobin content may vary widely according to the patient and the oxygenator priming technique used, this factor must also be taken into account in selecting the perfusion rate. Figs. 88 and 89 show the family of curves relating perfusion rate to body

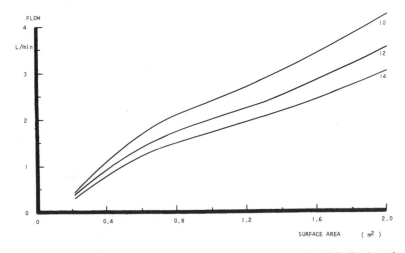

Fig. 89. Chart indicating the perfusion rate (in L./min.) as a function of the body surface (in sq. m.) in man. The figures appended to each curve correspond to the hemoglobin content of the blood. The body surface area can be computed from height and weight by using the nomogram at the lower part of fig. 87. (Modified from Clark, 1958.)

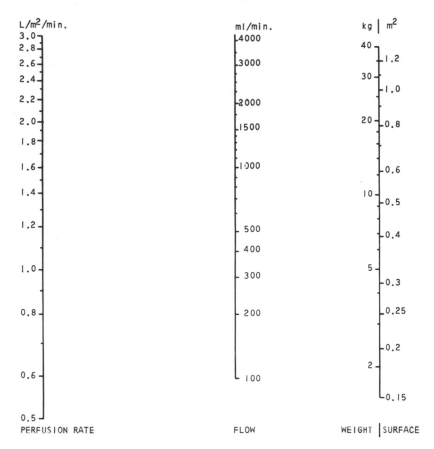

Fig. 90. Nomogram relating body weight (in Kg.) and surface area (in sq. m.) in the dog, to blood flow (in ml./min.) and perfusion rate (L./sq. m./min.). The scale on the left represents the relationship of weight to surface in mongrel dogs according to the formula

$$Surface\ area\ (m^2)\ =\ 0.012\ \sqrt[3]{(weight,\ Kg.)^2}$$

By joining the point corresponding to the weight of the animal on the left scale, to the point expressing the blood flow on the central scale, and extending the line to the right, one reads the perfusion rate in L./sq. m./min.

dimensions at various hemoglobin contents in man. According to these graphs, the ideal perfusion rate, in terms of ml./Kg./min., varies widely with the size of the patient: 105 ml./Kg./min. are needed for a 9 Kg. infant; 85 ml./Kg./min. are recommended for a 20 Kg. child; whereas 52 ml./Kg./min. would suffice for a 50 Kg. adolescent. The difference is less conspicuous when the perfusion rate is related to the body surface: the perfusion rate should amount to 2.4 L./sq. m./min. when the surface is around 0.5 sq. m. (18 to 24 months old baby); to 2.0 L./sq. m./min. when the surface is 1 sq. m. (about 8 years); 1.8 L./sq. m./min. in the average adult. Kirklin et al. (1957) recommend flow rates in excess of 2.2 L./sq. m./min. regardless of age. Senning (1959) does not take into account the expected oxygen uptake of the patient, but calculates the perfusion flow on the basis of 80 per cent of the cardiac output measured at catheterization, 14 Gm. per cent hemoglobin, 95 per cent arterial oxy-

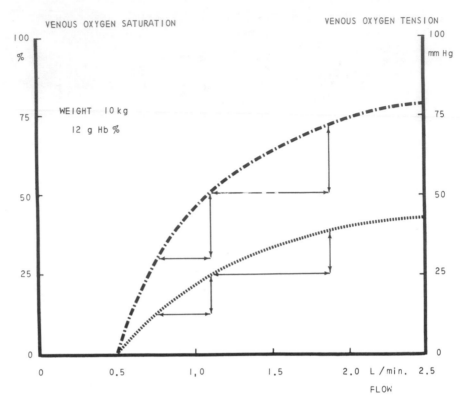

Fig. 91. Relationship between venous oxygen saturation (dash dot line; in per cent), venous oxygen tension (dotted line; in mm. Hg.) and perfusion flow (in L./min.). Modified from Clark (1958).

gen saturation and 65 per cent venous oxygen saturation. The concept of "optimal flow rate" has been reviewed by Clark (1958), Kirklin et al. (1958), Andersen (1958) and Margulis (1959).

No perfusion charts have been worked out for dogs, despite the extensive use of this animal in the laboratory. Fig. 90 merely relates the extracorporeal blood flow to the weight or the surface of the dog, so as to express the perfusion rate in terms similar to those used in man and to permit comparisons between animals of different sizes. The main reason for the lack of acceptable perfusion charts is the uncertainty as to the basal cardiac output of the dog. Unless one works with very well trained animals, anesthesia is necessary. Most experimental studies on cardiac output in dogs fail to standardize and keep constant the most important factor of variation, namely the level of anesthesia. Melrose, et al. (1953) have remarked that even the most skilled anesthetist finds it difficult to regulate the depth of narcosis so as to make consecutive determinations of the cardiac output identical. Using Nembutal, oxygen uptake may vary by a factor of 1.8 during a one hour perfusion (Clark, 1958). Our own experience with chloralose anesthetized animals perfused for ten hours demonstrates that a perfusion flow of 100 ml./Kg./min. certainly suffices to maintain metabolic equilibrium at normal body temperature. This flow, which corresponds to 2.2 L./sq. m./min. in 15 to 16 Kg. dogs (fig. 91), should thus be sufficient to meet the animal's oxygen requirements.

There are obvious limitations to the use of perfusion charts: First, they are based on average values for oxygen needs, around which there is a considerable scattering, particularly in the young age group. Another criticism concerns the arbitrary choice of venous blood oxygen saturation. Fig. 91, again borrowed from Clark (1958), shows how venous oxygen saturation and venous oxygen tension vary with the perfusion rate, assuming a steady oxygen consumption. The suggested perfusion rate, according to fig. 88, assuming a 50 per cent venous oxygen saturation, amounts to 1.1 L./min. To raise the venous saturation to 70 per cent, one would have to perfuse 1.8 L./min. By contrast, venous oxygen saturation falls to 30 per cent, and oxygen tension plunges towards zero if the perfusion rate is reduced to 0.75 L./min.

These figures illustrate the difficulty of expressing the extracorporeal flow in various organisms in comparable terms, and also illustrates the variations encountered in experimental and clinical work. It should be clear that perfusion rates, even expressed in terms of ml./Kg./min. or L./sq. m./min., do not fully define the situation when the weight or surface (or average weight or surface) is not indicated. Table 4 represents merely an attempt to settle quantitatively what is meant by the commonly used expressions of "normal flow," "high flow," "medium flow," "low flow" and "azygos flow."

Summarizing

The oxygen requirements of the normothermic organism under light general anesthesia are the same as those under strictly basal conditions. Since the standard values for basal metabolism in the classic tables are up to ten per cent too high and since the temperature of the organism always drops a little during perfusion, the oxygen requirement calculated on the basis of body dimensions is about 20 per cent larger than that actually needed. Based on standard oxygen needs, the blood perfusion rate required can be calculated and presented in the form of charts. Limitations of perfusion charts stem from the large scatter around the average values for oxygen needs and the necessity for an arbitrary selection of venous blood oxygen saturation.

PERFUSION FLOW AND ACTUAL OXYGEN UPTAKE

Since in principle the oxygen need of an organism depends on its size only, one would expect the actual oxygen uptake during perfusion to remain the same over a fairly wide range of blood flow rates. The tissues would extract the oxygen they need from the blood available to them simply by widening or narrowing the arteriovenous oxygen difference.

In reality, there are considerable discrepancies among the experimental results concerning tissue oxygen extraction in dogs (fig. 92). Paneth, et al. (1957), observed that the oxygen uptake in the extracorporeal circuit reaches a plateau as soon as the perfusion rate amounts to 40 ml./Kg./min. or more. This opinion was confirmed by Beer et al. (1959), who stated that the oxygen uptake is constant regardless of the perfusion rate for all values of blood flow exceeding 35 per cent of the normal cardiac output. At variance with the previous results, Clowes et al. (1958), Andersen and Senning (1958), Cheng et al. (1959), and Starr (1959) calculated that in experimental animals, the oxygen uptake increases almost linearly from 50 per cent of the control at perfu-

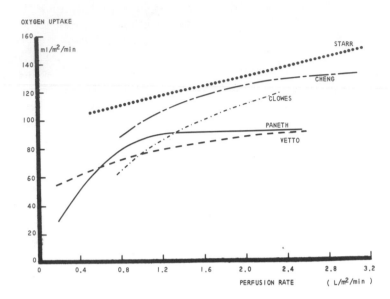

Fig. 92. Variations in oxygen uptake (in ml./sq. m./min.) according to the perfusion rate (in L./sq. m./min.) during total heart–lung bypass in the dog. The data published by Starr (1959), Cheng, et al. (1959); Clowes, et al. (1958); Paneth, et al. (1957); and Vetto, et al. (1959), have been transcribed on a common scale. (See details in text.)

sion rates in the order of 30 ml./Kg./min. (0.6 L./sq. m./min.), to 85 to 100 per cent of the control when the flow reached 100 ml./Kg./min. (2.2 L./sq. m./min.).

These contradictory results are partially explained by variations in temperature during lengthy perfusions, the depressant effect of some of the drugs used (anesthetics, muscular relaxants) and by the experimental difficulties involved in measuring gas exchange in an extracorporeal circuit. As demonstrated by Vetto et al. (1959), oxygen consumption rates during cardiopulmonary bypass are often inconstant and tend to increase with time. It is therefore questionable whether a steady state of oxygen uptake is ever reached during perfusions at low flow rate. A single arteriovenous difference is not a reliable basis for the determination of oxygen uptake for a long period. Furthermore, indirect measurements of oxygen uptake, calculated from flow, arterial oxygen content and venous oxygen content, compound the experimental errors involved in these three determinations. In this respect, direct measurements of oxygen uptake, using an oxygenator directly connected to a spirometer (Cheng et al., 1959) have a higher degree of accuracy.

There are a few pertinent data available in man because conditions in the operating room do not lend themselves easily to metabolic experimentation. Moffitt et al. (1959) studied a series of patients, each of whom was perfused at a flow rate corresponding to about one half of the resting cardiac output measured during heart catheterization a few days before the operation. The venous oxygen saturation during bypass was practically the same as that during catheterization. This would mean that the oxygen consumption is markedly reduced during cardiopulmonary bypass, even if one takes into account that oxygen uptake under so-called resting conditions may exceed the basal metabolic rate. However, careful physiologic studies performed on selected patients by the same team indicate that oxygen consumption during perfusion remains within the normal range (McGoon et al., 1960). Using flow rates approximating basal cardiac output, Starr (1959) occasionally found values of oxygen uptake exceeding the oxygen requirements expected on the basis of Clark's perfusion charts (figs. 88 and 89).

There is at present no direct experimental evidence for a decrease in tissue oxygen *requirements* during total body perfusion. Data showing a decrease in oxygen *uptake* are inconclusive as long as the constancy of temperature, arterial blood pH and buffer base is not ascertained simultaneously. Restriction of oxygen *supply* to the tissues may be caused by a number of incidental factors such as failure of the artificial lung to achieve full arterialization of the blood, hemodilution or insufficient flow rates. That the organism can survive on a limited oxygen supply does not mean that its requirements are fully covered. In fact, during the period of decreased oxygen uptake, the perfused organism lives partly under anaerobic conditions and incurs an oxygen debt, which must be paid off at a later time.

As pointed out by Schneider (1959), isolated organs, and consequently the organism as a whole, can live under anaerobic conditions for a limited period. Glycolysis or phosphocreatin catabolism then produce some energy, which, however, does not suffice to maintain full functional activity for more than a short time. The delay preceding the appearance of signs of suspended or depressed function varies from organ to organ, depending upon energy expenditures, energy reserves, rate of glycolysis, type of function, and similar factors. However, the organ can be fully revived as long as its energy expenditures do not drop below a limit Schneider calls "metabolism of preservation." For some organs, this "metabolism of preservation" represents as little as 15 to 20 per cent of the metabolism of activity. Therefore, one can conceive that a living organism could survive for quite a long time on a decreased oxygen uptake, provided that compensation is facilitated by an abundant supply during the period of recovery. To again use Schneider's terminology (1953), reduced oxygen consumption during total body perfusion is more likely to be a "hypoxydosis,"—the condition of decreased oxygen distribution, than a "hypochreosis,"—the condition of decreased oxygen need.

Suggestions that an organism's oxygen requirement may be supply-dependent have been advanced from time to time (Chance, 1959; Vinitskaya and Volinsky, 1960) since the original speculations of von Hösslin (1888). In the case of newborn mammals, the actual oxygen requirement may be actually decreased in the presence of decreased supply: this phenomenon, however, is not found in all species. In the human, Bing et al. (1947) have reported that patients with decreased effective pulmonary blood flow also display a lowered oxygen consumption. Their finding suggests that a permanent decrease in overall metabolic processes may result from prolonged hypoxemia. Whether this applies to normothermic perfusions is by no means proven. For the time being, it is safe to assume that the oxygen requirement of a perfused organism equals that measured under basal conditions, and one should therefore calculate the perfusion flow on this basis.

Summarizing

In principle the oxygen uptake of an organism may be expected to remain constant over a wide range of perfusion flow rates, as long as the tissues can extract whatever oxygen they need. However, most experimental findings indicate a decrease in oxygen uptake with decreasing perfusion rates. It appears that during periods of decreased oxygen supply the perfused organism lives partly under anaerobic conditions and incurs an oxygen debt which must be paid back at a later time. As long as the energy expenditure of the individual tissues does not fall below the "metabolism of preservation", the organism can actually be fully revived. Nevertheless, it is safer to use perfusion flow rates commensurate with an oxygen uptake equaling that of the body under basal metabolic conditions.

ACID-BASE BALANCE

The occurrence of acidosis in organ perfusion (Bjørk, 1948) or total body perfusion (Dennis, et al., 1951) has been noted since the beginning of the extracorporeal circulation era. Early reports (Spreng, et al., 1953; Miller, et al., 1953; Cohen, et al., 1954) pointed to a fall in arterial blood pH of 0.20 to 0.30 units during the period of heart–lung bypass and the hours following the procedure. The changes in plasma CO_2 content or CO_2 tension were rather erratic. Owing to the complexity of the metabolic factors involved in total body perfusion (anesthesia, skeletal muscle activity in the perfused organism, artificial respiration before and after bypass, ventilation of the artificial lung with pure oxygen, shifts in body temperature), numerous theories arose to explain the development of this acidosis. Around 1956, however, it was realized that the common denominator for the disturbances of acid-base balance brought about by extracorporeal circulation was *metabolic acidosis*, compensated or not by *respiratory alcalosis*. Kirklin et al. (1956) reported that low or decreasing blood flows were associated with progressive decreases in blood pH, while at higher flows, the pH remained relatively stable. Levowitz, et al. (1956) discussed the desirability of a low arterial pCO_2 to counteract the acidosis. DeWall et al. (1956a) observed that a moderate plasma bicarbonate depression regularly occurred during total body perfusion. This depression was accompanied by an elevation of blood lactic acid, whereas values for pH did not depart greatly from normal. It was then clearly established that the acidosis associated with heart–lung bypass procedures was of hypoxic origin, and developed because the perfusion failed to distribute as much oxygen as the tissues required. Consequently, a partly anaerobic catabolism was called upon to cover the energy requirements of the organism. "Hypoxic acidosis" at the cellular level resulted in the blood picture of metabolic acidosis during and after artificial perfusion.

In experimental work, it was proven that low perfusion rates were the most common cause of metabolic acidosis (Kolff, et al., 1956a; Diesh, et al., 1957; Craoford, et al., 1957b; Gammelgard, et al., 1957; Bell, et al., 1957; 1958; Pontius, et al., 1958; Varco, et al., 1958; Elliott and Callaghan, 1958b, 1959; Norlander, et al., 1958; Kashchevskaia, 1958; Paladino, et al., 1958; Jicha, et al., 1959; Moraes, et al., 1960a; Pezzoli, et al., 1960).

The lower the perfusion flow, the more marked was the fall in buffer base. The decrease in pH was not so impressive simply because some compensation was brought about by hyperventilation. When hyperventilation was prevented by maintaining a constant CO_2 tension in the artificial lung, the blood pH fell much below 7.0 (Pontius, et al., 1958; Clowes, et al., 1958). (These observations support the demonstration by Astrup (1956, 1961) and Peirce (1960b) that the reduction in blood pH is proportional to the accumulation of "nonrespiratory" acids, provided the CO_2 tension is kept constant.) It remained for Paneth, et al. (1957), and Clowes, et al., (1958) to demonstrate that the development of metabolic acidosis was directly related to the deficit in oxygen uptake during perfusion. In carefully planned experiments, Loeschke, et al. (1959), found that, when the perfusion rate was diminished from 100 ml./Kg./min. to 50 ml./Kg./min., the oxygen uptake decreased by 1.3 ml./Kg./min., or about 20 per cent of the control value. Simultaneously however, the whole blood buffer base decreased on the average by 2.6 mEq./L. These changes were partially reversible when high blood flow was restored. No acidosis occurred when the venous oxygen saturation was maintained at sufficiently high levels to permit adequate oxygen extraction by the tissues (Clowes and Neville, 1957; DeWall, et al., 1957a; Matthews, et al., 1958; Zenker, et al., 1958; Starr, 1959; van Eck, 1960). The greater the anoxia, the more the anaerobic end products that were formed. Coffin and Ankeney, (1960) observed that the rise in blood lactate and pyruvate was stoechiometrically related to the fall in plasma bicarbonate. To take into account the fluctuations in plasma bicarbonate caused by changes in ventilation, Litwin, et al. (1959) related blood lactate concentration to the plasma pH/HCO_3^- ratio. (The relationship of plasma pH to bicarbonate based on changes in carbonic acid concentration is linear. Therefore the proportional changes in pH and HCO_3^- due to ventilation are eliminated if one considers the pH/HCO_3^- ratio.) Using this type of plot, they found that blood lactate concentration was directly proportional to plasma $H+$ concentration and inversely proportional to plasma HCO_3^- concentration. They also observed that the increase in blood lactate during perfusion was directly proportional to the fall in venous saturation caused by the procedure.

Ballinger, et al. (1961) remarked that increased lactate levels are only an indication of anaerobic metabolism, since lactate also accumulates during hyperventilation (Papadopoulos and Keats, 1959) or when the pH or blood glucose are artificially raised. Such factors can be present during cardiopulmonary bypass, and therefore one cannot ascribe the rise in blood lactate to anaerobic metabolism alone. A way out of this dilemma has been indicated by Huckabee (1958), who proposed the term "excess lactate" to include only that lactate produced by anaerobic metabolism, and derived a formula for its calculation. Using this approach, Ballinger, et al. (1961) observed that under ideal conditions, patients undergoing heart–lung bypass do not develop a metabolic acidosis secondary to anaerobic metabolism. However, when flow rates are less than optimal, there is a prompt rise in lactate produced anaerobically. Correction of the factors causing decreased blood flows leads to a fall of excess lactate. As pointed out by Jervell (1928), there is a maximal rate at which the liver can remove anaerobic metabolites in the presence of sufficient oxygen. It is possible to exceed this rate by increasing the rate of lactate formation. It is presumably this mechanism which leads to the formation of an increased amount of lactic and pyruvic acid during perfusion at inadequate flow rates, in a manner somewhat comparable to what happens during heavy muscular exercise.

The establishment of an oxygen debt during perfusion requires compensation after perfusion. Alpert, et al. (1958) demonstrated that the oxygen missed in a period of severe hypoxia is directly correlated with the excess consumption during recovery. There has been no direct study as to the payment of oxygen debt incurred because of inadequate tissue perfusion during cardiopulmonary bypass. Vetto, et al. (1959) expressed the opinion that the debt paid was smaller than the anticipated deficit. Yet the patients who are unable to maintain a high cardiac output after bypass fail to clear the accumulation of acid metabolites, develop hypotension together with acidosis and finally die (Mendelsohn, et al., 1957, 1959; Clowes, et al., 1958; Vaysse, 1959; Boyd, et al., 1959; Clowes and Del Guercio, 1960; Hartmann, et al., 1960). Those who survive compensate for the acid products in the blood by a proportional fall in buffer base. Consequently, they display low plasma CO_2 tension together with subnormal pH (Gammelgard, et al., 1957; Zenker, et al., 1958; Peirce and Dabbs, 1959). Even in high flow perfusions where metabolic acidosis does not develop, there is a fall in arterial pH and CO_2 tension one hour after the procedure (McGoon, et al., 1960). The administration of sodium bicarbonate has been advocated to assist the intrinsic defense mechanism (Crafoord, et al., 1957b; Ito, et al., 1957; Beer and Loeschke, 1959). Usually however, the organism is able to handle the excess of fixed acids by itself when the circulation has regained stability (Keats, et al., 1958; Reed and Kittle, 1958; Mendelsohn, et al., 1959).

Besides inadequate flow rates, other perfusion factors which limit the amount of oxygen distributed to the tissues have been recognized: (1) insufficient saturation of the arterial blood (Pontius, et al., 1958; Clark, et al., 1958; Magovern, et al., 1959); (2) dilution of the blood with saline, resulting in a decreased oxygen carrying capacity (Kaplan, et al., 1958); (3) hyperventilation of the blood in the artificial lung, resulting in a shift of the oxygen dissociation curve towards a region less favorable to oxygen release from the oxyhemoglobin to the tissues (Malette, 1958); (4) arterial hypotension resulting, even at relatively high flow rates, in underperfusion of those organs which exhibit the highest vascular resistance (Andersen and Senning, 1958; Paladino, et al., 1958; Beer, 1959).

Some factors indirectly associated with the perfusion tend to obscure and also to aggravate the picture of metabolic acidosis. Chief among these is that blood used to prime the oxygenator develops a considerable degree of metabolic acidosis while standing at normal body temperature prior to bypass (Mendelsohn, et al., 1957). Measurements on blood collected in the same manner as that used for bypass show a fall of 0.11 pH unit at the end of four hours of incubation at body temperature. However small this pH fall may seem, the underlying accumulation of lactate due to anaerobic glycolysis is of the order of 16.5 mg. per 100 ml. of blood per hour of incubation (Beer, 1959). The amount of acid metabolites in the priming blood may account for half of the lactate levels measured at the end of perfusion (Beer, 1959; Beer and Loeschke, 1959; Mendelsohn, et al., 1959). These data emphasize the necessity of delaying up to the last moment the warming and recirculation of the blood within the oxygenator. When needed, the addition of sodium bicarbonate to the priming blood will limit the fall in plasma bicarbonate during subsequent perfusion (Bucherl, et al., 1959; Gutelius and Dobell, 1960).

Anesthetic techniques also occupy a key position in the genesis and control of metabolic disturbances during perfusion (Keats, et al., 1958). Underwood, et al. (1960) demonstrated the role of residual muscular activity in increasing the oxygen requirement of a perfused organism and pointed to the usefulness of muscle relaxants in cardiopulmonary bypass procedures. Another important factor to consider is the hypocapnia intentionally produced by hyperventilation of the lungs prior to perfusion. Some investigators believe that the harmful consequences of the tide of acid metabolites brought by the priming blood and low perfusion rates can be prevented if the patient is hyperventilated prior to bypass (DeWall, et al., 1956a; Kolff, et al., 1956; Mendelsohn, et al., 1957; Keats, et al., 1958). Unfortunately hyperventilation alone gives rise to some degree of metabolic acidosis, as pointed out by Pontius, et al., (1958),

Henneman, et al. (1958) and Papadopoulos and Keats (1959). A sudden fall in pH occurs if CO_2 is permitted to reaccumulate at a later stage (Dobell, et al., 1960). Litwin, et al. (1959) observed that those animals with the most severe degree of respiratory alkalosis prior to perfusion also show the highest blood lactate concentration at the end of perfusion. It therefore seems preferable to maintain the ventilation of the anesthetized organism before perfusion as close to normal as possible.

During cardiopulmonary bypass, respiratory alkalosis can also lead to increased lactate levels when the CO_2 washout in the artificial lung exceeds the metabolic CO_2 production (Melrose, et al., 1953). An arterial CO_2 tension below 25 mm. Hg. results in increased cerebrovascular resistance. If the mean arterial pressure is not maintained at a normal level, the cerebral blood flow diminishes markedly, as demonstrated by Beer, et al. (1959). Hypocapnia during bypass can be prevented in a variety of ways: the one most favored in clinical perfusions is ventilation of the artificial lung with an oxygen–carbon dioxide mixture instead of using pure oxygen. According to the various schools, carbon dioxide in the range of 1.5 to 6 per cent is employed. The partial pressure of CO_2 in the gas phase sets a minimum below which the arterial CO_2 tension cannot go, regardless of the volume of ventilation. This relieves the heart–lung machine operator of most worries about gas flow. However, it is obvious that the same result can be obtained using pure oxygen, provided that the gas flow is adapted to the metabolic production of CO_2. Most artificial lungs employ unnecessarily high gas flows. Some of them, particularly the disc and bubble oxygenators, can be equally well maintained with 100 per cent oxygen at lower flow rates (Clark, et al., 1958; Loeschke, et al., 1959; Viles, et al., 1960). Whether the decrease in blood trauma associated with a lower gas flow justifies the inconvenience of a closer control of the ventilation of the artificial lung remains to be appreciated under practical conditions.

Finally, it has been suggested that exclusion of the pulmonary circulation could be a cause of lactic acid accumulation, since according to Lochner (1957a, b) the lung may participate in the catabolism of lactic acid. No direct proof for such a mechanism during heart–lung bypass has yet been brought forward.

In conclusion, when attention is directed to all of the above mentioned factors, no acidosis is developed during the extracorporeal circulation procedure itself (Norlander, et al., 1958). The pH can be controlled within 0.04 units (Clark, et al., 1958). A mild decrease in the arterial blood CO_2 content and CO_2 tension occurs, mainly as a result of general anesthesia and manual hyperventilation (McGoon, et al., 1960). These observations suggest that cardiopulmonary bypass plays no role in the genesis of an acidosis when flows are adequate. Because the heart is not always able to cope fully with its task immediately after bypass, or because mild hypoxic acidosis develops first in the intracellular compartment and requires some time to manifest itself in the plasma, disturbances are often restricted to the postoperative period. Therefore control of the patient must be extended to the period after bypass, particularly in the case of long range perfusions.

Summarizing

Total body perfusion is usually accompanied by some degree of metabolic acidosis, often compensated by an extra elimination of carbon dioxide. Acidosis is caused by underperfusion of the tissues invoking a partly anaerobic catabolism. In addition to cellular hypoxia from inadequate perfusion rates, the following factors can also contribute to metabolic acidosis: (1) anesthesia and thoracotomy as such; (2) accumulation of acid metabolites in the priming blood as a consequence of glycolysis; (3) accumulation of acid metabolites as a consequence of arterial hypotension; (4) increase in the plasma lactate levels prior to perfusion as a consequence of hyperventilation. The oxygen debt incurred during heart–lung bypass can be paid back after the cessation of the extracorporeal circulation provided the circulation returns to normal.

ELECTROLYTES AND WATER BALANCE

The accumulation of fixed acids in blood during and after cardiopulmonary bypass has prompted studies of electrolyte shifts associated with perfusion. The picture reported is often complicated by factors independent of the perfusion itself, such as preoperative metabolic acidosis due to overzealous administration of ammonium chloride and organic mercurial diuretics, respiratory alkalosis caused by hyperventilation just prior to perfusion, or dilution of the patient's blood with saline or citrated blood used for priming the extracorporeal circuit. Nevertheless, it appears possible to draw the main lines in the picture of electrolyte change from numerous scattered observations and a few more complete studies such as those of Litwin, et al. (1959).

With respect to *anions* organic acids, such as lactate and pyruvate, increase as byproducts of anaerobic processes, under the conditions we have just discussed. Lactate increases are in the order of 2 to 5 mM./L./hr. of perfusion (DeWall, et al., 1956; Paneht, et al., 1957; Clowes, et al., 1958; Litwin, et al., 1959; Coffin and Ankeney, 1960). Plasma pyruvate levels rise 0.1 to 0.5 mM./L./hr. of perfusion in the estimates of different authors (Dennis, et al., 1951; Stuckey, et al., 1956; Coffin and Ankeney, 1960). Pyruvate levels above 0.5 mM./L. carry an ominous prognosis (Spreng, et al., 1952). Moderate increases in plasma chloride levels, usually insignificant from the clinical standpoint, have been observed by Stephenson, et al. (1957), Crafoord, et al., (1957b); DeWall, et al. (1959) and Litwin, et al. (1959). Decrease in bicarbonate levels is customary in heart–lung bypass procedures: the extent depends largely upon the metabolic conditions before and during perfusion (Norlander, et al., 1958; Litwin, et al., 1959). It is small (1 to 3 mEq./L./hr.) in subjects hyperventilated before bypass and perfused at high flow rates, because the initial level is already low; it can be more pronounced (1 to 10 mEq./L./hr.) in normally ventilated subjects perfused at medium and high flow rates, because bicarbonate is called upon to a larger extent to compensate for fixed acid production and to maintain a constant pH; loss becomes conspicuous (6 to 10 mEq./L./hr.) in low flow perfusions or when the patient has been treated preoperatively with ammonium chloride (Clowes, et al., 1958; Norlander, et al., 1958; Callaghan, et al., 1958; Litwin, et al., 1959; Peirce and Dabbs, 1959; DeWall, et al., 1959; Elliott and Callaghan, 1959; Bucherl, et al., 1959; Loeschke, et al., 1959). Inorganic phosphate increases during perfusion by 3 to 4 mg. per cent (Crafoord, et al., 1957a; Clowes, et al., 1958). Changes in the "undetermined" anions (including such ions as proteins, organic phosphates and sulfates) are usually in the direction of a decrease (Litwin, et al., 1960).

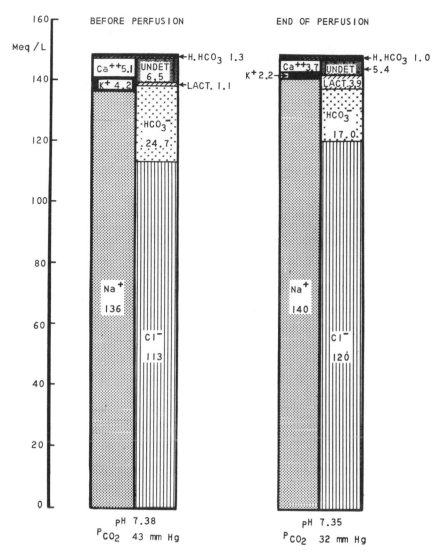

Fig. 93. Alterations in plasma electrolyte levels caused by total body perfusion at high flow rates. (Redrawn from Litwin (1959).)

With respect to *cations*, the plasma concentration in sodium displays clinically insignificant variations, either in the direction of a slight increase (Newman, et al., 1955; Crafoord, et al., 1957b; Litwin, et al., 1959) or of a slight decrease (Sturtz, et al., 1957b; Clowes and Del Guercio, 1960). There is often slight to marked depression of the potassium level at the end of bypass (Crafoord, et al., 1957; Callaghan, et al., 1958; Litwin, et al., 1959). DeWall, et al., (1957) reported an increase of serum potassium in cyanotic patients, unless perfused at high flow rates. Elevated serum potassium levels associated with massive hemolysis or recirculation of blood in the oxygenator (Burton, et al., 1960) are no longer a serious problem. The usual hypokalemia (2 to 3 mEq./L.), which may lead to the development of cardiac arrhythmias, is fortunately accompanied by a corresponding decrease in plasma calcium levels (Litwin, et al., 1959; Clowes and Del Guercio, 1960) so that the effects of hypokalemia and hypocalcemia on the myocardium tend to cancel each other. The use of citrated or EDTA blood for priming the extracorporeal circuit severely depresses the ionized calcium level, unless adequate amounts of calcium salts are simultaneously injected (Soulier, 1958; Brown and Smith, 1958; Smith, et al., 1959).

The overall picture of electrolytes change is schematized in fig. 93. As observed by Litwin, et al., (1959), the biochemical changes associated with medium and low flow rate perfusion bear a striking resemblance to those seen under conditions of respiratory alkalosis. The reason may be that in "hypoxic" tissue acidosis, the acid load appears first in the intracellular compartment. Thus the extracellular compartment is more alkaline than the intracellular compartment, as happens in respiratory alkalosis. Hence the electrolyte changes in plasma may be expected to be the same in both conditions. Since the acid load is being buffered first in the intracellular compartment, the drop in plasma bicarbonate and pH observed during perfusion might represent only a portion of the free hydrogen ion formed. This would help to explain why, with the short periods of perfusion usually employed, acidosis is often more marked after than during the procedure.

Little is known about the influence of the perfusion as such on the *water balance* of the organism. Sturtz, et al. (1957a, b) presented data which suggest a striking increase in insensible water loss during the operation, probably from the exposed moist surfaces of the pleura and pericardium. Each patient had a slightly low water concentration in the serum immediately after perfusion, an observation confirmed by other investigators (Litwin, et al., 1959; Clowes and Del Guercio, 1960). The data of Crafoord, et al. (1957b) suggest that water and sodium retention develops in the period immediately following perfusion. In view of the depressed kidney function which often occurs in perfusion procedures (*see* Chapter XV), one should be careful not to overload the patient with water in the immediate postoperative period (Crafoord, et al., 1959; Lyons, et al., 1960; Scott, 1960). Otherwise edema and even heart failure may result. Investigation of variations in body fluid compartments during and after long term cardiopulmonary bypass are presently being carried out in our laboratory. They indicate a moderate increase in the volume of extracellular fluid and total body water after ten hours of perfusion despite the maintenance of a subnormal urine flow.

Summarizing

The normal electrolyte and water balance is altered during and after heart–lung bypass either by the perfusion itself or by various medications and extraneous factors. On the *anionic* side, lactate, pyruvate, inorganic phosphate and chloride levels in plasma usually increase, while bicarbonate is decreased. On the *cationic* side, plasma sodium levels increase, but potassium levels are depressed. Since the hypokalemia is accompanied by hypocalcemia, their effects on myocardial excitability tend to cancel each other. Water is lost from exposed surfaces during open-chest perfusions. However, perfused organisms tend to retain water during lengthy procedures so that edema may result.

OXYGEN TOXICITY

Around 1957, it was suggested by two leading groups that oxygen toxicity was the cause of sudden death among perfused patients in the early postoperative periods (Penido, et al., 1957; Kolff, 1958; Ito, et al., 1958; Effler, et al., 1959). Overarterialization of the blood in the artificial lung, resulting in arterial blood oxygen tensions far above the normal values, was thought to be responsible for disturbances in tissue metabolism and CO_2 transport which finally led to irreversible cerebral damage. The basis for a toxic effect of high oxygen tensions was mainly observation of this clinical syndrome under conditions where the plasma oxygen content was extremely high. The maintenance of arterial oxygen tensions, as monitored by a polarographic electrode, within the range of normal was followed by the disappearance of this dreaded complication of perfusion.

It must be pointed out that the abovementioned evidence is only inferential and that there is little ground for regarding as toxic the arterial oxygen tensions attainable when pure oxygen under *atmospheric* pressure is used in the artificial lung. "Oxygen poisoning" classically refers to two cardinal manifestations observed in organisms submitted to very high oxygen tensions: convulsions (the "Paul Bert effect"), and pulmonary irritation (the "Lorrain Smith effect"). In a review of the clinical literature, Fleisch (1958) discusses complications associated with long term oxygen therapy, which have little bearing on the difficulties encountered in short-term heart–lung bypass. Circulatory abnormalities are not apparent during pure oxygen breathing unless pressures far above atmospheric are used (Lambertsen, et al., 1955). Oxygen poisoning in the biological literature (Dickens, 1946; Donald, 1947; Gerschman, et al., 1954; 1959; Bauereisen, et al., 1958) refers to biochemic disturbances and bioelectrical defects, similar in many respects to those caused by x-irradiation and possibly mediated by the formation of oxidizing free radicals. They occur only in tissues or animals breathing pure oxygen under pressure above atmospheric. Clark, et al. (1958) have reported a large series of human perfusions in which the arterial oxygen tensions were of the order of 600 mm. Hg. No untoward effect could be detected and the patients survived the procedure. However, on the basis of redox potential measurements in tissues perfused with blood from an artificial lung, Hyman (1959a) has speculated that damage to cytochrome-oxidases and other enzymatic systems may occur from high oxygen tensions. The present status of the question can be summarized as by Kolff, et al. (1960): no deleterious effect from the high oxygen tensions encountered during total body perfusion has yet been demonstrated. However, overoxygenation does not occur in nature and it is unlikely that the human organism has defense mechanisms against it. Since it provides no obvious benefit to the organism and is a source of potential dangers, it should rather be avoided.

Most of the difficulties ascribed to oxygen toxicity are related to faulty ventilation of the artificial lung (Sanger, et al., 1959) or to the release of gas bubbles in the arterial blood stream. The possibility of gas bubble embolization in a perfused organism exists even if one assumes that the blood leaving the extracorporeal circuit does not contain any bubbles. Many mechanisms could be responsible. The most likely occurs when blood equilibrated with high oxygen tensions enters an organism which is relatively warmer—supersaturation may then cause the release of microbubbles from the plasma (Jordan, et al., 1958b). However, according to the observations of Donald and Fellows (1959), a temperature difference of 17°C. is required for bubbles to be liberated in a sustained, steady stream, and the release follows a delay of many minutes. Other physical factors which affect the formation of gas bubbles in an organism have been thoroughly analyzed by Harvey, et al. (1944a, b, c), and Harris, et al. (1945), and recently reviewed by Ross (1959). The formation of bubbles in a liquid is closely allied to the presence or absence of small invisible gas masses called gas nuclei. Gas nuclei are usually attached to hydrophobic areas or stabilized in surface cracks. They are also present on dust or particles suspended in a liquid. It is possible that multiplication and expansion of gas nuclei rather than supersaturation is the most important factor in bubble formation following artificial oxygenation and heating. Still another mechanism has been suggested by Salisbury (1956), namely bubble formation through cavitation at the tip of the arterial infusion cannula where high flow velocities are reached. However, according to experiments by Ross (1959), cavitation strong enough to release gas bubbles implies a ratio of blood flow to cannula size far larger than is actually encountered in perfusion procedures.

Whether gas bubbles are introduced in the blood stream during its passage through the extracorporeal circuit, or are released only after the blood has entered the arterial system, the resulting danger is the same. It is not possible to review here all aspects of microbubble embolism, as intriguing as some observations may be. Early experiments with bubble oxygenators suggested that gas embolism was the cause of unexplained neurologic damage after extracorporeal circulation (Maloney, et al., 1958; Schmutzer, et al., 1958; Jordan, et al., 1958b). Using the same perfusion equipment, others were unable to demonstrate gas embolism (Willman, et al., 1958; Heimbecker, 1958; Landew, et al., 1960). There is also no agreement among the values reported as the lethal dose of oxygen deliberately injected into an artery. The reason for these discrepancies are numerous:

(1) The site of injection should be standardized because the occlusion of cerebral and coronary vessels is much more critical than capillary blockade in other organs (Fries, et al., 1951);

(2) The danger of gas embolism depends greatly upon the nature of the gas, CO_2 being almost harmless and oxygen much better tolerated than air (Harkins and Harmon, 1934; Oppenheimer, et al., 1959; Kunkler and King, 1959);

(3) The danger of oxygen embolism is reduced if the patient has previously been denitrogenized;

(4) Small amounts of surface tension reducing substances, such as the silicones used in extracorporeal circulation techniques, markedly reduce the risk involved from gas embolism (Eiseman, et al., 1959);

(5) Finally, the average size of the bubble itself is the most critical factor affecting its disappearance time in a desaturated liquid environment. Consequently, the actual risk of gas embolism is proportional to the diameter of the bubbles.

The formulae proposed by Epstein and Plesset (1950) and Pattle (1960) for the lifetime of a spheric bubble, stationary in an infinite amount of liquid can be simplified as follows for the case of an oxygen bubble in arterial blood:

$t = R^2 \times 10$,[4] where t is the disappearance time in seconds and R the radius of the bubble in mm (Gertz, et al., 1960). From this formula, one can calculate that bubbles with a radius below 0.1 mm. should disappear within two minutes. The oxygen bubbles observed by Landew, et al. (1960) did not last more than 15 to 25 seconds in the blood stream, which accounts for their lack of toxicity.

Summarizing:

Oxygen toxicity has been implicated in the sudden death of perfused patients in the postoperative period. However, arterialization of blood by exposure to pure oxygen under normal atmospheric pressure does not seem to exert harmful effects, despite the high arterial oxygen tensions which are encountered. Most difficulties ascribed to oxygen toxicity are actually related to faulty ventilation of the artificial lung or to the release of gas bubbles in the arterial blood stream.

XV. Effects of Perfusion on Organs

Although the *total* blood flow to a patient is controllable during extracorporeal circulation, the rate of perfusion of *individual* organs during total heart–lung bypass cannot be modified at will. As discussed in Chap. XIII, the maintenance of a total perfusion flow as close as possible to the normal provides the best approach to adequate distribution of blood to all parts of the body. This ideal state cannot always be reached, and therefore effects of perfusion on individual organs must first depend on a pure flow distribution basis. Secondly, hemodynamic characteristics of the artificial circulation, such as the position of the cannulae and the nature of the flow, influence some organs more than others. The same applies to the biochemical values of blood arterialized in an extracorporeal circuit, for instance, high oxygen tensions and low CO_2 tensions. Finally, because the handling of blood in man-made devices is not perfect and because hypoxia or embolism may occur, damage is primarily caused to those organs which are more sensitive. For all these reasons, the individual adaptation, performance and pathology of organ systems represents an important chapter in heart–lung bypass studies which Clowes (1960) has most ably reviewed. In view of the wealth of material in the literature of recent years, we shall restrict this chapter to the discussion of the most salient points.

BRAIN

Hypoxic tolerance: Ever since the demonstration by Sir Astley Cooper in 1836 that no signs of brain activity could be evoked after a few minutes of complete interruption of the blood supply to this organ, there has been concern about perfusion of the brain under all abnormal circulatory conditions. In the case of cardiac arrest, the cerebral function is the first to be irreversibly jeopardized by lack of oxygen. From this observation it was inferred that the brain would also be the first organ to suffer irreparable damage if blood flow and oxygen availability were markedly reduced.

Then it was found that very young animals resist arrest of the cephalic circulation longer than do adults (e.g., Kabat and Dennis, 1939; 1940; 1941). Noell and Schneider (1948) demonstrated that there is no irreparable damage to the brain as long as the venous oxygen tension does not drop below 20 mm. Hg. Summarizing a long series of experimental studies, Opitz and Schneider (1950) and Schneider (1953) concluded that there is no absolute parallelism between brain perfusion and oxygen distribution on the one hand, and the state of consciousness on the other. The irreducible "structural metabolism" required for keeping cerebral tissue alive amounts to only 20 per cent of what is needed for functional activity. Therefore, the brain can survive much longer with a minimal supply of blood than without any perfusion at all, a principle which was repeatedly confirmed in the pioneer years of extracorporeal circulation (Andreasen and Watson, 1952; Cohen, et al., 1953; Read, et al., 1956). Schneider and his associates also established that the revival time of the brain (longest period of circulatory arrest compatible with survival) is about ten minutes, twice as long as the revival time of the organism as a whole. Observations that the brain cannot survive circulatory arrest for more than three or four minutes (e.g., Carrel, 1914; Heymans, et al., 1937; Fauteux, 1947) are explained by the inability of the heart to maintain normal pressures in the early recovery period, thus the ischemia of the brain is prolonged considerably beyond the recognized duration of circulatory arrest (*see* Chap. II). Reviewing the literature on the subject, Hirsch, et al. (1957a, b), Dawes, et al. (1959), Bunec (1960) and Malméjac and Malméjac (1960) analyzed the factors which cause discrepancies in experimental data on the revival time of the brain and that of the organism as a whole. They are: (*1*) persistence of a minimal, unrecognized perfusion during the ischemic period, due to collateral circulation; (*2*) progressive drop in the temperature of the non-perfused organ or organism, requiring consideration of the protective effect of hypothermia; (*3*) insufficient head of pressure for perfusion during the recovery period, resulting in unrecognized prolongation of the ischemic period; (*4*) beneficial effect of cerebral "lavage" by solutions containing neither oxygen, nor glucose, probably due to the flushing out of toxic products of ancrobic metabolism.

Cerebral circulation: Cerebral blood flow in man amounts normally to 51 ml./min./100 Gm. of brain, or approximately 15 per cent of the basal cardiac output (Lassen, 1959). Under experimental conditions, cerebral blood flow is determined largely by four factors: (*1*) arteriovenous pressure difference (mean arterial pressure minus venous or cerebrospinal fluid pressure); (*2*) blood viscosity; (*3*) CO_2 tension in the arterial blood; (*4*) O_2 tension in the venous blood or cerebrospinal fluid (as the closest, easily obtainable approximations to cerebral tissue oxygen tension). Little is known concerning the exact location of changes in cerebrovascular resistance, and how and when they are mediated. However, a general rule was expressed by Bovet, et al. (1960): "The chemical (active) regulation is characterized by a high sensitivity of the cerebral vessels to the chemical and humoral agents and prevails when the functional and the metabolic activities of the central nervous system are elevated. The hydrostatic (passive) regulation is on the contrary, characterized by variations in the cerebral blood flow which are dependent on changes in the arterial pressure, and is predominant under conditions of depressed metabolic and functional activity of the central nervous system."

Halley, et al. (1958) found, in agreement with the aforementioned rule, that the cerebral blood flow during extracorporeal circulation is dependent essentially on the mean systemic blood pressure. Therefore, cerebral blood flow is close to normal at high perfusion rates (even above the control values in recent experiments by Ankeney and Viles, 1961) and decreases proportionately as the perfusion rate is decreased. For reasons which are still unclear, the cerebral oxygen consumption falls abruptly with the onset of extracorporeal circulation and is maintained constant thereafter, regardless of fluctuations in flow, by widening of the arteriovenous oxygen difference. When the head of pressure for brain perfusion is low, compensation can be brought about by an increase in total perfusion flow, by vasoconstriction elsewhere, or by filling the vascular system with blood. Increase in total perfusion flow has already been discussed (Chapter XIII). Vasopressor agents administered during extracorporeal circulation produce a striking increase in cerebral perfusion with correspondingly decreased flow through the kidneys, intestine and extremities (Halley, et al., 1959b). The advantages of a rise in blood pressure obtained by overtransfusion are partially overcome by the simultaneous increase in venous pressure (Patrick, et al., 1958) which tends to reduce the driving pressure across the brain (the spinal fluid pressure follows the variation of the superior vena cava pressure). The detrimental effects of an impairment to venous drainage from the brain have been stressed by Theye, et al. (1957), who recognized functional changes in brain activity at the time of caval cannulation or when manipulation of the heart produced a kinking at the tip of the venous catheter.

Changes in blood viscosity are of limited importance in the regulation of cerebral blood flow during normothermic perfusions. However, increased viscosity may contribute to the increased cerebrovascular resistance observed during hypothermia.

Fluctuations in oxygen and carbon dioxide tensions, as occur in artificial circulation procedures, are known to affect cerebral vasomotion. A decrease in O_2 tension and an increase in CO_2 tension result in a fall in cerebrovascular resistance, thereby augmenting the proportion of the total blood flow diverted to the brain. Conversely, an increase in O_2 tension and a decrease in CO_2 tension tend to diminish brain perfusion. In general, the effects of the factors reducing cerebral blood flow are not so pronounced as the effects of factors which tend to increase flow (Patrick, et al. 1958). During heart–lung bypass at low flow rates, hypoxia by causing cerebral vasodilation provides some degree of brain protection. Brain tissue oxygen tensions are the last to fall below the control values when the organism is underperfused (Schwartz, et al., 1958). Bloor, et al. (1958) observed that animals maintain a normal cerebral oxygen tension through a 50 per cent fall in mean arterial pressure caused by graded hemorrhage. In unanesthetized persons, clinical signs of cerebral hypoxia become evident when the cerebral blood flow falls to about 60 per cent of the control value (Lassen, 1959). Consciousness is lost when the oxygen tension of cerebral venous blood reaches 20 mm. Hg., and at this level, cortical electrical activity also disappears abruptly. Thews (1960) has recently calculated that the oxygen tension in the part of the cerebral tissue receiving the least supply is normally around 17 mm. Hg. The oxygen tension in the cerebrospinal fluid, which approximates the mean oxygen tension of the brain (Bloor, et al., 1961), may provide a convenient means for studying cerebral oxygen tensions during human perfusions.

It would be hazardous to rely on hypoxic vasodilation to maintain oxygenation of the brain at low extracorporeal flow rates since underperfusion leads to metabolic acidosis, which in turn is compensated by a loss of bicarbonate base and results in lowered CO_2 tension, a factor leading to cerebral vasoconstriction. A lowering of the CO_2 tension must also be considered during perfusion at high flow rates because hyperventilation of the artificial lung sometimes results in hypocapnea and alkalosis. Malette (1958) demonstrated that the cerebral tissue anoxia resulting from hyperventilation is due mainly to the Bohr effect and only to a small degree to cerebral vasoconstriction.

Neurologic disturbances: Signs of temporary or permanent neurologic damage after otherwise successful cardiopulmonary bypass have been reported often (e.g., Helmsworth, et al., 1952a; Clowes, et al. 1954; Reed and Kittle, 1958a, b; Ehrenhaft and Claman, 1961). They have been ascribed to particulate emboli such as fibrin or to gas emoblism either from a bubble oxygenator (Diesh, et al., 1957; Gianelli, et al., 1957; Maloney, et al., 1958), or from improperly designed coronary suction devices (Miller and Albritten, 1960). Antifoam emboli (*see* Chapter III) and fat emboli (Adams, et al., 1960) have also been detected. In other hands, however, similar perfusion equipment did not cause any recognizable damage (Hodges, et al., 1958; Heimbecker, 1958; Willman, et al., 1958a; Zuhdi, et al., 1959). Autopsy and histologic examination often fail to indicate the exact cause of brain damage in patients or animals who obviously die from neurologic complications after cardiopulmonary bypass. The blood–brain barrier breakdown test of Hodges, et al. (1958) is an attempt to establish objectively whether or not cerebrovascular permeability is affected by artificial perfusion. Fluorescein injected into the blood stream should not stain brain tissues unless they are damaged. This test has proven useful for experimental evaluation of perfusion techniques. However, there is no unanimity as to its interpretation (Fries, et al., 1957); it is not specific for the trauma caused by heart–lung machines (Story, et al., 1958) and is subject to numerous pitfalls (Broman, et al., 1961).

In the search for intravital signs of brain damage caused by perfusion, ophthalmoscopic observation of retinal vessels (Kevorkian, 1957; Redo, 1958) has been found to provide some insight into the cerebral circulation and it may be possible by this means to recognize cerebral air embolism. In the dog the state of relaxation of the nictitating membrane is correlated with the degree of functional activity of the brain (Guastavino, et al., 1958, 1959d). The triad of negative palpebral reflex, completely relaxed nictitating membrane and open lids constitutes a very ominous sign. A staggering gait is commonly encountered in experimental animals after perfusion. There is no agreement as to whether it constitutes a minor sign of neurologic damage or is merely related to operative trauma in the inguinal area (Landew, et al., 1960; Lesage, et al., 1961) or the use of barbiturates as anesthetic agents.

Electroencephalogram: Because of its sensitivity to significant decreases in brain oxygen supply, and because it can be used continuously without causing any harm to the subject, the electroencephalogram (EEG) is the best available technique for monitoring brain activity during and after heart–lung bypass. As early as 1944, Opitz and Palme were able to correlate the oxygen tension of blood issuing from the brain with the wave frequency of the electroencephalogram in the deeply hypoxic range. In 1954, Clowes, et al. first reported on the use of the EEG during extracorporeal circulation. They noted little deviation from the preperfusion tracings in those animals which were maintained at normal arterial pressure throughout the procedure. Waves of low amplitude and frequency were observed in the frankly hypotensive animals who subsequently died. The correlation between the severity of the EEG changes and the prognosis in experimental animals was subsequently confirmed by Owens, et al. (1956), Beaussart, et al. (1959), and Margulis and Ostrovsky (1960). A slight depression of the frequency of the EEG has been consistently observed in successful, long-term perfusions (Hopf, et al., 1961).

Most of the knowledge about electroencephalographic changes has been gathered in human perfusions. In a large series of patients perfused at low flow rates, Matthews, et al. (1957) frequently observed severe depression of EEG activity with an early loss of rapid activity, and replacement by high voltage, slow delta waves which later flattened to a point where no electrical activity could be recognized. These extreme alterations were correlated with inadequacy of the perfusion flow. However, they did not affect the awareness of the patient after the perfusion, nor the final outcome of the operation, probably because the underlying hypoxia was of short duration. With relatively high flow rates, the clinical experience of Theye, et al. (1957), and Hodges, et al. (1958) indicated that for the most part normal EEG patterns were predominant during and after heart–lung bypass. The most frequent alterations appeared at the time of venous cannulation, at the onset of perfusion or when the superior vena cava was inadvertently compressed during perfusion. The depression which coincided with the beginning of extracorporeal circulation was explained by the lower temperature of the priming blood and relative hypothermia of the brain. Decrease in cerebral blood flow caused by obstruction of the superior vena cava accounted for most other disturbances, as confirmed by Brechner, et al. (1959), Trede, et al. (1959), and Paton, et al. (1960). The EEG alterations included replacement of the low amplitude, high frequency pattern, characteristic of light anesthesia, with high amplitude, low frequency waves. The changes were transient and disappeared after resumption of unimpaired flow. The authors viewed the appearance of an abnormal pattern with alarm, since normal EEG are maintained even with moderately deficient perfusion of the brain. Studies by Walter, et al. (1958), Owens, et al. (1958), Stephen, et al. (1959), Kavan, et al. (1959a,b), Bark (1960), and Adelman and Jacobsen (1960) showed few significant alterations in the EEG pattern during successful perfusions. In conflicting reports, Mirabel, et al. (1957) and Davenport, et al. (1959) found an abnormal EEG in the majority of their patients. The beginning of bypass was marked by the appearance of slow, high amplitude waves superimposed on the previously existing rhythm. In case of more marked alterations, the background pattern became less apparent and even disappeared. Throughout the remainder of the perfusion, the EEG was unlike that recorded prior to bypass.

Torres, et al. (1959) pointed to the high percentage of abnormal electroencephalograms and neurologic findings that exist in patients with heart disease prior to surgical treatment. This observation alone makes it difficult to generalize about the association of EEG changes with artificial circulation. Scurr (1958) considered deterioration of the EEG pattern as indicative of a fall in cerebral blood flow below a safe level. Yet Kirklin, et al. (1958b) have occasionally observed a normal EEG in the presence of a grossly inadequate brain perfusion, and Cliffe, et al. (1959) have called attention to the fallacy of regarding a return to normal of the EEG after a period of cerebral anoxia as necessarily indicating recovery. Methods of grading deterioration of the EEG (Hudson, 1958; Davenport, et al. 1959; Hopf, et al. 1961) are arbitrary and find little acceptance outside the immediate circle of their proponents. Not everybody would agree that "the nonspecific summation of the physiologic and metabolic processes as expressed by the electrical activity of the brain is an excellent gauge for judging from moment to moment the immediate state of neurologic viability of a subject during and after employment of a pump-oxygenator" (Owens, et al. 1958). There remain presently two schools of thought concerning the usefulness of the EEG during heart–lung bypass. The greater number of investigators regard it as a "dependable and sensitive monitor of brain oxygen supply" (Adelman and Jacobsen, 1960) and rely on it for judging the adequacy of brain perfusion. The other investigators stress that the EEG cannot pinpoint intrinsic deficiencies in artificial oxygenation and circulation, that its warning gives little information concerning the final outcome of the procedure, and that one should not wait until alterations occur before recognizing the hemodynamic or metabolic defects which are causing changes in the EEG pattern.

Summarizing:

Among all organs, the brain is the first to stop functioning from lack of oxygen in case of circulatory arrest. Irreparable damage results after a few minutes. However, the brain can survive much longer with a minimal supply of blood than without any perfusion at all. During extracorporeal circulation adquate cerebral blood flow is attainable provided that mean arterial pressure is kept in the normal range and drainage through the superior vena cava is not obstructed. In the case of low flow perfusion, decrease in blood oxygen tension enhances brain perfusion by decreasing cerebrovascular resistance, and this protects the brain to some extent. Neurologic damage after perfusion is usually explained by cerebral hypoxia, or embolism of fibrin fragments, gas bubbles, antifoam or endogenous fat. The electroencephalogram is the most widely used monitor of cerebral function during and after heart–lung bypass, although the information it provides is not directly related to the adequacy of cerebral function.

HEART

Coronary flow: Gregg and Sabiston (1956) summarize the factors controlling coronary flow as follows: "Flow will vary directly with the effective perfusion pressure head (aortic or central coronary pressure minus right atrial pressure) and with the size or mean bore of the coronary bed. The bore of the coronary bed is regulated to increase flow by changes in the intrinsic smooth muscle of the coronary vessels as mediated by nervous, humoral and metabolic influences (active coronary vasodilatation) and by a passive or mechanical mechanism arising from myocardial contraction during systole (passive dilatation)."

During total cardiopulmonary bypass, the effective pressure head driving blood across the coronary vascular bed is usually equal to mean aortic pressure, since the right heart cavities are either open to atmospheric pressure for surgical purposes, or vented into the low pressure pulmonary vascular bed. The coronary blood flow, measured as the outflow in the isolated right heart cavities, increases proportionately with mean arterial pressure and total perfusion flow (Lenfant, et al., 1957; Case, et al., 1958; Willman, et al., 1958b; Cortesini, et al., 1959). The coronary pressure–flow relationship is nearly linear in the range of perfusion rates used clinically. At perfusion rates approximating basal cardiac output, coronary flow equals that measured under normal conditions: 46 ml./min.100 Gm. heart in the average (Glenn, et al., 1958) or between four and seven per cent of extracorporeal flow (Read, et al., 1957a; Glenn, et al., 1958). However, there is little increase in coronary flow for further increments in total body perfusion (Case, et al., 1958), and the coronary flow tends to reach a plateau, possibly because aortic pressure also levels off at extremely high perfusion rates. At the other end of the scale, the proportion of blood passing through the myocardium increases as total perfusion flow is reduced below 30 ml./Kg./min., thereby favoring the heart over other organs in the presence of impending hypoxia (Read, et al., 1957a). At constant extracorporeal flow rate, adrenergic agents in large doses increase coronary flow tremendously (Maraist and Glenn, 1952; Glenn, et al., 1958). This is caused at least partially by the rise in aortic pressure and by preferential distribution of the blood to the coronary vascular bed in the face of peripheral vasoconstriction. A marked increase in coronary flow has also been observed with relatively small doses of 1-norepinephrine, ranging from 2 to 5 mmg./Kg. (Laurent, et al., 1959).

The main potential factor in coronary vasomotion during total cardiopulmonary bypass is hypoxia. At constant extracorporeal flow rates, there is already a modest increase in coronary flow as arterial blood saturation falls from normal to 70 per cent. Below this point, the coronary flow increases rapidly (Maraist and Glenn, 1952), sometimes by a factor of three to five. Since anoxia limited to the coronary vascular bed produces the same effect, the mechanism which induces vasodilation must be a local one. As shown by Lord, et al. (1958), flow returns promptly to normal if the period of hypoxia is short. If it exceeds a few minutes, however, vasodilation persists long after hypoxia has been relieved, together with a decreased arteriovenous oxygen difference (Glenn, et al., 1958). In other words, the estimated flow debt is very much overpaid (Coffman and Gregg, 1960).

Another determinant of coronary blood flow which is modified by cardiopulmonary bypass is related to passive changes in size of the coronary vessels which accompany the mechanical events of cardiac contraction. During bypass, left ventricular systolic pressure varies widely according to the nature of the operation performed, the type of cardiac rhythm, and the presence or absence of "emptying beats" (occasional left ventricular ejections). According to Case, et al., (1958) there is a marked increase in coronary flow associated with a rise in left ventricular systolic pressure. Under their experimental conditions, however, the aortic pressure rose concomitantly with ventricular pressure. Thus, it cannot be decided whether the observed increase in coronary flow was caused by a more marked passive dilation, by an increase of pressure head across the coronary vascular bed, or by an increased requirement for oxygen when the total tension developed by the myocardium was increased. Using a gravity arterial infusion system, Kunlin, et al. (1952) observed that maximal coronary arterial inflow occurs during diastole, a fact which is at variance with many classic observations. We have found no report of the use of modern phasic flowmeters to study the cyclic variations in coronary flow during heart–lung bypass. Ventricular fibrillation, when induced in the presence of a relatively normal coronary flow, is usually followed by a rise in flow (Glenn, et al., 1958). When it occurs in the presence of large coronary flows, as caused by hypoxia for instance, no further increase in flow occurs.

Myocardial metabolism: Although blood flow through the walls of the empty beating heart during total body perfusion at high flow rate is essentially the same as that reported for the normally functioning heart, the oxygen use of the myocardium is decreased to 60 to 70 per cent of the control value (Willman, et al., 1958b; Salisbury, et al., 1959a). At variance with these results, Wallace, et al. (1960a, b, 1961) have found the metabolic demands of the beating, non-working heart to be the same as or greater than those of the normally beating heart. The factors which affect oxygen uptake of the beating heart muscle during cardiopulmonary bypass have not been sufficiently elucidated. In fact, there is presently a controversy among physiologists as to the determinants of myocardial oxygen uptake under normal circulatory conditions. Numerous empiric correlations have been derived between oxygen use of the heart muscle on the one hand, and left ventricular pressure, aortic pressure, area under the aortic pressure curve, mean difference between aortic and right atrial pressure, or between aortic and left ventricular pressure curves, myocardial tension, myocardial work and similar parameters of cardiac function on the other side. The fundamental question, however, as to whether oxygen use at the tissue level determines the coronary blood flow, or the amount of oxygenated blood distributed determines the metabolism of the heart, is still unanswered (Alella, et al., 1955; Braunwald, et al., 1958; Feinberg, et al., 1958). It appears doubtful that correlation analysis, which does not recognize that the experimental errors of measurement are of a different order for different parameters, and that many of the relationships involved are not linear, will ever solve the dispute. It must also be kept in mind that according to Laplace's law, the size of the ventricular cavities, and consequently the distension of myocardial fibers, is the primary (and most often forgotten) determinant of cardiac energy expenditure. Therefore it is somewhat futile to discuss the details of oxygen uptake by the beating heart under conditions of total heart–lung bypass. The subject of cardiac metabolism in the fibrillating and arrested heart is considered in Chapter XVII.

Cardiac action: The heart rate is usually slowed during complete cardiopulmonary bypass (Lenfant, et al., 1957). In the experience of other authors, however (Salisbury, et al., 1959a, b), the heart rate does not change materially. The physiologic mechanism of this relative bradycardia are not clear. A fall in temperature of the pacemaker area, the cessation of normal tension of the atrial walls, relative hypoxia of the cardiac muscle or of the carotid sinus have all been advocated. Spohn, et al. (1958) reported a peculiar phenomenon of "accrochage" between the heart rate and the pump rate at the inception of bypass, with one systole for each second pressure cycle of the pump. Heart block as a consequence of injury to the conduction system is primarily a surgical problem and as such is beyond the scope of this book.

Ventricular fibrillation is a common occurrence during cardiopulmonary bypass. This arrhythmia is not particularly ominous in its implications when the circulation is supported by a pump-oxygenator. Without going so far as considering it "a simple cosmetic defect in the electrocardiogram" (Gollan 1959a), it must be stated that ventricular fibrillation is in most instances easily reversible under open-chest conditions. It can even be reversed in closed-chest animals provided that the oxygen requirements of the fibrillating heart have been satisfied by the artificial perfusion (Bell and Beretta, 1959; Kuhn, et al., 1960a, b). The factors responsible for ventricular fibrillation, besides direct stimulation of the myocardium, are usually those which fit the "short refractory period" theory of Burn (1960a, b): hypoxia, hypoglycemia, high potassium levels.

The adequacy of blood flow and oxygen distribution to the heart during cardiopulmonary bypass is proven by the experiments of Stirling, et al. (1957). Using Starling's "ventricular function curve" technique, these authors did not observe any impairment in right ventricular function after 30 minutes of total body perfusion at flow rates ranging between 0.3 and 1.7 L./sq. m./min. Only at extremely low perfusion rates (below 0.3 L./sq. m./min.) did ventricular function show definite impairment. The same evidence of unaltered cardiac function with respect to the left ventricle was obtained by Willman, et al. (1959b), and Waldhausen, et al., (1960). Direct measurements of myocardial contractile force by the strain gauge arch technique (Darby, et al., 1958; Lee, et al., 1958; Bloodwell, et al., 1960; Goldberg, et al., 1960) also demonstrate that cardiopulmonary bypass does not of itself cause any significant depression of ventricular function. The myocardial weakness sometimes manifested after perfusion by inability of the heart to support the circulation can usually be traced to the following specific causes: Hypoxic damage in case of insufficient coronary perfusion (Wesolowski, et al., 1952); shunting of a large portion of the cardiac output through the widely dilated coronary vascular bed after myocardial hypoxia, resulting in a picture somewhat similar to hypovolemic shock (Glenn, et al., 1958); impairment of cardiac function following incisions of the ventricular wall (Stirling, et al., 1957); gas embolism in the coronary vascular bed (Helmsworth, et al., 1952, Benjamin, et al., 1957); myocardial damage caused by improper technique of cardiac arrest (*see* chap. XVIII); hypervolemic or obstructive distension of the heart resulting from inadequate drainage of blood (Sanger, et al., 1959). A study of deaths associated with heart–lung bypass procedures indicates that in adults cardiocirculatory complications make up the most common cause (Hackett, et al., 1961). Histologic observations related by Helmsworth, et al. (1959) reveal only minute alterations in cardiac tissues after successful perfusions. However, animals dying after long-term perfusion consistently show rather diffuse subendocardial and subepicardial hemorrhages with ecchymotic areas scattered over both ventricles (Andersen and Hambraeus, 1961). On the other hand, perfusion is known to cause myocardial edema under unfavorable conditions (Salisbury, et al., 1961). It is thus possible that the cardiocirculatory shock which leads to death after apparently successful perfusion might be associated with myocardial alterations.

Coronary perfusion: When the base of the aorta is open for surgery of the aortic valves, the ascending aorta must be clamped. Consequently, coronary perfusion is impaired and the heart soon goes into anoxic arrest. To prevent myocardial ischemia, techniques of coronary perfusion directly from the pump-oxygenator have been devised. Perfusion of the coronary ostia requires special cannulae (Gregg and Shipley, 1944; Eckstein, et al., 1951; Roe, 1858; Kay, et al., 1958b; Shumway, 1959; Headrick, et al., 1959; Littlefield, et al., 1960) to insure equal perfusion of all regions of the myocardium. It can be carried out for prolonged periods in animals and in patients with consistent survival (Mendelsohn, et al., 1959). Other investigators have demonstrated the feasibility of retrograde perfusion of the myocardium through the coronary sinus (Blanco, et al., 1956; Salisbury, et al., 1956; Gott, et al., 1957c, d; Massimo, et al., 1958a, b; Micozzi, et al., 1959a). A flow rate approximating 50 per cent of the normal coronary perfusion rate can be reached before too much blood leaks into the ventricular cavities through the Thebesian vessels. In the dog, most of the blood distributed by retroperfusion goes to the left heart, thereby limiting the usefulness of the technique (Gott, et al., 1957c, d; Shumway, 1959). In man the distribution is fortunately more even, since the right ventricular myocardium also remains pink (Lillehei, et al., 1958; DeWall, et al., 1958). Recently, Sabiston, et al. (1959) and Talbert, et al. (1960) made the striking observation that the beat of the isolated heart can be maintained for hours by perfusion of the coronary vascular bed with oxygen in the gaseous state, either direction or in a retrograde fashion (*see* Chapter II). This may well open new avenues of approach to the problem of cardiac support during heart–lung bypass.

Electrocardiogram: The electrocardiogram (ECG) is usually recorded during and after heart–lung bypass, because it provides a simple and atraumatic method of displaying and following the cardiac function. Its main merit is that it gives prompt warning of impending asystole or arrhythmias (Adelman and Jacobson, 1960). If one excludes disturbances related to the pathologic conditions for which human subjects undergo total body perfusion, and the alterations caused by operative manipulations (Fraser and Ressall, 1958), the ECG changes are usually minimal (Zimmerman, et al., 1958; Deuchar and Muir, 1959; Kavan, et al., 1959a, b; Aschenlova, et al., 1960). Some of the changes recorded may be explained by the anesthesia, others are related to changes in serum potassium or calcium levels, particularly in long term perfusions. Alterations suggestive of anoxia are uncommon in perfusion procedures unless the heart is arrested, and they often fail to warn of grave hemodynamic alterations until the situation is far advanced and sometimes irreversible. Consequently, for monitoring the adequacy of oxygen supply during cardiopulmonary bypass, the electrocardiogram is not very useful.

Summarizing:

During heart–lung bypass coronary blood flow is usually proportional to mean aortic pressure and consequently to the artificial perfusion rate. The proportion of flow passing through the heart muscle increases relatively as total blood flow is reduced to very low levels because of hypoxic coronary dilatation. Although blood flow through the walls of the empty, beating heart during bypass may be the same as that of the normally functioning heart, the oxygen uptake of the myocardium is only 60 to 70 per cent of the normal value. Heart–lung bypass by itself does not cause any significant depression of ventricular function. However, myocardial weakness can be caused by factors which often accompany bypass, such as myocardial hypoxia, cardiotomy, coronary gas embolism, overdistension of the heart and faulty surgical repair. Electrocardiographic changes are minimal during properly executed perfusion procedures. Ventricular fibrillation does not carry particularly ominous implications when the circulation is artificially supported and it can be easily reversed on most occasions.

LUNGS

By definition, the lungs are excluded from the circulatory system during total heart–lung bypass. However, the anatomic and physiologic relations between the lesser and the main circulation are such that exclusion of the pulmonary vascular bed is not absolute. It is therefore important to recognize the particular patterns of blood circulation in the lungs to understand the functional disturbances which may be observed.

Collateral circulation: The blood supply to the lungs is of dual origin: the largest volume is distributed under low pressure through the pulmonary artery, whereas a small and, under ordinary conditions, almost negligible amount is delivered at high pressure through the bronchial arteries. During total heart–lung bypass, occlusion of the central veins prevents the systemic blood from entering the right heart cavities and proceeding across the pulmonary vascular bed. If coronary venous return to the right heart cavities is also drained to the outside, the only remaining source of lung perfusion is the "collateral blood flow" entering through the bronchial arteries. Salisbury, et al. (1957) observed that 0.5 to 1 per cent of blood perfused into the aorta is distributed to the lungs via the bronchial arteries. Their estimate has been confirmed by Helmsworth, et al. (1959) and Auld, et al. (1960). Mean systemic arterial pressure, acting as the head of pressure for bronchial circulation, is the main determinant of bronchial flow. Other controlling factors have been recognized; the collateral blood flow to the lungs is directly proportional to systemic venous pressure and inversely proportional to the pulmonary artery pressure. Bronchial flow increases with high concentrations of carbon dioxide in the inspired air, but decreases when ventilatory action is arrested. Collapsed lungs have a minimal bronchial flow (Salisbury, et al., 1957; Weil, et al., 1957; Pezzoli and Pulin, 1957). From the above considerations, it is obvious that during cardiopulmonary bypass at high flow rates, the collateral blood flow to the lungs is not reduced below the normal value, but possibly enhanced (Moersch and Donald, 1959; Micozzi, et al., 1960b; Cortesini, et al., 1960). If no escape for the bronchial venous blood returning through the pulmonary veins into the left atrium and ventricle is provided by a septal defect and opened right heart cavities, blood will accumulate in the left ventricle until enough ventricular distension is developed to bring about an "emptying" beat into the aorta. When the heart is fibrillating, or arrested, accumulation of bronchial venous blood can be accommodated for a while in the lesser circulation, since the pulmonary vascular bed has been emptied of its content during the initial phase of heart–lung bypass. Later on, left atrial distension develops which in turn leads to pulmonary edema and to interstitial hemorrhage. Due to this blood pooling in the lungs, a remarkable amount of blood is denied to the extracorporeal and systemic circulation, and the deficit must be made up by the addition of blood to the extracorporeal circuit (Muller, et al., 1958).

Difficulties associated with collateral blood flow to the lungs do not occur in all perfusions. First, they are associated with long-term bypass since the accumulation of blood is obviously dependent upon the duration of the perfusion. Second, they are more likely to appear under clinical conditions characterized by an increase in collateral blood flow (Lillehei, et al., 1957; Muller, et al., 1958). Difficulties also develop when heart–lung bypass is prolonged after closure both of a septal defect and of the cardiotomy incision, because the "escape valves" are suppressed (Littlefield, et al., 1958a), or conversely, when external perfusion is prematurely stopped before the left ventricle is able to support the circulation alone (Littlefield, et al., 1958b). Other factors causing pulmonary venous and left atrial distension could be closure of the azygos vein, which normally drains a part of the bronchial venous return, or the maintenance of a high systemic venous pressure, which reverses the flow of blood through the intact azygos and bronchial veins from the systemic into the pulmonary veins. Finally, in conditions associated with narrowing of proximal pulmonary arterioles, "high pressure" bronchial blood could be prevented from refluxing freely into the pulmonary arterial bed, thus inducing another mechanism of local hypertension and hemorrhage. From the review of these mechanisms, it is clear that no other measure is as efficient in preventing pulmonary parenchymal changes associated with pulmonary hypertension as is proper decompression of the left atrium by a drainage catheter (Kolff, et al. 1958, 1960).

Coronaro-pulmonary flow: In open-heart procedures, the coronary venous return is drained towards the extracorporeal circuit and is thus prevented from entering the pulmonary vascular bed. During cardiopulmonary bypass with an unopened, beating heart, the coronary venous blood accumulates in the right heart cavities, is expelled into the pulmonary vascular bed, and returns to the left ventricle together with the bronchial blood. Next it is ejected by "emptying beats" into the root of the aorta, from where it provides part, if not all, of the coronary arterial supply. Since the lungs usually are not ventilated during a bypass procedure, this blood remains venous in character despite its passage through the lungs. Consequently, the myocardium becomes cyanotic, electrocardiographic alterations develop and vasodilation of the coronary vascular bed tends to induce a vicious cycle by promoting a larger coronary flow. This particular type of circulation is called "coronaro-pulmo-nary" circulation (Lopez-Bello, et al., 1958). The main ill effects are myocardial hypoxia and ventricular fibrillation, which can be prevented by ventilating the lungs or by draining the right heart cavities. When the heart is fibrillating or arrested, the cardiac cavities and the pulmonary vascular bed form essentially a common chamber (Bell, 1959). The mitral, tricuspid and pulmonary valves are incompetent, but aortic valves are kept shut by the pressure prevailing in the aorta. Provided the pulmonary artery is not occluded, a retrograde, left-to-right blood flow through the pulmonary bed can be observed. Unless the right and left atrium are drained, an accumulation of blood leads to pulmonary hemmorrhage.

Pulmonary function: A reduction in the diffusion capacity of the lung after cardiac operations involving heart–lung bypass has been demonstrated by Schramel, et al. (1959). Cardiopulmonary bypass alone, without thoracotomy, did not cause a consistent reduction in pulmonary diffusion capacity. The relative contribution of alveolar membrane damage and altered pulmonary circulation could not be established.

Studies of respiratory mechanics also give some indication of pulmonary damage. According to Guastavino, et al. (1959c,d), there is a progressive loss of the lung distensibility as perfusion goes on. Pulmonary compliance tends to return towards normal when normal circulation is restored, the degree of recovery depending upon the duration of bypass. As a possible cause for increased stiffness of the non-perfused lungs, Guastavino, et al. (1960) have called attention to the accumulation of blood from the bronchial vessels, which leads to vascular stasis and structural modifications. Tissue anoxia due to the absence of ventilation may also play a role. They do not believe that the decreased compliance observed during cardiopulmonary bypass is accounted for by the marked diminution in blood volume circulating in the pulmonary vascular system, as compared to normal conditions. In their experience the stiffness of the lungs was the same regardless of the amount of pulmonary blood flow which they could artificially establish. These results are somewhat at variance with those of Lewin, et al. (1960) who reported that in experiments involving separate perfusion of the lungs during cardiopulmonary bypass, a decrease of the pulmonary blood pressure and of the pulmonary blood volume below normal caused an increase in peak insufflation pressures. This observation was interpreted to indicate a decreased pulmonary compliance caused by the reduction in pulmonary blood content.

During cardiopulmonary bypass for surgical purposes, it is convenient to keep the lungs motionless. If ventilation is continued, pressure changes are produced which increase the bronchial to pulmonary artery collateral flow (Salisbury, et al., 1957; Muller, et al., 1958). One procedure consists of filling the lungs with a mixture of oxygen and an inert gas and then gently inflating and deflating them at intervals of several minutes to prevent atelectasis (Patrick, 1957; Moffit and Theye, 1959). Others do not use inert gas and keep the lungs motionless. Kottmeier, et al. (1958) reported that periodic lung inflation prevents peribronchial hemorrhages. Whatever procedure is used, it is prudent to remember that sudden inflation of the lungs may elicit stretch reflexes which result in peripheral vasodilation and systemic hypotension (Salisbury, et al., 1959c; Bianconi and Green, 1959; Coleridge and Kidd, 1960). It is also important to adapt the ventilation to the volume flow of blood through the lungs so as to maintain normal gas tensions in the pulmonary venous blood (Cartwright, 1960b).

Pulmonary damage: Pulmonary congestion and edema have been encountered since the beginning of artificial perfusion procedures (e.g., Miller, et al., 1953). Dodrill (1958) described a particular type of pulmonary complication associated with heart–lung bypass which he held responsible for a fatal out-come in a sizable proportion of perfused patients. This syndrome, character-ized by cyanosis and hypercapnia, displayed a random distribution of areas of alveolar collapse in the lungs as its main pathologic feature. The only micro-scopic abnormality was thickening, distortion and fragmentation of the elastic fibers in the alveoli. The etiology of these alterations remained unknown. Kottmeier, et al. (1959) described patch pulmonary collapse and peribron-chial hemorrhages in animals sacrificed at different time intervals after cardio-pulmonary bypass. None of the animals ventilated during the perfusion showed these pulmonary changes. Muller, et al. (1958), and Kolff, et al. (1958) described pulmonary edema and gross hemorrhages associated with failure to prevent adequate drainage of the cardiac cavities during bypass. Cartwright, et al. (1960a, b) stressed that the physiologic integrity of the lungs is most closely guarded when the ventilation-perfusion ratio of the excluded lungs is maintained within a physiologic range. Nevertheless a postperfusion syn-drome, characterized by dark, congested lobes or segments with focal zones of collapse and parenchymal hemorrhage, is still observed occasionally despite the most careful management of the perfusion. Baer and Osborn (1960) sug-gested that it may be caused by denaturation and destruction of blood ele-ments, since it is also observed in partial perfusion procedures in closed-chest animals. This observation recalls the finding by Daly, et al. (1954), of peri-arterial hemorrhages with accumulation of polymorphonuclear leucocytes in terminal pulmonary vessels, during the course of long perfusions. Tomin, et al. (1961) recently reinvestigated this aspect of the problem and observed that leucocytes migrate in large numbers toward pulmonary arterioles and capil-laries at the onset of cardiopulmonary bypass. Such studies provide a clue to the etiology of the pulmonary complications of perfusion procedures, which still account for a considerable proportion of the mortality, particularly in infants.

Summarizing:

The anatomic and physiologic relations between the lesser and main circu-lation are such that the pulmonary circulation is not completely excluded dur-ing total heart–lung bypass. The pulmonary alterations observed reflect the importance of the bronchial circulation, and, to a lesser degree, of the coro-nary circulation, to the temporarily isolated lungs. Adequate right and left ventricular drainage are key factors in avoiding pulmonary damage due to overdistension. A better understanding of the physiopathology of the lungs during bypass is dependent on a more complete knowledge of the diffusion function of the lungs, the metabolism of the lungs, and the reflexogenic rela-tions between the lesser and main circulation.

KIDNEYS

Hypoxic tolerance: The kidneys are the first organs to be impaired in their function when general circulatory conditions begin to deteriorate. It has often been observed that renal function is arrested when the arterial pressure drops below a critical value. This does not mean that the kidneys incur irreparable damage. On the contrary, the kidneys can tolerate complete ischemia for a very long period (about 90 minutes). Suppression of the arterial blood flow to the kidneys for a period of 150 minutes is almost uniformly fatal. However, low flow perfusion (7 ml./Kg./min.) with arterialized blood is sufficient to maintain urine secretion and permit the animal to survive without evidence of renal damage (Bounous, et al., 1960a, b). Polarographic studies of oxygen tension in kidney tissues (Schwarta, et al., 1959) do not indicate any impressive decrease at flow rates as low as 40 ml./Kg./min. Oxygen saturation in the renal venous blood falls progressively as the perfusion flow is reduced (Brown, et al., 1958b). Thus the renal oxygen uptake is maintained on the normal level despite marked decreases in renal blood flow (Halley, et al., 1959b).

Renal function: The vulnerability of the kidneys, together with their ability to recover their secretory function provided a minimal blood supply is maintained during the period of relative ischemia, explains most of the features of renal function during and after cardiopulmonary bypass.

Jongbloed (1953) already noted a decrease in urine production during prolonged experimental perfusions. Beall, et al., (1957) and Crafoord (1958) reported transient depression of renal function in humans perfused at low flow rates. Beall, et al. (1957), Morris, et al. (1957; 1958) and Ottolenghi and Drago (1958) observed that a total perfusion flow of 35 ml./min./Kg. was sufficient to maintain renal blood flow and glomerular filtration rate at around 25 per cent of the control values, and prevented the development of ischemic damage. Experimental observations by Senning, et al. (1960) demonstrate that renal function (measured as renal plasma flow, glomerular filtration rate and electrolyte excretion) is significantly depressed during extracorporeal circulation, even at high flow rates. The extent to which kidney function is affected appears to be dependent upon the prevailing perfusion flow or arterial pressure, and is not influenced by previous settings of the perfusion flow at other levels. There is a 50 per cent decrease in the volume of urine production at flow rates in the range of 100 ml./Kg./min. Decrease of extracorporeal flow is followed by a disproportionately large drop in apparent effective renal blood flow. In a conflicting report, Repogle and Gross (1960) indicate that there is nothing in extracorporeal circulation that precludes relatively normal renal hemodynamics. At perfusion rates approximating the normal cardiac output (3.2 to 3.4 L./sq. m./min.) the renal plasma flow closely approximates normal control values. At perfusion rates of 1.8 to 2.0 L./sq. m./min., a rapid decline in renal plasma flow occurs after the onset of perfusion. These data explain previous reports by the same group (Watkins, 1958) which stated that within five minutes after starting bypass effective renal blood flow completely halted. This striking change may occur despite minimal disturbances in acid-base balance and an adequate arterial pressure. It has been recently documented (Finsterbusch, et al., 1961) by renal arteriography that morphologic alterations consisting of narrowing, and loss of normal curvature of renal arteries are most marked during the first 30 minutes of extracorporeal circulation. Perfusion through a subclavian instead of a femoral artery, and administration of low molecular weight dextran, help to minimize these troubles.

Direct measurements of renal blood flow during extracorporeal circulation were reported by Reemtsma, et al. (1958), and Halley, et al. (1959). Renal blood flow decreases markedly during total body perfusion; and this is not closely correlated with systemic arterial pressure. This increased renal vascular resistance is enhanced considerably by adrenergic agents. Jontz, et al., (1960) claimed a linear relationship between total body perfusion on the one hand, and arterial pressure and renal blood flow on the other. Their conclusions are probably limited to the range of perfusion flows in which the observations were made.

Renal damage: Renal complications during and after extracorporeal circulation are relatively common in experimental perfusions and after long-term perfusions in man (Finsterbusch, et al., 1961). Brull and Louis-Bar (1957), speculated that localized renal vasoconstriction may be caused by serotonin released from disintegrated platelets. This hypotheses is supported by the experiments of Sarajas, et al. (1959), who established an extracorporeal arteriovenous shunt through a tubing specially intended to damage blood elements. As a result of blood corpuscle trauma 5-hydroxytryptamine and adenosine triphosphate were released. Concurrently, the urinary excretion of 5-hydroxytryptamine was markedly increased, while that of 5-hydroxyindolacetic acid (usually the main excretory product of serotonin) was, for unknown reasons, decreased. The animals exhibited pathologic changes typical of lower nephron nephrosis. Glomerular and tubular structures were not regularly affected; the lesions were often reversible, and the animals usually survived (Sarajas and Saure, 1960). According to Frick (1960), the release in extracorporeal circuits of serotonin, a substance with antidiuretic properties, with simultaneous reduction of urinary output, suggest that serotonin plays a role in renal hemodynamics during heart–lung bypass procedures. The liberation of adenosine triphosphate must also be taken into consideration since this substance releases antidiuretic hormone from the posterior pituitary (Dexter, et al., 1954).

Summarizing:

Reduced renal blood flow and glomerular filtration is an almost constant finding in cardiopulmonary bypass procedures. The lower the perfusion rate, the more marked is the functional impairment of the kidneys. Nevertheless, the kidneys can tolerate relative ischemia for a very long period without incurring permanent damage. Substances released by destruction of blood elements may play an important role in renal hemodynamics. Owing to their low threshold of sensitivity to minimal disturbances, kidney function studies are exceedingly useful in the assessment of different perfusion techniques.

LIVER AND SPLANCHNIC AREA

Cardiopulmonary bypass procedures may be consistently successful in terms of survival and yet involve a number of subtle functional or organic alterations of which we are not yet aware. The possibility of liver damage must be considered in view of the sensitivity of this organ to hypoxia. In fact, interest in the effect of total body perfusion on the liver has been stirred up by two lines of observations: the development of splanchnic congestion in experimental animals subjected to prolonged heart–lung bypass, and the transient alterations of hepatic function tests in some patients submitted to extracorporeal circulation procedures.

Splanchnic congestion: Splanchnic congestion has long been observed as a premonitory sign of circulatory failure in unsuccessful perfusions Many explanations have been proposed, ranging from overtransfusion to stasis, bacteremia, endotoxin shock, transfusion reaction, defibrination of blood, impairment of the oxidative metabolism in the body tissues at large, liver anoxia, respiratory and metabolic acidosis. Portal venous pressure nearly always exceeds inferior caval pressure by 3 to 5 mm. Hg. During the first minutes of bypass, it often rises to high levels (15 to 25 mm. Hg.), and comes back to normal later (Andersen, et al., 1958). Portal hypertension, accompanied by accumulation of blood in the splanchnic area, also accounts for arterial hypotension occurring at a late stage in the perfusion of dogs (Quintero, et al., 1959). It probably results from the closure of hepatic venous sphincters as a consequence of acidosis or other noxious stimuli elicited by artificial perfusion. The same mechanism has been used to explain the increased hepatic vascular resistance and the pooling of blood in the capillary sinusoids consistently observed in dogs by Ankeney and Viles (1960). Direct approaches to the problem of splanchnic congestion have been attempted by various means. Schwartz, et al. (1959) were unable to find any clear pattern of liver tissue oxygen tension changes as the perfusion flow rate was varied over a wide range. By direct observation of mesenterial vessels, Schönbach, et al. (1958, 1959) ascertained that the circulation is stopped in many capillary beds when the mean arterial pressure drops below 50 mm. Hg., an observation substantiated by Ogata, et al. (1960) and Takeda (1960). The same authors used plethysmographic techniques to measure the amount of blood trapped in the omentum at the inception of bypass and in the period thereafter. Capillary blood sequestration was much more pronounced when nonpulsatile perfusion flows were employed.

Measurements of blood flow and oxygen uptake in the splanchnic area have been reported by different groups with somewhat conflicting results. When comparing the data of such experimental studies, it must be stressed that the authors have often measured different aspects of blood flow in the splanchnic area: hepatic arterial flow (HAF); portal venous flow (PVF); or hepatic venous flow (HVF). Hepatic venous flow is made up of the hepatic arterial and the portal venous circulation (HVF = HAF + PVF). The blood oxygen content has been measured in different locations: hepatic artery (HAO$_2$); hepatic vein (HVO$_2$); portal vein (PVO$_2$); or superior mesenteric vein (MVO$_2$ = PVO$_2$). Consequently, the values calculated for oxygen uptake may relate to intestinal oxygen consumption: PVF $\times$ (HAO$_2$ − PVO$_2$) or liver oxygen consumption, (HAF $\times$ HAO$_2$) + (PVF $\times$ PVO$_2$) − (HVF $\times$ HVO$_2$). The best estimates of hepatic venous flow (or "total hepatic blood flow") in the dog under normal circulatory conditions range around 30 ml./Kg./min., which is about 25 per cent of the systemic blood flow, and is approximately equal to the renal blood flow. Of the total hepatic blood flow, 80 per cent is contributed by the portal circulation and only 20 per cent by the hepatic artery according to direct measurements by Selkurt and Brecher (1956). Oxygen consumption in the splanchnic area represents about one-fourth of the overall body oxygen uptake. Twenty per cent of this is accounted for by the gut, while 80 per cent is consumed in the liver.

There may be many pitfalls in attempts to uncover the adaptations of such a complex mechanism to the conditions of total body perfusion. Difficulties arise from: (1) The use of the dog as an experimental animal; (2) The disturbances of splanchnic circulation caused by anesthesia and surgical maneuvers; (3) The delicacy of venous outflow collection techniques for measuring regional flow (the type of connection of the outflow catheter, the resistance of the venous line and the level of the collection reservoir are all critical factors); (4) The presence of channels for collateral circulation; (5) The necessity for carrying calculation in multiple stages for measuring some of the parameters, resulting in a progressive loss of accuracy and significance.

Among individual reports, Reemtsma, et al. (1958), and Halley, et al. (1959b) found that intestinal blood flow and intestinal oxygen uptake increased above control values during cardiopulmonary bypass at flows around 50 ml./Kg./min. Injection of an adrenergic agent in dosages producing a pronounced rise in systemic arterial pressure markedly decreased the intestinal flow. Jontz, et al. (1960), at variance with the former results, found a reduction in portal flow at low perfusion flow rates (40 and 60 ml./Kg./min.), but values comparable to control when the body was perfused at 80 ml./Kg./min. In their experience, the splanchnic area received a greater share of the aortic flow during heart–lung bypass (at any flow rate) than under control conditions. It is not known whether or not the fact that the spleen was spared might have influenced the results. Measuring hepatic venous outflow, Andersen, et al., (1958) observed a marked reduction during bypass at very low perfusion rates, but little change from control values at the highest perfusion rates. However, the control values were already rather low. The most complete study of splanchnic perfusion during bypass was reported by Waldhausen, et al. (1959a), who determined hepatic arterial inflow and hepatic venous outflow, calculating portal flow from the difference. During bypass at very high perfusion rates, total hepatic blood flow remained essentially normal. It fell markedly when the perfusion rate was reduced and was less than a third of the control value when a minimal perfusion rate was employed. Hepatic arterial flow decreased less conspicuously than did portal venous flow, and consequently, the contribution of the hepatic artery to liver perfusion increased from 20 to 42 per cent while the extracorporeal rate was reduced from 2.8 to 1.0 L./sq. m./min. The hepatic artery kept supplying an almost constant amount of oxygen to the liver parenchyma, whereas the portal venous blood, becoming more and more desaturated, could not deliver its share.

Further calculations on the data of Waldhausen, et al. (1959a) reveal that intestinal oxygen uptake is not decreased when the extracorporeal flow rate is reduced, as previously found by Halley, et al. (1959b). If these data are significant, they point to the risk of equating blood stagnation, as observed directly in mesenteric vessels at low perfusion rates, with decreased metabolic support. The interpretation of much data concerning mesenteric circulation is made difficult by the scarcity of information concerning the effect of hypoxia and hypercapnia on vasomotor tone in that area. CO_2 exerts a vasodilating action on the mesenteric vasculature. On the other hand, local anoxia, as induced by occlusion of the artery or vein supplying a segment of intestine, brings about a reduction in flow after restoration of free passage for the blood (Turner, et al., 1959). Obviously, more information is needed to solve some puzzling questions of regional circulation during heart–lung bypass.

Functional disturbances: The hepatic chromoexcretory function is depressed during and immediately after a period of extracorporeal circulation (Andersen, et al., 1958). Crafoord, et al. (1957b), and Snyder, et al. (1958) both observed an elevation of serum glutamic oxalacetic transaminase in patients submitted to total body perfusion. In dogs, Andersen, et al. (1958), found a significant difference in lactate level between portal and hepatic venous blood, and concluded that the ability of the liver to remove lactate from the blood is preserved.

Pathologic examinations (Kottmeier, et al., 1959) revealed congestion of the abdominal viscera in all animals submitted to perfusion. Whether this finding is related to the intestinal bleeding which may occur after perfusion (Miller, et al., 1953) is not clear. Occult gastrointestinal bleeding has been occasionally detected during the postoperative phase in humans (Kreel, et al., 1960). Yet splanchnic congestion is conspicuously absent in the large majority of patients who die after extracorporeal circulation procedures. The existence of a sphincteric or throttle mechanism in the hepatic veins of the dog make it difficult to compare experimental animal data to clinical data.

Summarizing:

The relative sensitivity of the liver to hypoxia may result in subtle functional alterations which are not easily recognized after cessation of the perfusion. Since the dog is more prone to splanchnic congestion than is man, experimental findings are not necessarily applicable to clinical conditions. In dogs portal hypertension is frequently observed after the beginning of bypass. It is contributed to by acidosis and other noxious stimuli resulting in closure of liver venous sphincters which do not exist in the human. There seems to be no reduction in splanchnic flow during heart–lung bypass, as long as extracorporeal flow rates are kept high. If the perfusion rate is reduced, the hepatic artery keeps delivering an almost constant amount of blood and oxygen to the liver while the portal venous blood becomes much less abundant and more desaturated. At low perfusion rates oxygen extraction by the gut may jeopardize the oxygen supply to the liver.

OTHER ORGANS

Blood flow through the skin has not been investigated. The occurrence in some patients of areas of alopecia following total body perfusion suggests that there may indeed be some disturbances of blood supply to the skin. There is little more information about the mucosae. Schönbach, et al. (1958) observed the conjunctional vessels of perfused animals by capillaroscopy. They estimated that a flow rate amounting to 80 ml./Kg./min. insures a regular perfusion of all capillary beds examined. Striated muscle was examined by Schwartz, et al., (1959) and found to maintain oxygen tensions above the control level at perfusion rates exceeding 60 ml./Kg./min. Flow in the hindleg of the dog during total cardiopulmonary bypass does not bear any evident relationship to the aortic head of pressure, nor to the total perfusion flow rate (Reemtsma, et al., 1958; Halley, et al., 1959b). Plethysmographic studies of the extremities (Graf, et al., 1959; Takeda, 1960) reveal that blood flow is already reduced prior to perfusion probably owing to anesthesia. High flow rates are needed to maintain normal blood distribution throughout the organism. The oxygen consumption of the perfused hindlimb is decreased despite maintenance of normal flow rates (Hottinger, et al., 1960).

The endocrines are likely to be affected by the perfusion procedure, although very little has been reported on this subject. Schönbach, et al. (1958) observed histologically the picture of "stress" in the adrenals and in the thyroid. Mittelman, et al. (1959) studied the changes in steroid metabolism associated with perfusion and reported a definite drop in both plasma levels and urinary excretion during the procedure, with an increase afterwards. Dilution with priming blood was one factor. Changes in the vascular bed of the adrenal gland may have been another cause. The possibility of anterior pituitary depression or accelerated destruction of ACTH during perfusion could not be excluded. Belisle, et al. (1960) found an increase in levels of plasma epinephrine and norepinephrine during perfusions at very low flow rates. This observation led them to speculate on the role of adrenergic amines in the rebound phenomenon (the increase in arterial pressure and cardiac contractile force) upon termination of procedures characterized by systemic hypotension.

Summarizing:

Little is known about the perfusion of the skin, mucosae or skeletal muscle during heart–lung bypass. The extremities as a whole probably receive less than their usual share of blood. Endocrine response to artificial perfusion is still poorly understood.

XVI. The Control of Adequacy
of Perfusion

Cardiopulmonary bypass is such a formidable intrusion into the mechanisms of homeostasis that monitoring of a few key parameters is necessary for maintenance of viable conditions (Hudson, 1959). Any discussion of techniques available for verifying the adequacy of perfusion procedures should begin with a plea for simplicity and for a clear understanding of the type of information actually needed. It is only too apparent that some monitoring devices have been transferred from the experimental laboratory into the operating room merely by routine or tradition. Quite often, the inclusion of metering devices in the extracorporeal circuit is prompted solely by a desire for accumulating quantitative answers to future questions about perfusion techniques.

There are different approaches to the control of heart–lung machines, and it would be presumptuous to pretend that any one is intrinsically superior to another. Because of previous laboratory experience, one investigator may concentrate on hemodynamic measurements, and estimate blood oxygen saturations by visual inspection. Another may not measure vascular pressures, relying on accurate analysis of blood gas tensions to ascertain the adequacy of perfusion. Still another will be satisfied with evidence that the organism as a whole, or individual organs such as the brain or the heart, receive their share of oxygen; he will disregard as unessential the details of oxygen distribution. The operator of a high capacity, large-prime oxygenator enjoys a relatively wide margin of maneuverability in case of technical errors. Therefore, he may feel that he can ignore complicated controls and rely only on his own judgment. On the other hand, the opinion prevails that "feedback controls are necessary for uniformly safe operation of low-prime machines at adequate flow volumes" (Watkins, et al., 1960). This chapter is devoted to the theoretic background on which the choice of monitoring techniques should be made in order to perform the best possible perfusion.

THE IDEAL PERFUSION

The ideal perfusion is that which best replaces the action of the heart and lungs while these organs are excluded from the circulation. Theoretically, the ideal perfusion is defined by physiologic values of all measurable parameters of homeostasis. In practice, there must be exceptions, for example for parameters such as pulse pressure or clotting time, which in the present state of technology still need to be altered. For those, the concept of ideal perfusion must be extended by accepting complete return to normal after perfusion as a criterion of functional integrity.

The hemodynamic, metabolic and organic signs of ideal perfusion can be listed as follows:

1. Hemodynamic signs: (*a*) the perfusion flow rate must equal the basal cardiac output to insure a wide margin of safety in the metabolic support of the tissues; (*b*) the mean systemic arterial pressure must be maintained above 70 mm. Hg., to provide enough head of pressure to all vascular beds; (*c*) the central venous pressure must be kept between 5 and 15 mm. Hg. because low venous pressure results in instability of venous drainage towards the extracorporeal circuit, and high venous pressure endangers cerebral and hepatic function; (*d*) the total body blood volume must be decreased at the onset of perfusion, as the central blood volume is temporarily stored in the extracorporeal circuit, and restored to its original level upon termination of the heart–lung bypass procedure.

2. Metabolic signs: (*a*) the oxygen content of the arterial blood must be maintained above 18 volumes per cent by avoiding undue dilution of blood with saline or plasma expanders; oxygen saturation must be maintained between 95 and 100 per cent while avoiding extremely high oxygen tensions, which possibly increase the risk of gaseous embolism; (*b*) venous oxygen saturation must remain above 70 per cent, or the venous oxygen tension above 40 mm. Hg., to make sure that enough oxygen has been made available to the tissues to cover even unanticipated requirements; (*c*) arterial blood pH must be kept between 7.35 and 7.45, or brought within that range if the initial values are abnormal; (*d*) arterial carbon dioxide tension must remain between 32 and 42 mm. Hg. before, during, and after perfusion, to avoid the risks of hypo- and hyperventilation in both the natural and artificial lungs; (*e*) the volumes of the extracellular and intracellular fluid compartment must remain constant; (*f*) there should be no shift of electrolytes from the vascular tree into adjoining compartments, so that the levels of various electrolytes in plasma are not affected by the procedure.

3. Organic signs: (*a*) a normal electroencephalogram should be observed throughout the perfusion; (*b*) excretory function of the kidney should remain unaltered by the artificial conditions created by the procedure; (*c*) the blood cells should not decrease in number, functional capacity or life expectancy, and the plasma proteins should not be removed or denatured to any extent; (*d*) cardiac and pulmonary functions, which are purposely interrupted during total heart–lung bypass, should promptly return to full efficiency once the perfusion is discontinued.

Temperature specifications have been purposely omitted from the above list of criteria. The first experimental and clinical perfusions were carried out with great attention to maintenance of a constant body temperature. This point does not appear as important now as formerly thought. While it is presently recognized that no benefit, and indeed only difficulties, are to be expected from hyperthermia, a moderate fall in body temperature is almost unavoidable in so-called "normothermic" perfusions, and does not induce any harmful consequences. Nowadays, the main reason for keeping the organism at normal temperatures is so that the above-mentioned criteria can be applied, and easy comparison made with the so-called physiologic state. As we shall see in chap. XIX, other criteria must be defined for hypothermic perfusions.

Summarizing

Despite wide differences of opinion as to how this goal is best achieved, the ideal perfusion is generally accepted as that which most adequately replaces the normal action of the heart and lungs while these organs are excluded. Total body perfusion involves considerable impairment of homeostatic mechanisms. Artificial maintenance of certain physiologic parameters, representative of hemodynamic, metabolic and organic activities during perfusion, is therefore required to make sure that viable conditions are maintained.

THE MONITORING DEVICES

Now that the ideal values of physiologic parameters during perfusion have been defined, let us examine how the common and certain less common laboratory devices can be used to ascertain them.

1. Hemodynamic signs: (*a*) The perfusion flow is measured on the venous side, on the arterial side, or on both sides of the extracorporeal circuit. In both places, the metering device can be a flowmeter (Chapter XI) or a precalibrated, occlusive pump (Chapter VIII). Since as much blood usually enters the oxygenator at its venous end as leaves at the arterial end, one flowmeter is sufficient.

(*b*) The arterial blood pressure is measured either directly, or indirectly. In the first case, an artery must be entered and connected to an electrical or mechanical manometer (Strain gauge manometers are mostly commonly used for this purpose). For indirect measurements one may use the conventional pressure cuff methods, or as suggested more recently, the tracing obtained from an ear oximeter (Bloom, et al., 1960) or from a finger impedance plethysmograph. An indirect indication of arterial blood pressure can also be obtained by recording the pressure in the arterial infusion line. Since the drop of pressure across the arterial cannula bears a constant relationship to flow, a correction factor can be worked out for estimating mean arterial pressure from the pressure measured in the extracorporeal circuit.

(*c*) Venous pressure is measured in the superior vena cava, in the inferior vena cava, or in both. Since the two caval beds are separated during complete bypass, the values may be different. Some authors consider pressure measurement in the superior vena cava as mandatory, since venous hypertension, which impairs cerebral perfusion can then be prevented or corrected. Others monitor the pressure only in the inferior vena cava because most of the blood drained to the outside comes from the lower part of the body, and the pressure there must be controlled to maintain a smooth extracorporeal drainage. Measurement of central venous pressure is important at the end of the perfusion because this is an aid in re-establishing the body blood volume at the optimal level.

(*d*) Body blood volume measurements during bypass are difficult to obtain and to interpret (Chapter XIII). The use of scales on the platform of which the organism is placed permits instantaneous measurements but this is limited to experimental perfusions. Plasma volume or red cell volume determinations serve to ascertain that the organism is neither overtransfused, nor undertransfused. Measurements of extracellular fluid and total body water permit the recognition of edema generated by the perfusion.

2. **Metabolic signs:** (*a*) Blood oxygen saturation can be measured constantly or intermittently by passing a fraction of the blood stream through a cuvette oxymeter. The usually accepted view is that during heart–lung bypass the venous saturation carries more significance than does the arterial, since it reflects the oxygen available to the tissues. After bypass the arterial saturation is more important because it indicates whether or not the lungs have recovered their normal function.

(*b*) Blood oxygen tension can be monitored directly with a polarographic electrode. Measurements on the arterial side provide information as to the functioning of the artificial lung, while values on the venous side reflect the adequacy of perfusion at the tissue level.

(*c*) Blood pH is monitored on the arterial side to ascertaining changes in acid-base balance (Clark, et al., 1958; Kamm, 1959; Edmark, 1959; Loeschke, et al., 1959). The pH is often used to reflect the level of fixed acids in the blood. Taken alone, however, it may be misleading, since the arterial blood pH is far more sensitive to the ventilation of the artificial lung than to acid metabolites released from hypoxic tissues. In fact, relative hyperventilation may mask partially or completely the effect of metabolic acidosis upon arterial blood pH.

(*d*) To avoid camouflaged acidosis, some indication of blood CO_2 content or tension must be obtained. Direct measurements of CO_2 tension can be made by using the newly developed CO_2 electrodes (Severinghaus and Bradley, 1958; Gertz and Loeschke, 1958). An indirect estimate can be obtained by measuring with an infrared analyzer the CO_2 tension in the gas leaving the artificial lung (Leigh, et al., 1961). For each type of oxygenator, a blood flow–gas flow range can be defined in which CO_2 tensions in the gaseous phase closely reflect the arterial blood values.

(*e*) In the gas phase, the total volume flow of oxygen can easily be measured with a gas flowmeter (usually of the rotameter type). Little attention is devoted to total "ventilation" of the artificial lung, and most heart–lung machines provide an unnecessary hyperventilation, which then requires compensation by the addition of CO_2 to the inflowing oxygen. The availability of accurate gas flowmeters and of CO_2 analyzers permits restriction of the flow of pure oxygen without incurring the risk of either hyper- or hypoventilation.

(*f*) Carbon dioxide elimination by the artificial lung can be calculated if one knows the minute-ventilation and the CO_2 tension of the gas leaving the oxygenator. Direct measurements of oxygen uptake in an extracorporeal lung can be obtained by ventilating the artificial lung with oxygen in a closed circuit provided with a CO_2 absorber and a spirometer (*see* chap. IV).

(*g*) The temperature of the blood is usually measured in the extracorporeal circuit. Body temperature determinations present some problems, because the rectal temperature during bypass sometimes reflects the temperature of the blood in the aorta rather than the mean body temperature. Esophageal temperature, which is also commonly employed, is subject to similar pitfalls.

(*h*) Although the day is probably not far away when ions, such as sodium, potassium and calcium can be monitored (Clark, 1959), there is still no practical way of doing it at present and probably not enough knowledge of the permissible variations to utilize this information.

3. Organic signs: (*a*) Brain activity is monitored by the electroencephalogram. Once the technical difficulties associated with measurements in an operating room filled with electrical apparatus are mastered, the EEG offers some insight into the functional state of the brain during perfusion.

(*b*) Electrocardiographic recordings are commonly obtained although the practical information they provide during heart–lung bypass is limited.

(*c*) Kidney function during heart–lung bypass is usually estimated solely by measurement of urine flow. Little practical information is gained from such observations.

(*d*) Polarographic techniques are sometimes employed in the experimental laboratory to follow variations in tissue oxygen tensions and to reach conclusions concerning the oxygen availability in the tissues. These techniques are ticklish and are subject to considerable drift over a period of time, so that the results are mainly qualitative.

Summarizing

Many common laboratory procedures are employed to monitor physiologic variables during heart–lung bypass. Hemodynamic orientation is gained by determining perfusion flow rate, the arterial and venous pressures and the body blood volume. Information about the metabolic status can be obtained by measuring the blood oxygen saturations, tensions, and pH, the arterial CO_2 tension, the oxygen uptake of the artificial lung and the body temperature. Organic signs can be checked with the electroencephalogram, the electrocardiogram and similar techniques.

TECHNIQUES OF CONTROL

There is merely a difference of degree between the "ideal" perfusion, defined by normal values of all measurable physiologic parameters, and the "well tolerated" perfusions actually carried out. Since all the vital signs, hemodynamic as well as metabolic, are closely interdependent in a perfused organism, there is no need to measure them all. The monitoring of a few key factors is, for practical purposes, sufficient to infer the behavior of the others. The question is then to decide which parameters should be measured during heart–lung bypass (Wood, et al., 1959). The investigator is torn between the desire for complete biologic information and the common sense warning that the more numerous and complex the controls, the more likely are the instrumental and human failures. On the one hand, he may feel safer if he has the opportunity to check a variety of vital signs. On the other hand, there is a point of diminishing return when the patient is so cluttered up by pickup devices that the actual perfusion is delayed or impaired, or when the heart–lung machine has so many dials that the operator can hardly read and understand them all before the need for mechanical support of the circulation is actually over. Gollan (1959) has vividly described a natural evolution in many surgical centers. First, there is a "spectacular mob scene in the operating room" and the "intimidating complexity of the heart–lung machine with controls and monitoring devices resembling the dashboard of an atomic submarine"; later, when the group has gained enough experience, one witnesses the return of "the entire technical exhibit of flowmeters, oximeters, pH meters, carbon dioxide analyzers and polarographs to the clinical physiologist."

There are positions intermediate between these two extremes. One solution of the dilemma of apparent safety versus complexity is to make the controls automatic, so as to eliminate delays and errors due to the human factor (Edwards and Bosher, 1960). The Convair heart–lung machine (Kamm, 1959) is probably the most sophisticated step in this direction since it senses and eventually corrects any deviations in oxygen saturation, pH and temperature of the arterialized blood, and closely controls pressure in the arterial line, the perfusion flow rate and the volume of blood in the extracorporeal circuit. However, Watkins, et al., (1960) have pointed out that "although monitoring devices and feed back controls may appeal to workers in this field, it is safer to avoid such controls where automatic functioning based upon the design of the mechanical device permits elimination of a complex monitoring mechanism."

Another solution to the control problem, and the most widely accepted in clinical circles, is to monitor only those parameters which have been empirically found useful for operating the heart–lung machine. The choice of parameters varies from school to school. According to Stewart, et al. (1960), three vascular pressures (arterial, superior caval and inferior caval), the electrocardiogram and blood as well as body temperature supply adequate information. Another group (Hale, 1960) adds the electroencephalogram and pH measurements to the list. Still another group (Waldhausen, 1959) relies upon measurements of the perfusion flow rate and ascribes less importance to the measurement of vascular pressures. Some authors stress the importance of blood pH and gas tension measurements (Clark, et al., 1958; Bucherl and Trede, 1959; Loeschke, 1960; Montgomery, et al., 1960; Race, et al., 1960). Unless an electronic brain takes over the integration of all these elements of information and translates them into action on the controls of the machine, an intelligent operator is needed to decide upon the course of the perfusion. Up to now, control techniques in artificial maintenance of circulation and respiration have largely been developed on an empiric basis. Nonetheless, a rational approach must be favored because it provides the only means of making a correct decision in new, unforeseen or hazardous circumstances.

The first type of rational approach is to make sure that the organism receives an adequate perfusion flow, and that the ventilation of the artificial lung provides for efficient oxygenation and CO_2 removal. This approach constitutes in fact the background of most controlling techniques used. It is obvious that, if a volume of arterialized blood somewhat in excess of the basal body requirement is continuously distributed to the organism, the vascular pressures *must* remain within safe limits, the individual organs *must* receive their share of oxygen and the blood oxygen tensions *must* be within the range of normal. Provided gas flow through the artificial lung is adequately adapted to the blood flow, the CO_2 balance will be maintained, too. If a small percentage of CO_2 is added to the oxygen entering the artificial lung, the gas flow can be boosted without risk of hyperventilation. On this basis, some proponents of high flow perfusions have achieved the highest degree of simplification in the monitoring of heart–lung machines by renouncing all blood pressure and gas tension measurements and relying simply on the accurate knowledge of the perfusion flow.

A second type of rational approach is to establish the blood gas concentrations (arterial and venous) which are sufficient for adequate tissue gas exchange. The most refined presentation of this concept of control was made by Montgomery (1960). A somewhat similar, but less detailed exposition can be found in Loeschke (1959). Not by coincidence, both authors have derived their analyses from experience with a rotating disc oxygenator because such factors as blood flow, gas flow and efficiency of gas transfer (disc speed) can easily be singled out using this type of machine. However, the same control can be achieved with a bubble oxygenator by varying the bubble size, or the ratio of large bubbles to small bubbles, as already pointed out by Clark (1958), or the percentage of oxygen, carbon dioxide or nitrogen in the inflowing gas.

The key to this approach is monitoring the position of the arterial and venous points on a P_{O_2}—P_{CO_2} diagram (fig. 94) and making appropriate adjustments of blood flow, gas flow, and efficiency of gas exchange. As stated by Montgomery, the arterial point lies on the straight dotted line, which is the O_2—CO_2 diffusion ratio line (*slope = $-1/20$*). This line and, consequently, point "a" on the line moves upwards with an increase in CO_2 production by the perfused organism but downwards with an increase in the flow rate of gas through the artificial lung. The slope of the line, along which the arterial point moves up and down, is given by the particular equilibrating efficiency at which the oxygenator is actually working (Equilibrating efficiency is defined here as the ratio of arterial oxygen tension to gas oxygen tension in the equilibration chamber. In simplest terms, it is dependent upon the length of time that a given amount of blood is exposed to the atmosphere of the artificial lung. In the disc oxygenator, the equilibrating efficiency is proportional to the speed of the discs and inversely proportional to the rate of blood flow.) Thus the arterial point can be moved to the right by an increase in disc speed (increase in efficiency), while it would move to the left with an increase in extracorporeal flow (decrease in efficiency). If the observer is able to measure continuously the arterial oxygen tension and the carbon dioxide tension (or the arterial pH since in that range iso-pH lines are approximately horizontal), he has a complete definition of the arterial point, and can correct it, if necessary, by appropriate adjustment of gas flow or rate of rotation of the discs. With the arterial point fixed in this manner, he knows that the venous point lies somewhere along the blood respiratory exchange ratio line (0.80 in fig. 94). Then to fix the venous point ("v̄"), he only needs to measure the oxygen tension of venous blood. If the oxygen uptake of the organism increases, the venous point will move to the left along the respiratory exchange ratio line, while, if perfusion flow increases, the venous point will be displaced to the right. In summary, the perfusion flow rate will be regulated according to the position of the venous point, while ventilation and disc speeds will be modified according to the position of the arterial point. In this way it is possible to manage an adequate perfusion without exact knowledge either of the oxygen uptake of the organism, or of the perfusion flow rate. Perfusion control by maintenance of venous and arterial gas tensions within the range of normal should prove ideal under the conditions in which hemodynamic parameters and organic signs such as the elec-

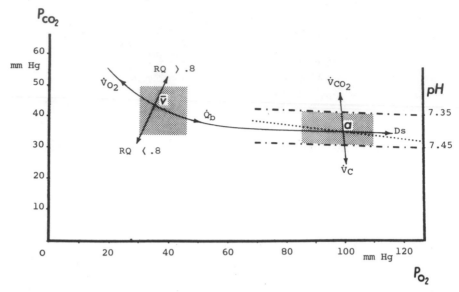

Fig. 94. P_{O_2}—P_{CO_2} diagram used for monitoring of total body perfusion with a rotating disc oxygenator. The arterial point (a) and the venous point (v̄) are determined by the oxygen and carbon dioxide gas tensions in arterial and mixed venous blood, respectively. The shaded rectangles indicate the permissible variations in the blood gas tensions. The transverse black line is that corresponding to a respiratory quotient (R.Q.) of 0.8. Iso-pH lines (dot-dash lines) are almost horizontal in the range of arterial blood pH considered. The straight dotted line is the O_2/CO_2 diffusion ratio line. $\dot{V}_{O_2}$ = oxygen uptake per minute. $\dot{V}_{CO_2}$ = carbon dioxide elimination per minute. $\dot{Q}_b$ = blood flow rate. $\dot{V}_C$ = ventilation of artificial lung. (See details in text and in Montgomery, 1960, from which this graph was modified.)

troencephalogram are difficult to interpret, as for example, during hypothermia. However, a theoretically inclined observer with a good understanding of physiology is required for best results.

A last rational approach to the problem of control is that of making sure the organism's gas exchange during perfusion is indeed what it should be. This technique calls for measuring oxygen uptake of the organism during a control period before perfusion, then to perfuse it at such a flow rate that the oxygen uptake equals the control value. The most practical way of doing this is to connect an airtight artificial lung in a closed circuit with a spirometer and a blower (*see* fig. 16). Then a continuous recording of oxygen uptake is obtained which can easily be compared to control values. A gas flowmeter and a CO_2 meter used simultaneously permits one to measure the CO_2 elimination parameter of the respiratory gas exchange ratio. Since the ultimate aim of perfusion is to provide satisfactory tissue gas exchange, this technique gives an answer to the important question of the adequacy of perfusion. This has been worked out in our laboratory, along the lines previously proposed by Shen, et al. (1931), Staub (1931), and Jongbloed (1952). Disc and membrane oxygenators lend themselves particularly well to measurements in the gas phase because of their compactness and because they can easily be made leakproof. The main advantages of this technique are simplicity and low cost. Each organism is its own control. The drawback is that oxygen uptake is temperature dependent. Hypothermia is therefore not the ideal field for this particular application.

Summarizing

In the control of heart–lung bypass procedures one must choose between the technical difficulty of obtaining complete biologic information and the common sense observation that the more numerous the monitoring devices, the greater is the likelihood of instrumental and human failure. Since all vital signs, hemodynamic as well as metabolic, are interdependent, not all need be measured. One practical solution to the control problem is to monitor only those parameters which empirically have been found useful in the operating room, such as arterial, superior caval and inferior caval pressures, the electrocardiogram, the electroencephalogram, and blood and body temperatures. A more rational approach is to ascertain that quantities of well arterialized blood in excess of the basal body requirements are distributed to the organism. Then other measurements can be omitted for simplicity. Another rational approach is based on the principle that normal oxygen and carbon dioxide tensions in arterial and venous blood reflect normal tissue gas exchange. Blood flow rate, gas flow rate and efficiency of extracorporeal gas exchange are adjusted accordingly. A last rational approach is to be sure that over all gas exchange during perfusion is the same as before perfusion. This can be done by connecting an airtight artificial lung to a closed circuit spirometer and using a CO_2 meter for instantaneous recording of the carbon dioxide elimination.

XVII. Hematologic Problems

"In its natural form within the circulatory system, blood is in kinetic equilibrium between formation and senescence. The end products of cellular disintegration may not only stimulate new cell growth, but also serve as the actual building blocks. Thus, when any blood is diverted through an extracorporeal circuit, no matter how transiently, two things occur: the body sacrifices other tissue stores as it steps up production, and the amputated blood promptly begins to autolyze as it changes from a kinetic to a static state" (Tullis, 1958).

Blood is obviously the first tissue to be concerned in extracorporeal circulation, and the one most altered by the passage from normal to artificial maintenance of the circulation and respiration. In fact, blood damage was the major obstacle to survival up to the time heparin was first applied to external perfusion techniques (Gibbon, 1937). Denaturation of blood remains one of the major difficulties confronting the unlimited extension of extracorporeal circulation, despite considerable progress in the control of the clotting mechanisms, the reversal of anticoagulation and the prevention of damage to corpuscular elements. It is therefore important to study in some detail the specific problems of blood handling in extracorporeal circuits.

COLLECTION OF PRIMING BLOOD

Because of the need for large amounts of fresh blood to fill the extracorporeal circuit, blood procurement is an important problem in heart–lung bypass procedures. According to the type of oxygenator and the size of the patient, a volume varying between one and five liters is required. The priming blood is mixed with the patient's own blood so that after the perfusion, between 30 and 70 per cent of what remains in the circulatory system is foreign blood. It is therefore important that the priming blood be of the highest quality.

In most surgical centers blood is collected a few hours before use in plastic bags or siliconized bottles which usually contain 1500 to 2500 units of heparin per 500 ml. of blood (Taux and Magath, 1958). To ease the burden imposed on the blood bank on the morning of surgery, some centers have extended the procurement of heparinized donor blood to 16 to 24 hours before surgery (Abbott, et al., 1958, 1960). In this case, dextrose (30 to 60 ml. of a 5 per cent solution) must be added to the preservative solution and the blood is stored at 4°C. until a short time before use. Since metabolic processes continue at a reduced rate under refrigeration, misgivings have been expressed about a possible drop in the platelet count (Perkins, et al., 1958; Kirby, 1958; Mocchi and Cascone, 1958), a loss in heparin activity (Fantl and Ward, 1960), a marked increase in plasma potassium (Lobpreis, et al., 1960), a slight increase in spontaneous hemolysis and in mechanical fragility of the red cells (Fleisch, 1960a), the development of metabolic acidosis (Gutelius and Dobell, 1960) and a more severe postoperative anemia when the donor blood has been drawn the day before surgery (Cooley, et al., 1958b). Nevertheless, it is felt that these drawbacks are more than compensated for by the convenience of unhurried processing of the priming blood.

Because heparinized blood is difficult to keep more than 24 hours, other anticoagulant solutions have been investigated. A great deal of experimentation has been conducted with exchange columns, but it has usually been found that treatment with resins not only removes calcium and magnesium, but also traps most of the platelets. Furthermore, the survival time of erythrocytes, once retransfused, does not exceed one week. McLaughlin, et al. (1960) recently reported that alterations in pH and electrolytes present in stored blood can be reverted by passage over suitable anion-cation exchange resins. New avenues for preservation of blood are opened up by this observation. Actually, the removal of calcium by chelating agents has been found practicable by Brown and Smith (1958). Edathanil calcium-disodium (EDTA) as such is unsuitable for use. By the addition of magnesium chloride, however, a EDTA-magnesium complex is formed which is a satisfactory anticoagulant. Since the amount of EDTA bears a well defined relationship to the calcium content of the blood, it is important that the container be very closely filled to the level indicated by the manufacturer. Blood preserved with EDTA should be used within five days of collection. For this purpose, EDTA-Mg blood is converted into heparinized blood by the addition of 1500 to 2000 USP units of heparin. After thorough mixing, 1.67 mM. of calcium ion in about 5 ml. is added to each unit of blood either in the form of calcium chloride or of calcium gluconate. The blood then has all the characteristics of heparinized blood. The chief disadvantages of EDTA blood are a depression of antihemophilic globulin and factor V levels, a marked increase in the plasma potassium content and a slight degree of hemolysis (Smith, et al., 1959; Kittle and Eilers, 1960). Nevertheless, it has proven reliable and safe in the hands of its proponents.

Citrated blood still offers real possibilities. At the beginning of the clinical heart–lung bypass era, it was rejected because of its "toxicity" to the myocardium (Dennis, et al., 1951a, b; Cookson, et al., 1954; Senning, 1955; Hubbard, et al., 1956; Ludbrook and Wynn, 1958; Dixon, 1958) and the occurrence of hemolysis and hemorrhage after transfusion (Soulier, 1958; Sarkar, et al., 1959; Noble and Abbott, 1959). Citrate must be added to blood in excess, thus putting an overwhelming metabolic load on the organism —a single unit of blood drawn into a standard ACD solution contains enough citric acid to add 27 mM. of fixed acid to the body. Hypocalcemia also interferes with myocardial contractility as well as with muscular innervation at the neuromuscular junction. Thus citrate increases the risk of cardiac irregularities or arrest and may impair the arteriolar contraction necessary for control of hemorrhage. Finally, citrate binds calcium and magnesium, thus leading to depletion of bivalent cations which are essential for intermediate carbohydrate metabolism. For all these reasons, regular bank blood preserved with ACD solution (a mixture of citric acid, sodium citrate and dextrose) usually is reserved for slow transfusions after a bypass procedure. Recently, however, it has been found that the acute toxicity of large doses of citrate can be reversed by calcium salts (Shellito, et al., 1959). After addition of heparin, the effects of ACD are neutralized by injecting 20 to 27 mEq. of calcium ion into the container (Foote, et al., 1960), as is done with EDTA blood. Larger heparin dosage is possibly desirable to counteract the antiheparin effect of calcium. Clinical perfusions have been performed using ACD blood converted by calcium and heparin with essentially the same results as with heparinized blood (Lobpreis, et al., 1960; Zuhdi, et al., 1960c). The metabolic acidosis due to citrated blood should disappear within two minutes of the start of perfusion (Foote, et al., 1960). Citrate is partly metabolized and partly excreted in the urine (Ludbrook and Wynn, 1958).

ACD blood is still the most satisfactory perfusate for a medium length period of preservation (Fleisch, 1960a). CPD (citrate-phosphate-dextrose) solution does not alter the pH so much as ACD, but it does increase potassium and ammonium levels to a larger extent (Gibson, et al., 1957). The introduction of ACDI (acid, citrate, dextrose, inosine) as a preservative may not only extend the useful period of preservation, but may also exert a protective effect on the red cell during the conventional period of storage (Gabrio, et al., 1956; Donati, 1957, 1959; Rubinstein, et al., 1958, 1959; Schmitt and Schmidt, 1959). Adding CO_2 to the container enhances the qualities of citrate solution (Nashat, et al., 1961). A very slow, controlled rotation of the blood containers during the period of preservation also contributes to the viability of the blood elements (Frei and Fleisch, 1961). Pretreatment of the donors with vitamin E should increase the mechanical resistance of the red cells to the trauma inflicted in the extracorporeal circuit (Meyer-Wegener, 1960). If the citrate action upon the myocardium can be prevented by the addition of the correct amount of calcium and if the acid load of the preservative solution is adequately compensated, the main objection to citrated blood will be its relatively high dilution and, consequently, its decreased oxygen carrying capacity. This drawback loses its importance with the high flow rates presently recommended for normothermic perfusions and may actually prove beneficial in hypothermic perfusions. A renewed acceptance of citrated blood is therefore not excluded.

Summarizing

Utmost care must be observed in the collection of blood for priming the extracorporeal circuit since 30 to 70 per cent of the donor blood remains in the patient's circulation after bypass. Priming blood is usually collected a few hours before perfusion and preserved with heparin. It is permissible to store heparinized blood up to 24 hours in order to ease the burden on the blood bank. At present, the removal of calcium by chelating agents deserve consideration as a practical method. Citrated blood which was found toxic in early clinical experience with cardiopulmonary bypass still offers interesting possibilities. It can be preserved much longer than any other blood, and can be made suitable for use in a heart–lung machine by the addition of heparin and calcium salts.

CONTROL OF THE CLOTTING MECHANISM

During cardiopulmonary bypass the clotting mechanism should ideally be controlled to the point where coagulation is fully inhibited, yet in a way which is easily reversible after perfusion. Heparin is the only drug used at the present time for this purpose because it is remarkable nontoxic and its action, which is primarily antithrombic, can easily be kept under control. The doses quoted in the literature range between 1 and 10 mg. per Kg. of body weight. Most satisfactory results are seemingly obtained with 2 to 3 mg./Kg., administered intravenously just prior to the insertion of the venous cannulae.

Expression of the dose in terms of mg. is becoming increasingly misleading, since the activity of heparin is tested by biologic assay and the requirement of the United States Pharmacopia have recently been modified. While one mg. of heparin (0.1 ml. of most of the commercially available solutions) once corresponded to 100 international units (I.U.), the USP XIII now requires a minimum of 130 I.U./mg. However, no maximum concentration or activity which manufacturers can offer has been set. Most available solutions contain 1000 I.U./ml. or 10 mg./ml. Since manufacturers are in a position to produce heparin with an activity close to 200 I.U./mg., considerable caution must be exercised when exact comparisons of dosages are to be made.

Many methods have been devised for the assay of heparin in blood: isolation and colorimetric dosage (Bassiouni, 1954); titration with graded concentrations of protamine

(Allen, et al., 1949; Leroy, et al., 1950; Perkins, et al., 1956; Hurt, et al., 1956; Guendel, 1955; Satter, 1961), or assessment of some form of coagulation time (Jaques, 1939; Monkhouse, et al., 1953; Blomback, et al., 1955; Peden and McFarland, 1959; Rothnie and Kinmonth, 1960a; Fantl and Ward, 1960). According to Warren and Wysocki (1958), a carefully performed coagulation time provides the best estimate of blood heparin levels. Blomback, et al. (1955, 1959) found that in a system with a constant amount of thrombin and an excess of heparin co-factor, the coagulation time is a function of the heparin concentration (table 5). There is considerable variation in coagulation time for the same heparin concentration among different individuals, although correlation in the same individual is very good.

Table 5. Relationship between plasma heparin concentration and coagulation time, after Blomback, et al. (1959).

I.U. HEPARIN/ML PLASMA	COAGULATION TIME (IN MIN)	
	Range	*Mean*
0.2..........1.2	10'–19'	13'
1.2..........2.6	17'–46'	30'
2.6..........3.6	47'–180'	104'
3.6..........4.8	>180'	

The duration of heparin effect depends on the rate of removal of heparin from the circulation (Jaques, 1939). The plasma levels decrease markedly during the first two hours, and then at a much slower rate, since at levels below 1 I.U./ml. the rate of clearance is proportional to the concentration. Eiber and Danishefsky (1958) observed that the rate of clearance increases sharply as the initial dose is raised above 2 mg./Kg. Thus, excessively high doses of heparin should not prolong the physiologic effects materially. Senning (1959) indicates that after intravenous administration of 4 mg./Kg. of heparin, the initial concentration in plasma ranges from 4.6 to 7.6 I.U./ml. The rate of disappearance of active heparin from the blood is then approximately 50 per cent per hour (Andersen, et al., 1959; Olsson, et al., 1959). Heparin is transferred from the blood to a number of possible sites. Most of it is taken up in the liver or in the lungs. An appreciable portion passes directly through the kidneys into the urine (Eiber and Danishefsky, 1958). Some is inactivated by a heparinase (Cho and Jacques, 1956), or is adsorbed at the surfaces of the red blood cells (von Kaulla and Henkel, 1952). The portion which has been taken up by the tissues is excreted in the urine over a period of several days. From these observations, it is obvious that additional heparin must be given if the perfusion is prolonged. In our experience, an initial dose of 2 mg./Kg., supplemented at the rate of 1 ml./Kg. every hour, provides a satisfactory, yet easily reversible anticoagulation for a 10-hour period of extracorporeal circulation.

After the perfusion, it is necessary to restore the clotting mechanism to normal by neutralizing the action of heparin. This can be done either with protamine (Chargraff and Olson, 1937; Jaques, et al., 1938; Jorpes, et al., 1939; Tocantins, 1943; Parkin and Kvale, 1949) or with hexadimethrine bromide, more generally known as Polybrene (Preston, et al., 1953, 1956; Weiss, et al., 1958). The amount of protamine needed for the neutralization of heparin after cardiopulmonary bypass varies between 75 per cent (Levowitz, et al., 1956; Anderson, et al., 1959), 100 per cent (Cooley, et al., 1957; Wulff, et al., 1959) and 120 per cent (Bencini, et al., 1957c; Gross and Holemans, 1961) of the total dose of heparin employed. With increasing time after heparin administration, progressively less protamine is needed. Polybrene is employed in the same dosage as protamine. Both drugs must be diluted and given slowly because hypotensive reactions are not uncommon. Rather than relying on empiric rules of thumb for heparin neutralization, many prefer to inject the amount of antagonist as indicated in each individual case by plasma heparin titration, so as to arrive directly at the correct dosage (Hurt, et al., 1956). Neutralization by both drugs is maximal within five minutes of administration and usually sustained (Keats, et al., 1959). Polybrene produces somewhat fewer side effects than protamine, and its potency is more uniformly standardized. It is preferred by most investigators (Keats, et al., 1959; Lillehei, et al., 1960; Blumberg, et al., 1960; Rothnie and Kinmonth, 1960b; Bittard, et al., 1960) although others (Andersen, et al., 1960) see no superiority of one drug over the other. Since both protamine and Polybrene possess some anticoagulant effects of their own, caution must be exercised in the face of slight abnormalities in clotting time (10 to 18 minutes) persisting after heparin neutralization. There is a danger that protamine (or Polybrene) inhibition of clotting will be interpreted as insufficient neutralization of heparin. In such cases, further administration of protamine can only prolong the coagulation time instead of shortening it. It should also be recalled that heparin activity is related to platelet concentration (Conley, et al., 1948; Gross, et al., 1956). In the presence of severe thrombocytopenia, more protamine is needed to neutralize heparin after perfusion (Allen, 1958).

After perfusion some authors (e.g., Salisbury, et al., 1955; Levowitz, et al., 1956; Effler, et al., 1956; Dodrill, et al., 1957; Beer and Loeschke, 1959) have observed the phenomenon of "heparin rebound," a return of blood noncoagulability. They state that one hour or later after satisfactory heparin neutralization the clotting time is again increased but can be restored to normal by further administration of protamine. This phenomenon has not been clearly explained and is rarely observed at the present time. It is possible that protamine is more rapidly metabolized than heparin, thus "uncovering" a heparin excess, or that heparin is slowly released from unneutralized "stores" somewhere in the body. Confusion of the "heparin rebound" phenomenon with overdosage of protamine or progressive depletion of certain coagulation factors is not easy to avoid. Finally, the possibility that a new anticoagulant substance is produced by the body has been suggested by von Kaulla and Swan (1958). It is unfortunate that the term "heparin rebound" has been used lately for the return of blood noncoagulability after apparent heparin neutralization because it was first applied to a period of hypercoagulability following prolonged heparin therapy (Cate, et al., 1954). It is probably best not to use this term at all.

In recent years, following scattered reports of protracted bleeding after dextran infusions, attention has been called to the anticoagulant properties of low molecular weight dextran. This substance was found to be a satisfactory anticoagulant for heart–lung bypass procedures by Wade and Vickers (1958). It prevents sludging, or intravascular aggregation of red cells, much more effectively than does heparin (Lofstrom and Zederfeldt, 1959; Dahlback, et al., 1959; Fajers and Gelin, 1959) and also may prevent the disturbances of capillary circulation which still limit the extension of normothermic and hypothermic perfusions.

For the time being, total body perfusion requires that the blood be made noncoagulable in the circulatory system as well as in the extracorporeal circuit. The day can be envisioned when anticoagulation will be limited to the extracorporeal circuit, as is already the case in some forms of external dialysis (Gordon, et al., 1956a,b; Anderson and Kolff, 1959; Scribner, et al., 1960; Teschan, et al., 1960). Blood would then be heparinized as it is drained from the organism into the oxygenator circuit, and heparin would be neutralized by a suitable antagonist as the blood re-entered the vascular system. Since practical difficulties contraindicate the application of this technique to total body perfusion, the discussion of "regional" or "extracorporeal" heparinization is beyond the scope of the present textbook.

Summarizing

The clotting mechanism during perfusion is controlled by heparin, which has primarily an antithrombic activity. Coagulation time, which becomes longer with increasing dosages of heparin, provides the best estimate of heparin levels. The duration of heparin effect depends upon the rate of removal of heparin from the circulation. After heart–lung bypass, the clotting mechanism is restored either with protamine or hexadimethrine bromide (Polybrene). Since these drugs possess some anticoagulant effects of their own, overdosage must be avoided.

EFFECTS OF PERFUSION ON BLOOD

Some degree of blood denaturation can be detected in all heart–lung bypass procedures. The denaturation bears a direct relationship to the duration of the perfusion and the volume flow of blood handled. Unfortunately, an analysis of the factors responsible for blood damage by the various elements of the extracorporeal circuit is not easy because most of the studies have been made during human or animal perfusions, so that clearance of the damaged blood and other compensations by the organism intervene. Strictly speaking, testing should be performed in vitro by recirculating the same amount of blood under the same mechanical, thermal and biochemical conditions as prevail during in vivo perfusions. Comparing the two parallel sets of data, one should then be able to distinguish the blood damaging action of the artificial circulation and respiration procedure from the responses of the living organism. However, formidable difficulties still confront the design of useful in vitro experiments, because it is hard to keep blood in viable condition for more than a few hours at normal body temperature. Most available data therefore come from in vivo perfusions.

1. Erythrocytes: destruction of red cells occurs during perfusion. Hemoglobin is liberated into the plasma and transported first in a protein-bound form, and then in a free unbound state as plasma binding capacity is exceeded (Lathem and Worley, 1959). Protein-bound hemoglobin disappears slowly from circulating plasma. Free hemoglobin is removed at a faster rate by the reticuloendothelial system, by the kidneys and by transformation into methemalbumin in the blood. During cardiopulmonary bypass, hemolysis seldom reaches the level at which it would interfere with the normal production of urine or would be responsible for vasomotor failure. When all organic functions have been protected by the use of high perfusion rates, free hemoglobin is cleared within a few hours after the end of the procedure, as indicated by studies utilizing intravenous injections of hemoglobin solutions (Lichty, et al., 1932; Ottenberg and Fox, 1938; Fairley, 1940; Gilligan, et al., 1941; Maluf, 1949). Study of possible factors responsible for hemolysis reveals the following:

(a) Most of the erythrocyte destruction during extracorporeal circulation procedures is caused by the pumps and constricted passages in the circuit (McCaughan, et al., 1957; Bucherl, 1959).

(b) The extent of destruction varies with the material of which the tubing and the pump-oxygenator parts are made. In general, the smoother the walls, the less the hemolysis produced (Bucherl, 1957; Stewart and Sturridge, 1959).

(c) For any given tube size, there is a critical velocity of flow which, if exceeded, produces hemolysis (see chap. XII).

(d) Excessive suction with foaming in the cardiotomy suction line is the most important single factor producing hemolysis in open-heart procedures (McCaughan, et al., 1958).

(e) Sustained high pressures applied to the blood are not detrimental. Intermittent positive pressure is more likely to produce hemolysis (Chevret and Besson, 1958; Bjørk and Rodriguez, 1959).

(f) In bubble oxygenators with large gas flow through minute orifices, the shearing force of bubble formation may be responsible for hemolysis (Gott, et al., 1957a, b; Merendino, et al., 1957; Ferbers and Kriklin, 1958; Bucherl, 1959).

(g) Occlusive pumps produce hemolysis by shearing action on the squeezed red cells, whereas unocclusive pumps are prone to cause blood damage by turbulence (Hodges, et al., 1958; Leonards and Ankeney, 1958; Snow and Coulson, 1960).

(h) Overheating of blood can cause severe hemolysis (Ham, et al., 1948).

(i) Storage of heparinized blood before use increases its liability to destruction (Allen, 1958; Stewart and Sturridge, 1959; Fleisch, 1960).

(j) Dilution of the blood with physiologic solutions decreases the liability of destruction (Moraes, et al., 1960).

In human perfusion procedures, hemolysis usually remains well within acceptable limits. The exceptional occurrence of massive hemolysis can be traced to accidental factors such as incompatible transfusion (Kirklin, et al., 1956), overheating of the blood (Clowes, 1960) or leaching of toxic components out of plastic tubes (Keith, et al., 1961). Although hemolysis is usually harmless, it is important that it be monitored in perfusion procedures because it provides the most sensitive index of blood trauma and a good criterion for comparison of different pump-oxygenators. Unfortunately, there are marked discrepancies among the methods of quantitating plasma hemoglobin in clinical laboratories. Deceptively low values are obtained when the determination of plasma hemoglobin levels is based upon the amount of a single derivative of hemoglobin; all possible derivatives should be measured. Determination of plasma hemoglobin after its transformation into cyanmethemoglobin and

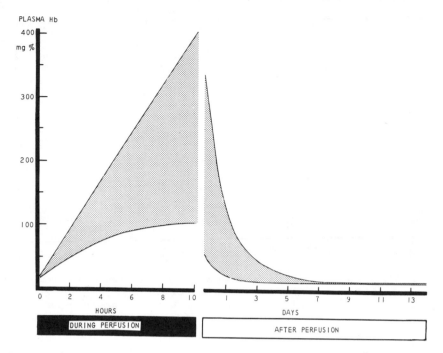

Fig. 95. Hemolysis as a function of time during and after cardiopulmonary bypass. Abcissa: time in hours and in days. Ordinate: plasma hemoglobin, in mg. per 100 ml. The upper curve depicts the linear increase in plasma hemoglobin levels which is usually observed. The lower curve shows how plasma hemoglobin levels tend to level off when the rate of hemolysis does not markedly exceed the clearance capacity of the organism. The dotted area between the two curves represents the range of variation expected with modern heart–lung machines. (Details in text.)

cyanmethemalbumin provides the most reliable assessment of the hemolysis which occurs in perfusion procedures (Fleisch, 1960b). Meanwhile, the various determinations should be compared with only extreme caution.

Under conditions of constant blood flow, gas flow and temperature, in vitro experiments indicate that hemolysis increases linearly with time for the first few hours, then at a progressively faster rate as the blood cells lose viability. In vivo a linear increase (fig. 95) is observed (Andersen and Hambraeus, 1961; Brinsfield, et al., 1961). In the clinical experience of DeWall, et al. (1959), the rate of liberation of hemoglobin into plasma amounted to 1.56 mg./100 ml./min., or 94 mg./100 ml./hr. This exceeds by far the rate of clearance of plasma hemoglobin, which has been estimated to 5 mg./100 ml./hr. (Ferbers and Kirklin, 1958). In exceptional circumstances, when the rate of hemolysis is kept to a minimum, by the use of a well adjusted perfusion equipment and low flow rates, and in the presence of a large volume of diuresis, the plasma hemoglobin levels tend to reach a plateau after 10 to 15 hours of perfusion (Brinsfield, et al., 1961). Plasma hemoglobin levels ranging between 30 and 150 mg. per cent are usually reported at the end of human perfusions of about one hour duration. Some authors have noticed an elevation in plasma hemoglobin which reaches a maximum 12 hours after the cessation of bypass, and a persistently elevated level during the first three to five postoperative days. Since a single injection of hemoglobin is cleared from the dog's plasma within 12 hours, these findings imply a continued intravascular hemolysis in the postperfusion period.

From the plasma hemoglobin levels noted at the end of bypass, one can easily calculate that less than one per cent of the erythrocytes are destroyed under ordinary condi-

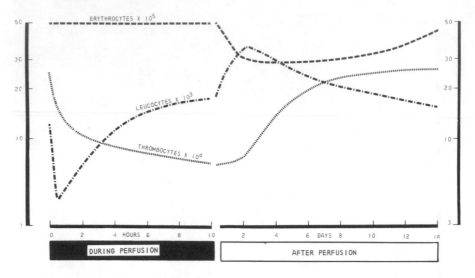

Fig. 96. Variations in the erythrocyte, leucocyte and platelet counts during and after cardiopulmonary bypass. Abscissa: time in hours and days. Ordinate: cell counts per cu. mm., plotted on a logarithmic scale. Owing to differences in the mechanical and biochemical resistance of the different formed elements, and to different time courses of the compensating mechanisms involved, variations in erythrocyte, leucocyte and platelet counts do not parallel each other.

tions of perfusion. The red cell count and the hematocrit therefore remain unchanged (fig. 96). However, this statement does not hold true for the postperfusion period. In fact, there is a considerable body of evidence to indicate that much more red cell destruction occurs after than during perfusion. Follow-up studies in patients who have not received blood transfusions after perfusion usually reveal the "first week anemia," a drop in blood hemoglobin levels of 3 to 5 Gm. per cent which reaches a maximum after seven to ten days (Abbott, et al., 1958; Kreel, et al., 1960). Finding a progressive drop in hematocrit in the presence of normal blood volume confirms this view. An increase in the endogenous formation of carbon monoxide in the days after bypass also suggests an accelerated destruction of erythrocytes (Ibring, 1959). Studies with tagged red cells have well established the fact that the ultimate survival time of erythrocyte is shortened when they have been circulated through a pump-oxygenator; the precise timing and the responsible mechanisms are still under debate, however. Hewitt, et al. (1957) stated that the surviving intact red cells of a perfused subject have a normal postperfusion survival time, at least in the first two to four weeks. Brown and Smith (1958), however, observed a rapid disappearance of donor red cells beginning about 20 days after perfusion. This sudden late drop was accounted for by antibodies provoked in some recipients by the lesser antigenic blood group difference because this abnormal response did not occur when blood from the pump-oxygenator was returned to the original donor. Burke and Gardner (1959) note that the apparent chromium half-life of canine erythrocytes is reduced less when the extracorporeal circuit is primed with autologous blood instead of homologous blood. They conclude that both antigenic factors and blood trauma are responsible for the shorter survival time of erythrocytes after perfusion. Clowes (1960) found that the radioactivity counts of subjects perfused with tagged red cells increases over the liver and spleen to a maximum on the seventh to tenth day. The same phenomenon occurs when an aliquot of the same blood is transfused into a compatible recipient, indicating also an abnormally reduced viability of the red cells.

The trauma responsible for the abnormally short survival time of red cells subjected to extracorporeal circulation is probably of a complex nature. No significant change in osmotic fragility has been observed (Iankovskii, et al., 1939; Abbott, et al., 1958). The mechanical resistance of the erythrocytes measured according to Shen, et al. (1944) is also said to be unchanged. This last statement, however, may reflect the inadequacy of the method used, since more recent techniques (Fleisch and Fleisch, 1960) consistently reveal an increase in mechanical fragility of the red blood cells in the first 14 days after perfusion. It should not be forgotten that the pump-oxygenator itself subjects the red cells to a violent test of mechanical resistance. Consequently, the technique used for measuring mechanical resistance may fail to reveal an increased fragility during extracorporeal circulation in vitro or in vivo (Conne, et al., 1960; Brinsfield, et al., 1961), simply because the weaker and older cells are destroyed in the extracorporeal circuit. On the other hand, the fragility of the red cells is conspicuously increased after bypass (fig. 97) because numerous red cells have a low resistance to trauma. However, their destruction in vivo does not exceed the clearing capacity of the organism. Consequently normal levels of plasma hemoglobin are observed when blood is carefully sampled.

In recent years, the trauma to blood during clinical perfusions has been reduced to the point that the same priming blood can safely be used for two consecutive operations (Gross, 1959; Keith, et al., 1960; Sakakibara, 1960; Swan and Paton, 1960; Paton, et al., 1961). Nevertheless, destruction of red cells remains a subject of major concern when long-term perfusions are to be employed. One possible solution was suggested by Dodrill, et al. (1957), who proposed giving an exchange transfusion prior to heart–lung bypass, to save some of the patient's own blood for later transfusion. While most clinicians agree that the advantage gained does not warrant the added complexity of the procedure, Dodrill's suggestion should not be disregarded as a means of preventing postperfusion anemia. Bone marrow stimulation and the appearance of nucleated red cells in the peripheral blood stream has been noted after 10 hours of perfusion (Brinsfield, et al., 1961). This suggests that with improved techniques reactive mechanisms might some day be able to compensate for the increased red cell destruction in the extracorporeal circuit.

2. Leucocytes: Little is known about the effect of artificial circulation on the function and viability of the leucocytes. Melrose, et al. (1953), Stephenson, et al., (1956), Brown and Smith (1958), Craafoord (1958) and DeWall, et al. (1959) reported a decrease in the white cell count during perfusion, followed by an increase after perfusion. Using a membrane oxygenator, Kolff, et al. (1956a) found no change or a slight increase during perfusion and a marked increase after perfusion. It appears that the initial drop is caused by the traumatic effects of the pump-oxygenator and is therefore less conspicuous with the best machines, while the secondary rise one to four hours after the start of perfusion reflects the reaction of the organism. The leucocytosis is usually observed after the bypass is finished because clinical perfusions are short. However, the secondary rise of white cells also appears during perfusion (fig. 97) when the procedure is of extended duration (Anderson, 1961; Brinsfield, et al., 1961). The initial decrease in leucocyte count is primarily at the expense of mature granulocytes and mononuclear cells, while the subsequent increase is due mainly to immature granulocytic elements. The appearance in the peripheral blood of very young and atypical cells such as myelocytes and promyelocytes is not uncommon (Iankovskii, et al., 1939). There is no conspicuous change in the number of eosinophils. From the end of perfusion up to 10 to 12 days later, the leucocytosis persists even in the absence of infection. Stimulation of myeloid elements of the bone marrow has been directly observed at the end of long-term perfusions (Brinsfield, et al., 1961).

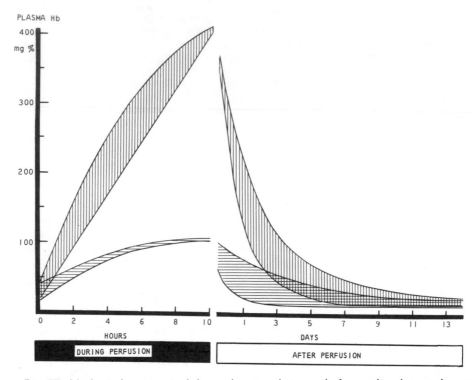

Fig. 97. Mechanical resistance of the erythrocytes during and after cardiopulmonary bypass. Abscissa: time in hours and days. Ordinate: Plasma hemoglobin in mg. per 100 ml. The mechanical resistance of the erythrocytes is assessed in the following way: a blood sample is obtained and plasma hemoglobin is measured in one aliquot. Another aliquot is submitted to a standardized trauma, then its plasma hemoglobin is measured. The difference between the two plasma hemoglobin values is a function of the mechanical fragility of the cells. In the figure, each striped band is limited by two curves: The lower one represents plasma hemoglobin levels, as in fig. 95. The upper one represents plasma hemoglobin levels after standardized trauma. The difference between the two curves (striped area) indicates the mechanical fragility of the erythrocytes. Results have been represented for the most favorable (horizontal stripes) and the least favorable (vertical stripes) conditions encountered during perfusion. From the changes in width of the striped bands, it would appear that mechanical fragility apparently decreases during perfusion and that the highest values are observed two to four days after perfusion. (Details in text.)

Since leucocytes undergo degradation during artificial circulation, one would expect the release of a number of proteolytic enzymes, notably pepsin, cathepsin, trypsin, lysozyme and desoxyribonuclease (fig. 98). It remains to be determined whether or not these enzymes participate in the postoperative oozing and hemorrhaging, which is sometimes encountered after perfusion, as for instance by digesting the mucoproteins deposited on the sutured surfaces.

3. Thrombocytes: A decrease in the platelet count of the order of 50 to 70 per cent is a consistent finding during extracorporeal circulation. Levels down to 50,000 cu. mm. are reported (Osborn, et al., 1956; Levitskaia, et al., 1958; DeWall, et al., 1959; Tucci, et al., 1959). The major drop occurs within the first 5 to 15 minutes (Kirby, 1958; Penick, et al., 1958), followed by a more gradual decrease. In long-term perfusions reduction in the number of circulating platelets may be compensated for by the release of new ones (Brins-

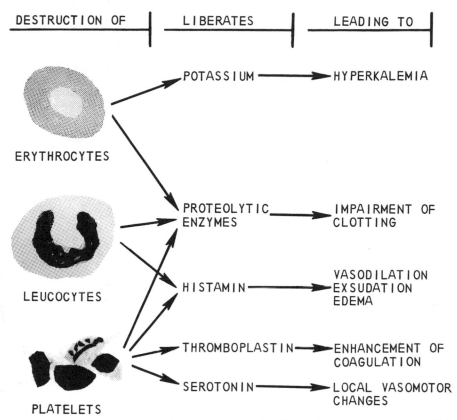

DESTRUCTION OF   LIBERATES   LEADING TO

POTASSIUM ⟶ HYPERKALEMIA

ERYTHROCYTES

PROTEOLYTIC ENZYMES ⟶ IMPAIRMENT OF CLOTTING

HISTAMIN ⟶ VASODILATION EXSUDATION EDEMA

LEUCOCYTES

THROMBOPLASTIN ⟶ ENHANCEMENT OF COAGULATION

SEROTONIN ⟶ LOCAL VASOMOTOR CHANGES

PLATELETS

Fig. 98. Physiologically active substances which can be liberated by destruction of formed blood elements in an extracorporeal circuit. (Modified from Marggraf, 1958.)

field, et al., 1961), so that the counts tend to remain fairly constant after about five hours (fig. 97). After bypass the platelet count is usually depressed for four to five days (Crafoord, 1958; Kreel, et al., 1960) and then returns to normal.

Thrombocytopenia results from platelet deposition on foreign surfaces (Morrow, et al., 1957; Perkins, et al., 1958) or from any activation of the coagulation system (Osborn, et al., 1956). It bears no evident relation to the type of oxygenator used nor to the duration of perfusion. Massive transfusion of stored bank blood aggravates it. Marked thrombocytopenia is sometimes related to inadequately cleaned equipment (Perkins, et al., 1958). One should remember that the platelets, present in the blood at the end of perfusion may be largely donor platelets with a short survival time. However, it seems unlikely that simple thrombocytopenia is responsible for the bleeding tendency sometimes encountered after perfusion.

The platelet count decreases quite rapidly in the presence of heparin in vitro (Kirby, et al., 1958; Aepli, 1960). This effect is less apparent when heparin is administered in vivo. During extracorporeal circulation procedures the platelet count drops sharply when inadequate quantities of heparin are used. Heparin exerts a direct effect on the surface of the platelets so as to render them less sticky (Mocchi and Cascone, 1958). Another hazard to consider is the antiheparin effect of platelets (Allen, 1958b). If a fairly pronounced fall in the platelet count occurs for any reason, the quantity of heparin required to maintain anticoagulation is considerably reduced. This may increase bleeding resulting from a specific dosage of heparin and therefore an increased amount of protamine is required to restore normal coagulability. Platelets serve not only as a link in the clotting mechanism but also as a substrate for thrombin. The role of the numerous platelet factors is still not clearly established (Luscher, 1960). Possible harmful effects of serotonin release have been discussed in chap. XV.

4. Plasma proteins and coagulation factors: The major blood proteins do not appear to be seriously affected by viviperfusion. In the early experience with extracorporeal circulation, Stephenson, et al. (1956) reported an average decrease in plasma protein levels of 1.4 Gm. per cent, primarily at the expense of the albumin fraction. This decrease was frequently large enough to cause a reversal of the albumin-globulin ratio. Parola, et al. (1958a), however, were unable to observe changes in blood protein content or in the distribution of albumin and globulin in most of their cases. Considerable change in the electrophoretic distribution of lipoproteins was noted, possibly due to the presence of heparin (Cruz, et al., 1960).

Perkins, et al. (1958) and Gerbode, et al. (1958) noted a negligible loss of fibrinogen in human and experimental perfusions despite earlier reports by the same group (Osborn, et al., 1955) of hypofibrinogenenia after bypass. There was also no decrease of fibrinogen in the experiments of Penick, et al. (1958a). Other authors have reported decreases in fibrinogen values ranging from 5 to 50 per cent (Brown and Smith, 1958; Wright, et al., 1958; Parola, et al., 1958a; Senning, et al., 1959b; Semb, 1959a; Sanger, et al., 1959; Wulff, et al., 1959). In such cases fibrinogen transfusions are indicated after bypass (Allen, 1958b; Nilsson and Swedberg, 1959; Gross and Holemans, 1961), although the formation or release of new fibrinogen into the plasma is a rather rapid phenomenon (Raderecht, 1958). Decreased fibrinogen levels, and the possibility of a "defibrination syndrome" (DeWall, et al., 1959) with abnormal hemorrhage and neurologic damage are often assumed when deposits of amorphous material are noted in filters, joints and other parts of extracorporeal circuits (Stokes and Gibbon, 1950). However, according to Gadboys, et al. (1960), this clot-like material is composed predominantly of fragmented erythrocytes. The same authors mention that the fibrinogen concentration of adequately heparinized blood is unaffected by severe degrees of agitation. The formation of a very loose fibrinogen-heparin complex has been noted by Godal (1960).

Despite all anticoagulants, blood has a tendency to clot outside of its natural intravascular environment (Allen, et al., 1957). Wright, et al. (1958), and Holemans, et al. (1960a, b) noted an increase in prothrombin, factor V and antihemophilic globulin (AHG) during the initial phase of perfusion. Thereafter prothrombin concentration fell as did platelet, fibrinogen and AHG levels. A depletion of a number of other individual clotting factors such as factors VII, IX and plasminogen has been reported as the perfusion goes on (Penick, et al., 1958a, b; von Kaulla and Swann, 1958a, b; Hoeksema and Mustard, 1959; Nilsson and Swedberg, 1959). These observations support the concept that intravascular clotting is activated during perfusion, possibly when inadequate amounts of heparin are used. The depression of platelet counts, of AHG titer and poor prothrombin consumption have been considered as fairly sensitive indices of this reaction. This depression also results in an increase in fibrinolytic enzyme activity sufficient to impair clotting for several hours (von Kaulla and Swan, 1958a; Wulff, et al., 1959).

The problem of postperfusion hemorrhage and the return to normal blood coagulation are extensively discussed in the literature. According to many published reports (Bencini, et al., 1957; Allen, 1958; Mondini and Ziliotto, 1958; Wright, et al., 1959; Perkins, et al., 1959; Crosby, 1959; Tucci, et al., 1959; Wulff, et al., 1960; Rothnie and Kinmonth, 1960a; Lillehei, et al., 1960; Hougie, 1960; Levitskaya, 1960; Holemans, 1960; Gross and Holemans, 1961), postoperative bleeding no longer appears to be a major problem in clinical perfusions. The above mentioned authors conclude that the most obvious cause of postoperative bleeding is failure to neutralize heparin. Less obvious is the fact that coagulation is activated by heparin with resulting depletion of some of the coagulation factors. A debated cause of postoperative bleeding is the excessive administration of protamine or Polybrene to the point at which the clotting time is prolonged by the heparin antagonist. Bleeding associated with severe thrombocytopenia is only caused by improperly cleaned circuits. Low flow perfusion and sustained peripheral hypoxia aggravate the tendency to bleed. Finally, the need for meticulous hemostasis in any extracorporeal circulation procedure must be recognized by the surgeon.

Protracted bleeding is not the sole expression of clotting disturbances following extracorporeal circulation. Intravascular thrombosis may result from activation of the clotting mechanism. Though less frequent and less widely recognized than are hemorrhagic tendencies, thrombosis was early described as a complication of extracorporeal blood handling by Mustard and Chute (1951) and Helmsworth, et al. (1952). In our laboratory we have occasionally observed extensive caval thrombosis between the second and the fifth day after successful long-term perfusions. The etiology of this insidious complication is still open to speculation; investigators may have to consider possible alterations of the vascular lining by physical or chemical trauma (Shimamoto, et al., 1960a, b) and the role of the autonomic nervous system on the physiological clotting mechanisms (Tereschenko, 1960; Kudriashov and Kalishevskaia, 1960; von Kaulla, et al., 1960).

Summarizing

All extracorporeal circulation procedures traumatize the blood to some extent. Physical factors such as squeezing, turbulence, foaming, temperature fluctuations and foreign surfaces weaken or destroy platelets, leucocytes and red cells. It is also impossible to handle blood in extracorporeal circuits without activation of the clotting complex. Enzymes and other substances liberated by cell or protein degradation, may cause vascular disturbances and impair the coagulation mechanism. Therefore any extracorporeal circulation procedure requires skilled navigation between the Charybdis of premature clotting in the external circuit and the Scylla of intractable bleeding in the organism after termination of the perfusion.

BLOOD PROBLEMS IN DOGS

Experimental heart–lung bypass studies and trials of new perfusion devices are usually performed on dogs. One assumes that the results obtained in the animal laboratory have direct clinical application. This is only true within certain limits because human blood and dog blood are not exactly alike. The species difference is reflected in significant differences in the normal values for plasma sodium, chloride and some of the proteins (Carr and Schloerb, 1959). Dog blood also clots much more readily than does human blood (Didisheim, et al., 1959) and dog erythrocytes are more fragile than are human erythrocytes (Schermer, 1958). The poor nutritional background of "normal" dogs is frequently reflected in some degree of anemia and hypoproteinemia. The most important point to stress, however, is that problems of blood handling, blood compatibility and blood transfusions are much less understood and possibly more complex in dogs than they are in humans. Dog blood is far more susceptible to trauma in an extracorporeal circuit than is human blood. In some modern heart–lung machines human blood is treated so gently that it can be re-used in a second perfusion or for later transfusions in the same or other patients. On the contrary, simple exposure of canine blood to the oxygenation process in an artificial heart–lung machine causes marked denaturation. Dramatic results occur when this blood is transfused into healthy dogs: apnea, hypotension progressing towards peripheral circulatory collapse and intractable bleeding are the more obvious signs of the reaction (Penick, et al., 1958a). Lability of canine blood is the factor responsible for many of the initial failures when a new group of investigators starts to work with perfusion techniques. In one respect, this may be considered beneficial since investigators who have mastered the difficulties involved in handling dog blood may well be on firmer ground when they attempt human application (Mondini and Ziliotto, 1958).

The problems of blood incompatability in dogs are illustrated by the reaction to, and the outcome of, rapid isovolemic exchange-transfusions of homologous blood in animals not previously transfused. No matter how elaborate are the cross-matching techniques employed, the procedure results in a high incidence of transfusion reactions (30 to 60 per cent and a significant mortality (10 to 20 per cent) according to the studies of Maher, et al. (1956, 1958), Cruz and Baumgarten (1958) and Dow, et al. (1959, 1960b). Furthermore, severe reactions are encountered in attempting a second perfusion in the same dog or in utilizing as donors animals who have survived an earlier perfusion. The toxic pattern of transfusion reaction in dogs is characterized initially by hypotension, bradycardia and respiratory depression (Maher, et al., 1958). To this triad of conspicuous signs, others must be added: rise in portal venous pressure, hepatic congestion and sequestration of blood in the splanchnic area (Dow, et al., 1960). Participation of the central nervous system in the reaction is indicated by the experiments of Glants (1959). Cruz and Baumgarten (1958) describe two types of hypotension: one immediate, the arterial pressure falling within 10 minutes after the onset of the blood exchange; and another delayed, the blood pressure fall beginning after a latent period of 20 to 30 minutes. In some animals the pressure remains low for at least two hours. In others, spontaneous recovery is observed during that period. The cases that do not recover go into true shock with the venous oxygen saturation falling to exceedingly low levels. Few animals survive more than 24 hours. Those animals which recover do not show any apparent sequelae and they are alert and lively by the following day.

There may be more than a single incompatible factor in dog blood since transfusion reactions are observed with washed, saline-suspended erythrocytes as well as with plasma alone. The presence of an antigen-antibody framework in dog blood is quite well established. Melnick, et al. (1936, 1937) and Young, et al., (1952) have described more than 10 blood groups in dogs based on antigens contained in their erythrocytes. The blood groups have been arbitrarily identified as A, B, C, D, in the order of discovery but they bear no known relationship to antigens present in man or in other animals. Factor A is present in 63 per cent of dogs, and C antigen has been recognized in 90 per cent of them. Only seven per cent of dogs exhibit a single erythrocyte type. Antigenicity is particularly associated with erythrocytes of the A and C types. Cells of the A type undergo agglutination and hemolysis when transfused into dogs of the A-type. Young and his associates concluded that the routine use of A-dogs as donors should eliminate most transfusion hazards, and that cross-matching techniques would probably add little to the safety of transfusion. Unfortunately, the experience of Maher, et al. (1958) and Cruz, et al. (1958) has not supported this concept. Routine use of A-donors without cross-matching caused transfusion reactions in more than half of the dog pairs observed. Using cross-matching only, there were still seven reactions in a series of 14 compatible cross-matches. Typing data associated with cross-matching procedures did not increase the reliability of the prediction. The term "blood group," which is usually applied to red cell antigens, is now extended to include white cell and platelet antigens, plasma antigens, and possibly, antigens to the very hemoglobin within the red cells (Joysey, 1959). Using this terminology, transfusion reaction may be said to cause the acute circulatory collapse which follows homologous plasma infusion in normal animals (Hamilton, et al., 1947) and in adrenalectomized dogs maintained on desoxycorticosterone acetate (Baker and Remington, 1958).

Bloody diarrhea and edematous swelling of the face are associated with hemodynamic signs, suggesting histamine release by homologous plasma. The role of histamine in reactions to plasma transfusion is also hinted at by the experiments of Bliss and Walker (1959), who injected dogs intracutaneously with their own plasma and plasma from other dogs. More free histamine was found in the skin injected with homologous plasma than in the skin injected with autologous plasma. Diphenhydramine prevented the collapse following plasma infusion (Baker and Remington, 1958). Piperoxan, an adrenergic blocking agent, was the only drug found to prevent major reactions to exchange transfusions in the experience of Maher, et al. (1958). Diphenhydramine and porto-caval anastomosis minimized "anaphylactoid" response according to Dow, et al., (1960). Atrophine, antihistamines, cortisone and adrenocorticotrophic hormone did not exert any protective effect.

Transfusion reactions occurring at the beginning of a heart–lung bypass procedure in a dog are likely to be obscured by the hemodynamic changes brought about by the perfusion itself. The former are recognized solely when the blood exchange is performed at a relatively slow rate under isovolemic conditions prior to the cardiopulmonary bypass itself. Indeed, circulatory support by a pump-oxygenator is the best therapy for transfusion reactions since blood flow and gas exchange are thus maintained during the acute phase. Failure to recognize transfusion reactions at the beginning of bypass is frequently caused by a poor volume control because the circulatory collapse is less evident when the animal is allowed to take up blood from the extracorporeal circuit. The protection offered by a markedly increased body blood volume may also explain why reactions are less pronounced when transfusion is given to normovolemic dogs than when a transfusion is given to reestablish normal blood volume in hypovolemic animals.

In view of the difficulties associated with transfusions reactions in dogs, special measures must be taken whenever blood volume control is of importance and survival is desired. Autogenous blood can be used to prime the extracorporeal circuit if the volume of blood required does not exceed 600 ml. (Maher, et al., 1958; Henrotin, et al., 1958; Galletti and Salisbury, 1959). In the authors' laboratory, this simple procedure has limited hypotensive reactions to less than five per cent of extracorporeal circulation procedures. The dogs are bled into ACD containers one to two weeks prior to the perfusion procedure and permitted to recover spontaneously from the ensuing anemia. Just before perfusion the citrated blood is slowly given intravenously while arterial blood from the heparinized animal is used to fill the extracorporeal circuit. When the animal cannot be kept for many days before perfusion, heparin-dextrose or EDTA-Mg containers are used. Five hundred to 600 ml. of blood are first withdrawn, then replaced by an equivalent amount of citrated blood from the blood bank. The animal is given one to four days to recover from the anesthesia and possibly from a transfusion reaction. Surprisingly enough, only two dogs out of 40 died following this preparatory procedure, despite the marked hemodynamic disturbances brought about by sequential, instead of simultaneous, exchange-transfusion of homologous blood. The high rate of recovery may be due to one or a combination of many details of the procedure: (a) The use of chloralose anesthesia which is more likely than barbiturates to preserve intact the homeostatic pressure mechanism. (b) Exsanguination from a central vein within three to five minutes. (c) Immediate transfusion of blood stored in the ice-box, resulting in a moderate hypothermia. (d) No collection of blood before an adequate dose of heparin has been given to the donor. (e) Sterile collection and immediate transfer of the blood to the ice-box.

Homologous blood must obviously be used when large amounts are needed to prime an extracorporeal circuit. Careful anesthesia and proper cannulation are essential to obtain the largest possible volume of blood from sacrified animals (Kletschka, et al., 1959; Kellogg, et al., 1959). Since reactions are more likely when the blood of several donors is pooled, as is apparent in the experience of Dow, et al. (1960b), we resort in our laboratory to one chronic donor for each perfusion procedure. A large healthy dog can give five per cent of its weight in blood (enough to prime most of the circuits) and recover from the blood loss. The donor is anesthetized with chloralose, heparinized, and a wide catheter is advanced into a central vein. When everything is ready for the heart–lung bypass procedure, the donor is bled directly into the pump-oxygenator and the perfusion begins immediately. Thus blood temperature and chemical qualities are not affected by a waiting period. The donor receives 1000 ml. of cold five per cent dextrose, the first half very quickly, the second half more slowly. Recovery is usually uneventful. If there is a pronounced transfusion reaction when the recipient goes on bypass, the donor is discarded. If there is none, the donor can be used again three weeks later, provided attention is paid to proper care and nutrition.

Summarizing

Dog blood is far more delicate than human blood because its cells are more fragile and it clots more readily. Canine blood which has circulated in a heart–lung machine causes apnea and circulatory collapse when transfused into healthy dogs. Transfusion reactions characterized by hypotension, bradycardia and respiratory depression are also frequent at the beginning of heart–lung bypass in dogs although they are often obscured by hemodynamic changes brought about by the perfusion itself. Use of autogenous blood for priming extracorporeal circuits minimizes these difficulties.

XVIII. Induced Cardiac Arrest

Since survival despite complete respiratory arrest startled biologists in the early phase of heart–lung bypass development, deliberate arrest of the heart beat appeared to many as doubly foolhardy. Indeed, it was not until total body perfusion became an established clinical procedure that surgeons actually tried to stop the heart. As the correction of increasingly complicated cardiac lesions was attempted, the need for a dry, motionless operative field became apparent. Human hearts were successfully arrested and restarted before much was known about the problems involved. After an initial period of enthusiasm, grounds for misgivings appeared. Little help was obtained from physiologists who could only confess abysmal ignorance of the cardiac contractile mechanism. It now remains to fill the gap between theory and practice and to document the invaluable experience gained in operating rooms with results tediously gathered in the animal laboratory.

PHYSIOLOGIC PRINCIPLES

The ideal of a pink, quiet, flaccid and dry heart with which the surgeon would most like to deal is not within easy reach. The obvious advantages of clinical cardioplegia, or induced cardiac arrest, are those of an organ in which the details of a defect can be most clearly recognized and repaired. Also important are a decrease in operative blood loss, the suppression of regurgitant flow across an incompetent aortic valve, and the reduction in blood trauma which results from a less extensive use of coronary suction equipment (Kolff, et al., 1957). The chief objection is based on the difficulty of recognizing interferences with the conduction system or a distortion of intracardiac structures when the heart is arrested. The surgeon is also unable to functionally evaluate the correction of valvular lesions. Overdistension of the flaccid cardiac muscle and trapping of air in its cavities, with the risk of coronary embolism, can be prevented by suitable measures. Yet the major problem remains:—Is it possible to interfere with the contractile mechanism of the heart without involving structural damage?

Ideally, the action of a cardioplegic maneuver or drug should be selective on the heart, easily reversible and directed to the triggering mechanism rather than to the energy building process. In practice, it is impossible to be absolutely selective because the heart is connected to the rest of the vascular system by a number of reflex pathways. Drugs which will simply switch the heart on and off are not available. Most drugs also have actions elsewhere which must be taken into account. The heart cannot be arrested without compromising its metabolism to some extent, yet it is preferable to slow down the entire chain of energy building processes rather than any one step, since there are too many alternate metabolic pathways which otherwise permit the contractile process to be shunted around the blocked step. There are three main approaches to arresting the normal heart beat: (1) induction of another type of mechanical activity; (2) massive vagal stimulation reducing the rate of discharge of the pacemaker; (3) use of cardiac "depressant" drugs or metabolic inhibitors (Shumway, 1959; Redo, 1959).

Deliberately induced ventricular fibrillation does not completely arrest all mechanical activity of the heart muscle. The relative quietness is, however, sufficient for most surgical purposes, and the situation is clinically familiar. Cholinergic drugs, acetylcholine or cholinesterase inhibitors, are able to stimulate the vagi so strongly that the sinus node discharge ceases. Sustained stimulation is, however, difficult to maintain because of the abundance of esterase in plasma and tissues and, in any case, "escape" of cardiac automatism tends to occur. Steroid-like alkaloids of the veratridine type could conceivably be used because they chemically stimulate coronary receptors resulting primarily in vagal stimulation and secondarily in sinus node inhibition through a vago-vagal reflex. However, peripheral vasodilation is also part of the response, so that their application seems precluded. Among cardiac "depressant" drugs, only inorganic ions, potassium and magnesium, have been used. Sudden increases in the extracellular level of these ions disturbs the movement of potassium and possibly of calcium across the cellular membrane and consequently, alter the depolarization process and arrest the synchronized contraction of the muscle fibers. Nonspecific myocardial "depressant" drugs, as barbiturates in large doses would be, have too many other effects to be considered seriously. Metabolic inhibition by acute anoxia is actually employed, although it destroys the contractile machinery if unduly prolonged. Cold provides the least harmful approach to induced cardiac arrest because it decreases the energy requirement while the energy supply is turned off. Nevertheless, all cardioplegic techniques which do not include coronary perfusion with oxygenated blood are likely to cause cellular damage and should be assumed guilty until proven innocent. Electrocardiographic patterns are deliberately induced which, in other circumstances, would be regarded as ominous. Despite the changed prognosis, their pathophysiologic significance remains the same. Therefore cardiac arrest should be attempted only by those who have become proficient in artificial support of the circulation.

Summarizing

Knowledge of the physiologic processes involved in deliberately arresting the heart is very scanty. Cardioplegic techniques should be selective on the heart, easily reversible and aimed at the triggering mechanism rather than at the energy building process. Cardiac activity can be arrested through induction of ventricular fibrillation, by massive vagal stimulation by cholinergic drugs, or by "depressant" drugs such as potassium and magnesium. Metabolic inhibition by anoxia or cold is also employed. All procedures which do not involve coronary perfusion while the heart beat is turned off are limited in scope.

METHODS OF INDUCING CARDIAC ARREST

1. Ventricular fibrillation: Deliberately induced ventricular fibrillation had been proposed originally as a method for preventing air embolization during surgery on the open heart (Senning, 1952, 1955; Glenn and Sewell, 1953). Fibrillation is induced by electrical stimulation and provides a relatively quiet operative field. Since coronary circulation is not impaired, but rather is enhanced (Maraist and Glenn, 1952), myocardial oxygen requirements are well taken care of. Thus, normal rhythm and adequate cardiac function are easily restored upon termination of the fibrillation. Fibrillatory arrest has been used by Oselladore, et al. (1957) and Bencini, et al. (1958c) with satisfactory results. According to Glenn, et al. (1960), the chief disadvantages of this technique are as follows: Coronary venous blood interferes with visibility and must be removed; the state of mild contraction of the ventricles interferes somewhat with exposure of intracardiac structures; finally, the well perfused normothermic heart tends to revert spontaneously to an organized beat. Glenn and his associates devised a source of DC current and an electrode which keep the heart in a state of fine fibrillation by sustained electrical stimulation. Fibrillation can be terminated by electrical shock or by the injection of a potassium salt, followed by cardiac massage and perfusion with oxygenated blood. Ventricular fibrillation can be induced by a number of chemicals which inhibit myocardial metabolism, as reviewed by Burn (1960), but none of these appears to be as convenient as electrical stimulation.

2. Potassium arrest: Ringer (1883) made the original observation that the myocardium of an isolated heart is depressed by the addition of potassium to the perfusing fluid. Later, Winckler, et al. (1938) reported the progressive electrocardiographic changes associated with increasing plasma potassium concentrations in dogs. With concentrations of 5 to 7 mEq./L., the T wave was altered. Intraventricular block was observed at 10 mEq./L. and asystole occurred at 14 to 16 mEq./L. Melrose, et al. (1955) considered using potassium-induced arrest to reduce myocardial damage due to hypoxia during aortic occlusion. In isolated mammalian hearts, a concentration of 1 to 2 mg. of potassium citrate per ml. of perfusing fluid was required. The demonstration by Kolff and his associates (1956b) that cardiac action in dogs could be restored after potassium arrest led to the first clinical application (Effler, et al., 1956). The aorta was clamped and 10 to 150 ml. of a 2.5 per cent solution of potassium citrate were injected via the root of the aorta into the coronary vessels. After removal of the aortic clamp, oxygenated blood flushed the potassium away and the heart usually reverted to normal sinus rhythm. Kolff, et al. (1957b), Baker, et al. (1957) and Wasserman, et al. (1959) discussed the relative efficacy of potassium chloride vs. potassium citrate. The experience of the Cleveland Clinic group (Effler, et al., 1957, 1958; Kolff, et al., 1957a) was summarized by Sones (1958): there was a return to satisfactory cardiac activity in 72 out of the first 75 patients.

The safe duration of potassium induced cardioplegia depends on many factors. Arrythmias are less apt to occur when the procedure is not unduly prolonged. Kolff, et al. (1956) reported consistently successful reversal after periods up to 23 minutes. According to Helmsworth, et al. (1959), the duration of arrest should not exceed 30 minutes. Allen and Lillehei (1957) and Lillehei, et al. (1957) restricted potassium arrest to the most difficult surgical cases and deferred the decision as to its use until after the heart was opened. Gerbode and Melrose (1958) gave detailed directions regarding the solution for injection, the equipment, and the induction of arrest as well as the methods of avoiding left ventricular distension and of restoring the heart beat. Harschbarger, et al. (1958) emphasized the importance of maintaining a high perfusion flow in the resumption of cardiac action, while Burroughs and Donald (1956), Ross, et al. (1958) and Glenn and Holswade (1961) called attention to the necessity of venting the arrested heart to avoid overdistension and subsequent myocardial failure. Laboratory and clinical experience has been described by numerous other workers (Weiss, et al., 1957; Dubost, et al., 1958; Cianciarullo, et al., 1959; Piskorz, et al., 1959; Bertho, 1960). Dodrill and Takagi (1960) have improved the condition of the heart after arrest by the addition of adenosine triphosphate to potassium citrate. Continuous coronary perfusion with oxygenated blood containing 15 mEq./L. of potassium made it possible for Headrick, et al. (1959) to extend the period of cardiac arrest up to three hours.

3. Magnesium arrest: The plasma magnesium concentrations associated with depression of the cardiac conduction system were determined by Smith, et al. (1939). According to Engbaek (1952) magnesium blocks energy transfer within individual myofibrils. Bass, et al. (1958) showed that small doses of magnesium induce coronary vasodilation without affecting cardiac contraction, while higher doses depress the amplitude of contraction. Magnesium alone proved to be an unsatisfactory cardioplegic drug (Merrit, et al., 1958). However, when combined with potassium and neostigmine it is effective in reducing the amount of potassium required for cardioplegia (Young, et al., 1956; Sealy, et al., 1957; 1958). A 0.81 per cent solution of potassium citrate can be used instead of the usual 2.5 per cent when combined with 2.41 per cent magnesium sulfate and 0.001 per cent neostigmine methylsulfate. Neostigmine brings about a slow heart rate in the immediate washout period. Atrioventricular dissociation is sometimes present but ventricular fibrillation is not a problem. This technique has been used mainly in combination with hypothermia.

4. Hypocalcemic arrest: Cardiac arrest produced by massive transfusions of citrated blood is a well established clinical entity. The high potassium and low calcium levels in citrated blood both tend to produce cardiac standstill during transfusion (Leveen, et al., 1959). The same hypocalcemic mechanism can be used to bring about cardiac standstill by means of coronary perfusion with sodium citrate, as performed by Riberi and Shumaker (1958). Clark, et al. (1959) used an exchange resin to remove calcium from the arterial blood stream. Continuous perfusion of the coronary vascular bed with blood of low calcium, but normal potassium level allowed them to maintain cardioplegia for 45 minutes without evidence of myocardial damage in the recovery period.

5. Acetylcholine arrest: Intracardiac administration of acetylcholine stops the isolated, perfused heart for a short period (Fröhlicher, 1945). However, Bjørk (1948) was unable to bring about cardiac arrest in situ by coronary infusion of acetylcholine. Using extremely large doses of this cholinergic drug (about 10 mg./Kg. of body weight) Lam, et al. (1955, 1957a,b, 1958) and Sergeant, et al. (1956) reported that cardiac action first slowed down, then an atrioventricular block resulted followed by almost complete arrest, with an occasional ectopic beat. The cardioplegic action of acetylcholine was never as rapid nor as complete as that of potassium citrate. Whereas potassium affects the heart muscle fibers directly and prevents response to any stimulus, the action of acetylcholine is restricted to the impulse forming and conducting tissue (Purkinje tissue), so that a stimulus applied directly to the myocardium may still produce a contraction (del Missier, et al., 1957). Release of aortic occlusion, resulting in coronary perfusion with oxygenated blood usually restores an organized beat to the acetylcholine arrested heart, although abnormal rhythms and even ventricular fibrillation can supervene (Caluzzi and Ciocallo, 1958). According to Holle, et al. (1959), perfusion of the coronary vascular bed with artificial cholinesterase permits a smoother return to sinus rhythm and satisfactory blood pressure.

Acetylcholine induced arrest has been successful in the hands of its proponents and in the experience of others (Mondini, et al., 1956; Goffrini, et al., 1957; Piskorz, et al., 1959). It was employed, with retrograde perfusion of the coronary vascular bed, for surgery of the aortic valves by DeWall, et al. (1958). It has proven useful in association with hypothermia (Moulder, et al., 1956; Brockman and Fonkalsrud, 1958) and therefore has been investigated during hypothermic perfusion of isolated hearts (Benforado, 1958; Merchant and Ranade, 1959). A combination of acetylcholine, adenosin-monophosphoric acid and novocain was used in hypothermic dogs by Herbst, et al. (1958a, b), without obvious advantages over acetylcholine alone. In the experience of other workers (Cooley, 1958), acetylcholine in the recommended dose often failed to produce complete arrest. When it did so, it was after such a long latent period that the arrest might have been caused by anoxia.

6. Anoxic arrest: A heart deprived of oxygen first shows signs of myocardial "suffering" and irritability, then goes into arrest within a few minutes. The anoxic tolerance of the myocardium is rather limited. At normal body temperature, the safe limit of anoxic cardiac arrest in dogs, while the systemic circulation is being supported by a pump-oxygenator, is of the order of 25 to 35 minutes (Wesolowski, et al., 1953a; Clowes and Neville, 1954; Cass, 1959). In many cases sinus rhythm returns but a sufficient cardiac output and acceptable blood pressures are not restored. Although anoxic arrest develops more slowly than does drug induced arrest, the safe period provided in human perfusions (up to 10 minutes) is long enough to satisfy many surgeons (Cooley, et al., 1958). A lower incidence of ventricular fibrillation is noted than is the case with potassium arrest (Nunn, et al., 1959; Dubourg, et al., 1959) and anoxic arrest can be reinstated intermittently during long-term operations.

7. Hypothermic arrest: The hypoxic tolerance of the myocardium is extended by hypothermia. In his classical experiments Gollan (1954) reported survival after cardiac arrest of one hour's duration in dogs cooled close to 0°C. Gollan and Nelson (1957) found that a slowly beating heart could safely be deprived of its coronary flow for 33 minutes at 20°C. At the same temperature, the period of myocardial ischemia could be prolonged to one hour if cardiac arrest was induced with potassium citrate. Peirce, et al. (1959) also combined hypothermia with potassium induced cardioplegia. In the experience of Berne, et al. (1958a,b), animals undergoing potassium arrest followed by infusion of cold blood into the coronary arteries had the most satisfactory postoperative course. However, recent data by Sealy, et al. (1959b) suggest that periods of complete circulatory standstill cannot greatly exceed 60 minutes at temperatures of 10°C. or lower. Otherwise, ventricular fibrillation occurs possibly because the myocardial metabolism, though reduced by the cold and asystole, is still sufficient to cause irreversible damage to the cells if oxygen deprivation is continued beyond 60 minutes.

Hypothermic cardioplegia seems the best approach to cardiac arrest available at the present time. It makes the addition of chemical agents unnecessary and avoids most of the hazards of anoxic arrest (Lillehei, et al., 1958; Bjørk and Fors, 1961). According to Shumway, et al., (1959), selective, local hypothermia of the heart makes it possible for the myocardium to endure at least one hour of anoxia during cardiopulmonary bypass with blood at normal temperature. The usual duration of pump-oxygenator support after release of aortic occlusion is of the order of 20 minutes. Decompression of the left atrium is essential for the prevention of cardiac distension and to bring about maximal cooling of the heart. Despite a contradictory report by Kenyon, et al. (1959), Urschell, et al. (1959), Bernhard, et al. (1960, 1961), and Bjørk (1961) found that coronary perfusion with Ringer's solution at 2°C. and topical application of cold saline to the external surface of the heart provide the most dependable technique of cardiac arrest. It is rapidly produced, easy to maintain and sinus rhythm is easily restored. Uniformity of cardiac cooling is important to prevent arrythmias.

Summarizing

The procedures devised for surgical cardioplegia include: (*1*) ventricular fibrillation, induced and terminated by an electrical shock; (*2*) potassium arrest by coronary injection of potassium citrate or chloride, which prevent depolarization of the heart muscle fibers; (*3*) magnesium arrest which serves mainly to lower the dose of potassium required for bringing about cardiac standstill; (*4*) hypocalcemic arrest by coronary perfusion with sodium citrate in order to unbalance the normal calcium-potassium ratio in the extracellular space; (*5*) acetylcholine arrest, which affects impulse formation and conduction; (*6*) anoxic arrest by coronary occlusion in order to temporarily deprive the myocardium of its blood supply; (*7*) hypothermic arrest by generalized cooling of the organism or by local cooling of the heart only, thus slowing myocardial metabolism.

MORPHOLOGY, FUNCTION AND METABOLISM OF THE ARRESTED HEART

After the initial enthusiasm over the conveniences of induced cardiac arrest, its drawbacks have become increasingly apparent. Despite resumption of normal sinus rhythm with some pumping activity during the early recovery period, the heart which has been arrested is not always able to return to a fully normal function. From a review of the pertinent literature, it appears that this functional incapacity must be ascribed partly to the drugs used and partly to the myocardial anoxia which accompanies most types of arrest.

1. Morphology: Kaplan, et al. (1958) reported that half of their animals died of heart failure after potassium arrest. Rigor of the ventricle and irreversible fibrillation could be prevented by adequate drainage of the left heart chambers. Nevertheless, histologic examination revealed myocardial damage (focal areas of necrosis) which was not present to the same extent when arrest for the same length of time was induced by hypoxia alone (Helmsworth, et al., 1959). This same group described myocardial damage due to topical application of potassium citrate solutions in isolated atrial pouches (Helmsworth, et al., 1958b). High concentrations of potassium were observed in blood samples drawn from the left atrium during potassium induced arrest, as compared to the slight rise observed in anoxic and acetylcholine arrest (Helmsworth, et al., 1958a). Studies with radiopotassium revealed an uneven distribution of potassium within the heart (Kaplan, et al., 1958; Kaplan and Fisher, 1960). The greatest concentrations were found in the middle third of the ventricular septum, which might explain the persistent arrythmias which frequently follow potassium arrest. From the study of washout curves, potassium appeared to be distributed in two compartments—a vascular space easily flushed and another space from which elimination was slower. Re-establishment of the normal intracellular and extracellular potassium equilibrium appeared largely beyond control. Reynolds, et al. (1958), Antipov (1960) and Tountas, et al. (1960) studied microscopically functioning capillary beds in the beating and in the potassium arrested heart of the dog. In arrested hearts, the erythrocytes appeared swollen and rounded or packed in clumps in the capillaries. A weakening of the connective tissue elements of the myocardium, more marked with longer periods of arrest, was also apparent. The myocardial picture in man, following cardiac arrest induced by potassium citrate, was described by McFarland, et al. (1960). The lesions consisted of multiple, sharply circumscribed microscopic areas of necrosis usually encountered in the central portion of the ventricular myocardium. The necrotic fibers were swollen, their cytoplasm is either hyalinized, or granular; neither cross striation, nor longitudinal fibrils could be recognized. Such lesions were already apparent in a patient who died less than two hours after induction of cardiac arrest. In these observations, capillaries, small arterioles and connective tissue within the lesion appeared to be unaffected. These criteria allow one to distinguish the lesions of potassium induced arrest from other types of myocardial necrosis, as are seen in acute infarcts, and in association with potassium deficiency or noradrenalin. Electron microscope observations on the morphology of the heart muscle after arrest have recently been reported in great detail by Löhr (1960) and Löhr, et al. (1960).

2. Function: Functional studies of the influence of potassium-induced arrest on myocardial contractility in dogs and in human beings were reported by Darby, et al. (1958). By direct measurements of myocardial contractile force, they found that after recovery from cardioplegia and cardiotomy, the heart was still capable of performing the same amount of work as before. Unfortunately, this conclusion has not been confirmed by subsequent studies. The right and left ventricle are not equally sensitive to hypoxia (Szekeres, et al., 1958). Gehl (1959) has shown that after potassium arrest, the right heart recovers faster than the left heart. After three to four minutes of perfusion of the coronary arteries, the right ventricular output may be such as to precipitate left heart failure. Using ventricular function curves, Weirich, et al. (1960) and Willman, et al. (1959), observed a severe myocardial depression after 30 minutes of arrest by various pharmacologic agents. Arrest with potassium citrate for only 20 minutes causes significant myocardial depression. The deleterious effects of prolonged arrest are less marked with hypothermia (Cooper, et al., 1959a; Willman, et al., 1961a) and can be prevented by prophylactic administration of digitalis (Cooper, et al., 1960; Willman, et al., 1960b).

In the experience of Waldhausen, et al. (1960), both potassium citrate and acetylcholine result in severe depression of myocardial function when the period of arrest exceeds 10 minutes. Continuous aortic occlusion for 10 or 20 minutes is responsible for only moderate impairment of function, and intermittent aortic occlusion totaling 30 minutes in duration causes no significant depression. Similarly, Kusunoki, et al. (1960), found a depression of myocardial function of 50 to 70 per cent of control values when measured 15 minutes after the end of arrest regardless of the cardioplegic technique used. Partial recovery occurs following an additional 15 minutes of perfusion. Prolongation of cardioplegia results in greater depression of myocardial function and further delay in recovery. Hypothermia to 25°C. partially protects the heart rendered hypoxic for 15 minutes. In comparison with other methods, anoxic-hypothermic cardioplegia results in the least cardiac depression and the best return of myocardial function.

In concluding this review of functional studies after cardioplegia, it seems relevant to ascribe the minor discrepancies among the observations of the various authors to the difficulties inherent in the measuring techniques employed. Ventricular function studies, while allowing a rough quantitation of the maximum performance of the heart, require some time to be carried out. Since myocardial depression after cessation of cardioplegia tends to disappear as time goes on, the ventricular function curves obtained vary according to the time at which they are measured. Direct measurements of cardiac contractile force make possible continuous assessment of myocardial function; however, changes in ventricular size often preclude direct comparisons, or necessitate difficult corrections. Nevertheless, from the body of information available, it appears that at normal temperature any cardiac arrest procedure involves some depression of myocardial function. If cardioplegia is prolonged over 10 minutes, the depression may be sufficient to render the heart unable to support the full load of the circulation when normal coronary circulation is re-established. Hypothermia, by reducing the energy requirement of the heart, permits an extension of the period of myocardial hypoxia.

3. Metabolism: Metabolic studies of cardioplegia must be traced back to Rohde (1910), who first observed that the oxygen requirement of the arrested heart is significantly less than that of the beating, empty heart. Gregg (1958) estimated cardiac oxygen uptake to eight to ten ml./100 Gm. of left ventricle per minute under normal conditions. During ventricular fibrillation, Senning (1952) found values close to 4 ml./100 Gm./min. Berglund, et al. (1957) compared the oxygen uptake of the myocardium during potassium induced arrest and that during ventricular fibrillation. They found oxygen uptake decreased markedly during arrest, while during ventricular fibrillation oxygen usage varied widely, sometimes even exceeding that of the working state. Dealing with the closed-chest animal, Beuren, et al. (1958) found no statistically significant difference in oxygen usage between the empty beating heart, the fibrillating heart and the arrested heart. In all of these preparations the oxygen uptake was between 20 and 30 per cent of the control values. However, McKeever, et al. (1958) found that oxygen usage of the myocardium was reduced to only half in ventricular fibrillation, and to one quarter during arrest. The higher values in the fibrillating heart, together with the marked scattering of results, were related to the type and forcefulness of the fibrillation. The heart arrested with acetylcholine (Willman, et al., 1958b) or by perfusion with hypocalcemic blood (Clark, et al., 1959) was also characterized by an oxygen uptake reduced to 25 per cent of the control. Lately, independent studies by Hoffmeister, et al. (1959) and Greenberg, et al. (1960) yielded

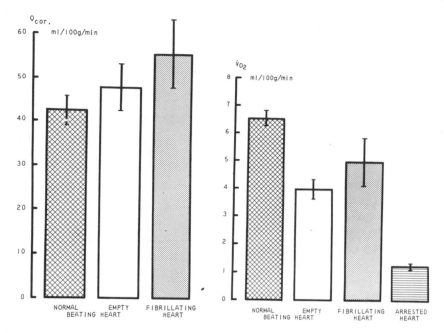

Fig. 99. Comparative values of coronary blood flow (Q_{cor}, in ml./100 g./min., left graph) an myocardial oxygen uptake ($\dot{V}_{O_2}$, in ml./100 g./min., right graph) in the normal beating heart, in the empty beating heart during cardiopulmonary bypass, in the fibrillating heart and in the arrested heart. The vertical lines represent ± one Standard Error. (Modified from data of Hoffmeister, et al., 1959.)

surprisingly similar results (fig. 99): The oxygen uptake decreases progressively from the normal beating heart to the fibrillating heart, the empty beating heart and the potassium arrested heart. In the empty beating heart, there is a linear relationship between oxygen uptake and heart rate, with a heart rate = zero intercept close to the values obtained in the arrested heart. The authors conclude that overall oxygen usage by the heart includes an uptake for resting activity, one for maintaining the contractions, and one for external work.

Glucose is the primary subtrate for metabolism in the isolated, perfused, beating or arrested heart (Jesseph, et al., 1958; Winterscheid, et al., 1958; Ernst, et al. (1959). Glucose utilization by dog myocardium increases markedly during bypass and increases still further during elective cardiac arrest (Ikins, et al., 1959). Progressive glycogen depletion, therefore, characterizes prolonged asystole (Conn, et al., 1959); the lactic acid content of the myocardium rises, together with a fall of pH in the vascular bed of the arrested heart. The readily available storehouse of high energy phosphate contained in phosphocreatine drops to low levels within 20 minutes of standstill (Gott, et al., 1959; Michal, et al., 1959). Adenosindiphosphate (ADP) remains low and constant, indicating that ADP is recharged to adenosintriphosphate (ATP), probably by glycolysis and phosphocreatine breakdown. The loss of glycogen, phosphocreatine and ATP is minimized under hypothermic conditions (Gott, et al., 1960).

Some form of metabolic support for the heart after reversal of induced asystole has been advocated by many authors. Hall, et al., (1960) suggest that hypertonic glucose, together with insulin, may have some merit in providing the myocardium with a readily available source of glycogen. This follows the practice of Mavor, et al. (1957), who utilized a 50 per cent glucose-insulin mixture injected intravenously as an adjunct to cardiac massage in restoring the action of potassium arrested hearts under conditions of general hypothermia. Fructose was used instead of glucose by O'Brien and Guest (1959) with similar results. Mephentermine sulfate enhances cardiac contractility after potassium arrest (Cooper, et al., 1959). The problems of cardiac recovery are most ably discussed by Cicero, et al. (1959).

Summarizing

Although the heart resumes normal sinus rhythm and some pumping activity after standstill, it is not always able to return to completely normal function. Cardiac arrest can result in myocardial damage as evidenced by numerous microscopic areas of necrosis. Ventricular function curves and contractile force decline markedly after arrest periods lasting longer than 20 minutes. Hypothermia partially protects the heart from the depression resulting from standstill. The arrested heart still has considerable metabolic requirements (about one-fourth of the normal heart). Glucose is the primary substrate for the metabolism of the isolated, perfused, beating or arrested heart.

XIX. Hypothermia by Means of Extracorporeal Circulation

Hypothermia as an aid to cardiac surgery developed directly from the work of Bigelow, et al. (1950). As pointed out by Delorme (1955), Bigelow's fundamental observation was that the oxygen consumption of the warm-blooded animal can be reversibly lowered by hypothermia without an oxygen debt being incurred. This reduction in tissue oxygen demand brought about by cooling prompted the idea that low flow perfusion might be usefully associated with hypothermia. At first, it seemed that "extracorporeal cooling" would combine the difficulties of the two procedures rather than their advantages (Lillehei, et al., 1957). However, expanding knowledge of the physiology of hypothermia (Delorme, 1953; 1955; Ross, 1955; Dripps, 1956; Taylor, 1959; Gollan, 1959a, b) has refuted this pessimistic forecast. At the present time, the fall in blood temperature observed in most perfusion procedures is no longer feared, but rather deliberately facilitated by heat-exchange devices. Light (33 to 35°C.), moderate (26 to 32°C.), and deep (0 to 20°C.) hypothermia are commonly used in clinical practice. A review of the numerous studies dealing with hypothermic perfusions would exceed the scope of the present textbook. Attention will therefore be limited to the physiologic principles which are needed for understanding the references to hypothermia made in other chapters.

BLOOD STREAM COOLING VERSUS PERIPHERAL COOLING

J. F. Heymans (1921) introduced blood stream cooling as a method in physiologic research. Using a glass cannula inside a water jacket to link a carotid artery to a jugular vein, and using the heart of the animal as a pump, Heymans was able to cool the organism by perfusion with refrigerated blood. Boerema, et al. (1951), Delorme (1952), Gollan, et al. (1952), Peirce and Polley (1953), Senning (1954), Mazzoni and Baisi (1954) pioneered the way of extracorporeal cooling of the circulation as a means of inducing hypothermia. Recovery was found to be possible after the animal's temperature had been lowered to 0°C. (Gollan 1954; Kenyon and Ludbrook, 1957). Clinically, Brock and Ross (1955) used a simple extracorporeal shunt for blood stream cooling, while Sealy, et al. (1957a) first combined immersion hypothermia with cardio-pulmonary bypass, then for convenience added a heat exchanger to their extracorporeal circuit.

The rapid drop in blood temperature, the saving on caloric exchange and the unique distribution of hypothermia induced by blood stream cooling were already noted by early investigators. However, several years of systematic study were required to obtain a clear picture of the characteristics of "core cooling" by extracorporeal circulation of blood, as opposed to "peripheral cooling" by immersion in ice water or by other means. The significant advantages of *blood stream cooling* can be summarized as follows (Peirce, et al., 1958a, b):

(1) Since the blood is cooled just before returning it to the arterial tree, those organs having the highest perfusion rate (kidney, heart, brain and liver) manifest the most marked drop in temperature. Since these are also the organs with the highest oxygen uptake, a small caloric exchange suffices to produce a large decrease in oxygen demand. Meanwhile, the great bulk of the organism (skin, muscle and bone), which has a relatively low metabolism, is not cooled appreciably. Because of local temperature differences, core cooling is more efficient than is peripheral cooling in terms of the caloric exchange required for achieving a given metabolic depression. In fact, the overall heat transfer during blood stream cooling may be as little as one third of that required for bringing the entire organism to the same central temperature by immersion in ice water.

(2) The heat "stored" in (or rather not removed from) the nonvital areas of the body greatly facilitates the rewarming process. When the central temperature does not drop below 28 to 30°C., it is not even necessary to warm the blood returning from the extracorporeal circuit in order to reverse the hypothermia. Spontaneous heat exchange with the environment provides enough calories for a smooth return of the temperature to the near physiologic range.

(3) The temperature gradients in the organism during core cooling are the reverse of those associated with peripheral cooling since the internal organs are the first to be cooled when the heat exchanger is activated, and the first to be rewarmed when heat transfer is reversed in the extracorporeal circuit. Therefore the inherent difficulties of immersion hypothermia, namely the delay of central temperature change as well as the downward temperature drift occurring after cessation of external cooling no longer exist with blood stream cooling. The central temperature rises as soon as refrigeration is discontinued, yet it can be maintained at the desired level for as long a period as required.

(4) As recognized by Dill and Forbes (1941) and Bigelow, et al. (1950), external cooling requires a level of anesthesia deep enough to prevent reflex shivering and muscle tremor. Otherwise the oxygen demand rises considerably and the increased heat output by the organism prolongs the cooling procedure beyond practicable limits. Furthermore the shivering response leads to exhaustion and entails a prohibitive mortality. Boerema, et al. (1951) and Delorme (1952) introduced the method of blood stream cooling in order to circumvent the highly coordinated and efficient reaction of the organism elicited by the hypothalamus, the adrenals, and the thyroid in response to stimulation of peripheral end organs by cold. In fact, rapid blood stream cooling does not induce shivering so that only minimal anesthesia is required for starting the procedure. Thereafter cold narcosis becomes operative. During the rewarming phase, internally cooled animals regularly

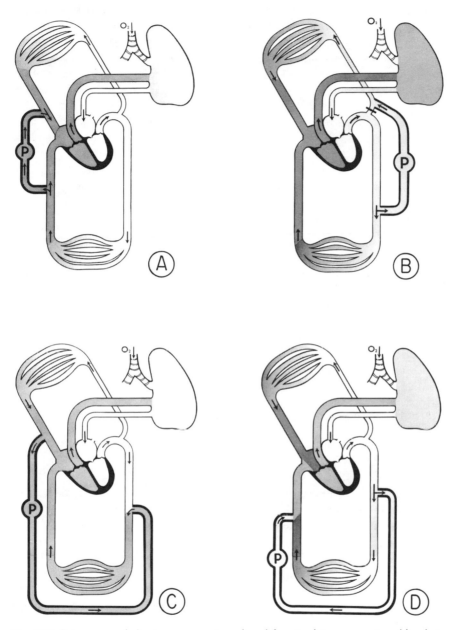

Fig. 100. Extracorporeal shunt arrangement employed for circulatory support or blood stream cooling.

A. Veno-venous pumping: blood is transferred from one vein into another after undergoing oxygenation or heat exchange in the extracorporeal shunt line.

B. Arterio-arterial pumping: blood is transferred from one artery to another, or from the central end to the peripheral end of the same artery.

C. Veno-arterial pumping: venous blood is drained into the extracorporeal shunt and infused under pressure into the arterial tree.

D. Arterio-venous pumping: blood is transferred from artery to vein. The pump (P) serves primarily as a metering device. and can be omitted shiver when their central temperature approaches 28° to 30°C., and this reaction greatly facilitates the return to normal conditions.

(5) Blood stream cooling is usually associated with generalized vasodilation and intravascular pooling of blood. However, the degree of anesthesia, the partial pressures of oxygen and carbon dioxide, and species differences must be taken into account to explain discrepancies among published data as to the degree of temperature depression required to induce vasodilation, and the extent of the vasomotor reactions. Externally cooled animals can maintain a higher arterial pressure than internally cooled animals at the same temperature and blood flow, because baroreceptor mechanisms are continuously stimulated by afferences from the periphery (Brendel, 1961). This observation is consistent with the concept that spinal vasomotor reflexes are less easily depressed by cold than central regulatory mechanisms.

Summarizing:

Hypothermia can be induced by cooling the blood stream in an extracorporeal circuit (core cooling) or by immersion of the body in ice-water (peripheral cooling). Blood stream cooling entails a larger metabolic saving than does peripheral cooling because the blood preferentially reduces the temperature in those organs which normally have the highest blood flow and the largest oxygen consumption—the kidney, heart, brain and liver. Rewarming occurs most quickly in the vital organs, returning them to normal function earlier than the less important ones. Anesthesia can be kept at a minimum because of the absence of reflex shivering during the cooling phase. Shivering during rewarming contributes to the reestablishment of normal temperature conditions.

MODES OF BLOOD STREAM COOLING

Different methods for blood stream cooling have been devised, all of which offer certain advantages and suffer from certain drawbacks in terms of efficiency, simplicity and safety.

1. Arterio-venous pumping: Arterial blood pumped by the heart itself into a vein (fig. 100, D), after passing through an external shunt and a heat exchanger, illustrates the simplest approach to central hypothermia and the least traumatic to blood. Its use was pioneered by Boerema, et al. (1951), Delorme (1952) and Ross (1954a, b). Because the size of the arterio-venous shunt must be small to prevent circulatory collapse, caloric exchange is slow. The hypothermia achieved is also self-limiting, since flow through the heat exchanger depends upon cardiac contraction, so cooling ceases as the cardiac action becomes weak.

2. Arterio-arterial pumping: Arterio-arterial pumping (fig. 100, B) through a cooling device interposed in an extracorporeal shunt is primarily intended for selective cooling of a single organ. Nevertheless, the cooled venous blood returning from the perfused organ eventually brings about a more general hypothermia. Arterio-arterial cooling has been primarily directed at the brain both in experimental animals (Parkins, et al., 1954; Buster, et al., 1958; Brendel, et al., 1958; Ross, 1959b) and in patients (Kimoto, 1956; Sakakibara, et al., 1958). Using the heart as a pump, it has the same conveniences and limitations as does arterio-venous cooling. Selective brain cooling induces a marked hypotension and some decrease in ventilation and oxygen uptake. When used in conjunction with circulatory arrest for cardiac surgery, its use is limited by the vulnerability of the spinal cord, heart and liver to anoxia.

3. Veno-arterial pumping: Veno-arterial pumping (fig. 100, C), with a mechanical pump in the shunt line in addition to the heat exchanger, was proposed by Ross (1954a) to complement the cooling initially started by arterio-venous pumping. It was hoped that this would maintain a sufficient pressure in the aorta, at a level of hypothermia where the cardiac action is usually too weak to prevent hypotension. Thus, the aortic valves could be kept shut and coronary gas embolism from air trapped in the left ventricle after cardiotomy avoided. Ross also noted that the contractions of the heart were much more forceful when given this kind of assistance. During veno-arterial pumping, the volume of blood available for oxygenation in the lungs is decreased since part of the venous blood is transferred directly into the arterial tree. Consequently, veno-arterial pumping must be limited to low flows in order to avoid hypoxic disturbances before the oxygen demand of the organism is sufficiently lowered. The rate of cooling obtained is, therefore, slow.

4. Veno-venous pumping: Veno-venous cooling and rewarming with the aid of a pump (fig. 100, A) and of a heat exchanger in the shunt line was suggested by Taddei, et al. (1954) and Ross (1955, 1959) as a simple technique for bringing about central hypothermia in the operating room. It allows the surgeon to defer his choice between simple hypothermic circulatory arrest and mechanical support of the circulation by a pump-oxygenator until the chest has been opened and the diagnosis confirmed. If hypothermia alone is decided upon, blood is circulated from the superior vena cava to the inferior vena cava through a refrigerated cooling coil for a period of about 45 minutes. Meanwhile, the surgeon prepares the great vessels which are clamped when the desired temperature is reached. During the period of circulatory arrest, the heat exchanger is changed over in preparation for rewarming. Return to normal temperature is then initiated in the extracorporeal shunt line. Veno-venous pumping has the advantages of simplicity and safety, but its limited efficiency restricts its use to light or moderate hypothermia. To maintain a normal arterial pressure during the cooling process, the administration of an adrenergic drug is often found necessary.

5. Autogenous lung oxygenation: In order to bring about deep hypothermia, it is necessary to take over the function of both ventricles by mechanical means. If, at the same time, the lungs are perfused to maintain gas exchange, the procedure is called autogenous lung oxygenation (*see* fig. 12). In this way, the cooling process can be continued in the presence of a non-functioning heart, adequate gas exchange can be maintained in the lungs, rewarming can be started when desired and normal cardiac action can be restored at the most appropriate moment (Drew, et al., 1959). Autogenous lung oxygenation under conditions of deep hypothermia and circulatory arrest was developed by Shield and Lewis (1959) and Holt, et al. (1960), in Chicago and Drew, et al. (1959), in London. Drew and Anderson (1959) successfully introduced the procedure into clinical practice. The American authors first used a system of bilateral cardiac bypass and bilateral cooling. Now they resort to a single efficient heat exchanger in the left sided circuit. The English investigators start the perfusion with a left heart bypass circuit incorporating the heat exchanger. They substitute a pump for the right ventricle when the heart appears unable to handle all the blood draining into the right atrium. Then, during the rewarming process, they first use a bilateral bypass, then stop the "right ventricle" pump after the heart has been resuscitated and appears able to sustain the circulation. The left heart bypass is terminated shortly thereafter. Hypothermic autogenous oxygenation combines the advantages of adequate gas exchange with a small priming volume requirement. It accomplishes what other investigators obtain by the combination of hypothermia and low-flow cardiopulmonary bypass. It is still questionable whether or not the inconveniences of additional cannulation for autogenous oxygenation outweighs the technical complexity and the additional blood trauma introduced by an artificial gas exchange device.

6. Partial heart–lung bypass: Used for blood stream cooling, partial heart–lung bypass (*see* fig. 3) combines the hemodynamic support provided by veno-arterial pumping with the additional virtue that oxygenated blood is infused into the arterial tree. The procedure is undoubtedly more complex and more traumatic to blood than is simple veno-arterial pumping. Yet, it provides full metabolic support during the period of cooling and rewarming regardless of the rate of heat exchange. Maintenance of acceptable conditions is also possible, should the heart weaken or fibrillate. Cooling by partial heart–lung bypass makes possible the use of peripheral cannulation. Thoracotomy and other major surgical procedures can be delayed until after induction of hypothermia, a convenience which might be life-saving in patients with a failing circulation. The blood from the extracorporeal circuit must be returned by a catheter long enough to deliver it into the aortic arch; otherwise, purely regional cooling occurs. The flow rate is limited by the size of the catheters which can be introduced into peripheral veins (*see* chap. XII) and by the increasing blood viscosity as the temperature goes down. It follows that partial heart–lung bypass is most appropriate when cooling is to be done slowly (Enerson, et al., 1960). When circulatory arrest is the ultimate aim of the procedure, partial bypass requires a longer duration of extracorporeal circulation for cooling and rewarming than does total bypass.

7. Total heart–lung bypass: Drainage of all venous blood into the extracorporeal circuit requires thoracotomy for adequate venous cannulation. The arterialized blood can be returned at any point in the arterial tree since there is no output of the left ventricular output which might keep the upper part of the body from perfusion with cooled blood, as happens with partial bypass. The entire period of extracorporeal circulation can be used for heat exchange and, since high flow rates are obtained, cooling and rewarming are extremely rapid. Thus, the central temperature is lowered with a minimum caloric exchange because there is almost no time for the tissues at the periphery to participate in the cooling. Ideally, the blood flow rate selected should provide adequate metabolic support at all temperatures. Therefore, the flow should be high at the beginning, then gradually decreased as hypothermia is achieved and later again progressively increased as rewarming progresses. Actually continuing variation of flow rate is not easy to carry out, and in most instances a constant blood flow is maintained during the period of perfusion. It follows then that, when low flows are used from the beginning, the cooling must be done rapidly to depress the metabolism before the organism has incurred a significant oxygen debt.

Summarizing:

Each mode of blood stream cooling has its advantages and drawbacks. Arterio-venous pumping through the action of the heart is simple but the cooling ceases as the heart weakens. Arterio-arterial pumping is useful for selective cooling of an organ but eventually lowers the entire body temperature and depresses the heart upon which the pumping depends. Veno-arterial pumping using a mechanical pump maintains aortic pressure but tissue hypoxia results when too much venous blood is pumped into the arterial tree. Veno-venous pumping allows cooling for diagnostic thoracotomy, so that the decision can be made subsequently as to whether or not a pump oxygenator is needed for the contemplated operation. Autogenous lung oxygenation combined with mechanical pumping makes possible efficient and safe hypothermia but necessitates extensive cannulations. Cooling during partial or total heart–lung bypass provides full hemodynamic and metabolic support of the organism but is technically more complex than the aforementioned procedures.

TEMPERATURE, GAS EXCHANGE AND AND PERFUSION FLOWS

Regional differences in temperature during blood stream cooling were already apparent in the experiments of J. F. Heymans (1921). However, the flow of blood through the arterio-venous shunt was small as compared to the cardiac output and, therefore, no large difference could develop. When pumps were introduced into the extracorporeal shunt so as to make the cooling process independent of the animal's own circulation, temperature differences of more than 20°C. between different parts of the body were reported (Gollan, et al., 1955a, b; Peirce, et al., 1956, 1958a, b; Shield and Lewis, 1959), Peirce, et al. (1960) studied in detail the cooling rate of various organs during partial and total heart–lung bypass. Their results, schematized in fig. 101, show that an efficient heat exchanger provides a wide temperature difference between the incoming venous blood and the outgoing arterial blood, a difference which is reversed during the rewarming phase of the cycle. The internal organs are refrigerated rapidly, in the order: kidney-heart-brain-liver, as would be expected considering their normal share of perfusion flow. The rectal temperature continues to fall slowly even after the warming process is initiated and fails to reflect mean body temperature. The esophageal temperature is somewhat more informative.

The shaded area in fig. 101, bounded by lines depicting the temperatures of arterial and venous blood, affords an easy estimation of the caloric exchange. As is expected in a heart–lung bypass procedure, the temperature of the arterial blood is lower than that of the venous blood during cooling, and higher during rewarming. The product of the arterio-venous temperature difference times the extracorporeal flow rate times the specific heat

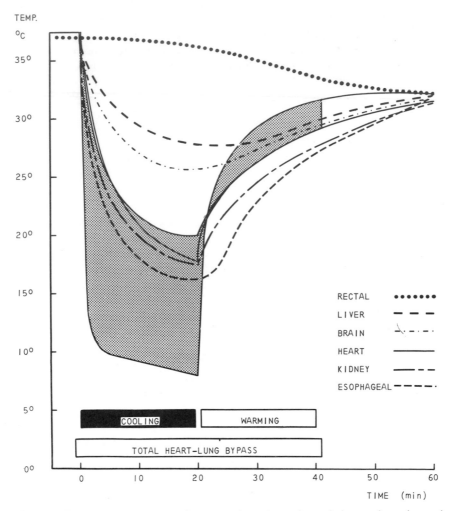

TEMP.
°C

RECTAL ••••••
LIVER – – –
BRAIN ⨉ – ⋅ –
HEART ——
KIDNEY — —
ESOPHAGEAL – – – ⋅

COOLING   WARMING

TOTAL HEART-LUNG BYPASS

TIME (min)

Fig. 101. Temperature variation in the rectum, liver, brain, heart, kidney and esophagus during blood stream cooling and rewarming. The shaded area is limited by lines depicting the temperatures of venous and arterial blood. (Details in text.) (Modified from Peirce, et al., 1960.)

of blood equals the number of Calories removed by the heat exchanger during the cooling phase, or added during the warming phase. The specific heat of blood is usually taken as 1.00, although blood with a normal hematocrit has an actual value of only 0.86 (Mendlowitz, 1948). In fig. 101, assuming a perfusion flow of 0.5 L./min. and a mean arteriovenous temperature difference of 12°C., the heat removed in 20 minutes of cooling amounts to 120 Calories. Using immersion hypothermia instead of core cooling, at least 400 Calories would have to be extracted in order to bring about a 20°C. fall in temperature of the heart in a 20 Kg. organism. During the warming phase fewer calories need be added by the heat exchanger than were removed during the cooling phase, as illustrated by the much smaller shaded area between the arterial and venous temperature curves. Again assuming the perfusion flow to be 0.5 L./min. and the mean arterio-venous temperature difference to be 3°C., the heat added during 20 minutes of warming amounts to 30 Calories. This low value is due in part to the fact that heat-exchangers are less efficient for warming than for cooling, owing to the smaller temperature gradient permissible between blood and heating fluid (*see* Chapter XI). The fact that heat is drawn into the blood from the warmer peripheral organs and from the environment also accounts for decreased heat transfer in the extracorporeal circuit. Finally, shivering speeds the rewarming process. Since the final temperature of the organism is of the order of 32°C. and its weight 20 Kg., the net caloric loss at the end of the procedure is on the order of 100 Calories. Yet, a similar antimetabolic effect of cold on the central organs by way of peripheral hypothermia would have required the extraction of 400 Calories, and a considerable expense of time and effort in the rewarming phase. It must be stressed that measurements of temperature variation, and the calculations based thereon, are necessarily crude. The rates of cooling and rewarming depends upon the extracorporeal flow rate. Lower flows make possible more accurate temperature determinations, but defeat one of the purposes of blood stream cooling, namely the minimizing of heat transfer by conduction from adjacent tissues. Since no single temperature is representative of the entire organism, or for that matter of any single organ (Fisher and Fedor, 1961; Peirce, 1961b), multiple temperature readings are necessary. Esophageal temperature is often used as a convenient index of central temperature. However, deceptively low values are observed when the tip of the sensing element leans against the esophageal wall close to the aorta. Rectal temperature may also give abnormally low values when a short femoral cannula is used for arterial infusion and the rectal sensing element happens to be influenced by the temperature in the iliac vessels.

Consideration of a chart of temperature variations during blood stream cooling (*see* fig. 101) suggests that the oxygen demands of a perfused organism are never constant, a circumstance which makes indirect measurements by a reverse Fick computation questionable. It would probably be better to measure directly the overall oxygen uptake during the cooling and warming phases, and to ascertain the oxygen saving by comparison with a control oxygen uptake measured before hypothermia. Meanwhile, it is best to follow the practice of experienced workers in this field in maintaining the venous oxygen saturation (or tension, or content) within or above physiologic limits. In fact, any of these venous oxygen values rise markedly if blood flow is constant while temperature is depressed (Brown, et al., 1958b). The arterio-venous difference in oxygen tension narrows progressively and venous oxygen tension at times exceeds the arterial oxygen tension of a normothermic subject breathing air. As Gollan (1959a) puts it, one deals then with an animal without venous blood. Although highly unphysiologic, this state appears to be perfectly innocuous, particularly since there has been no evidence of oxygen toxicity (*see* Chapter XIV) under conditions encountered so far in experimental perfusions.

Compared with normothermic perfusions, hypothermic perfusions make possible the use of lower flow rates without resulting in hypoxia and metabolic acidosis. On the basis of Clark's estimates of oxygen need and perfusion requirements at normal body temperature (*see* Chapter XIV), Gollan (1959) calculated the optimal flow rate at lower body temperatures. As a rule of thumb, it can be stated that the oxygen demand of the organism is decreased to about one half at 30°C., one third at 25°C., one fifth at 20°C., and one sixth at 10°C. Although there are no extensive data concerning oxygen requirement in deep hypothermia, it seems that below 10°C. the metabolism does not decrease to negligible levels (Adolph, et al., 1958). Complete circulatory standstill is not tolerated beyond 60 to 90 minutes even at temperatures below 10°C. (Sealy, et al., 1959b). This might indicate that the oxygen demand, though greatly reduced, is still large enough to cause irreversible damage if oxygen deprivation is continued beyond limits. On the other hand, it is easier to resuscitate the heart after low flow perfusion without oxygenation than after complete circulatory standstill (Lesage, et al., 1959), a fact which points out the possibility that some "washing out" of metabolites may be even more urgently needed than is distribution of oxygen to the tissues.

In the preceding paragraphs, it was tacitly assumed that the decreased oxygen uptake during blood stream cooling merely reflects the hypometabolic effect of hypothermia, and has not been influenced by inadequate perfusion of certain portions of the vascular bed, leading to the accumulation of an oxygen debt. This assumption must be scrutinized, since under conditions of deep peripheral hypothermia, blood flow ceases in many small vessels (Lynch and Adolph, 1957). Löfström (1959) emphasized the concept of cell aggregation with interruption of blood flow in peripheral hypothermia, a condition which can be prevented by the addition of low molecular weight dextran (*see* chap. XVII). No direct observations of small peripheral vessels during blood stream cooling have been reported. From studies with radioactive indicators, Gollan (1955b, 1959a) concluded that it was necessary to dilute blood with physiologic solutions to bring about complete mixing with the tracer at low temperature. However, the stability of arterial and venous pH during cooling and rewarming is an argument against inadequate perfusion of certain areas in the circulatory system, which should result in a tide of acid metabolites when the region of stasis is again perfused. A possible beneficial effect of lowering the hematocrit may be related to the fact that this compensates for increased blood viscosity as the temperature goes down.

Hypothermia affects gas transfer in many complex ways (Brewin, et al., 1956; Boere, et al., 1957; Severinghaus, 1959). With regards to *oxygen* the following condition exists: (*1*) The metabolic demand for it is diminished. (*2*) Its solubility in body fluids is increased considerably, being approximately doubled at 20°C. (*3*) Since the temperature goes down and the pH goes up, the oxygen dissociation curve is shifted to the left making less oxygen available to the tissues at a given tension, and causing the hemoglobin to be more completely saturated in the artificial lung. With regards to *carbon dioxide:* (*1*) Metabolic production falls and its solubility in biologic fluids increases with hypothermia. (*2*) Because pH is increased and pK is also increased merely by cooling the blood, the blood CO_2 tension decreases while CO_2 content remains constant. (*3*) Since blood CO_2 tension is decreased, less carbon dioxide is eliminated per unit of time if ventilation and blood flow through the artificial lung are kept constant. (*4*) In practice, the situation is made even more involved by some degree of metabolic acidosis which is difficult to avoid in perfusion procedures. Metabolic acidosis tends to depress the arterial pH elevated by cooling. To compensate for this, more CO_2 elimination is necessary.

In view of this complexity it is not surprising that CO_2 and pH data reported from blood stream cooling procedures vary widely (Peirce, et al., 1958b; Holt, et al., 1960). Rather than analyzing them in detail, it may be more useful to call attention to Severinghaus' attempt (1959) to define normal ventilation during hypothermia: "Either pH or P_{CO_2} might arbitrarily be held constant, but the observation of the rapid changes in both pH and P_{CO_2}, when a sample of blood is cooled (anaerobically) detracts from the rationality of using them. It is more reasonable to propose that normal ventilation is that in which carbon dioxide elimination equals its rate of metabolic production as cooling progresses. This definition has several characteristics: (*1*) Blood carbon dioxide content remains constant; (*2*) pH rises in vivo at the same rate as in blood cooled in vitro, i.e., by 0.0147 U/°C.; (3) alveolar and arterial P_{CO_2} fall at the same rate as in blood cooled in vitro, reaching 22.9 mm. Hg. at 25°C. However, if metabolic acidosis occurs, pH fails to rise much and extra carbon dioxide is eliminated. If ventilation is unchanged, P_{CO_2} after a period of elevation due to freed body stores, will return to the same level as in the absence of metabolic acidosis. Finally, then, it would appear that the P_{CO_2} should be used to define normal ventilation; not that CO_2 should be constant, but that it should fall as the P_{CO_2} does in blood cooled in vitro. In the absence of metabolic acidosis, carbon dioxide elimination would keep pace with its metabolic production."

This 'normal' ventilation, as defined by Severinghaus, is not necessarily the best ventilation for assuring protection of the circulation in hypothermia. In fact, it may be more beneficial for the organism to retain some CO_2, since at low temperatures CO_2 exerts a protective effect on several biologic functions ("Giaja" effect, 1940). For this purpose, the P_{CO_2} must be higher and the pH lower than is the case when CO_2 elimination equals metabolic production. The question remains to be settled experimentally. It would be valuable if an investigator attempted to use modern techniques for continuous monitoring of CO_2 tension in blood or 'alveolar' gas from the artificial lung to regulate ventilation of the artificial gas exchange device during hypothermia.

Summarizing:

Blood stream cooling results in marked regional temperature differences in the body because organs with the greatest perfusion flow are the first to reach the lowest temperatures. The caloric exchange of core cooling and rewarming is more efficient than that of peripheral cooling and rewarming for the same degree of metabolic depression. Since oxygen requirements during blood stream cooling cannot be predicted accurately, the safest procedure is to maintain venous oxygen tension, or saturation, within the normal range. The dynamics of CO_2 exchange are considerably altered at low temperature, and it might be beneficial for the organism to accumulate some CO_2 during hypothermia.

HEART AND CIRCULATION AT LOW TEMPERATURE

Decreased heart rate, prolongation myocardial contraction and relaxation period, lowered arterial pressure and slightly elevated venous pressure were the simple hemodynamic signs which first suggested that death from hypothermia was related to cardiocirculatory failure (Bigelow, et al., 1950). With peripheral cooling the high incidence of ventricular fibrillation at temperatures below 28°C. entailed a prohibitive mortality rate and contributed to an aura of fear concerning the condition of the heart. Investigations performed in the last ten years justify a more optimistic outlook. It has been conclusively demonstrated that myocardial function in light and moderate hypothermia is at least adequate for the amount of work required from the heart under such conditions (Berne, 1959). In deep hypothermia induced by peripheral cooling, the cardiovascular system is involved in a vicious cycle because some blood circulation is needed to raise the central temperature while a rise in central temperature is required to start the heart again after cooling is terminated. Nowadays it is rather easy to restart the circulation by using a pump-oxygenator. By virtue of the protection afforded by extracorporeal circulation ventricular fibrillation "has lost its deadly scare and is not more than a cosmetic defect of the electrocardiogram" (Gollan, 1959a).

The cardiodynamics of hypothermia by blood stream cooling combine the features of immersion hypothermia with those of normothermic perfusion procedures, with the added complexity introduced by unequal cooling of different vascular beds. We shall briefly summarize some pertinent points. For the most complete presentation available at the present time, the reader is referred to the reviews by Berne (1959), Gollan (1959a, b), Dubost, et al. (1960; 1961), Kenyon (1961), Cooper (1961) and Darbinian and Portnoy (1961).

The heart rate decreases as the central temperature falls. The relationship is not linear because the slowing effect of cold is less pronounced at low temperatures (Gollan, 1959b). In the absence of ventricular fibrillation the heart usually ceases its organized beat between 15°C. and 10°C., although occasional contractions are still observed between 5°C. and 10°C. When hypothermia is not so deep, asystole is easily brought about by aortic occlusion or by deliberate cessation of the perfusion. The hypothermic, arrested heart is small and firm. Its metabolism is reduced to a bare fraction of the normothermic requirements. However, its tolerance to hypoxia remains limited, as evidenced by the present impossibility of resuscitating a heart which has been arrested for more than 90 minutes. Provided that no hypoxic damage has occurred, restarting the arrested heart during the rewarming phase does not present a difficult challenge. If ventricular fibrillation occurs, it is usually stopped by electric defibrillation, potassium arrest or recooling of the heart. Above 25°C., the heart can be expected to take over some of the circulatory load since its intrinsic performance is increased as compared to normothermia (Brown and Cotten, 1954; Goldberg, 1958; Covino and Beavers, 1958).

The relationship between perfusion flow, mean arterial pressure and body blood volume during hypothermic heart–lung bypass is very complex. Experimental perfusions are usually conducted at constant flow rates and a constant central venous pressure is maintained. Considering the expected decrease in oxygen demand, the flow rate selected at the start of perfusion is subnormal; therefore, the "control" arterial pressure at normal body temperature is low. As the temperature goes down, the mean arterial pressure is maintained, or decreased slightly, while the vascular system takes up a considerable volume of blood from the extracorporeal circuit to maintain the same venous pressure (Lindberg, 1959; Pierucci, et al., 1960). Calculated total peripheral resistance scarcely changes between 38°C. and 10°C., regardless of the flow rate used (Oz, et al., 1960; Lopez-Belio, et al., 1960). Considering that across this temperature range, the blood viscosity increases by about 60 per cent, it appears that blood stream cooling at constant flow rate entails a marked vasodilation. Oz, et al. (1960) estimated that 85 per cent of the control blood volume must be added in order to maintain at 10°C. the high perfusion rate selected at 38°C. This increase in blood volume is not accompanied by an increase in hematocrit (Pierucci, et al., 1960) and is partly reversible during rewarming.

The practical significance of these results is not yet clear. Some reservation is indicated due to the fact that the data have been obtained in the dog, which has a high capacity for blood pooling in many abnormal circumstances. Also these results still have not been verified in man. The maintenance of high extracorporeal flow rates in the presence of markedly decreased tissue metabolism also entails some biochemical changes in the blood which could partly account for the observed vasomotor response. Finally high perfusion rates and pressures at low temperatures represent a considerable departure from the usual hypothermic conditions, characterized by low cardiac output and hypotension (Brendel, et al., 1958). Below 22°C., high extracorporeal flow rates may precipitate heart failure, because the ability of the heart to eject the excessive coronary and thebesian flow is limited and severe dilation may result (Gollan, 1959a). Berne (1954) demonstrated that cold induces a decrease in coronary resistance either by a direct effect on the coronary vessels or possibly by retarding the rate of destruction of a vasodilator substance. Whether or not other vascular beds behave in the same manner is still unknown. Reliable measurements of the flow-pressure relationship during artificial perfusion (Chapter XIII) and detailed studies of the distribution of blood flow among different vascular beds (Chapter XIII) at different temperatures are still to be reported.

Summarizing:

During hypothermia the heart rate decreases, myocardial contraction and relaxation periods are prolonged, arterial pressure is markedly lowered, while venous pressure rises slightly. Nevertheless, myocardial function is adequate for the reduced work demands. In extreme hypothermia the heart stops beating but can still be damaged by anoxia if the circulation is arrested for more than 60 to 90 minutes. Cooling causes an increase in blood viscosity and a dilation of the peripheral as well as of the coronary vessels.

XX. Assisted Circulation

The availability of blood pumps and of artificial gas exchange devices has prompted their use not only for fully replacing the function of the heart and lungs, but also for supplementing that function in case of failure of these organs. Circulatory assistance by a pump-oxygenator was first considered as an aid to surgery in order to support patients who otherwise would not have been able to withstand the operation (Dogliotti and Constantini, 1951; Aird, et al., 1954). It was also utilized in nonsurgical cases for the purpose of pure respiratory (Helmsworth, et al., 1952b) or circulatory assistance (Newman, et al., 1955). Published reports on applications in man of assisted circulation techniques are still scanty (Stuckey, et al., 1957; Harken, 1958; Dickson, et al., 1959c; Peirce, et al., 1961). The limited success obtained, while encouraging further clinical trials, has indicated the necessity of documenting the actual degree of assistance provided by these mechanical systems. This can hardly be done as long as so little is known about the reaction of the normal organism to a parallel circulation supplementing that carried by the heart. When gas exchange and blood pumping occur simultaneously in the natural organs and in artificial devices, the hemodynamic and metabolic conditions are far more complex than those during complete substitution of the heart and lungs. In fact, the information available is so scarce that many workers still consider hazardous the intermediate period of *partial* heart–lung bypass which immediately precedes and follows *total* heart–lung bypass. Rather than attempting to manage the state of competition between the heart and the pump-oxygenator, they prefer to make the partial bypass period as short as possible, and face the relatively well understood problems of total body perfusion or normal circulatory conditions, despite the advantages which a gradual weaning of cardio-respiratory assistance would sometimes offer.

Theoretically at least, mechanical assistance to the failing heart can be envisioned as being carried on for far longer periods of extracorporeal circulation than is presently the case in open–heart surgery. Thus the problems of blood denaturation in artificial circuits, solved to a degree sufficient for surgical bypass procedures, again come into the foreground. All partial extracorporeal circulation procedures are definitely limited in scope by the requirements of vessel isolation and the hazards of blood handling. Since circulatory assistance can be applied for short periods only, its use is limited to pathological states which are potentially reversible. Generally, it should be reserved for cases in which all avenues of conservative treatment have been exhausted. It is not uncommon to encounter clinical situations in which a primary hemodynamic defect leads to metabolic disturbances which in turn affect detrimentally the function of the circulatory system. When such a vicious cycle becomes established, it is often impossible to break it by drugs or other conventional means. Mechanical assistance to the circulation can then be advised as a powerful measure for tiding the patient over a transient period of cardio-respiratory failure in the hope that recovery will allow termination of the procedure.

Mechanical pumping and/or extracorporeal gas exchange provide the support needed while the underlying process responds to conventional treatment, or until the affected function recovers spontaneously.

According to the nature of the disease encountered, the main clinical signs can be hemodynamic, respiratory, or both simultaneously. It is, therefore, convenient to classify the various modes of assisted circulation as intended primarily for circulatory support (veno-arterial pumping, selective left or right ventricular bypass, synchronized ventricular assistance), for metabolic support (veno-venous oxygenation, arterio-venous oxygenation, extracorporeal dialysis) or for both simultaneously (partial heart–lung bypass).

CIRCULATORY SUPPORT

The following methods have been designed to support primarily the flow and pressures in the circulatory system. They do not substantially aid the metabolism of the organism.

1. Veno-arterial pumping: Venesection and intra-arterial transfusion are therapeutic adjuncts to the treatment of heart failure, but neither of these can be employed over any length of time because of the marked alterations in blood volume they entail. It thus seemed reasonable to associate the two procedures in order to combine their advantages and to eliminate their main drawback (Connolly, et al., 1958a). A simple vein-to-artery shunt provided with a mechanical pump drains unoxygenated blood from the venous system and injects it under pressure into the arterial tree (*see* fig 100, C). Results have been indeed favorable in acute right heart failure caused by pulmonary artery obstruction, partly because some of the venous blood is shunted around the stenosis thus relieving the dilated right ventricle, partly because aortic root pressure is raised, affording increased coronary blood flow and more forceful cardiac contractions. Further studies by the same group (Connolly, et al., 1960; Storli, et al., 1960) substantiated the point that veno-arterial pumping can restore a normal coronary perfusion following acute constriction of the pulmonary artery or of the aorta below the left subclavian artery. Reed (1961) used veno-arterial pumping to support the circulation during the period of acute right heart failure following pulmonary embolism.

Dickson, et al., (1959b) developed a very commendable system for veno-arterial pumping. Their circuit (*see* fig. 102) is completely closed thus decreasing the risk of air embolism and contamination, and also preventing marked changes in the patient's blood volume by exsanguination into the extracorporeal circuit. Dickson, et al., (1959a; 1960) reported that in normal animals cardiac output is reduced by the volume pumped into the extracorporeal circuit. Total body perfusion thus remains unchanged. The diastolic and mean aortic pressures are slightly elevated while pulse pressure decreases owing to the diminished cardiac output. The brain and heart are supplied with fully oxygenated blood from the left ventricle, while the liver and kidneys receive some venous blood from the extracorporeal circuit without apparent impairment of function. According to Hamer, et al. (1959), the oxygen saturation of the venous blood in the shunt line does not decrease until the extracorporeal flow rate exceeds 30 ml./Kg./mn. It still averages 62 per cent when the flow in the shunt line is of the order of 60 ml./Kg./min. The average CO_2 tension and buffer basis remain within normal limits. Such results are quite surprising since they can hardly be explained without postulating a relative increase in pulmonary

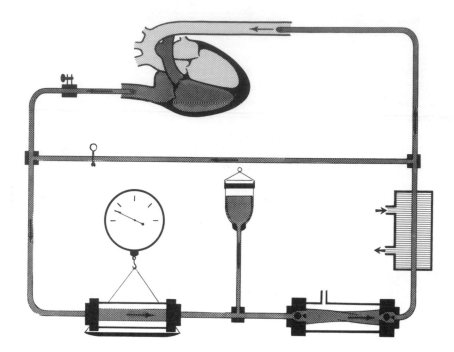

Fig. 102. Apparatus for veno-arterial pumping according to Dickson, et al. (1959). Blood from the superior vena cava drains into a thin walled collecting chamber enclosed in a transparent case which is suspended from scales. A ventricle pump of the Hufnagel type (see fig. 52, C) infuses the blood into a femoral artery after passage through a heat exchanger (right). The plastic bag in the center and the shunt between the venous and arterial lines serve to prime the circuit and to eliminate air bubbles.

blood flow, or a decrease in the oxygen requirement of the organism. At variance with Hamer's data, Rutherford and Swan (1960) and Ashbaugh, et al. (1961) found it necessary to infuse sodium bicarbonate into dogs submitted to veno-arterial pumping in order to prevent the appearance of metabolic acidosis. Veno-arterial pumping does not cause major damage to the formed elements of the blood or to the coagulation mechanism. It has been tolerated for as long as 52 hours in the dog and for 26 hours in man (Hamer, et al., 1959).

There has been much discussion as to the circulatory assistance actually provided by veno-arterial pumping (Wyman, et al., 1959). Apparently using the same technique as Connolly, et al. (1958a), Kuhn, et al. (1959, 1960) were unable to produce any rise in proximal aortic pressure and hence in coronary blood flow in normal animals and in others with coronary embolism. However, an increase in proximal aortic pressure could be obtained by compartmentalizing the circulation by means of balloon obstruction of the lower abdominal aorta. The pressure was maintained when venous blood from the shunt line was then used to perfuse the arterial tree below the level of obstruction. These results point out the necessity for increasing the resistance to ventricular ejection in order to elevate aortic arch pressures and coronary flows in the presence of an unchanged body blood volume. The authors do not say whether the same result could be obtained by hypervolemic perfusion so as to make the remaining cardiac output, for a given extracorporeal flow, larger than it would be under normovolemic conditions. Salisbury, et al. (1960a, b) evaluated the effects of veno-arterial pumping after inducing acute right-sided or left-sided cardiac failure in dogs. They found that the abnormal hemodynamic pattern of right heart failure was restored to normal by veno-arterial pumping. In the case of left heart failure, systemic arterial pressure was increased and the left ventricle contracted more forcefully. However, left atrial pressure increased as did left ventricular diastolic pressure so that finally the signs of failure became more, rather than less, apparent. To explain these unexpected results, the authors suggested various mechanisms: increase of regurgitant flow across the aortic valve; reflex systemic vasodilation caused by left ventricular distension; and increase in stiffness of the cardiac muscle engorgement of the coronary circulation. Salisbury's conclusions were supported by the experience of Patt, et al. (1960): in dogs with fresh or recent coronary occlusion, veno-arterial pumping promptly induced a state of irreversible shock.

At present there is general agreement as to the usefulness of veno-arterial pumping in right heart failure but considerable controversy as to its effects in left heart failure. One possible source of confusion resides in the varying ratios of extracorporeal shunt flow to the remaining cardiac output. The higher the flow in the shunt, the more depressed is the cardiac output as well as the distribution of oxygen to the tissues, regardless of the high "total perfusion flow" achieved. The fact, that in Connolly's and Kuhn's experiments veno-arterial pumping appeared beneficial when the aorta was partially or totally occluded, also suggests that the heart and the brain must in all cases be provided with arterial blood.

Clinically, veno-arterial pumping was used by Harken (1958), Dickson, et al. (1959c) and Damman (1960) in a few isolated cases. Pulmonary edema could be cleared within a matter of minutes. No obvious improvement in peripheral edema was observed. The best results were obtained in assisted perfusion in preparation for or concommitant with cardiac surgery. Other cases did not clearly benefit from the procedure. The explanation may be that in the case of long-term assistance the remarkable simplicity of veno-arterial pumping does not compensate for its inherent metabolic limitations. Ashton and Rains (1960) employed veno-arterial pumping in an attempt to maintain circulation through the smaller distal vessels of an ischemic limb while the main artery was occluded during the insertion of a vascular graft.

2. Right or left ventricular partial by-pass: Selective bypass of one ventricle by a mechanical pump is more a procedure of substitution than simply one of assistance. By this means blood is diverted around a failing ventricle or a stenotic outflow tract with minimal disturbance of normal blood pathways. Pulmonary blood flow and systematic perfusion flow are thus returned to their control level. Unilateral ventricular bypass is the procedure that provides the least questionable help to the failing heart since it relieves distended cavities by extracorporeal drainage and fulfills the mechanical function which the bypassed ventricle is unable to perform without producing any metabolic deviation of its own.

There are few experimental studies devoted to unilateral ventricular bypass which are focused on this aspect of circulatory assistance. Partial *right* heart bypass (*see* fig 10) should be of help in patients with pure right ventricular failure, as for instance, in case of acute pulmonary embolism. The effects of partial *left* heart bypass (*see* fig. 11) have been compared by Ballsbury, et al. (1960), to those of veno-arterial pumping in different forms of experimentally induced cardiac failure. The former offered all the advantages of veno-arterial pumping, namely increase in aortic pressure and in coronary flow together with obvious relief of elevated left atrial and left ventricular diastolic pressures. The quick disappearance of left heart overdistension brought about by left atrial drainage into the extracorporeal circuit, followed by infusion of the arterialized blood into some part of arterial tree makes this the procedure of choice in a few selected cases (Clauss, et al., 1959; Edmunds, et al., 1961; Muto, et al., 1961). However, the applicability of partial left heart bypass is generally limited by the necessity of opening the chest for purposes of cannulation. Its clinical usefulness will therefore be restricted to preoperative support of surgical patients. It may also be useful in the few medical cases in which a diagnosis can be made with certainty and where considerations of expected benefit due to temporary restoration of normal perfusion conditions outweigh the risks of general anesthesia and preparative surgery.

3. Synchronized ventricular assistance: Providing assistance to the arterial circulation by means of a pump, the action of which is synchronized with the cardiac cycle, was devised and proposed by Harken (1958). The pump is a single-ended diverticulum connected to the arterial tree. Blood is aspirated into this ectopic artificial "ventricle" as the heart goes into systole, and is returned with a pulsatile pattern during diastole, while the aortic valves are closed. The purpose is to permit the heart to eject against less resistance by having the artificial ventricle suck in blood during systole, and to maintain a normal perfusion of the tissues by returning the blood to the arterial tree in the intervals between cardiac contractions. An ingenious countercycling device, triggered by the patient's electrocardiogram was devised for proper timing of the alternating aspiration and ejection of the artificial ventricle. The pump used (the "arterial counterpulsator") (*see* fig. 52 F) can put out a stroke volume of up to 75 ml. at rates synchronized to any landmark of the electrocardiogram. The pulse pressure pattern in the aorta can be altered in almost any conceivable way, providing every variation from true assistance to the left ventricle to marked competition with its function. This procedure is still in its infancy, and only a few reports of its actual use are available (Clauss, et al., 1961; Watkins and Duchesne, 1961; Willman, et al., 1961).

Boucek and Murphy (1960) recently designed a programming system which directs a pump to inject drugs selectively into the coronary arteries during diastole. Murphy (1961) has also described a cardiac programmer to trigger an arterial pump. Much more sophistication in the monitoring of vascular pressures and a better understanding of their variations in disease are still needed before the capacities of these machines can be fully exploited.

Summarizing:

There are three methods primarily aimed at maintaining flow and pressures in the vascular system. Veno-arterial pumping simply drains blood from the venous system and transfers it under pressure into the arterial tree. The arterialized blood ejected from the left ventricle supplies the heart and brain, while venous blood from the extracorporeal shunt perfuses the lower half of the body. This procedure can relieve right sided heart failure but its action on left heart failure is questionable. Partial bypass of the right or left ventricle can be used to shunt blood around a failing ventricle or a stenotic outflow tract. Despite the necessity of opening the chest, such unilateral ventricular bypass may be valuable in selected cases. Synchronized ventricular assistance is provided by an "artificial ventricle" or pump connected to a major artery. During systole, blood is drawn from the artery into the pump, thereby lowering the resistance to cardiac ejection. During diastole the blood is reinfused into the arterial tree.

METABOLIC SUPPORT

In contrast to the methods aimed primarily at hemodynamic support of the organism, the following three techniques mainly support the metabolism.

1. Veno-venous oxygenation: Veno-venous pumping (*see* fig. 100 A) has been used extensively for blood stream cooling (*see* chap. XIX). Since blood is drained from and infused into the same segment of the vascular system, the sites of drainage and of infusion must be as widely separated as possible. Hemodynamically speaking, the procedure should have no effect on pressures or flows as long as it does not affect the body blood volume. However, hypotension occurs fairly often in long term veno-venous pumping, possibly because of increased sensitivity of the cardiac output to small variations in systemic blood volume in artificially perfused organisms. In the field of circulatory assistance, veno-venous pumping is useful only if it includes an artificial gas exchange device in the shunt line. Veno-venous pumping then supplements the pulmonary oxygen uptake and carbon dioxide elimination by delivering to the right heart blood which has already been partially oxygenated. It is, therefore, a "complementary oxygenation" procedure (Battezatti, et al., 1953) and can be used as an adjuvant in the treatment of patients suffering from severe hypoxemia.

Inferior to superior vena caval pumping has been studied experimentally by Krasna, et al. (1960). With the assistance of complementary oxygenation the animals showed marked improvement in their venous and arterial saturations which had previously been depressed by low oxygen mixture breathing. Clinically, Helmsworth, et al. (1952b) reported striking relief of cyanosis, dyspnea and orthopnea during such a procedure in a patient with marked impairment of respiratory function. Arterial oxygen saturation and pH rose, while plasma CO_2 tension again approached normal. Unfortunately, the improvement did not persist once the procedure was terminated. Rygg (1958) used venovenous oxygenation for as long as 20 hours with essentially the same results. At the present time, the future of complementary oxygenation utilizing veno-venous pump appears limited to patients with stable circulatory systems, and in whom the temporary relief of respiratory difficulties may offer a chance of survival during a period in which recovery of pulmonary function is brought about by other means.

2. Arterio-venous oxygenation: an arterio-venous shunt, with or without a pump to serve as a metering device, can be employed for blood stream cooling (*see* fig. 100 D). For purposes of circulatory assistance, this is a burden. However, metabolic support is provided if one resorts to the drastic solution proposed by Zeller (1908), and Potts, et al. (1951) for extracorporeal gas exchange: the aorta was connected to an external gas exchange device (homologous lung) and blood having been oxygenated outside the body was returned to the caval veins. Dogs could be kept alive for three hours without the use of their own lungs by this procedure of functional pulmonary bypass.

Our laboratory experience with arterio-venous oxygenation suggests that the cardiac output is markedly enhanced by the shunting procedure. Despite the low arterial oxygen tension prevailing when the animal rebreathes from the closed bag, no serious acidosis develops, provided the perfusion flow is sufficiently high and the extracorporeal oxygen uptake equals the control pulmonary oxygen uptake. Survival is easily obtained after as long as six hours of perfusion. No blood pump is required to regulate the flow if the extracorporeal circuit is not open to atmospheric pressure. Using a membrane lung with a fixed blood content and a proper resistance to the shunt flow, the hemodynamics of the systemic circulation is not too much disturbed and the blood trauma is minimal. One can, therefore, envision prolonged arteriovenous oxygenation without a blood pump for clinical situations which are characterized by inadequate pulmonary gas exchange in presence of a relatively stable circulation.

3. Extracorporeal dialysis of toxic substances (the "artificial kidney") is not within the scope of this book. However veno-venous or arterio-venous pumping can be associated, for the purpose of circulatory assistance, with dialyzing, ion exchange or ultrafiltration devices. For instance, Moore, et al. (1961) described a treatment of hyperkalemia utilizing extracorporeal circulation of blood through exchange resin columns, and Nakamoto (1961) reported on the use of the artificial kidney for the removal of edema fluid in cardiac patients by ultrafiltration. It should also be mentioned that for purposes of circulatory assistance, external dialysis can be combined with any pumping device which provides hemodynamic support. The artificial heart-lung-kidney suggested by Salisbury (1954) was actually used by Hyman (1959b) to prevent a drop in pH or a rise in blood lactic acid during total body perfusion. The insertion of an artificial kidney into the pump-oxygenator circuit provides additional metabolic safeguard in long-term perfusions. It also offers tantalizing opportunities for maintaining the plasma equilibrium of a number of ions and small molecules which otherwise cannot be monitored directly. Up to now, one of the main deterrents to the combination of external dialysis with circulatory assistance techniques has been added complexity due to the artificial kidney circuit. The increasingly widespread use of membrane lungs (*see* chap. VII) foreshadows development of devices featuring membranes for gas exchange combined with membranes for solutes exchange.

Summarizing:

Veno-venous pumping through an artificial gas exchange device allows a "complementary oxygenation" for hypoxemic patients. Arterio-venous oxygenation may be thought of when the circulation is stable enough to support the hemodynamic consequences of an arterio-venous shunt. Extracorporeal dialysis offers remarkable possibilities for maintaining a biochemically stable environment during perfusion procedures.

CIRCULATORY AND METABOLIC SUPPORT BY PARTIAL HEART–LUNG BYPASS

Experience shows that techniques aimed either at hemodynamic or metabolic assistance alone are often incapable of relieving the complex disturbances characteristic of heart and circulatory failure for any prolonged period. The reason for this is that one must be able to supplement, to varying degrees, the respiratory as well as the circulatory function of the patient. Often the degree of support required changes independently for each function. There-

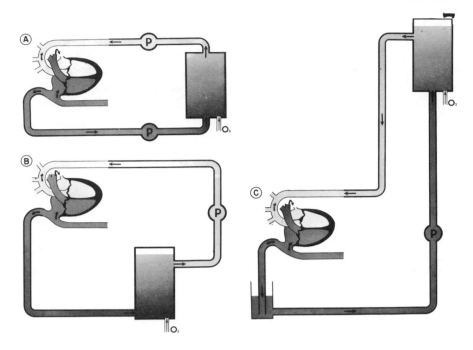

Fig. 103. Circuits used for partial heart–lung bypass.

A. Completely closed system with pump drainage and pump infusion.
B. Gravity venous drainage into an artificial lung open to atmospheric pressure followed by pump infusion into the arterial system.
C. Gravity venous drainage and gravity arterial infusion. The oxygenator is suspended at a height above heart level sufficient to overcome arterial pressure. The pump serves only to raise the blood from the level of the collecting reservoir to the level of the oxygenator.

fore, only a circuit which offers extracorporeal gas exchange together with hemodynamic support can be considered truly satisfactory. Ideally, the most beneficial conditions for circulatory assistance are provided by *partial* heart–lung bypass (*see* fig. 3) or "parallel blood circulation" as it was originally called by Brukhonenko in 1929. It offers the same hemodynamic support, in terms of flows and pressures, as does veno-arterial pumping, with the added advantage that the extracorporeal flow rate can be increased to a high level without endangering oxygenation of the tissues. There is no need to keep the body blood volume constant but it can be increased or decreased if an advantage is to be expected from such alteration. When the particular disturbances is primarily metabolic, the blood in the extracorporeal circuit can be hyperventilated or equilibrated with any appropriate gas mixture. In case of an acute emergency, such as ventricular fibrillation or cardiac arrest in the course of the perfusion, the extracorporeal flow rate can be increased so as to support the organism fully and give time for reestablishing cardiac action (Kuhn, et al., 1960a, b).

Consideration of the extracorporeal circuit arrangement makes it easy to understand how partial heart–lung bypass can fulfill the requirements of simultaneous hemodynamic and metabolic assistance to the perfused organism.

There is continuous drainage of a fraction of the central venous blood into an artificial gas exchange device, followed by reinfusion of the arterialized blood into the aorta or one of its branches. Venous drainage is facilitated by any kind of suction device: pump (*see* fig. 103, A), vacuum-reservoir or gravity (*see* fig. 103, B). Extracorporeal flows of the order of 50 per cent of the control cardiac output can easily be attained with a single catheter advanced into the chest through a peripheral vein. The problem of venous collapse is much less critical than is the case in total heart–lung bypass, as one does not attempt to remove all of the blood flowing in the venous system. Arterial infusion can be carried out by a pump or even by simple gravity (*see* fig. 103, C) provided the oxygenator is suspended at the height above the patient's level needed to overcome mean arterial pressure and the resistance of the arterial cannula (Galletti, et al., 1960).

The femoral artery is the most adequate portal of entry for blood from the extracorporeal circuit, since emboli, which might occasionally be present, are prevented from reaching the heart and brain directly. Instead, blood from the extracorporeal circuit is filtered in the capillary bed of the lower half of the body. The problems of selecting the site of venous drainage also deserves special scrutiny. When blood is drained from the inferior vena cava and reinfused into the femoral artery, the perfusion involves predominantly the lower part of the body. Since the pulmonary venous return ejected by the left ventricle perfuses mainly the upper part of the body where the oxygen requirements are relatively high, oxygen saturation in superior caval blood tends to fall to rather low levels. Meanwhile, the arterialized blood from the artificial lung perfuses the lower part of the body where oxygen extraction is not as great as in the upper part. Consequently within a few hours, wide differences in blood oxygen and carbon dioxide content develop between the upper part and the lower part of the body, and the metabolic assistance afforded by the extracorporeal circuit becomes less and less effective. To prevent this, venous drainage for partial heart–lung bypass must be from the superior vena cava or one of its tributaries. For practical purposes, the external jugular vein is satisfactory.

Summarizing:

Partial heart–lung bypass provides the most beneficial assistance to the circulation by combining hemodynamic and metabolic supports. It involves continuous drainage of part of systemic venous return into an artificial gas exchange device, followed by reinfusion of the arterialized blood into a large artery. Various circuits are available for this purpose.

EFFECTS OF PARTIAL HEART–LUNG BYPASS ON THE CIRCULATION

The effects of partial heart–lung bypass on vascular pressures and flows result from a complex inter-relationship among extracorporeal flow rate, cardiac output and body blood volume. The main features of this adaptation have been investigated under a variety of experimental conditions (Galletti and Salisbury, 1959; Salisbury, et al., 1959a, b; Galletti and Brecher, 1960; Hopf and Galletti, 1961; Galletti, 1961), and can be summarized as follows:

(*1*) When body blood volume is held strictly constant, cardiac output varies inversely with extracorporeal flow rate so that the total amount of arterial blood distributed to the circulation remains nearly the same over a wide range of extracorporeal flow rates.

(*2*) When no special precaution is taken to keep the body blood volume constant, there is a tendency for blood to shift from the organism into the external circuit as the extracorporeal flow rate is increased, and to come back into the vascular system as the rate of artificial perfusion is diminished.

(*3*) The perfused organism is extremely sensitive to variations in blood volume. It reacts markedly to small transfusions or withdrawal of small amounts of blood, which would barely affect the normal circulatory system. At constant extracorporeal flow rates, shift of blood into the organism causes an increase in cardiac output; blood shift into the external circuit results in a decrease in cardiac output.

(*4*) Changes in arterial pressure closely reflect changes in total perfusion flow (cardiac output plus extracorporeal flow). When extracorporeal flow is modified without changes in the body blood volume, and thus without change in the total perfusion flow, mean aortic pressure remains constant, regardless of the relative sizes of the left ventricular and pump-oxygenator contributions. The pulse pressure, however, decreases with decreased cardiac output. The mean central venous pressure is slightly decreased by increases in extracorporeal flow. Right ventricular systolic pressure and pulmonary arterial pressure are consistently and progressively diminished with increments of size in extracorporeal flow which correspond to decrements in pulmonary blood flow. Left atrial pressure is always significantly decreased when the bypass circuit carries more than 25 per cent of the total perfusion flow.

(*5*) There is no evidence of systemic vasomotion when the total perfusion flow rate is maintained constant, although the relative contributions of the left ventricle and of the heart–lung machine are varied. The meaning of the concept of "peripheral resistance" under conditions of partial heart–lung bypass is probably limited, because ejection of blood under pressure occurs from two sites simultaneously and the pattern of flow in the aorta and main arteries is largely unknown. Calculated pulmonary resistance increases during partial heart–lung bypass as would be expected with reduction in pulmonary blood flow in the absence of vasomotion.

(*6*) The pattern of capillary circulation does not appear to change from the normal in organs which have been scrutinized. Sludging of red cells and blockage of capillary networks, as observed in various pathologic conditions, can sometimes be reversed by partial heart–lung bypass, owing probably to the higher head of pressure provided at the arterial level (Bor, et al., 1961).

(*7*) Heart rate usually slows down as more and more blood is carried by the extracorporeal circuit. This relative bradycardia is associated with a fall in central venous pressure and in right ventricular pressure and may be interpreted as an extended "Bainbridge effect." Conversely, the heart rate usually accelerates when pulmonary blood flow, and as a result, cardiac output is permitted to increase as extracorporeal flow rate decreases. Since there is no concomitant change in arterial pressure, the changes in heart rate cannot be ascribed to a carotid sinus mechanism. Changes in heart rate are not consistently observed in open-chest animals, nor in those which are deeply anesthetized.

(*8*) When partial heart–lung bypass brings about a reduction in cardiac output out of proportion to the decrease in heart rate, the left ventricular pressure pulse tracing often shows mechanical alternance. Every other left ventricular systole shows no ejection phase. Aortic pressure remains constant during the ineffective systole and consequently the aortic pulse rate is reduced to one half. There is no change in the electrocardiographic sequence nor in the right ventricular pressure pattern. Left ventricular mechanical alternation is noted when the stroke volume of the right ventricle is insufficient to fill the left ventricle after passage of the blood through the pulmonary vascular bed. Two contractions of the right ventricle are needed to pump enough blood into the left heart cavities to bring about left ventricle ejection. This situation is easily recognized with auscultation, or by comparing the peripheral pulse rate to the electrocardiographic rate. It is not of especially ominous significance, although it does warn that total perfusion flow may be too low.

(*9*) Partial heart–lung bypass is associated with no electrocardiographic alterations except with bradycardia. Though not bearing a direct relationship to the perfusion, modifications caused by myocardial hypoxia, hyperkalemia, right ventricular overload, marked temperature variations or mechanical stimulation by intracardiac catheters are occasionally observed.

(*10*) The myocardial oxygen consumption is not consistently affected by the redistribution of total systemic flow between the left ventricle and the extracorporeal circuit. There is usually no decrease in oxygen consumption of the myocardium, as measured by coronary sinus outflow studies, as long as the left ventricle carries more than half of its control output. When extracorporeal flow represents more than 50 per cent of the total perfusion flow, myocardial oxygen consumption will decrease in some cases. In others, it remains fairly constant as long as there is any left ventricular output at all. Variations in coronary blood flow and coronary venous oxygen content are also somewhat unpredictable. The inconsistencies of these results are probably related to variability of the effect of partial heart–lung bypass upon the size of the heart in open-chest animals.

(*11*) There is no general agreement over the effects of partial heart–lung bypass upon the work of the heart. Since the energy expenditure of the empty, beating, non-ejecting heart is undoubtedly decreased as compared to that of the normal heart (*see* fig. 99), one would expect a diminished work load on the myocardium associated with the decrease in cardiac output. Generally speaking, however, cardiac work does not decrease unless heart rate, mean aortic pressure (and, consequently, left ventricular pressure) and heart size are decreased. The effect of partial bypass on each of these parameters depends upon the experimental conditions chosen. The decrease in cardiac output and in right ventricular pressures, which always accompany partial heart–lung bypass, have no obvious effect upon the energy expenditure of the myocardium (Salisbury, et al., 1959a, b; 1960; Gerfin, et al., 1960). It is probably pointless at the present time to elaborate further upon the effects of partial heart–lung bypass upon cardiac "work" or "efficiency." However, a note of caution should be added concerning the intemperate use of statistical methods in this field and the multiplication of "indices" which carry no more meaning, and considerably less statistical significance, than do the directly measured parameters. It must also be appreciated that cardiac work may be decreased under certain experimental conditions, but that the functional state of the myocardium will not be "improved" by this, unless metabolic support of the heart is relatively increased at the same time (Katz, et al., 1955; Salisbury, et al., 1959a).

Summarizing

The effects of partial heart–lung bypass on vascular pressures and flow result from a complex relationship among extracorporeal flow rate, cardiac output and body blood volume. The sum of cardiac output and extracorporeal flow rate remains unchanged when the body blood volume is kept constant. If the body blood volume varies, blood shifts between the organism and the extracorporeal circuit lead to variable hemodynamic conditions. Mean arterial pressure does not change as long as the organism receives from the heart and the pump-oxygenator as much blood as under control conditions. Information available on cardiovascular reflexes, myocardial oxygen consumption and work load is insufficient and partly conflicting.

EFFECTS OF PARTIAL HEART–LUNG BYPASS ON ORGANS

Partial heart–lung bypass involves not only the bodily functions with which it is immediately concerned, namely circulation and gas exchange, but it also affects all other processes which may be modified by a redistribution of blood flow, such as the cerebral, renal and thermoregulatory functions. Consequently, before being able to recommend partial heart–lung bypass as a therapeutic procedure, its side effects must be thoroughly investigated in the normal organism. The results of such studies are reported here.

1. Lungs: When pulmonary blood flow is reduced, spontaneously breathing dogs tend to ventilate less. Tidal volume is much more affected than is respiratory frequency (Hopf, et al., 1961). Depression of ventilation is progressively more marked as extracorporeal flow increases and is particularly obvious when considered in terms of *alveolar* ventilation rather than of *total* ventilation. Providing no changes in body blood volume occur during the perfusion procedure, oxygen uptake in the lungs also decreases in a stepwise fashion as the extracorporeal flow rate increases. The overall oxygen uptake of the organism (natural plus artificial lung) remains nearly constant.

Despite the decrease in pulmonary ventilation as expressed in absolute terms, a state of relative hyperventilation prevails in the lungs because ventilation does not decrease so much as does pulmonary blood flow. This relative hyperventilation expresses itself in an increased alveolar ventilation/pulmonary perfusion ratio ($\dot{V}_A/Q$) and also in the pulmonary gas exchange ratio (R_E). Consequently, blood passing through the lungs becomes more "arterialized" and higher oxygen tensions and lower carbon dioxide tensions are found than normally would be expected. Oxygen tensions have not actually been measured, but CO_2 tensions in alveolar gas and in pulmonary venous blood are reported to fall with increases in extracorporeal flow rates (Haab, et al., 1960). At pulmonary blood flows below 30 per cent of the control value, increasingly larger alveolar-arterial CO_2 tension differences develop, indicating that the underperfused lung has lost some of its efficiency as a carbon dioxide exchanger. Uneven distribution of the blood as related to ventilation in the different regions of the lung may possibly account for the phenomenon. The effect of partial heart–lung bypass on alveolar diffusion and on respiratory mechanics has not as yet been investigated.

In a smooth partial bypass procedure characterized by maintenance of adequate tissue perfusion, the pH and CO_2 content of arterial blood barely change, regardless of the relative contributions of the left ventricle and pump-oxygenator. Thus, the procedure should have no specific metabolic consequences. During long-term perfusions, in which the level of anesthesia is not always maintained as constant as would be desirable, hypoventilation or hyperventilation may be encountered, and can be managed by suitable alteration of blood and gas flow through the artificial lung.

2. Brain: *A priori* any marked change in cerebral function during *partial* heart–lung bypass would not be expected because the brain is usually perfused with blood from the left ventricle. Hence, the risk of gas bubbles or other types of embolism is less pronounced than during *total* heart–lung bypass. Cerebral blood flow is probably well maintained in the presence of normal aortic and low venous pressures. No direct measurements of cerebral blood flow have yet been reported, nor has brain tissue oxygen tension been systematically investigated. The electroencephalographic pattern during partial heart–lung bypass was studied in detail by Hopf, et al. (1961). The pattern characteristic of light anesthesia is a constant finding. The frequency and, to a lesser extent, the voltage are slightly decreased during perfusion. They return to control values within a few hours after the procedure. The possible meaning of these changes is not clear. Careful observation of the tracings during and in the days following partial perfusion has not demonstrated any signs of cerebral hypoxia.

3. Kidney and Body Fluids: Experimental perfusion studies in our laboratory have shown that when there is no evidence of transfusion reaction and mean aortic pressure is adequately maintained, urine output remains in the range observed under anesthesia in the hours preceding bypass. Urine specific gravity is not significantly altered. Injection of hypertonic glucose is followed by a prompt diuresis. Sodium excretion in response to a saline load is also within normal limits (Veith and Thrower, 1959; Thrower, et al., 1960). Hematocrit and plasma osmolarity are not significantly altered. Animals perfused for ten hours show a slight increase in weight. Extracellular fluid volume and total body water are consistently augmented immediately after perfusion and for a period of 12 hours thereafter. Then, a massive diuresis eliminates the water retained in the organism (Galletti, 1961). Interestingly enough, animals perfused by means of simple gravity do not exhibit as marked an increase in weight after perfusion as do animals perfused at the same flow rate by means of an occlusive roller pump (Galletti, et al., 1960). There is place for considerable speculation concerning the occurrence of water retention in perfused organisms. Impairment to lymph flow by forced immobilization of the organism or reduction in arteriolar pulse pressure, increased capillary pressure with nonpulsatile flow, increased capillary permeability as a consequence of trauma to the blood or to the vascular elements by the repeated stress imposed by the pump cycle, leakage of fluid as a consequence of peripheral pooling and stasis, are all mechanisms which might come into play.

4. Liver and gastro-intestinal tract: To the best of our knowledge, no data are available on any modification of the liver function during partial heart–lung bypass. Hypoglycemia after 10 to 15 hours of perfusion in the dog may reflect a disturbance of hepatic function. A rise in portal venous pressure at the onset of perfusion was reported by Dow, et al. (1959), and found to be associated with the anaphylactoid reaction of massive blood transfusion. Gastrointestinal bleeding occasionally occurs after perfusion, but its pathogenesis is not known.

5. Blood: The traumatic effect of long-term extracorporeal blood handling today represents the main hurdle to more widespread clinical application. Hemolysis during the procedure itself is not a problem and plasma hemoglobin levels do not exceed 100 to 200 mg. per cent after ten hours of perfusion (Rutherford and Swan, 1960; Brinsfield, et al., 1961). Plasma hemoglobin levels seem to reach constant values during long-lasting perfusions, possibly because the renal threshold is exceeded. Hematocrit and red cell counts remain nearly constant. However, a marked hemolytic reaction begins a few hours after extracorporeal circulation is discontinued, and the hematocrit often drops to 25 per cent within two to four days after perfusion. A bright yellow coloration of the plasma is observed after a week in animals which otherwise look healthy. Red cell survival studies are urgently needed to further investigate this aspect of the problem. After an initial drop, the white cell count usually increases during perfusion and continues to increase for several days thereafter. The platelet count usually falls to levels ranging between 50,000 and 100,000/cu. mm. after a few hours of extracorporeal circulation and then remains fairly stable, possibly as a result of the equilibrium between destruction and new formation. Platelet counts start to increase two to three days after perfusion unless a clotting process is at work somewhere in the organism. Comparison of bone marrow smears obtained before and after partial heart–lung bypass reveal an increased activity of the bone marrow starting a few hours after the beginning of perfusion. Stimulation by an unknown factor is also revealed by the appearance of immature white cells and nucleated red cells in the blood stream.

Summarizing:

With a reduction in pulmonary blood flow, spontaneously breathing dogs ventilate less. However, the decrease in ventilation is not so great as the decrease in blood flow, resulting in relative hyperventilation at low pulmonary blood flows. The brain is well maintained during long-term bypass and the electroencephalogram shows no significant alteration. Kidney function is apparently little affected, yet water retention is a common finding after perfusions of long duration. Hematologic studies reveal that with presently available pump-oxygenators, blood trauma is still too severe to be fully compensated for by the organism.

RECENT DEVELOPMENTS IN PARTIAL HEART–LUNG BYPASS

1. Survival studies: According to Gibbon (1959a, b), partial bypass of the heart and lungs can be tolerated by animals for periods of four to five hours with a low mortality rate. This is substantiated by Galletti and Salisbury (1958, 1959) who observed a 90 per cent survival rate in 30 dogs perfused for three to five hours using a foam oxygenator and a gravity arterial infusion technique. At variance with the above authors, Fisher and Smyth (1959) reported an immediate mortality of 85 per cent when about 25 per cent of the cardiac output was carried by a bubble or disc oxygenator for a period of six hours. Lately, consistent long-term survival has been reported in animals partially perfused for 10 to 12 hours at flows of the order of 40 per cent of the cardiac output (Galletti, et al., 1960; Rutherford and Swan, 1960). It made no difference which oxygenator type and which perfusion technique was used—disposable bubble oxygenator with gravity venous drainage and arterial infusion, disc oxygenator with pump drainage and infusion, membrane oxygenator with gravity venous drainage and arterial infusion by a pump. Detailed studies of blood and body fluid changes will be needed to ascertain the possible superiority of any one system over another.

Up to now, the main difficulties encountered have been associated with blood trauma, temperature control and anesthesia. Some animals exhibit a marked "transfusion reaction" when a large amount of blood exchange is carried out at the start of perfusion. In a few instances when intravascular hemolysis and a marked drop in platelet and white cell counts are noted, the chance for survival appears jeopardized. Considerable attention must be devoted to the temperature regulating system in the extracorporeal circuit since few factors are as detrimental as accidental overheating. Also possible related to blood trauma is the occasional occurrence of caval thrombosis as the direct cause of death two to five days after perfusion. It is not clear whether thrombosis is initiated by insufficient heparinization, a too early reversal of anticoagulation after perfusion, localized trauma of the vessel wall by the tip of the venous catheter or a general alteration of the vessel wall under abnormal flow and pressure conditions. Anesthesia is obviously one of the most difficult problems. In our experience it should be light enough so that spontaneous respiratory and circulatory control will be maintained and that awakening will be complete within two to four hours after perfusion. The depression of the central nervous system and the deterioration of circulatory homeostasis observed by some investigators may be due to the continuing action of anesthetic substances.

2. Control of perfusion: The circuit for partial heart–lung bypass should be as simple as possible and require a minimum of cutdown and vessel isolation. In our experience, all the information needed for control can be obtained from the extracorporeal circuit and the patient's airways. Arterial and venous pressure are monitored with sufficient accuracy from the infusion and drainage lines. The extracorporeal flow rate must be known from calibration of the pump or by direct measurements. Measurement of oxygen uptake in the lung during the period of bypass, as compared with control values, provides information as to the adequacy of overall tissue perfusion. Determination of venous oxygen saturation or tension, and monitoring of CO_2 tension in the end-expiratory air and in the gas equilibrated with blood in the artificial lung, provide the simplest approach to metabolic control. The electrocardiogram may reveal some abnormalities, while the electroencephalogram serves mainly to control the level of anesthesia.

3. Assistance by partial heart–lung bypass: Since the early reports by Dogliotti (1951, 1952, 1958) and Costantini, et al. (1953b), of clinical application of partial heart–lung bypass, experimental attempts have been carried out in Italy to resuscitate animals subjected to drowning, electric shock or carbon monoxide poisoning (Dei Poli, et al., 1953b, c, d). Gollan and Meneely (1953), and Kuhn, et al. (1960) showed that it was possible to keep animals alive with ventricular fibrillation. Newman, et al. (1955) and Stuckey, et al. (1958) reported the successful use of partial heart–lung bypass in patients suffering from pulmonary edema and acute myocardial infarction. Bor, et al. (1959), and Bor and Rieben (1961) experimented with dogs in which acute heart failure was induced. The symptoms of failure could be corrected by an appropriate selection of flow and pressure conditions. In dogs made hypotensive by spinal anesthesia, Weiss, et al. (1960b) reported beneficial effects proportional to the extracorporeal flow rate and the amount of blood simultaneously transfused. Thrower, et al. (1960) attempted partial heart–lung bypass in animals with chronic congestive failure. They were unable to reverse any aspect of the clinical picture, and the animals died shortly thereafter. Experimental shock has been a convenient means for testing the effect of assisted circulation. Endotoxin shock is usually selected, because decreased venous return and fall in cardiac output are the primary circulatory disturbances (Weil, et al., 1956). Bor, et al. (1961) noted clear reversal of the hemodynamic signs associated with endotoxin shock. Survival studies are in progress to elucidate the ultimate value of circulatory assistance under acute conditions such as these.

Summarizing:

Recent developments in partial heart–lung bypass include consistent survival of dogs after 10 to 12 hours of perfusion. The main problems are associated with blood trauma, temperature control and anesthesia. In long-term perfusion, the physiologic measurements which are important in the control of the procedure can be obtained from the extracorporeal circuit and the patient's airways. Hemodynamic signs of acutely induced circulatory failure in dogs can be temporarily reversed by partial heart–lung bypass.

Concluding Remarks

The course of progress in the development of extracorporeal circulation, which we have attempted to survey in these 20 chapters, has extended over the past 70 years. Patient research in physiology and cross-fertilization from neighboring disciplines have finally carried perfusion procedure from the experimental laboratory to the operating room. All along the road, the obstacles encountered can be summarized in one word: trauma. It was trauma to the blood which first precluded extracorporeal handling for any length of time. It was trauma to the brain and to the heart which made early clinical perfusions so hazardous. It is still blood, brain or heart damage, associated with more subtle disturbances of the homeostatic equilibrium of the organism, which presently limits safe application of perfusion techniques to a few hours.

With the aim of preventing trauma, investigators in the field of artificial circulation have often shared one common principle of design: that of closely imitating nature. A century of development in technologic physiology suggests that this ideal might be mistaken. Indeed pumps and oxygenators whose behavior most closely resembles the natural processes are not unquestionably the best, and actual perfusion of living beings reveals how disappointingly small are the differences among various types of heart–lung machines in terms of blood handling. Should the present state of affairs lead to the "heretical" conclusion that following nature is not always the best approach? Is it possible that the natural state of the organism merely represents one set of conditions which are admirably adapted to each other and that intrepid investigators in the course of time will find another set of conditions which is even better suited to the preservation of life? Are we approaching the Faustian era in which a combination of artificial machines will cooperate in maintaining man in his normal state? No one knows the answer to these questions, but contemplating them may lead to an upsurge of imaginative solutions.

Most observations gathered in the course of artificial perfusion procedures can be explained in terms of classic physiology, and most newly established facts require no other discussion than that based upon the development of accepted principles. Superstitions born of the awe of initially frightening procedures, such as the maintenance of circulation by mechanical pumps, the arrest of the heart, and the cessation of pulmonary gas exchange, have been dispelled one after another. The more *physiologic* the perfusion conditions, the *closer to normal* becomes the *reactivity of the organism*. "The perfused organism has lost its soul," the colorful image evoked by an early investigator in the field, is not true anymore. The large majority of clinical perfusions are now characterized by minimal deviation from normal physiologic conditions and by quick recovery. The progressive disappearance of the aura of "mystery" around extracorporeal circulation procedures and the considerate application of solid biophysical principles to the condition of the perfused organism have led to a more realistic appraisal of today's achievements and of tomorrow's hopes.

What will be the future of extracorporeal circulation techniques? In the field of cardiac surgery, a large scale comparison is under way between heart–lung bypass using the pump-oxygenator, and simple cardiac bypass using autogenous lung oxygenation. Clinical experience will tell whether low-flow hypothermic perfusion is definitely preferable to high-flow, normothermic perfusion. The trend is happily toward simplification of procedures. Yet, years of experience and follow-up study are needed before a clear answer can be obtained. In the field of medicine, regional perfusion for the treatment of localized cancer or infection has opened new therapeutic opportunities, but its actual contribution remains to be evaluated. Cardiopulmonary assistance by means of perfusion techniques is still in its infancy. Perfusion of organs or body parts severed from one organism for eventual transplantation into another organism is only now coming into consideration.

Regardless of the up and down swings of favor in evaluating clinical perfusions, one major fact is already firmly established: extracorporeal circulation, born in the hands of physiologists, nurtured and brought to maturity by surgeons, now returns to the research laboratory as a much improved tool. It can be applied over long periods without damaging the preparation. Many areas of investigation have been revived, and others have benefited from a completely new approach. Perhaps the most important contribution of perfusion techniques to physiological research resides in the fact that conditions of controlled flow can now be created. A preparation which features constant flow and variable pressures is more stable, and more easy to interpret, than one with constant pressures and variable flows. Controlled circulation can be surgically limited to one vascular bed, or carried simultaneously into two or more vascular beds. Thus, extracorporeal circulation techniques have made it possible to study at leisure the reflex interactions of artificially separated vascular beds and the reflex control of the heart isolated from the vascular system, upon the peripheral circulation. Quantification has become possible in the vastly unknown field of collateral circulation. Pulmonary physiology, limited for a long time to inquiry into the gas phase, can now be approached by varying at will circulatory conditions and the blood phase. Since powerful means of changing the organisms' equilibrium conditions have become available, the whole concept of homeostasis must undergo a thorough reappraisal. Hypothermia is being investigated to its extreme limits. Finally, immunologic and transplantation studies are offered a new avenue of approach. The historical development of extracorporeal circulation demonstrates that there is no barrier between basic and applied research: physiology and clinical medicine continue to complement each other.

Bibliography

The bibliography covers material which has been published up to April 30, 1961. It has been intentionally limited to publications dealing with physiologic and technical aspects of extracorporeal circulation. However, a fair amount of information is related in clinically oriented papers. For this reason, clinical publications are quoted as far as they contain pertinent material which cannot be found elsewhere.

For all contributions in English, French, German, Italian, Latin, Portuguese and Spanish, the titles are given in the original language. For the other papers, the title has been translated into English and the original language indicated by one of the following abbreviations: (*Bu*) Bulgarian; (*Chin*) Chinese; (*Cz*) Czech; (*Du*) Dutch; (*Fl*) Flemish; (*Hun*) Hungarian; (*Pol*) Polish; (*Rus*) Russian; and (*Se*) Serbian.

A

ABADZHIEV, P.: Current status of extracorporeal circulation in heart surgery with heart–lung apparatus. Khirurgiia (Sofiia) *11*, 601–613, 1958 (*Bu*).

ABBOTT, J. P., D. A. COOLEY, M. E. DE-BAKEY and J. E. RAGLAND: Storage of blood for open-heart operations. Surgery *44*, 698–705, 1958.

ABBOTT, J. P., J. B. RAGLAND, M. E. DE-BAKEY and D. A. COOLEY: Observations on blood drawn and stored for open-heart surgery. A study of 10 anticoagulant solutions. Amer. J. Clin. Path. *33*, 124–134, 1960.

ABEATICI, S., V. LAUGERI and T. DE NUNNO: Sulle possibilità di ossigenazione ematica attraverso membrane porose mediante soluzioni di perossido di idrogeno. Minerva chir. *13*, 860–868, 1958.

——, —— and ——: Etude expérimentale de l'oxygénation sanguine extra-corporelle par aérosol de peroxyde d'hydrogène (H₂O₂). Lyon Chir. *55*, 352–354, 1959a.

——, T. DE NUNNO and V. LAUGERI: Über die Verwendungsmöglichkeit des Wasserstoffsperoxyd für die künstliche Oxygenierung bei extrakorporalen Kreislauf. Thoraxchirurgie *6*, 536–541, 1959b.

——, ——, —— and M. QUERCI: Sulla somministrazione endevenosa di soluzioni di perossido d'idrogeno: prime applicazione cliniche. Minerva med. *50*, 654–656, 1959c.

ABRAMS, L. D., F. ASHTON, E. J. CHARLES,

A. L. D'ABREU, J. FEJFAR, E. J. HAMLEY, W. A. HUDSON, R. E. LEE, R. LIGHTWOOD and E. T. MATTHEWS: Total cardiopulmonary bypass in the laboratory. Lancet *1*, 239–243, 1958.

ADAMS, J. E., E. M. LANCE, B. F. MOORE and H. W. SCOTT, JR.: An autoclavable stainless steel modification of the stationary screen oxygenator. Surg. Forum *9*, 198–202, 1959.

——, G. OWENS, G. MANN, J. R. HEADRICK, A. MUNOZ and H. W. SCOTT, JR.: Experimental evaluation of Pluronic F 68 (a nonionic detergent) as a method of diminishing systemic fat emboli resulting from prolonged cardiopulmonary bypass. Surg. Forum *10*, 585–589, 1960.

ADELMAN, M. H. and E. JACOBSEN: Electroencephalography in cardiac surgery. Amer. J. Cardiol. *6*, 763–772, 1960.

ADOLPH, E. F., S. KLEM and L. B. MORROW: Reversible cessation of blood circulation in deep hypothermia. J. Appl. Physiol. *13*, 397–405, 1958.

AEPLI, R.: Action traumatique exercée sur le sang par les matières servant à la fabrication des appareils "coeur-poumons" Helv. Physiol. Pharmacol. Acta *18*, 119–135, 1960.

AIKEN, D. W.: A method of securing tubing connections in cardiopulmonary bypass equipment. J. Thor. Cardiov. Surg. *41*, 272–273, 1961.

AIRD, I., D. G. MELROSE, W. P. CLELAND and R. B. LYNN: Assisted circulation by pump oxygenator during operative dilation of the aortic valve in man. Brit. Med. J. *1*, 1284–1287, 1954.

ALBERS, C., W. BRENDEL, A. HARDEWIG and W. USINGER: Der intrapulmonale Gasaustauch in tiefer Hypothermie. Pflüger Arch. ges. Physiol. *266*, 394–407, 1958.

ALBERT, S. N., W. E. BAGEANT and C. A. ALBERT: Circulating blood volume measurements for cardiac surgery. Amer. J. Cardiol. *6*, 752–755, 1960.

——, ——, A. S. RUSSELL, F. H. SMALL, C. A. ALBERT and W. BRUNER, JR.: The value of routine blood-volume measurements in major surgical procedures. Anesth. Analg. *40*, 266–274, 1961.

ALBERTAL, G., R. H. CLAUSS, A. M. FOSBERG and D. E. HARKEN: Flowmeter for extracorporeal circulation. IRE Trans. Med. Electronics *ME-6*, 246–248, 1959.

——, ——, ——, W. J. TAYLOR and D. E. HARKEN: An improved electromagnetic flowmeter for extracorporeal circulation. J. Thor. Cardiov. Surg. *41*, 368–374, 1961.

ALELLA, A., F. L. WILLIAMS, G. BOLENE-WILLIAMS and L. N. KATZ: Interrelation between cardiac oxygen consumption and coronary blood flow. Amer. J. Physiol. *183*, 570–582, 1955.

ALETRAS, H. J., GARIBOTTI, E. KOLB, M. NOIRCLERC, J. OSORIO, W. TOMAZEWSKY, G. WILLIAM-OLSSON and A. SENNING: Pressure conditions in the pulmonary circulation during cardiac bypass by double pumps. J. Thor. Cardiov. Surg. *40*, 35–42, 1960.

ALLAN, A. J. G.: Wettability and friction of polytetrafluoroethylene film: effect of prebonding treatment. J. Polymer Sci. *24*, 461–466, 1957.

—— and B. ROBERTS: Wettability of perfluorocarbon polymer films: effects of roughness. J. Polymer Sci. *39*, 1–8, 1959.

ALLAN, R. S., G. E. CHARLES and S. G. MASON: The approach of gas bubbles to a gas/liquid interface. J. Colloid Sc. *16*, 150–165, 1961.

VAN ALLEN, C. M.: A pump for clinical and laboratory purpose which employs the milking principle. J.A.M.A. *98*, 1805–1806, 1932.

ALLEN, J. G.: (editor) Extracorporeal Circulation. Springfield, Ill.: Thomas 1958a.

——: Problems and questions on coagulation of blood arising from the use of extracorporeal circulation pumps and oxygenators. pp. 231–252 *In:* Extracorporeal Circulation,

J. G. Allen (editor) Springfield, Ill.: Thomas 1958b.

——, P. V. MOULDER, R. M. ELGHAMMER, B. J. GROSSMANN, C. L. MCKEEN, M. SANDERSON, W. EGNER and J. M. CROSBIE: A protamine titration as an indication of a clotting defect in certain hemorrhagic states. J. Lab. Clin. Med. *34*, 473–476, 1949.

——, ——, D. M. EVERSON, C. BASINGER, J. J. LANDY and D. J. GLOTZER: Physiology of intravascular coagulation in health and disease with reference to the safeguards and hazards of the prophylactic and therapeutic uses of heparin and Dicumarol. Surg. Clin. N. Amer. *37*, 1473–1506, 1957.

ALLEN, P., J. J. LEDERMANN and G. J. PEARL: Prevention of surgical heart block by the use of supravital stain. J. Thor. Surg. *38*, 37–61, 1959.

—— and C. W. LILLEHEI: Use of induced cardiac arrest in open heart surgery. Results in 70 patients. Minnesota Med. *40*, 672–676, 1957.

ALPERT, N. R., H. KAYNE and W. HASLETT: Relationship among recovery oxygen, oxygen missed, lactate production and lactate removal during and following severe hypoxia in the unanesthetized dog. Amer. J. Physiol. *192*, 585–591, 1958.

AMATUZIO, S., F. GRANDE and L. J. HAY: A natural occurring lipid that neutralizes heparin activity in blood. J. Lab. Clin. Med. *56*, 277–280, 1960.

AMBERSON, W. R., J. E. JACOBS, A. HISEY and J. V. MONKE: Blood substitutes and blood transfusion. Springfield, Ill.: Thomas, 1942.

——, J. J. JENNINGS and C. M. RHODE: Clinical experience with hemoglobin-saline solutions. J. Appl. Physiol. *1*, 469–489, 1949.

AMBRUS, J. L.: A simple heart-lung apparatus, not injurious to white cells and thrombocytes. Trans. Amer. Soc. Art. Int. Organs *1*, 98–101, 1955.

AMER, N. S., J. H. STUCKEY, B. F. HOFFMAN, R. R. CAPELETTI and R. T. DOMINGO: Activation of the interventricular septal myocardium studied during cardiopulmonary bypass. Amer. Heart. J. *59*, 224–237, 1960.

VAN AMERONGEN, C. J.: Influence of structures of elastomers on their permeability to gases. J. Polymer Sc. *5*, 307–332, 1950.

ANANEV, M. G., S. A. MUSHEGIAN, L. A. LEVITSKAIA, E. A. VAINRIB, E. A. FRID, IU. G. KESLOV and L. N. MARTYNEV: Apparatus of artificial blood circulation of the Scientific Research Institute for Experimental and Surgical Apparatus and Instruments and the experience with it. Eksp. Khir. *3*, 25–31, 1958 (*Rus*).

——, E. A. VAINRIB, S. A. MUSHEGIAN, E. A. FRID, L. N. MARTYNOV, IU. F. KESLOV and L. A. LEVITSKAIA: Improvement of the apparatus for the artificial blood circulation of the construction A.I.K. Eksp. khir. *4*, 3–8, 1959 (*Rus*).

ANDERSEN, M. N.: What is "Optimum flow rate"? Surgery *43*, 1020–1023, 1958.

——: Studies during prolonged extracorporeal circulation. J. Thor. Cardiov. Surg. *41*, 244–251, 1961.

—— and G. HAMBRAEUS: Physiologic and biochemical responses to extracorporeal circulation: experimental studies during four-hour perfusion. Ann. Surg. *153*, 592–598, 1961.

—— and A. SENNING: Studies in oxygen consumption during extracorporeal circulation with a pump-oxygenator. Ann. Surg. *148*, 59–65, 1958.

——, B. NORBERG and A. SENNING: Studies of liver function during extracorporeal circulation with low flow rate. Surgery *43*, 397–407, 1958.

——, M. MENDELOW and G. A. ALFANO: Experimental studies of heparin-protamine activity with special reference to protamine inhibition of clotting. Surgery *46*, 1060–1068, 1959.

——, —— and ——: A comparative study of heparin neutralization and the danger of blood clotting abnormalities with protamine and Polybrene. J. Thor. Cardiov. Surg. *39*, 613–618, 1960.

——, G. HAMBRAEUS, G. A. ALFANO and G. W. SCHENK, JR.: Distribution of splanchnic and peripheral blood flow during acute reduction in circulatory rate: Studies during total body perfusion. Ann. Surg. *153*, 477–482, 1961.

ANDERSON, A. and W. J. KOLFF: Artificial kidney in treatment of uremia associated with acute glomerulnephritis (with note on regional heparinization) Ann. Int. Med. *51*, 476–487, 1959.

ANDERSON, D. P.: Personal communication 1961.

ANDERSON, H. M. and J. C. TURNER: Preparation and the haemoglobin content of red cell ghosts. Nature (London) *183*, 112–113, 1959.

ANDERSON, R. M., D. P. ANDERSON and J. H. KAY: A filmer for the stationary

screen oxygenator. Surgery *42*, 896–897, 1957.

ANDREASEN, A. T.: Cross circulation. Brit. Med. Bull. *11*, 233–235, 1955.

—— and F. WATSON: Experimental cardiovascular surgery. Brit. J. Surg. *39*, 548–551, 1952.

—— and ——: Experimental cardiovascular surgery: Discussion of results so far obtained and report on experiments concerning donor circulation. Brit. J. Surg. *41*, 195–206, 1953.

ANDRES, R., K. L. ZIERLER, H. M. ANDERSON, W. N. STAINSBY, G. CADER, A. S. GRAYYIB and J. L. LILIENTHAL, JR.: Measurement of blood flow and volume in the forearm of man; with notes on the theory of indicator dilution and on production of turbulence, hemolysis and vasodilation by intravascular injection. J. Clin. Invest. *33*, 482–504, 1954.

ANKENEY, J. L. and P. H. VILES: The effect of extracorporeal circulation upon portal hemodynamics. Surg. Forum *11*, 228–229, 1960.

—— and ——: The effect of total body perfusion on carotid blood flow. Surgery *49*, 209–222, 1961.

——, —— and J. R. LEONARDS: A study of changes in peripheral flow and resistance as associated with total body perfusion. Surg. Forum *9*, 157–162, 1959.

ANREP, G. V.: A new method of cross circulation. Proc. Roy. Soc. (Biol.) *97*, 444–449, 1925.

ANTIPOV, B. V.: Patho-morphological investigations on the "dry" arrested heart in conditions of experimental application of artificial circulation. Arkh. Pat. *22*, 67–72, 1960 (*Rus*).

ARMENIO, S.: Il problema dell'ossigenazione extracorporea. Riforma Med. *67*, 972–974, 1953.

——: Biologic oxygenation of the blood for experimental and clinical extracorporeal circulation. J. Int. Coll. Surg. *21*, 768–771, 1954.

ARNULF, G.: Systematic coronary arteriography with acetylcholine cardiac arrest. Prog. Cardiov. Dis. *2*, 197–206, 1959.

ARTUSIO, J. F., B. E. MARBURY, D. B. VALENTINO and A. VAN POZNAK: Anesthesia for cardiac surgery. Surg. Clin. N. Amer. *41*, 327–338, 1961.

ARTZ, C. P.: Newer concepts of nutrition by the intravenous route. Ann. Surg. *149*, 841–849, 1959.

Ascheulova, E. N., L. V. Rosenstraukh and A. V. Trubetskoy: The study of electrocardiographic data and the uptake of oxygen by the myocardium during extracorporeal circulation. Eksp. Khir. 6, 38–42, 1960 (Rus).

Ashbaugh, D. G., B. C. Paton and H. Swan: Prolonged partial perfusion. Presented at the Scientific Assembly of the American Medical Association, New York, 1961.

Ashton, F. and A. J. H. Rains: Arterial perfusion in the lower limb as an aid to vascular surgery. Lancet, 1, 19–22, 1960.

Astrup, P.: A simple electrometric technique for the determination of carbon dioxide tension in blood and plasma, total content of carbon dioxide in plasma, and bicarbonate content in "separated" plasma at a fixed carbon dioxide tension (40 mm. Hg.). Scand. J. Clin. Lab. Invest. 8, 33–43, 1956.

——: A new approach to acid-base metabolism. Clin. Chem. 7, 1–15, 1961.

Auld, P. A., A. M. Rudolph and R. J. Golinko: Factors affecting bronchial collateral flow in the dog. Amer. J. Physiol. 198, 1166–1170, 1960.

Ausman, R. K. and J. B. Aust: A regional perfusion oxygenator. Surgery 48, 782–784, 1960.

——, S. J. Gemmill, J. B. Aust and C. W. Lillehei: Use of blood volume determinations in open heart surgery. Trans. Amer. Soc. Art. Int. Organs 7, 220–222, 1961.

Austen, W. G. and R. S. Shaw: Experimental studies with extracorporeal circuits as a method to enable surgical attack on thoracic aneurysms. J. Thor. Cardiov. Surg. 39, 337–356, 1960.

——, A. P. Monaco, G. S. Richardson, W. H. Baker, R. S. Shaw and J. W. Raker: Treatment of malignant pelvic tumors by extracorporeal perfusion with chemotherapeutics agents. New Engl. J. Med. 261, 1037–1045, 1959.

Autian, J. and A. J. Kapadia: A note on the leaching constituent from medical grade plastic tubings. Drug Stand. 28, 101–102, 1960.

B

Babskaya, Yu. E. and A. V. Pogosova: Changes in certain redox processes during extracorporeal circulation with the AIK apparatus. Eksp. Khir. 6, 53–55, 1960 (Rus).

Baer, D. M. and Osborn, J. J.: The postperfusion pulmonary congestion syndrome. Amer. J. Clin. Path. 34, 442–445, 1960.

Bahnson, H. T.: Characterisitcs of an ideal pump for extracorporeal circulation. p. 9 In: Extracorporeal circulation. J. G. Allen (editor) Springfield, Ill., Thomas, 1958.

——: Cardiopulmonary bypass. Amer. J. Surg. 96, 447–478, 1958b.

——, F. C. Spencer, R. A. Gaertner and D. W. Benson: Experiences with open-heart surgery during cardiopulmonary bypass in 270 cases. Amer. Surgeon 26, 227–235, 1960.

Bailey, C. P. and W. M. Lemmon: Current research in the surgery of ventricular septal defects. Amer. J. Cardiol. 5, 242–257, 1960.

——, T. J. E. O'Neill, R. P. Glover, W. L. Jamison and H. P. R. Ramirez: Surgical repair of mitral insufficiency. Dis. Chest 19, 125–141, 1951.

Bain, W.: The role of the liver and spleen in the destruction of the blood corpuscles. J. Physiol. (London) 29, 352–368, 1903.

Bain, W. H. and W. A. Mackey: Extracorporeal circulation. J. Roy. Coll. Surg. Edinburgh 5, 45–56, 1959.

Baker, C. H. and J. W. Remington: Acute circulatory collapse of the adrenalectomized dog following plasma infusion. Circulat. Res. 6, 294–300, 1958.

Baker, J. B. E., H. H. Bental, B. Dreyer, and D. G. Melrose: Arrest of isolated heart with potassium citrate. Lancet, 555–559, 1957.

Balint, P., Fekete, P. G. and Nagy, Z.: Das Verhalten des Minutenvolumens und der Nierendurchblutung bei arterieller Hypoxie. Pflüger Arch. Ges. Physiol. 271, 705–714, 1960.

Ballinger, W. F. II, Vollenweider, H., Pierucci, L., Jr. and Templeton, J. Y.: Anaerobic metabolism and metabolic acidosis during cardiopulmonary bypass. Ann. Surg. 153, 499–506, 1961.

Baltzer, V. and Bucher, K.: Problems des Gasaustausches in der Lunge. Helv. Physiol. Pharmacol. Acta 18, 193–197, 1960.

Baranov, Iu. N.: Linear speed of the blood supply to the organism during artificial circulation. Eksp. Khir. 4, 38–43, 1959 (Rus).

Barcroft, H.: Observations on the pumping action of the heart. J. Physiol. (London) 78, 186–195, 1933.

Barcroft, J.: The respiratory function of the blood. Cambridge, 1928.

—— and A. V. HILL: The nature of oxy-
haemoglobin, with a note on its molecular
weight. J. Physiol. (London) *39*, 411–428,
1909–1910.

BARD, P.: Medical Physiology, 10th Edition.
The C. V. Mosby Co., St. Louis, 1956.

BARK, J.: EEG bei Kreislaufunterbrechung
und künstlicher Perfusion. Thoraxchirurgie
7, 162–172, 1960.

BARNARD, C. N., R. A. DeWALL, C. W. LIL-
LEHEI and R. L. VARCO: Pre- and postoperative care for patients undergoing open
cardiac surgery. Dis. Chest *35*, 194–211,
1959.

——, M. B. McKENZIE and D. R. DE VILLIERS:
Preparation and assembly of the stainless steel sponge debubbler for use in the
helix reservoir bubble oxygenator. Thorax
15, 268–272, 1960.

BARRATT-BOYES, B. F., J. B. LOWE, W. J.
WATT, D. S. COLE and J. C. P. WILLIAMS:
Initial experiences with extracorporeal cir-
culation in interacardiac surgery. Brit.
Med. J. *2*, 1826–1831, 1960.

BARRER, R. M. and G. SKIRROW: Transport
and equilibrium phenomena in gas-elas-
tomer systems. I. Kinetic phenomena. J.
Polymer Sc. *3*, 549–563, 1948.

BARSAMIAN, E. M., S. W. JACOB and S. C.
COLLINS: A new pump-oxygenator. Surg.
Forum *11*, 234–235, 1960.

BARWELL, C. F. and M. A. FREEMAN: Sterilization by ethylene oxide. Lancet *1*, 917–
918, 1959.

BASS, P., I. MAZURKIEWICZ and K. I. MEL-
VILLE: Effects of magnesium on coronary
flow and heart action and its influence of
the responses to adrenaline and noradrenaline. Arch. Int. Pharmacodyn. *117*, 9–22,
1958.

BASSIOUNI, M.: The estimation of heparin and
similar substances in human blood and tissues using a combined biological and colorimetric method with paper electrophoretic
studies. J. Clin. Path. *7*, 330–335, 1954.

BATTEZZATI, M. and C. TADDEI: La perfusione della testa isolata in funzione della
cardiochirurgia a cuore esangue; ricerche
sperimentali. Minerva Chir. *8*, 925–934,
1953.

—— and ——: Descrizione di un apparecchio
per la circolazione extracorporea e per la
ossigenazione artificiale. Minerva Chir. *9*,
333–341, 1954.

——, —— and P. MOSETTI: Ricerche sperimentali sull' ossigenazione complementare.
Pat. Sper. Chir. *1*, 438–466, 1953.

BAUEREISEN, E., G. H. LIPPMAN, E. SCHU-
BERT and W. SICKEL: Bioelektrische Akti-
vität und Sauerstoff-Verbrauch isolierter
Potentialbildner und Sauerstoffdruck zwi-
schen 0 und 10 Atm. Pflüger Arch. ges.
Physiol. *367*, 636–648, 1958.

BAYLISS, W. M.: On the local reactions of the
arterial wall to changes of internal pressure. J. Physiol. (London) *28*, 220–231,
1902.

—— and E. A. MULLER: A simple, high speed
rotary pump. J. Scient. Instrum. *5*, 278–
279, 1928.

——, A. R. FEE and E. OGDEN: A method of
oxygenating blood. J. Physiol. (London)
66, 443–448, 1928.

BAZETT, H. C. and W. C. QUINBY: A new
method for cross circulation experiments,
with some observations on the nature of
pressor reflexes. Quart. J. Exp. Physiol. *12*,
199–226, 1919/1920.

BEALL, A. C., JR., D. A. COOLEY, G. C.
MORRIS, JR. and J. H. MOYER: Effect of
total cardiac bypass on renal hemodynamics and water and electrolyte excretion in
man. Ann. Surg. *146*, 190, 1957.

BEARD, J.: The anaesthetic management of
patients for extracorporeal circulation.
Proc. Roy. Soc. Med. *51*, 589–591, 1958.

BEAUSSART, W., M. RIBET, C. GAUTIER, J.
DECOULX, A. HASSOUM and A. SENNE-
VILLE: L'E.E.G. du chien au cours d'inter-
ventions chirurgicales à coeur ouvert avec
circuit extracorporel (C.E.C.) Rev. Neurol.
(Paris) *101:* 478–475, 1959.

BECK, A.: Zur Technik der Bluttransfusion.
Klin. Wschr. *2*, 1999–2001, 1924.

BEDNARIK, B. and M. VASCULIN: Experience
with extracorporeal circulation with bubble
oxygenator. Rozhl. Chir. *38*, 201–209, 1959
(*Cze*).

BEER, R.: Stoffwechselveränderungen während des extrakorporalen Kreislaufs. Thoraxchirurgie *6*, 360–369, 1959.

—— and G. LOESCHKE: Probleme bei Operationen mit extrakorporalem Kreislauf unter
besonderer Berücksichtigung der Anaesthesie. Anaesthesist, *8*, 70–76, 1959.

——, H. GEHL, H. G. BORST and M. SCHMIDT-
MENDE: Pathophysiologische Veränderungen bei Anwendung des extrakorporalen
Kreislaufs. I. Mitteilung: Gasstoffwechsel
und Säuren-Basengleichgewicht. Langenbeck Arch. Klin. Chir. *291*, 443–466, 1959.

BELAND, I. L., G. K. MOE and M. D. VIS-
SCHER: Use of aluminum metal in contact

with blood in perfusion systems. Proc. Soc. Exp. Biol. Med. *39*, 145–147, 1938.

BELISLE, C. A., E. F. WOODS, D. B. NUNN, E. F. PARKER, W. H. LEE JR. and J. A. RICHARDSON: The role of epinephrine and norepinephrine in rebound cardiovascular phenomena in azygos flow studies and cardiopulmonary bypass in dogs. J. Thor. Cardiov. Surg. *39*, 815–820, 1960.

BELL, A. L. L., JR. and H. FITZPATRICK: The influence of the rate of perfusion on physiologic responses during total body perfusion with the "bubble-type" oxygenator. Trans. Amer. Soc. Art. Int. Organs *3*, 24–28, 1957.

——, ——, E. ANDREAE, S. SHIMOMURA and R. PINGEON: The influence of the rate of perfusion on physiologic responses during cardiac bypass. Ann. Surg. *148*, 968–978, 1958.

BELL, J. R. and P. GROSBERG: Diffusion through porous materials. Nature (London) *189*, 980–981, 1961.

BELL, J. W.: Heart and lungs as a common chamber during extracorporeal support of fibrillating canine heart. Circulat. Res. *7*, 926–935, 1959.

—— and F. F. BERETTA: Prolonged ventricular fibrillation; an experimental study in the closed chest animal utilizing a pump oxygenator. J. Thor. Cardiov. Surg. *38*, 17–29, 1959.

BELT, A. E., H. P. SMITH and G. H. WHIPPLE: Factors concerned in the perfusion of living organs and tissues. Amer. J. Physiol. *52*, 101–120, 1920.

BENARD, H. and L. HENRY: Une nouvelle pompe pour perfusion. C. R. Soc. Biol. (Paris) *135*, 546–548, 1941.

BENCINI, A.: Un apparecchio ossigenatore e propulsore a scoppo sperimentale. Atti Soc. Med. Chir. *27*, 1, 1949.

—— and P. L. PAROLA: Un nuovo sistema per l'ossigenazione extracorporea del sangue. L'ossigenatore a spugna. Arch. Atti Soc. Ital. Chir. *2*, 572, 1956.

——, ——, G. TIBERIO, E. PETRELLA, P. FERRABOSCHI, A. AMBROSINI and G. BO-SELLI: Preliminary studies on the sponge oxygenator. Surgery *42*, 342–346, 1957.

——, ——, A. AMBROSINI, G. TIBERIO and P. FERRASBOSCHI: Studi sull'efficienza dell'ossigenatore a spugna. Minerva Chir. *12*, 1410–1413, 1958a.

——, ——, D. GALMARINI, E. PETRELLA and G. BOSELLI: Il problema del ripristino della coagulabilità del sangue dopo periodi di circolazione extracorporea. Minerva Chir. *13*, 1413–1415, 1958b.

——, ——, E. PETRELLA and P. FERRA-BOSCHI: Possibilità di utilizare la fibrillazione ventricolare indotta nella chirurgia del cuore esangue. Minerva Chir. *13*, 1416–1418, 1958c.

——, P. GALLI and S. SALVANESCHI: Possibilità di impiego dei siliconi antischiuma in medicina e in chirurgia e studio sulla tollerabilita di tale sostanze somministrate per via endovenosa in alcuni animali da esperimento. Biol. Lat. (Milano) *11*, 123–130, 1958d.

BENFORADO, J. M.: A depressant affect of acetylcholine on the idioventricular pacemaker of the isolated perfused rabbit heart. Brit. J. Pharmacol. *13*, 415–418, 1958.

BENICHOUX, R.: Position actuelle du problème de la chirurgie à coeur ouvert. Avantages de l'hypothermie profonde avec micro-oxygénateur. Rev. Med. Nancy *85*, 505–518, 1960.

BENJAMIN, R. B., C. E. TURBOK and F. J. LEWIS: Effect of air embolism in the systemic circulation and its prevention during cardiac surgery. J. Thor. Surg. *34*, 548–552, 1957.

BENVENUTO, R. and F. J. LEWIS: Influence of some physical factors upon oxygenation with a plastic membrane oxygenator. Surgery *46*, 1099–1106, 1959.

BERGLUND, E., R. G. MONROE and G. L. SCHREINER: Myocardial oxygen consumption and coronary blood flow during potassium-induced cardiac arrest and during ventricular fibrillation. Acta Physiol. Scand. *41*, 261–268, 1957.

BERKAS, E. M., D. J. FERGUSON, J. J. GARA-NELLA and R. L. VARCO: Studies in technique permitting prolonged cardiac venous inflow stasis. Surg. Forum *4*, 59–62, 1954.

BERLIN, R. and H. SANDRING: Increased suspension stability of blood after heparin administration. Acta Med. Scand. *169*, 369–372, 1961.

BERNATZ, P. E., J. W. DUSHANE and J. W. KIRKLIN: Surgical treatment of certain congential cardiovascular abnormalities in infants and children. Minnesota Med. *39*, 1–4, 1956.

BERNE, R. M.: The effect of immersion hypothermia on coronary blood flow. Circulat. Res. *2*, 236–242, 1954.

——: Cardiodynamics and the coronary circulation in hypothermia. Ann. N. Y. Acad. Sc. *80*, 365–383, 1959.

——, R. D. Jones and F. S. Cross: Oxygen consumption of the hypothermic potassium arrested heart. Proc. Soc. Exp. Biol. Med. *99*, 84–88, 1958a.

——, —— and ——: Myocardial hypothermia in elective cardiac arrest. J. Appl. Physiol. *12*, 431–436, 1958b.

Bernhard, W. F., H. F. Schwarz and N. P. Mallick: Intermittent cold coronary perfusion as an adjunct to open heart surgery. Surg. Gynec. Obstet. *111*, 744–748, 1960.

——, —— and ——: Elective hypothermic cardiac arrest in normothermic animals. Ann. Surg. *153*, 43–51, 1961.

Bertho, E.: Production of cardiac arrest by an electrolyte solution. A preliminary report. Canad. Med. Ass. J. *83*, 213–216, 1960.

Beuren, A., R. J. Bing and C. Sparks: Metabolic studies on the arrested and fibrillating perfused heart. Amer. J. Cardiol. *1*, 103–112, 1958.

Bhonslay, S. B., R. A. Deterling, Jr., H. W. Wallace and H. F. Rheinlander: Elective cardiac arrest (Experimental studies and a review of the literature). J. Cardiov. Surg. *2*, 168–175, 1961.

Bianconi, R. and J. H. Green: Pulmonary baroceptors in the cat. Arch. Ital. Biol. *97*, 205–315, 1959.

Bigelow, W. G., W. K. Lindsay and W. F. Greenwood: Hypothermia: its possible role in cardiac surgery: An investigation of factors governing survival in dogs at low body temperature. Ann. Surg. *132*, 849–866, 1950.

Binet, L. and C. Mayer: Technique nouvelle de perfusion sanguine. C. R. Acad. Sci. (Paris) *189*, 1330–1331, 1929.

Bing, R. J., L. D. Vandam and F. D. Gray, Jr.: Physiological studies in congenital heart disease. II. Results of preoperative studies in patients with tetralogy of Fallot. Bull. Johns Hopkins Hosp. *80*, 121–147, 1947.

Birkeland, S.: An evaluation of the circulation during cardiopulmonary bypass in dogs. Acta. Chir. Scand. *117*, 41–46, 1959.

Bischoff, T. L. W.: Beiträge zur Lehre vom Blute und der Transfusion desselben. Arch. Anat. 347–372, 1835.

Bittard, M., E. Remigy, J. Martin and R. Benichoux: La neutralisation de l'héparine au cours de la circulation extracorporelle. Expérimentation d'un nouveau produit anti-héparine. Rev. Med. Nancy *85*, 606–615, 1960.

Bittencourt, D., D. M. Long, Y. K. Lee and C. W. Lillehei: Intravital staining of the atrioventricular bundle with iodine compounds during cardiopulmonary bypass. Circulat. Res. *7*, 753–758, 1959.

Bjørk, V. O.: Brain perfusion in dogs with artificially oxygenated blood. Acta Chir. Scand. *96*, 1–90, 1948a.

——: An artificial heart or cardiopulmonary machine. Performance in animals. Lancet *1*, 491–493, 1948b

——: The use of "arterialized-venous" blood from a reservoir for short periods of open heart surgery in preference to hypothermia. Acta Chir. Scand. *111*, 285–291, 1956.

——: The principles for artificial oxygenation of blood. Acta Chir. Scand. *11*, 27–30, 1959.

——: An effective blood heart exchanger for deep hypothermia in association with extracorporeal circulation but excluding the oxygenator. J. Thor. Cardiov. Surg. *40*, 237–252, 1960.

——: Perfusion technic for surgery on the aortic valves. Ann. Surg. *153*, 173–182, 1961.

—— and B. Fors: Induced cardiac arrest. J. Thor. Cardiov. Surg. *41*, 387–394, 1961.

—— and G. Hultquist: Brain damage in children after deep hypothermia for open heart surgery. Thorax. *15*, 284–291, 1960.

—— and L. Rodriguez: The influence of high oxygen pressure on hemolysis. Acta Chir. Scand. *117*, 31–34, 1959.

Blanco, G. and C. P. Bailey: Experimental use of autogenous lung. Trans. Amer. Soc. Art. Int. Organs *5*, 157–161, 1959.

——, A. Adam and A. Fernandez: A direct experimental approach to the aortic valve. II. Acute retroperfusion of the coronary sinus. J. Thor. Surg. *32*, 171–177, 1956.

——, C. Oca, S. Laguna, L. E. Nunez, J. Schaeffer and C. P. Bailey: Autogenous lung oxygenation during cardiac bypass; experimental studies and clinical application in aortic valve surgery. Amer. J. Cardiol. *2*, 302–314, 1958.

——, ——, E. Rey-Baltar, H. T. Nichols and C. P. Bailey: Single catheter gravity drainage of the right atrium or right ventricle during total cardiac bypass. Dis. Chest *35*, 554–560, 1959.

Bliss, J. G. and J. D. Walker: Histamine release by homologous plasma in the dog. Canad. J. Biochem. Physiol. *37*, 371–375, 1959.

Blomback, B., Blomback, M. and P. Wallen: Détermination du taux de l'héparine dans le sang en cas de circulation extracorporelle au cours de la chirurgie cardiaque. Rev. Hemat. *10*, 45–53, 1955.

——, ——, P. OLSSON, G. WILLIAM-OLSSON and A. SENNING: Determination of heparin level of the blood (some observations on heparin elimination and correlation between heparin level and clotting time after intravenous injections). Acta Chir. Scand. *245*, 259–264, 1959.

BLOODWELL, R. D., L. I. GOLDBERG, E. BRAUNWALD, J. W. GILBERT, J. ROSS and A. G. MORROW: Myocardial contractility in man. Surg. Forum *10*, 532–535, 1960.

BLOOM, S. S., F. W. HELMSWORTH, JR., H. C. DODGE and E. L. BIRKMIRE: The ear oximeter as a circulatory monitor. III. The IR pulse as a guide to the selection of vasopressor drugs in cardiac surgery. Amer. J. Cardiol. *6*, 773–777, 1960.

BLOOR, B. M., R. D. FLOYD, K. D. HALL and D. H. REYNOLDS: A study of cortical oxygen tension during induced hypotension. Arch Surg. *77*, 65–74, 1958.

——, J. FRICKER, F. HELLINGER, H. NISHIOKA and J. McCURCHEN: A study of cerebrospinal fluid oxygen tension. Arch. Neurol. *4*, 37–46, 1961.

BLUM, L. and S. J. MEGIBOW: Exclusion of the dog heart by parabiosis. J. Mount Sinai Hosp., N. Y. *17*, 38–43, 1950.

——, —— and W. M. NELSON: A parabiotic blood pump. Surg. Forum *6*, 24–39, 1955.

BLUMBERG, J. B., L. C. WINTERSCHEID, D. H. DILLARD, R. R. VETTO and K. A. MERENDINO: The clinical use of polybrene as an antiheparin agent in open heart surgery. J. Thor. Cardiov. Surg. *39*, 330–336, 1960.

BLUEMLE, L. W., JR.: *In:* Discussion on blood pumps. Trans. Amer. Soc. Art. Int. Organs *4*, 80, 1958.

——, J. G. DICKSON, JR., J. MITCHELL and M. S. PODOLNICK: Permeability and hydrodynamic studies on the MacNeill-Collins dialyser using conventional and modified membrane supports. Trans. Amer. Soc. Art. Int. Organs *6*, 38–43, 1960.

BLUNT, J. W., JR.: Standards for surgical metals; thermal electromotive force as a practical property. Amer. J. Surg. *97*, 415–417, 1959.

BOCK, J.: Ein Apparat zu Infusionsversuchen. Arch. Exp. Path. Pharmakol. *57*, 117–182, 1907.

BOERE, L. A., N. DERLAGEN and D. KIERS: Hypothermia, its principles and biochemical disturbances. Arch. Chir. Neerl. *9*, 155–183, 1957.

BOEREMA, I., A. WILDSCHUT, W. J. H. SCHMIDT and L. BROEKHUYSEN: Experimental researches into hypothermia as an aid in the surgery of the heart. Arch. Chir. Neerl. *3*, 25–34, 1951.

——, N. G. MEYNE, W. K. BRUMMELKAMP, S. BOUMA, M. H. MENSCH, F. KAMERMANS, M. S. HANF and W. VAN AALDEREN: Life without blood (a study of the influence of high atmospheric pressure and hypothermia on dilution of the blood) J. Cardiov. Surg. *1*, 133–146, 1960.

BOR, N. M. and A. P. RIEBEN: Partial extracorporeal circulation in acute heart failure. Amer. J. Cardiol. *8*, 41–50, 1961.

——, P. F. SALISBURY, P. A. RIEBEN and C. E. CROSS: Influence of partial heartlung bypass on the failing heart. The Physiologist *2*, 13, 1959.

——, P. A. STEWART, Y. W. CHO and F. BIRKARDESLER: Flow and diameter changes in mesenteric capillaries of dogs in endotoxin shock. Trans. Amer. Soc. Art. Int. Organs *7*, 202–207, 1961.

BORNSTEIN, A.: Über Durchblutungsversuche an der überlebenden Hundeextremität. Arch. Exp. Path. Pharmakol. *115*, 367–382, 1926.

BORST, H. G.: Die künstlichen Oxygenatoren. Thoraxchirurgie *6*, 312–320, 1959.

——, R. BEER, H. GEHL, G. LOESCHCKE and M. SCHMIDT-MENDE: Pathophysiologische Veränderungen bei Anwendung eines extrakorporalen Kreislaufes. Langenbeck Arch. Klin. Chir. *291*, 467–481, 1959.

BOSHER, L. H.: Problems in extracorporeal circulation relating to venous cannulation and drainage. Ann. Surg. *149*, 652–662, 1959.

BOUCEK, R. J. and W. P. MURPHY, JR.: Segmental perfusion of the coronary arteries with fibrinolysin in man following a myocardial infarction. Amer. J. Cardiol. *6*, 525–533, 1960.

BOUNOUS, G.: Circolazione extracorporea in chirurgia. Minerva Cardioangiol. *6*, 493–507, 1958.

——, H. B. SHUMACKER, JR. and H. KING: Studies in renal blood flow: I. Some general considerations. Ann. Surg. *151*, 47–58, 1960a.

——, M. ONNIS, H. B. SHUMACKER and F. NASH: Renal autoregulation. Surg. Gynec. Obstet. *111*, 540–544, 1960b.

BOURGEOIS-GAVARDIN, M., L. W. FABIAN,

W. C. SEALY, I. W. BROWN, JR. and C. R. STEPHEN: Management of anesthesia and hypothermia for open-heart surgery with extracorporeal circulation. Anesth. Analg. *37*, 197–210, 1958.

BOURNE, G. and R. G. SMITH: The value of intravenous and intraperitoneal administration of oxygen. Amer. J. Physiol. *82*, 328–334, 1927.

BOVET, D., A. CARPI and M. VIRNO: Pharmacodynamic de la circulation cérébrale. Experientia *16*, 1–20, 1960.

BOYD, A. D., R. E. TREMBLAY, F. C. SPENCER and H. T. BAHNSON: Estimation of cardiac output soon after intracardiac surgery with cardiopulmonary bypass. Ann. Surg. *150*, 613–626, 1959.

BRACKEN, A., C. C. WILTON-DAVIES and F. E. WEALE: Ethylene oxide sterilization of a heart–lung machine. Guy Hosp. Rep. *109*, 75–80, 1960.

BRAUNWALD, E., S. J. SARNOFF, R. B. CASE, W. N. STAINSBY and G. H. WELSCH, JR.: Hemodynamic determinants of coronary flow: effect of changes in aortic pressure and cardiac output on the relationship between myocardial oxygen consumption and coronary flow. Amer. J. Physiol. *192*, 157–163, 1958.

BRECHER, G. A.: Venous return. New York: Grune & Stratton, 1956.

——, M. M. REYDMAN, M. FIER, B. L. BROFMAN and R. B. FREEMAN: Regulation of blood flow in cross-circulation for intracardiac surgery. Proc. Soc. Exp. Biol. Med. *89*, 134–138, 1955.

BRECHNER, V. L., R. O. BAUER, R. W. M. BETHUNE, R. E. PHILLIPS, E. M. KAVAN and J. B. DILLON: The electroencephalographic effect of arrested circulation in the normothermic human and dog. Anesth. Analg. *40*, 1–14, 1961.

——, E. M. KAVAN and J. B. DILLON: Electroencephalographic effect of compression of the superior vena cava during thoracotomy. J. Thor. Surg. *37*, 352–359, 1959.

BRECKLER, I. A., C. L. PORTNOFF and J. G. BITTERLY: An externally valved hydraulic cardiac substitute. J. Thor. Cardiov. Surg. *38*, 594–603, 1959.

BRENDEL, W., E. KOPPERMANN and R. THAUER: Der respiratorische Stoffwechsel in Narkose. Pflüger Arch. ges. Physiol. *259*, 177–206, 1954.

——, C. ALBERS and W. USINGER: Der Einfluss isolierter Veränderungen der Hirntemperatur auf Sauerstoffverbrauch, At-

mung und Kreislauf. Pflüger Arch. ges. Physiol. *268*, 8–9, 1958.

——, —— and ——: Der Kreislauf in Hypothermie; die einzelnen Kreislaufgrössen und ihre Koordination während der Auskühlung. Pflüger Arch. ges. Physiol. *266*, 341–356, 1958.

BREWIN, E. G., F. S. NASHAT and E. NEILL: Acid-base equilibrium in hypothermia. Brit. J. Anaesth. *28*, 1–2, 1956.

BRINSFIELD, D. E., M. A. HOPF, R. B. GEERING and P. M. GALLETTI: Hematological changes in long term perfusion. Submitted for publ. in J. Appl. Physiol.

BROCK, SIR R. and D. N. ROSS: The clinical application of hypothermic techniques. Guy Hosp. Rep. *104*, 99–113, 1955.

BROCKMAN, S. K. and E. FONKALSRUD: Experimental open heart surgery employing hypothermia, mecholyl arrest, and carotid perfusion. Surgery, *43*, 814–823, 1958.

—— and J. R. JUDE: The tolerance of the dog brain to total arrest of circulation. Bull. Johns Hopkins Hosp. *106*, 74–80, 1960.

BRODIE, T. G.: The perfusion of surviving organs. J. Physiol. (London) *29*, 266–275, 1903.

BROMAN, T., R. EDSTROM and O. STEINWALL: Technical aspects on dyes and radio-tracers in the determination of blood-brain barrier damage. Acta Psychiat. Neurol. Scand. *36*, 69–75, 1961.

BROWN, F., W. SEIDEL, V. MIRKOVITCH and R. LITTURI: Hemolysis caused by pumps at flow rates of two liters. Trans. Amer. Soc. Art. Int. Organs *7*, 350–354, 1961.

BROWN, I. W. JR., and W. W. SMITH: Hematologic problems associated with the use of extracorporeal circulation for cardiovascular surgery. Ann. Int. Med. *49*, 1035–1048, 1958.

——, W. W. SMITH and W. O. EMMONS: An efficient blood heat exchanger for use with extracorporeal circulation. Surgery *44*, 372–377, 1958a.

——, ——, W. G. YOUNG, JR. and W. C. SEALY: Experimental and clinical studies of controlled hypothermia rapidly produced and corrected by a blood heat exchanger during extracorporeal circulation. J. Thor. Surg. *36*, 497–505, 1958b.

——, C. H. WILMER, G. YOUNG, W. C. SEALY and J. S. HARRIS: A simple, expendable blood oxygen-gas exchanger for use in open cardiac surgery. Surgery, *40*, 100–112, 1956.

BROWN, T. G. and M. DE V. COTTEN: Responses to cardiovascular drugs during extreme hypothermia. J. Pharmacol. Exp. Therap. *110*, 8, 1954.

BROWN-SEQUARD, E.: Recherches expérimentales sur les propriétés physiologiques et les usages du sang rouge et du sang noir et leurs principaux éléments gazeux, l'oxygène et l'acide carbonique. J. Physiol. de l'Homme (Paris) *1*, 95-122, 353-367, 729-735, 1858.

BRUBACKER, D. W. and K. KAMMERMEYER: Separation of gases by plastic membranes —Permeation rates and extent of separation. Indust. Engin. Chem. *46*, 733-739, 1954.

BRUKHONENKO, S.: Appareil pour la circulation artificielle du sang des animaux à sang chaud. J. Physiol. Path. Gen. *27*, 12-18, 1929a.

——: Circulation artificielle du sang dans l'organisme entier d'un chien avec coeur exclu. J. Physiol. Path. Gen. *27*, 257-272, 1929b.

——: Application of the method of artificial blood circulation for reviving the organism. Vses. sezd fiziol. biokhimi farmak. dek. *6*, 667-674, 1937 (*Rus*).

—— and S. TCHECHULINE: Expériences avec la tête isolée du chien. I. Techniques et conditions des expériences. J. Physiol. Path. Gén. *27*, 31-45, 1929.

——, M. I. MARTSINKEVICH and S. A. PERESTERENIN: Some peculiarities for the temporary replacement of the functions of the heart and of the lungs, by the apparatus of artificial blood circulation. Tez. dokl. 2 Vseseizn konf. patofiziol. 51-52, 1956 (*Rus*).

BRULL, L.: A mechanical heart with coagulable blood. Science *111*, 277-278, 1950a.

——: Mechanical heart with coagulable blood. Arch. Int. Physiol. *58*, 321-328, 1950b.

—— and D. LOUIS-BAR: Toxicity of artificially circulated heparinized blood on the kidney. Arch. Int. Physiol. *65*, 470-476, 1957.

BRUNER, H. D. (editor): Methods in medical research. Vol. 8, Yearbook Publ. Chicago, 1960.

BUCHER, K. and F. GRUN: Zum Mechanismus des Gasaustausches in der Lunge. Ztschr. Naturforsch. *13B*, 748-752, 1958.

BUCHERL, E.: Extracorporaler Kreislauf mit künstlichem Herz-Lungensystem. Thoraxchirurgie *3*, 460-471, 1956.

BUCHERL, E. S.: In-vitro Untersuchungen zur Frage der Blutveränderungen bei Ver-

wendung einer künstlichen Lunge nach dem Gasdispersionsprinzip. Thoraxchirurgie *5*, 63-70, 1957.

——: How shall we regulate our perfusion volume during extracorporeal circulation. Minerva Chir. *13*, 1384-1385, 1958.

——: Der Einfluss physikalischer und chemischer Faktoren auf den Hämolysegrad menschlichen Blutes bei Gasdispersion. Thoraxchirurgie *6*. 327-336, 1959.

——: Die Hämodynamik während extracorporaler Zirkulation. Thoraxchirurgie *6*, 375-383, 1959.

——: Welche Kriterien bestimmen den Wert einer Herz-Lungen-Maschine? Thoraxchirurgie *7*, 101-108, 1960.

—— and M. TREDE: Praktische Bedeutung der Registrierung und Bestimmung biologischer Grössen bei extracorporaler Zirkulation. Langenbeck Arch. Klin. Chir. *292*, 660-666, 1959.

——, G. HORKENBACH and K. J. SCHMUTZER: Probleme des Säure-Basenhaushaltes während extrakorporalen Zirkilation. Thoraxchirurgie *6*, 505-515, 1959.

BULL, A. B., G. J. ROSSOUW, J. E. KENCH and C. N. BARNARD: The experimental use of Halothane in open-heart surgery with cardiopulmonary bypass. S. Afr. Med. J. *33*, 1097-1099, 1959.

——, J. OZINSKY and G. G. HARRISON: The clinical use of halothane anesthesia during cardiopulmonary bypass for open heart surgery. Brit. J. Anesth. *32*, 164-170, 1960.

BUNEC, D. F. M.: Survival of dogs following section of carotid and vertebral arteries. Proc. Soc. Exp. Biol. Med. *103*, 581-585, 1960.

BUNZL, A., A. S. V. BURGEN, B. D. BURNS, N. PEDLEY and W. G. TERROUX: Methods for studying the reflex activity of the frog's spinal cord. Brit. J. Pharmacol. *9*, 229-235, 1954.

BURKE, M. F. and R. E. GARDNER: Survival of red blood cells in dogs following total body perfusion. Surg. Forum *10*, 578-580, 1960.

BURN, J. H.: The cause of fibrillation. Brit. Med. J. *1*, 1379-1383, 1960a.

—— and S. HUKOVIC: Anoxia and ventricular fibrillation with a summary of evidence on the cause of fibrillation. Brit. J. Pharmacol. *15*, 67-70, 1960b.

BURNS, B. D., J. G. ROBSON and G. K. SMITH: The survival of mammalian tissues perfused with intravascular gas mixtures of oxygen and carbon dioxide. Canad. J. Biochem. Physiol. *36*, 499–504, 1958.

BURROUGHS, J. T. and D. E. DONALD: Some factors affecting recovery from stoppage of the heart and coronary flow during extracorporeal circulation. Circulation *14*, 917–918, 1956.

BURSTEIN, M. and J. P. BINET: Sur une irrigation artificielle du coeur et de l'encéphale, avec survie de l'animal après exclusion circulatoire momentanée des cavités gauches du coeur. C. R. Acad. Sci. (Paris) *231*, 883–884, 1950.

BURTON, S. D., S. ST. GEORGE and T. ISHIDA: Small volume perfusion system of the isolated rat liver. J. Appl. Physiol. *15*, 128–132, 1960.

BUSTER, C. D., B. C. PEVEHOUSE and H. J. McCORKLE: Cardiovascular changes associated with selective brain cooling in the dog. Surg. Forum *9*, 212–215, 1959.

BUTTERWORTH, R. F.: A device for producing realistic pulsation of a dead heart. J. Thor. Surg. *22*, 316–318, 1951.

BUTTON, L. N., W. F. BERNHARD and C. W. WALTER: In vitro oxygenation of fresh whole blood for arterial perfusion. Arch. Surg. *75*, 183–187, 1957.

C

CAHILL, J. J. and W. J. KOLFF: Hemolysis caused by pumps in extracorporeal circulation (In vitro evaluation of pumps). J. Appl. Physiol. *14*, 1039–1044, 1959.

CALLAGHAN, J. C., F. GERBODE, M. BIRNSTINGL and B. BELMONTE: Reservoir circulation without mechanical pumps for intracardiac surgery under direct vision. Surgical Forum, *6*, 150–154, 1956.

——, R. S. FRASER, J. DVORKIN and A. G. STEWART: The acid-base aspects of extracorporeal circulation. pp. 179–192 *In:* Extracorporeal circulation. J. G. Allen (editor). Springfield III.: Thomas 1958.

CALUZZI, F. and E. CIOCATTO: Der absichtliche Herzstillstand bei chirurgischen Eingriffen am blutleeren Herzen. Anaesthetist *7*, 354–359, 1958.

CAMPBELL, G. S., N. W. CRISP and E. B. BROWN, JR.: Maintenance of respiratory function with isolated lung lobes during cardiac inflow occlusion. Proc. Soc. Exp. Biol. Med. *88*, 390–393, 1955.

——, —— and ——: Total cardiac by-pass in humans utilizing a pump and heterologous

lung oxygenator (dog lungs). Surgery *40*, 364–371, 1956.

CANNON, J. A., LOBPRIES, E. L. and HERROLD, G.: Experience with new electromagnetic flow-meter for use in blood-flow determination in surgery. Ann. Surg. *152*, 634–647, 1960.

CAPPELLETTI, R. R., R. T. DOMINGO, C. DENNIS, N. S. AMER and J. H. STUCKEY: Plasma hemoglobin formulation during critically controlled studies in three pumping systems. Trans. Am. Soc. Art. Int. Organs *7*, 162–166, 1961.

CARMICHAEL, D. B.: Development of a heart–lung machine. J. Amer. Med. Wom. Assn. *14*, 502–504, 1959.

CARR, M. H. and P. R. SCHLOERB: Blood components in the dog: normal values. J. Lab. Clin. Med. *53*, 646–652, 1959.

CARR, E. A., JR., H. E. SLOAN, JR. and E. TOVAR: The clinical importance of erythrocyte and plasma volume determinations before and after open heart surgery. J. Nucl. Med. *1*, 165–173, 1960.

CARREL, A.: Experimental operations on the sigmoid valves of the pulmonary artery. J. Exp. Med. *20*, 9–18, 1914.

—— and C. LINDBERGH: The culture of whole organs, Science *81*, 621–623, 1935.

—— and ——: Culture of organs New York: Hoeber, 1938.

CARTER, D. and D. C. SABISTON: Myocardial metabolism during perfusion of the coronary circulation with gaseous oxygen. Surgery *49*, 625–628, 1961.

CARTWRIGHT, R. S. and W. E. PALICH: Simplified flow determination, volume control, and blood replacement in the rotating disc oxygenator. J. Thor. Cardiov. Surg. *39*, 624–628, 1960a.

—— and ——: An oxygenator for isolation-perfusion in the treatment of cancer. Arch. Surg. *80*, 506–507, 1960b.

——, T. P. K. LIM, U. C. LUFT and W. E. PALICH: A study of the physiological changes in the lungs during cardiopulmonary bypass. Surg. Forum *11*, 226–228, 1960a.

——, G. J. MAGOVERN and E. M. KENT: Cyanosis following cardiopulmonary bypass. Amer. J. Surg. *99*, 8858–90, 1960b.

CASE, R. B., H. FITZPATRICK, H. L. SACHS and P. KEATING: Total coronary flow and myocardial oxygen consumption during cardiopulmonary bypass in the dog. Trans. Am. Soc. Art. Int. Organs *4*, 172–177, 1958.

CASS, M. H.: Restoration of sinus rhythm

following elective cardiac arrest under hypothermia. Guy Hosp. Rep. *108*, 258–261, 1959.

—— and D. V. Ross: The evolution of a bypass technique using the lungs as an oxygenator. Guy Hosp. Rep. *108*, 237–244, 1959.

——, —— and D. G. Taylor: A single-pump bubble oxygenator. Lancet *2*, 621-622, 1958.

Cassie, A., A. Riddell and P. Yates: Hazard of antifoam emboli from a bubble oxygenator. Thorax *15*, 22–29, 1960.

Catchpole, L. A. and P. G. F. Nixon: A hand clamp for plastic tubing. Lancet *2*, 329, 1959a.

—— and ——: A labour saving plate for the Melrose heart and lung machine oxygenator. Lancet *2*, 329, 1959b.

Cate, W. R. Jr., R. N. Sadler, D. M. Seitzman and R. A. Light: Heparin rebound, a clinical and experimental study. Amer. Surgeon *20*, 813–819, 1954.

Chance, B.: Quantitative aspects of the control of oxygen utilization in regulation of cell metabolism. Boston, Little, Brown & Co., 1959.

Chargraff, E. and K. B. Olson: Studies on the chemistry of blood coagulation. VI. Studies on the action of heparin and other anticoagulants. The influence of protamine on the anticoagulant effect in vivo. J. Biol. Chem. *122*, 153–167, 1937/1938.

Cheng, H., T. Kusunoki, L. H. Bosher, R. B. McElvein and D. A. Blake: A study of oxygen consumption during extracorporeal circulation. Trans. Amer. Soc. Art. Int. Organs *5*, 273–276, 1959.

Chevret, R. and H. Besson: Quelques problemes poses par les circulations extracorporelles. Maroc med. *37*, 1314–1317, 1958.

—— and ——: Caracteristiques d'un coeurpoumon artificiel pour la chirurgie à coeur ouvert. Ann. Chir. (Paris) *13*, 1197–1201, 1960.

Cho, M. and L. B. Jaques: Heparinase. Preparation and properties of the enzyme. Canad. J. Biochem. Physiol. *34*, 799–813, 1956.

Churchill-Davidson, H. C.: Discussion on the extracorporeal circulation. Proc. Roy. Soc. Med. *51*, 579–581, 1958.

Cianciarulo, R., L. Sprovieri and C. Lenfant: Ventricular fibrillation in surgery with extracorporeal circulation and cardiac arrest: experimental study. Arq. Bras. Cardiol. *12*, 119–130, 1959.

Cicero, R., C. Mendez, J. Aceves and R.

Mendez: La recuperación del corazón después del paro por citrato de potasio. Arch. Inst. Cardiol. Mex. *29*, 421–439, 1959.

Clark, L. C., Jr.: Optimal flow rate in perfusion. pp. 150-163. *In:* Extracorporeal circulation. J. G. Allen (editor), Springfield, Ill.: Thomas 1958.

——: Blood gas exchange devices. IRE Trans. Med. Electronics *6*, 18–21, 1959.

——, F. Gollan and V. B. Gupta: The oxygenation of blood by gas dispersion. Science. *111*, 85–87, 1950.

——, F. Hooven and F. Gollan: A large capacity, all-glass dispersion oxygenator and pump. Rev. Scient. Instr. *23*, 748–753, 1952.

——, J. A. Helmsworth, S. Kaplan, R. T. Sherman and Taylor, Z.: Polarographic measurement of oxygen tension in whole blood and tissues during total bypass of the heart. Surg. Forum *4*, 93–96, 1953.

——, S. Kaplan, E. C. Matthews, F. K. Edwards and J. A. Helmsworth: Monitor and control of blood oxygen tension and pH during total body perfusion. J. Thorac. Surg. *36*, 488–496, 1958.

——, F. Berg, C. Lyons, S. Kaplan and W. S. Edwards: Continuous perfusion of the arrested heart with arterialized hypocalcemic blood. Surg. Forum *10*, 518–521, 1960.

Clauss, R. H., R. W. Buben and W. A. Altemeier: Selective redistribution of blood in the surgical treatment of aortic insufficiency. Ann. Surg. *150*, 586–594, 1959.

——, Birtwell, W. C., Albertal, G., Lunzer, S., Taylor, W. J., Fosberg, A. M. and Harken, D. E.: Assisted Circulation. I. The Arterial Counterpulsator. J. Thor. Cardiov. Surg. *41*, 447–458, 1961.

Cleland, W. P., and D. G. Melrose: The artificial heart–lung and its practical application to cardiac surgery. Brit. Med. Bull. *11*, 236–239, 1955.

——, A. J. W. Beard, H. H. Bentall, M. B. Bishop, M. V. Braimbridge, L. L. Bromley, J. F. Goodwin, A. Hollman, W. F. Kerr, E. B. Lloyd-Jones, D. G. Melrose and L. J. Telivuo: Treatment of ventricular septal defect. Brit. Med. J. *2*, 1369–1377, 1958.

Cliffe, P., C. Drew, G. Keen and D. B. Benazon: Observations on the electroencephalograph during experimental and clinical cardiopulmonary bypass. Thorax *14*, 97–103, 1959.

Clifton, E. E., C. Grossi and M. Siegel:

Hemorrhage during and after operation secondary to changes in the clotting mechanism. Physiology and methods of control. Surgery *40*, 37–51, 1956.

CLOSE, S. A., W. L. STUSEK, R. C. MEADE, D. LIPLEY and E. H. ELLISON: A method for determination of silicone (Antifoam) content of tissues. Surg. Forum *10*, 581–584, 1960.

CLOWES, G. H. A., JR.: Experimental procedures for entry into the left heart to expose the mitral valve. Ann. surg. *134*, 957–968, 1951.

——: Practical exposure to permit experimental surgical procedures within the left heart. Surg. Forum *2*, 235–240, 1952

——: Extracorporeal maintenance of circulation and respiration. Physiol. Rev. *40*, 826–919, 1960.

—— and L. R. M. DEL GUERCIO: Circulatory response to trauma of surgical operations. Metabolism *9* 67–81, 1960.

—— and W. E. NEVILLE: Experimental exposure of the aortic valve. Surg. Forum *5*, 39–45 1955.

—— and ——: Further development of a blood oxygenator dependent upon the diffusion of gases through plastic membranes. Trans. Amer. Soc. Art. Int. Organs *3*, 52–58, 1957.

—— and ——: Membrane oxygenator. pp. 81–100 *In:* Extracorporeal circulation. J. G. Allen (Editor). Springfield, Ill.: Thommas, 1958.

——, ——, A. HOPKINS, J. ANZOIA and F. A. SIMEONE: Factors contributing to success or failure in the use of a pump oxygenator for complete by-pass of the heart and lung, experimental and clinical. Surgery *36*, 557–579, 1954.

——, A. L. HOPKINS and T. KOLOBOW: Oxygen diffusion through plastic films. Trans. Amer. Soc. Artif. Int. Org. *1*, 23-24, 1955.

——, A. L. HOPKINS and W. E. NEVELL: An artificial lung dependent upon diffusion of of oxygen and carbon dioxide through plastic membranes. J. Thor. Surg. *32*, 630–637, 1956.

——, W. E. NEVILLE, G. SABGA and Y. SHIBOTA: The relationship of oxygen consumption, perfusion rate, and temperature to the acidosis associated with cardiopulmonary circulatory bypass. Surgery *44*, 220–223, 1958.

——, A. ALICHNIEWICZ, L. R. M. DEL GUERCIO and D. GILLESPIE: Relationship of postoperative acidosis to pulmonary and cardiovascular function. J. Thor. Cardiov. Surg. *39*, 1–22, 1960.

COFFIN, L. H. and L. ANKENEY: The effect of extracorporeal circulation upon acid-base equilibrium in dogs. Arch. Surg. *80*, 447–451, 1960.

COFFIN, J. D. and D. E. GREGG: Reactive hyperemia characteristics of the myocardium. Amer. J. Physiol. *199*, 1143–1149, 1960.

COHEN, M. and C. W. LILLEHEI: Autogenous lung oxygenator with total cardiac bypass for intra-cardiac surgery. Surg. Forum *4*, 34–40, 1954.

—— and ——: A quantitative study of the "azygos factor" during vena caval occlusion in the dog. Surg. Gynec. Obstet. *98*, 225–232, 1954.

——, R. N. HAMMERSTROM, M. W. SPELLMAN, R. L. VARCO and C. W. LILLIEHEI: The tolerance of the canine heart to temporary complete vena caval occlusions. Surg. Forum *3*, 172–177, 1953.

——, H. E. WARDEN and C. W. LILLEHEI: Physiologic and metabolic changes during autogenous lobe oxygenation with total cardiac bypass employing the azygos flow principle. Surg. Gynec. Obstet. *98*, 523–529, 1954.

COLERIDGE, J. C. G. and C. KIDD: Electrophysiological evidence of baroreceptors in the pulmonary artery of the dog. J. Physiol. (London) *150*, 319–331, 1960.

CONLEY, C. L., C. R. HARTMANN and J. S. LALLEY: Relation of heparin activity to platelet concentration. Proc. Soc. Exp. Biol. Med. *69*, 284–287, 1948.

CONN, H. L., JR., J. C. WOOD, and G. S. MORALES: Rate of change in myocardial glycogen and lactic acid following arrest of coronary circulation. Circulat. Research *7*, 721–727, 1959.

CONNE, G., C. HAHN, J. J. LIVIO, M. REBAGLIATE and F. SAEGESSER: Avantages et désavantages d'un oxygénateur à bulles "disposable" (appareil de Rygg-Kyvsgaard). Schweiz. Med. Wschr. *25*, 667–681, 1960.

CONNOLLY, J. E., M. B. BACANER, D. L.. BRUNS, J. M. LOWENSTEIN and E. STORLI: Mechanical support of the circulation in acute heart failure. Surgery *44*, 255-262. 1958a.

——, ——, ——, —— and ——: The effect of veno-arterial bypass on coronary blood flow. Arch. Surg. *81*, 58–60, 1960.

——, V. RICHARDS, E. J. HARRIS and S.HOL-

MAN: Total cardiopulmonary bypass using experimental intravenous oxygenation. Surg. Forum, *8*, 413–416,1958b.

COOKSON, B. A., and K. COSTAS-DURIEUX: The use of arterial transfusion as an adjunct to hypothermia in the repair of septal defects. Ann. Surg. *140*, 100–106, 1954.

——, —— and C. P. BAILEY: The toxic effects of citrated blood and the search for a suitable substitute for use in cardiac surgery. Ann. Surg. *139*, 430–438, 1954.

COOLEY, D. A., B. A. BELMONTE, M. E. DEBAKEY and F. R. LATSON: Temporary extracorporeal circulation in the surgical treatment of cardiac and aortic disease. (Report of 98 cases). Ann. Surg. *145*, 898–914, 1957.

——, ——, J. R. LATSON, and J. R. PIERCE: Bubble diffusion oxygenator for cardiopulmonary by-pass. J. Thor. Surg. *35*, 131–134, 1958a.

——, H. A. COLLINS, J. W. GIACOBINE, G. C. MORRIS JR., L. R. SOLTERO-HARRINGTON and F. J. HARBERG: The pump oxygenator in cardiovascular surgery: observations based upon 450 cases. Amer. Surgeon *24*, 870–882, 1958b.

——, J. R. LADSON and A. S. KEATS: Surgical considerations in repair of ventricular and atrial septal defects utilizing cardiopulmonary bypass. Surgery *43*, 214–225, 1958c.

COONS, R. E., A. S. KEATS and D. A. COOLEY: Significance of electroencephalographic changes occuring during cardiopulmonary bypass. Anesthesiology *20*, 804–810, 1959.

COOPER, A. : Some experiments and observations on tying the carotid and vertebral arteries and the pneumo-gastric, phrenic and sympathetic nerves. Guy Hosp. Rep. *1*, 457–475, 1836.

COOPER, K. E.: The circulation in hypothermia. Brit. Med. Bull. *17*, 48–51, 1961.

COOPER, T., V. L. WILLMAN, P. ZAFIRACOPOULOS and C. R. HANLON: Myocardial function after elective cardiac arrest during hypothermia. Surg. Gynec. Obstet. *109*, 423–426, 1959a.

——, ——, —— and ——: Use of cardiotonic agent (mephentermine) in myocardial depression due to potassium. Arch. Surg. *79*, 734–737, 1959b.

——, ——, —— and —— : Effect of prophylactic digitalization on myocardial function after elective cardiac arrest. Ann. Surg. *151*, 17–21, 1960.

CORDELL, A. R. and M. P. SPENCER: Electro-

magnetic blood flow measurements in extracorporeal circuits. IRE Trans. Med. Electronics, ME-6, 228–231, 1959.

—— and ——: Electromagnetic blood flow measurement in extracorporeal circuits: Its application to cardiopulmonary bypass. Ann. Surg. *151*, 71–74,1960.

——, —— and J. H. MEREDITH: Studies of peripheral vascular resistance associated with total cardiopulmonary bypass. I. Peripheral resistance under condition of normothermia and normotension. J. Thor. Cardiov. Surg. *40*, 421–427, 1960.

CORSSEN, G., G. W. EGGERS JR., J. R. DERRICK and C. R. ALLEN: Pharmacodynamic management of cardiac action during deep hypothermia. South. Med. J. *52*, 1009–1015, 1959.

CORTESINI, R., P. MICOZZI, M. MOGAVERO, P. NOVELLI and A. VENTURINI: Studio dell'ossimetria e del flússo coronarico durante la circolazione extracorporea e durante l'esecuzione dell'arresto cardiaco farmacologico. Arch. chir. Torace, *16*, 205–219, 1959.

——, F. TRANI, G. PEZZOLI and P. MICOZZI: Il ruolo del circolo bronchiale in chirurgia cardiaca. II. Cause delle alterazioni cardiopolmonari durante la circolazione extracorporea e loro prevenzione mediante la decompressione della cavità sinistre. Arch. Chir. Torace *17*, 69–86, 1960.

COSTANTINI, A., G. DE POLI, L. CALDAROLA, L. PIRONTI and C. BESSE: La nostra macchina cardiopolmonare. Minerva med. *44*, 1249–1254 1953a.

——, ——, ——, —— and ——: Presentazione di un caso clinico di circolazione sanguina extracorporea parziale. Minerva Med. *44*, 1272–1273, 1953b.

COULTER, N. A. JR. and J. R. PAPPENHEIMER: Development of turbulence in flowing blood. Amr. J. Physiol. *159*, 401–408, 1949.

COVINO, B. G. and W. R. BEAVERS: Changes in cardiac contractility during immersion hypothermia. Amer. J. Physiol. *195*, 433–436, 1958.

COWAN, R.: Physiological perfusion pump. J. Appl. Physiol. *4*, 695–697, 1952.

CRAFOORD, C. : Some aspects of the development of intrathoracic surgery. Surg. Gynec. Obstet. *89*, 629–637, 1949.

——: Operationen am offenen Herzen mit Herz-Lungen–Maschine (Stockholmer Modell). Langenbeck Arch. Klin. Chir. *289*. 257–266, 1958.

—— and E. JORPES: Heparing as a prophylactic against thrombosis. J. A. M. A. *116*, 2831–2835, 1941.

——, B. NORBERG and A. SENNING: Clinical studies in extracorporeal circulation with a heart-lung machine. Acta Chir. Scand. *112*, 220–245, 1957a.

——, —— and —— : Disturbances in fluid and electrolyte balance after extracorporeal circulation. Acta. Chir. Scand. *113*, 415–417, 1957b.

——, L. JOHANSSON, B. JONSSON, O. NOR-LANDER and A. SENNING: Klinische Erfahrungen mit extracorporalem Kreislauf. Langenbeck Arch. Klin. Chir. *292*, 709–710, 1959.

CRAIG, L. C. and W. KONIGSBERG: Dialysis studies. III. Modification of pore size and shape in cellophane membranes. J. Physical Chem. *65*, 166–171, 1961.

CREECH, O.: Recent advances in cardiovascular surgery. Surgery *47*, 500–519, 1960.

——, E. BRESLER, M. HOLLEY and M. ADAM: Cerebral blood flow during extracorporeal circulation. Surg. Forum *8*, 510–514, 1958.

CRESCENZI, A. A., P. C. HOFSTRA, A. DI-BENEDETTO, K. C. SZE, B. H. FOSTER, P. GLASS, C. L. CLAFF and P. COOPER: Development of a simplified membrane oxygenator. Trans. Amer. Soc. Art. Int. Organs *5*, 148–153, 1959.

——, ——, K. C. SZE, B. H. FOSTER, C. L. CLAFF and P. COOPER: Development of a simplified disposable membrane oxygenator. Surg. Forum *10*, 610–612, 1960.

CRISP, N. W. JR., G. S. CAMPBELL and E. B. BROWN, JR.: Studies on perfusion of human blood through the isolated dog lung. Surg. Forum *6*, 286–290, 1956.

CROSBY, W. H.: Problem of oozing during surgery. Anesthesiology *20*, 685–696, 1959.

CROSS, C. E., K. KATSUHARA, P. A. RIEBEN and P. F. SALISBURY: Edema of the heart muscle: A criterion for detecting oxygenator toxicity. Trans. Amer. Soc. Art. Int. Organs *7*, 185–186, 1961.

CROSS, F. S. and R. D. JONES: A new type of suction tip especially designed for intracardiac surgery. J. Thor. Cardiov. Surg. *41*, 412–415, 1961.

——, R. M. BERNE, Y. HIROSE and E. B. KAY: Description and evaluation of a rotating disc type reservoir-oxygenator. Surg. Forum *7*, 274–278, 1956a.

——, ——, ——, —— and ——: Evaluation of a rotating disc type reservoir-oxygena-tor. Proc. Soc. Exp. Biol. Med. *93*, 210–214, 1956b.

CROSS, S. B.: Some factors governing the efficiency of blood perfusion pumps. Quart. J. Exp. Phys. *42*, 386, 1957.

CRUISKSHANK, C. N. D., C. HOOPER, H. B. M. LEWIS and J. D. B. MACDOUGALL: The toxicity of rubbers and plastics used in transfusion-giving sets. J. Clin. Pathol. *13*, 42–50, 1960.

CRUICKSHANK, E. W. H.: A magnetic blood oxygenator. J. Physiol. (London) *82*, 26–32, 1934.

CRUZ, W. O., and A. BAUMGARTEN: Iso-hemodynamic transfusion followed by severe hypotension in normal dogs. Acta Physiol. Lat. Amer. *8*, 11–21, 1958.

——, A. C. OLIVEIRA and M. M. OLIVEIRA: Behavior of heparinized arterial blood on hemostasis in the dog hind-leg preparation. Amer. J. Med. Sci. *240*, 447–457, 1960.

D

DAGHER, I. K.: Pressure membrane oxygenator. J. Thor. Surg. *37*, 100–107, 1959.

DAHLBACK, O., L. T. DELANEY, L. E. GELIN, J. KUGELBURG, E. LINDER and S. E. NILSSON: A plasma substitute in extracorporeal circulation: an attempt to minimize the damage to the blood; a preliminary experimental report. Acta. Chir. Scand. *245*, 265–268, 1959.

DALE, H. H. and E. A. SCHUSTER: A double perfusion pump. J. Physiol. (London) *64*, 356–364, 1928.

DALY, I DE B. : A seven horse power Austin engine adopted as a blood pump. J. Physiol. (London) *77*, 36–37p, 1933.

——, P. EGGLETON, C. O. HEBB, J. L. LIN-ZELL and O. A. TROWELL: Observations on the perfused living animal (dog) using homologous and heterologous blood. Quart. J. Exper. Physiol. *39*, 29–54, 1954.

DARBINIAN, T. M. and V. F. PORTNOY: Deep hypothermia. Eksp. Khir. Anest. *1*, 52–61, 1961 (*Rus.*).

DARBY, T. D., E. F. PARKER, W. H. LEE, JR., and J. D. ASHMORE: The influence of cardiopulmonary bypass with cardiac arrest and right ventriculotomy on myocardial contractile force. Ann. Surg. *147*, 596–602, 1958.

DAVENPORT, H. T., G. ARFEL and F. R. SANCHEZ: The electroencephalogram in patients undergoing open heart surgery with heart-lung bypass. Anesthesiology, *20*, 674–684, 1959.

DAVENPORT, H. W.: The A B C of acid base chemistry - 4th ed. The University of Chicago Press, Chicago: 1958.

DAVIES, J. T.: The importance of surfaces in chemical engineering. Trans. Inst. Chem. Engineers *38*, 289–293, 1960.

——, I. M. RITCHIE and D. C. SOUTHWARD: Surface effects in a rotating disc contractor. Trans. Inst. Chem. Engineers *38*, 331–334, 1960.

DAWES, G. S., J. C. MOTT and M. S. SHELLEY: The importance of cardiac glycogen for the maintenance of life in foetal lambs and new born animals during anoxia. J. Physiol. (London) *146*, 516–538, 1959.

DAWSON, B., R. A. THEYE and J. W. KIRKLIN: Halothane in open cardiac operations: a technic for use with extracorporeal circulation. Anesth. Analg. *39*, 59–63, 1960.

DEBAKEY, M. E.: A simple continuous flow blood transfusion instrument. New Orleans Med. Surg. J. *87*, 386–389, 1934.

DEI POLI, G., L. CALDEROLA, L. PIRONTI and C. BESSE: Sulla circolazione sanguina extracorporea; Ricerche sperimentali. Minerva Med. *44*, 1255–1260, 1953a.

——, ——, V. FANTINO, C. ORECCHIA and E. PERAZZO: Il cuore-polmone artificiale quale mezzo di rianimazione degli elettrotraumatizzati. Minerva Med. *44*, 1261-1264, 1953b.

——, ——, C. ORECCHIA, E. PERAZZO and V. FANTINO: Il cuore-polmone artificiale quale mezzo eroico di rianimazione del'annegato. Minerva med. *44*, 1264–1270, 1953c.

——, ——, V. FANTINO, C. ORECCHIA and E. PERAZZO: Il cuore-polmone artificiale pue essere utilmente applicato a casi di avvelenamento da ossido di carbonio. Minerva Med. *44*, 1270–1272, 1953d.

DELORME, E. J.: Experimental cooling of the blood stream. Lancet *2*, 914–915, 1952.

——: Hypothermia in dogs. Technical Report ONRL-83-53, Office of Naval Research, Lond. 1953.

——: Hypothermia. Brit. Med. Bull. *11*, 221–225, 1955.

DEMETRAKOPOULOS, N. J., T. W. SHIELDS, and F. J. LEWIS: Experimental and clinical application of a pump for partial and total aortic bypass. J. Thor. Cardiov. Surg. *38*, 179–185, 1959.

DEMIKOV, V. P.: Experimental basis for replacement of the heart by a mechanical device in acute experiments. Biull. Eskp. Biol. Med. *32*, 22–24, 1951 (*Rus*).

DENNIS, C.: Certain methods for artificial support of the circulation during intracardiac surgery. Surg. Clin. N. Amer. *36*, 423–436, 1956.

—— and K. E. KARLSON: The multiple screen disc oxygenator, p. 69–80 *In:* Extracorporeal Circulation, J. G. Allen (editor) Springfield, Ill.: Thomas, 1958.

——, —— and D. SANDERSON: Pump-oxygenator to support the systemic circulation during the surgical approach to the heart. Presented before the 35th Clin. Cong. Amer. Coll. Surg. Chicago, 1949.

——, D. S. SPRENG JR., G. E. NELSON, K. E. KARLSON, R. M. NELSON, J. V. THOMAS, W. P. EDER and R. L. VARCO: Development of a pump oxygenator to replace the heart and lungs; an apparatus applicable to human patients and application to one case. Ann. Surg. *134*, 709–721, 1951a.

——, K. E. KARLSON, W. P. EDER, R. M. NELSON, F. P. EDDY and D. SANDERSON: Pump-oxygenator to supplant the heart and lungs for brief periods. Surgery *29*, 697–713, 1951b.

DEPRADE, P., R. LEFEBRE DES NOETTES, S. RICHARD and J. C. GOUNELLE: Analyse critique d'une méthode d'enregistrement continu du pH sanguin artériel. C. R. Soc. Biol. (Paris) *154*, 2033–2036, 1960.

DETTLI, L., F. FRUN and K. BUCHER: Probleme des Gasaustausches in der Lunge. Zur Bestimmung des permeationsfähigen Anteils der Kohlensäure in wässrigen Carbonatlösungen. Helv. Physiol. Pharmacol. Acta *13*, 32–41, 1955.

DEUCHAR, D. C. and F. H. MUIR: Electrocardiographic changes during cardiac operations performed with a pump oxygenator. Guy Hosp. Rep. *108*, 218–236, 1959.

DEVIN, R., E. JEAN and H. RICHELME: La chirurgie intracardiaque sous circulation extracorporelle; étude expérimentale et déductions cliniques. Marseille chir. *11*, 16–40, 1959.

DEWALL, R. A. and C. W. LILLEHEI: Design and clinical application of the helix reservoir pump-oxygenator system for extracorporeal circulation. Post-Grad. Med. *23*, 561–573, 1958.

——, H. E. WARDEN, V. L. GOTT, R. C. READ, R. L. VARCO and C. W. LILLEHEI: Total body perfusion for open cardiotomy utilizing the bubble oxygenator. J. Thor. Surg. *32*, 591–603, 1956a.

——, ——, R. C. READ, V. L. GOTT, N. R. ZIEGLER, R. L. VARCO and C. W. LILLEHEI: A simple, expendable, artificial oxygenator for open-heart surgery. Surg. Clin. N. Amer. *36*, 1025–1034, 1956b.

——, ——, J. C. MELBY, H. MINOT, R. L. VARCO and C. W. LILLEHEI: Physiological responses during total body perdusion with a pump-oxygenator. J.A.M.A. *165*, 1788–1792, 1957a.

——, C. W. LILLEHEI, R. L. VARCO and H. E. WARDEN: The helix reservoir pump-oxygenator. Surg. Gynec. Obstet. *104*, 699–710, 1957b.

——, V. L. GOTT, C. W. LILLEHEI and R. L. VARCO: The surgical treatment of stenotic or regurgitant lesions of the mitral and aortic valves by direct vision utilizing a pump-oxygenator. J. Thor. Surg. *35*, 154–190, 1958.

——, D. M. LONG, S. J. DEMILL and C. W. LILLEHEI: Certain blood changes in patients undergoing extracorporeal circulation. J. Thor. Surg. *37*, 325–333, 1959.

DEXTER, D., H. B. STONER and H. N. GREEN: The release of posterior pituitary antidiuretic hormone by adenosine triphosphate. J. Endocrinol. *11*, 142–159, 1954.

DICK, M.: The respiratory and circulatory responses to intravenous oxygen and their relation to anoxemia. Amer. J. Physiol., *127*, 228–231, 1939.

DICKENS, F.: The toxic effects of oxygen on brain metabolism and on tissue enzymes. I. Brain metabolism. Biochem. J. *40*, 145–171, 1946.

DICKSON, J. F. III, J. W. DOW, and N. A. J. HAMER: Prolonged veno-arterial pumping for circulation support. Trans. Amer. Soc. Art. Int. Organs *5*, 210–217, 1959a.

——, —— and ——: Prolonged venoarterial pumping for circulation support. Arch. Intern. Med. *106*, 639–646, 1960a.

——, N. A. J. HAMER and J. W. DOW: A system for veno-arterial pumping, Surgery, 288–291, 1959b.

——, ——, and ——: Veno-arterial pumping for relief of intractable cardiac failure in man. Arch. Surg. *78*, 418–421, 1959c.

——, —— and ——: The effects of venoarterial pumping for circulation support. Arch. Surg. *80*, 830–837, 1960b.

DIDISHEIM, P., K. HATTORI and J. LEWIS: Hematologic and coagulation studies in various animal species. J. Lab. Clin. Med. *53*, 866–875, 1959.

DIESH, G. , P. J. FLYNN, S. A. MARABLE, D. G. MULDER, K. J. SCHMUTZER, W. P. LONGMIRE, JR., and J. V. MALONEY, JR.: Comparison of low (azygos) and high flow principles of extracorporeal circulation employing a bubble oxygenator. Surgery *42*, 67–72, 1957.

DIETMANN, K.: Extracorporaler Kreislauf und künstliche Unterkühlung. Deutsch. Med. Wschr. *80*, 498–502, 1955.

DIETTERT, G. A., B. A. BERCU, W. H. DANFORTH, and E. E. PUND, JR.: A disposable screen oxygenator. Ann. Surg. *148*, 959–967, 1958a.

——, —— and T. B. FERGUSON: The use of a modified Gibbon-type pump oxygenator. I. Description of the apparatus. J. Thor. Surg. *35*, 416–420, 1958b.

DILL, D. B. and W. H. FORBES: Respiratory and metabolic effects of hypothermia. Amer. J. Physiol. *132*, 685–697, 1941.

DIXON, W. G.: Does tranfusion citrate cause hemorrage? Amer. Surg. *24*, 818–821, 1958.

DOBELL, A. R. C., J. R. GUTELIUS and D. R. MURPHY: Acidosis following respiratory alkalosis in thoracic operations with and without heart-lung bypass. J. Thor. Cardiov. Surg. *39*, 312–317, 1960.

DODRILL, F. D.: Experiences with the mechanical heart. J. A. M. A. *154*, 299–304, 1954.

——: The arterialization of blood with comment on two human perfusions. Trans. Amer. Soc. Art. Int. Organs *1*, 65–67, 1955.

——: The effects of total body perfusion upon the lungs. pp 327–335 *In:* Extracorporeal circulation, J. G. ALLEN (Editor), Springfield, Ill.: Thomas, 1958.

——, E. HILL and R. A. GERISH: Some physiologis aspects of the artificial heart problem. J. Thor. Surg. *24*, 134–150, 1952a.

——, —— and ——: Temporary mechanical substitute for the left ventricle in man. J. A. M. A. *150*, 642–644, 1952b.

——, ——, —— and A. JOHNSON: Pulmonary valvuloplasty under direct vision using the mechanical heart for a complete bypass of the right heart in a patient with congenital pulmonary stenosis. J. Thor. Surg. *26*, 584–597, 1953.

——, A. LUI, J. NYBOER, E. V. RIPPINGILLE and C. H. HUGHES: The arterialization of blood as it applies to the mechanical heartlung apparatus. J. Thor. Surg.*30*, 658–664, 1955.

——, N. MARSHALL, ——, C. H. HUGHES, H. J. DERBYSHIRE and A. B. STEARNS: The use of heart-lung apparatus in human cardiac surgery. J. Thor. Surg. *33*, 6–73, 1957.

—— and S. TAKAGI: The use of anaerobic energy in elective cardiac arrest. Surgery, *47*, 314–319, 1960.

DOGLIOTTI, A. M.: Clinical use of the artificial circulation with a note on intra-arterial transfusion. Bull. Johns Hopkins Hosp. *90*, 131–133, 1952.

—— and E. CIOCATTO: Les bases physiopathologiques de l'hypothermie et les possibilités de l'association hypothermie-circulation extracorporelle. Lyon Chir. *49*, 19–24, 1954.

—— and A. CONSTANTINI: Primo caso di applicazione all'uomo di un apparecchio di circulazione sanguinea extracoporea. Minerva Chir. *6*, 657–663, 1951.

——, G. DEI POLI and L. CALDAROLA: A cardiopulmonary machine for extracorporeal circulation of blood. J. Int. Coll. Surg. *22*, 107–114, 1954.

——, M. BATTEZZATTI, C. TADDEI, G. B. GEMMA, A. D. CATTANEO, R. WEISZ, B. TORCHIANA and V. BACHI: Circolazione assistita nell' uomo. V. Minerva Chir. *13*, 1454–1455, 1958.

DONALD, D. E. and E. A. MOFFITT: Studies in extracorporeal circulation III. The relation of blood flow and blood volume during extracorporeal circulation in man. Surg. Forum, *7*, 264–267, 1957.

—— and ——: Relation of temperature, gas tension and hydrostatic pressure to the formation of gas bubbles in extracorporeally oxygenated blood. Surg. Forum, *10*, 589–592, 1960.

——, H. G. HARSHBARGER, P. S. HETZEL, R. T. PATRICK, E. H. WOOD and J. W. KIRKLIN: Experiences with a heart-lung bypass (Gibbon-type) in the experimental laboratory: preliminary report. Proc. Mayo Clin. *30*, 113–115, 1955.

——, —— and J. W. KIRKLIN: Studies in extracorporeal circulation. II. A method for the recovery and use of blood from the open heart during extracorporeal circulation in man. Ann. Surg. *144*, 223–227, 1956.

DONALD, K. W.: Oxygen poisoning in man. Brit. Med. J. *1*, 667–672, and 712–717, 1947.

DONATI, M.: Osservazioni sulla conservazione del sangue mediante ACD + inosina. La trasfusione del sangue *2*, 33–40, 1957.

—— and G. ABOZZO: L'inosina nella conservazione dei globuli rossi prove in vitro. La Trasfusione del Sangue *4*, 57–64, 1959.

DONOVAN, T. J.: The uses of plastic tubes in the reparative surgery of battle injuries to arteries with and without intra-arterial heparin administration. Ann. Surg. *130*, 1024–1043, 1949.

DORSEY, A. E.: Control of foam during fermentation by the application of ultrasonic energy. J. Biochem. Microbiol. Techn. Engin. *1*, 289–295, 1959.

DOW, J. W.: In discussion of physiology of perfusion. pp. 220–221 *In:* Extracorporeal Circulation, J. G. Allen (editor), Springfield, Ill.: Thomas, 1958.

——, J. F. DICKSON, III, N. A. J. HAMER and H. L. GADBOYS: The shock state in heart-lung bypass in dogs. Trans. Amer. Soc. Art. Int. Organs *5*, 240–247, 1959.

——, —— and ——: Experimental evaluation of venoarterial pumping. A proposed technique for circulation support. Dis. Chest *38*, 323–331, 1960a.

——, ——, —— and H. L. GADBOYS: The effects of anaphylactoid shock from blood exchange on cardiopulmonary bypass in the dog. J. Thor. Cardiov. Surg. *39*, 457–463, 1960b.

DOYLE, J. E., A. E. MAC NEILL, R. ANTHONE and S. ANTHONE: Clinical application of new blood pump. Circulation *14*, 928, 1956.

DREW, G. E.: Profound hypothermia in cardiac surgery. Brit. Med. Bull. *17*, 37–42, 1961.

—— and I. M. ANDERSON: Profound hypothermia in cardiac surgery. Lancet, *1*, 748–750, 1959.

——, P. CLIFFE, C. F. SCURR, D. M. FORREST, D. J. PEARCE, P. A. KING, H. M. T. COLES, V. M. LEVEAUX and J. F. SILVA: Experimental approach to visual intracardiac surgery, using an extracorporeal circulation. Brit. Med. J. *2*, 1323–1329, 1957.

——, G. KEEN and D. B. BENAZON: Profound hypothermia. Lancet *1*, 745–747, 1959.

DRINKER, C. K., K. R. DRINKER and C. C. LUND: Circulation in the mammalian bone marrow. Amer. J. Physiol. *62*, 1–92, 1922.

DRIPPS, R. R. (editor): Physiology of induced hypothermia. Washington, D. C.: National Acad. Sc., Nation. Res. Council, 1956.

DUBBELMAN, C. P.: A perfusion pump of a capacity equal to that of the human heart. Acta Physiol. Pharmacol. Neerl., *2*, 157–179, 1951/1952a.

——: Attempts to construct an oxygenator for temporary replacement of the human lung. Acta Physiol. Pharmacol. Neerl. *2*, 320–348, 1951/1952b.

——: Experiments with an artificial heart-lung apparatus. Acta Physiol. Pharmacol. Neerl. *2*, 465–504, 1951/1952c.

DUBOST, C., and P. BLONDEAU: The association of the artificial heart-lung with deep hypothermia in open heart surgery. J. Cardiov. Surg. *1*, 85–93, 1960.

——, G. NAHAS, C. LENFANT, J. PASETECQ, J. GUERY, J. ROUANET, M. WEISS and R. HEIM DE BALSAC: Chirurgie à coeur ouvert sous circulation extracorporelle: Ensemble pompe-oxygénateur de Lillehei-DeWall. Poumon-Coeur *12*, 641–651, 1956.

——, C. LENFANT, I. PASSELECQ, I. GUERY, M. WEISS, P. BLONDEAU and R. HEIM DE BALSAC: La chirurgie des cardiopathies congénitales sous circulation extracorporelle: la place de l'arrêt cardiaque provoqué. Minerva Chir. *13*, 1385–1388, 1958.

——, P. BLONDEAU and A. PIWNICA: L'association du coeur-poumon artificiel et de l'hypothermie profonde dans la chirurgie à coeur ouvert. Cardiologia *38*, 158–171, 1961.

DUBOURG, G. F. FONTAN, D. COTTIN, H. BRICAUD and P. BROUSTET: Arrêt du coeur par anoxie en circulation extracorporelle. Sem. Hop. Paris *35*, 3081–3085, 1959.

DUCUING, J., A. ENJALBERT, H. ESCHAPASSE, J. MATHE, G. ESPAGNO, F. VAHDAT and A. GRAULLE: Notre expérimentation de la chirurgie du coeur ouvert avec le système pompe-oxygénateur de Lillehei-DeWall. Marseille Chir. *9*, 263–271, 1957.

DUNCAN, G. G., L. TOCANTINS and T. D. CUTTLE: Application in man of a method for continuous reciprocal transfer of blood. Proc. Soc. Exp. Biol. Med. *44*, 196–198, 1940.

DUSSER DE BARENNE, J. G.: Ueber den Einfluss der Blaehung der einen Herzkammer auf die Taetigkeit der anderen. Pflüger Arch. Ges. Physiol. *177*, 217–231, 1919.

E

ECKSTEIN, R. W., J. A. McEACHEN, J. DEMMING and W. B. NEWBERRY, JR.: A special cannula for determination of blood flow in the left common coronary artery of the dog. Science *113*, 385–386, 1951.

EDMARK, K.: Continuous blood pH measurement with extracorporeal cooling. Surg. Gynec. Obstet. *109*, 743–749, 1959.

EDMUNDS, L. H., AUSTEN, W. C., R. S. SHAW and S. KOZMINSKI: Clinical and physiologic considerations of left heart by-pass during cardiac arrest. J. Thor. Cardiov. Surg. *41*, 356–367, 1961.

EDWARDS, J. F. JR. and L. H. BOSHER, JR.: Application of closed loop servo control to cardiopulmonary bypass. Trans. Am. Soc. Art. Int. Organs *6*, 338–347, 1960.

—— and ——: Physiologically responsive closed loop servo in the control of cardiopulmonary bypass. Trans. Amer. Soc. Art. Int. Organs *7*, 175–179, 1961.

EDWARDS, W. S.: Improved technique of use of homologous lungs as an oxygenator. Trans. Am. Soc. Art. Int. Organs *3*, 43–45, 1957.

EERLAND, L. D.: Intracardialer Verschluss isolierter Ventrikelseptumdefekte mit Hilfe einer Herz-Lungen Maschine. Thoraxchirurgie *6*, 277–301, 1959.

——, R. BRINKMAN, C. R. RITSEMA VAN ECK, J. N. HOMAN VAN DE HEIDE and J. C. DORLAS: Extracorporeal circulation as an aid in direct vision intracardiac surgery. Proc. Koninkl. Ned. Akad. Wetenschap. *60*, 579–589 and 590–602, 1957.

EFFLER, D. B. and L. K. GROVES: Elective cardiac arrest with potassium citrate. pp. 459–465 *In:* Extracorporeal circulation, J. G. Allen (editor) Springfield, Ill. Thomas, 1958.

——, ——, F. M. SONES and W. J. KOLFF: Elective cardiac arrest in open-heart surgery. Report of three cases. Cleveland Clin. Quart. *23*, 105–114, 1956.

——, H. F. KNIGHT JR., L. K. GROVES and W. K. KOLFF: Elective cardiac arrest for open-heart surgery. Surg. Gynec. Obstet. *105*, 405–416, 1957.

——, W. J. KOLFF and L. K. GROVES: Complications peculiar to open heart surgery. Surgery *45*, 149–156, 1959.

EGDAHL, R. H.: The physiological basis of uncontrolled cross-circulation in dogs. Am. J. Physiol. *182*, 454–458, 1955.

EHRENHAFT, J. L. and M. A. CLAMAN: Cerebral complications of open-heart surgery. J. Thor. Cardiov. Surg. *41*, 503–508, 1961.

EIBER, H. B. and I. DANISHEFSKY: Fate of injected heparin. Trans. Am. Soc. Art. Int. Organs *4*, 152–156, 1958.

EICHOLTZ, F. and E. B. VERNEY: Conditions effecting perfusion of isolated mammalian organs. J. Physiol. (London) *59*, 340–344, 1924.

EISEMAN, B., B. J. BAXTER and K. PRACHUABMOH: Surface tension reducing substances in the management of coronary air embolism. Ann. Surg. *149*, 374–380, 1959.

ELDER, W. J.: Intravascular cannulae for use with an artificial kidney. Lancet *1*, 702, 1961.

ELLIOT, E. C. and J. C. CALLAGHAN: All plastic ventricle-type pump with tricuspid valves. Canad. J. Surg. *1*, 308–312, 1958.

—— and ——: Study of the effects of controlled cardiac output in thoracotomized dogs. Surg. Forum *9*, 189–192, 1959a.

—— and ——: Acid-base changes in dogs with and without extracorporeal circulation. Canad. J. Surg. *2*, 185–190, 1959b.

EMBLY, E. H. and C. J. MARTIN: The action of anesthetic quantities of chloroform upon the blood vessels of the bowel and kidney. With an account of an artificial circulation apparatus. J. Physiol. (London) *32*, 147–158, 1905.

ENERSON, D. M., F. SEBENING and J. F. NEVILLE JR.: Relationship of the selective cooling index to the rate of cooling with internal hypothermia. Surg. Forum *10*, 571–573, 1960.

ENGBAEK, L.: The pharmacological actions of magnesium ions with particular reference to neuromuscular and cardiovascular system. Pharmacol. Rev. *4*, 396–414, 1952.

ENGEL, H. C.: Demands made on a heart-lung machine. Act. Chir. Scandin. *112*, 429–433, 1956.

EPSTEIN, P. S. and J. PLESSET: On the stability of gas bubbles in liquid-gas solutions. J. Chem. Phys. *18*, 1505–1509, 1950.

ERICKSON, H. and S. HJORT: Discussion on the heart-lung machines. Act. Chir. Scandin. *112*, 442–444, 1956.

ERNST, E., A. NIEDETSKY and M. MAJNAL: Energiespeicherung bei rewersibler Arretierung des Herzens durch KCl. Act. Physiol. Acad. Sci. Hung. *16*, 71–76, 1959.

ESMOND, W. G. and R. A. COWLEY: Single use disposable disc oxygenator for open heart surgery. Am. Surgeon *24*, 685–688, 1958.

——, A. D. DEMETRIADES and R. A. COWLEY: A complete integrated pump-oxygenator system with disposable plastic disc oxygenators. Trans. Am. Soc. Art. Int. Organs *5*, 163–170, 1959.

——, J. R. STRAM, W. KURAD, J. CHYBA, S. ATTAR and R. A. COWLEY: Design and application of a disposable stainless steel blood heat exchanger with the integrated disposable plastic disc oxygenation system. Trans. Amer. Soc. Art. Int. Organs *6*, 360–367, 1960.

——, S. ATTAR, B. BAKER, J. CHYBA, A. D. DEMETRIADES and R. A. COWLEY: An improved 360° single roller spring-loaded blood pump. Trans. Amer. Soc. Art. Int. Organs *7*, 167–174, 1961.

VON EULER, U. S. and C. HEYMANS: An oxygenator for perfusion experiments. J. Physiol. (London) *74*, 2–3P, 1932.

F

FAGGELLA, M. L., M. N. ZUHDI, A. E. GREER, J. M. CAREY and J. A. SCHILLING: A method of eliminating air bubbles in a bubble-type oxygenator. Amer. J. Surg. *96*, 696–697, 1958.

FAIRLEY, H. B.: Metabolism in hypothermia. Brit. Med. Bull. *17*, 52–55, 1961.

FAIRLEY, N. H.: Fate of extracorpuscular circulating hemoglobin. Brit. Med. J. *2*, 213–217, 1940.

FAJERS, C. M. and L. E. GELIN: Kidney, liver, and heart-damage from trauma and from induced intravascular aggregation of blood cells: An experimental study. Act. Path. Microbiol. Scandin. *46*, 97–104, 1959.

FALOR, W. H., C. R. BOECKMAN and J. G. VALLEE: A modified DeBakey heart pump for use in extracorporeal circulation. Surgery *43*, 637–641, 1958.

FANTL, P. and H. A. WARD: Blood coagulation problems in open-heart surgery. Thorax *15*, 292–298, 1960.

FAUTEUX, M.: Chirurgie intracardiaque; arrêt temporaire de la circulation par occlusion des veines caves ou de l'artère pulmonaire comme temps préliminaire; étude expérimentale. Union Med. Canada *76*, 1036–1048, 1947.

FELIPOZZI, H. J., R. G. SANTOS and L. G. D'OLIVEIRA: Surgery under direct vision for the correction of pulmonary stenosis with intact ventricular septum. Surgery *41*, 227–235, 1957.

——, J. C. D'OLIVEIRA, S. PALADINO, A. B. LIMA, A. NICOLAI, R. G. SANTOS, J. S. PERFEITO, P. GERETTO, M. V. MARTIN and J. M. H. SOBRINHO: Correcao cirurgica do septo auricular sob controle da visao, com o emprego de um novo conjunto coracao-pulmao artificial. Revista Paulista de Medicina *52*, 157–168, 1958.

FERBERS, E. W. and J. W. KIRKLIN: Studies of hemolysis with a plastic sheet bubble oxygenator. J. Thor. Surg. *36*, 23–32, 1958.

FEINBERG, H., A. GEROLA, L. N. KATZ and E. BOYD: Effect of hypoxia on cardiac oxygen consumption and coronary flow. Amer. J. Physiol. *195*, 593–600, 1958.

FERUGLIO, G. and P. ZIGLIOTTO: Rilievi elettrocardiographici su animali sottoposti ad arresto cardiaco controllato mediante l'impiego di una miscela farmacologica nella chirurgia a cuore aperto. Minerva Cardioangiol. *7*, 518–524, 1959.

——, B. MIGUELI, S. CAMPUS and G. PANDOLFO: Studi sulla circolazione d'organo: determinazione simultanea del flusso coronarico, cerebrale e renale, della portata cardiaca e del consumo di O_2 del cuore, del cervello e del rene. Boll. Soc. Ital. Biol. Sper. *36*, 952–954, 1960.

FIELD, L. W., D. DE GRAFF and A. T. WALLIS: Constant output blood perfusion pump for use in cross transfusion experiments in small laboratory animals. J. Appl. Physiol. *12*, 142–144, 1958.

FINSTERBUSCH, W., D. M. LONG, R. D. SELLERS, K. AMPLATZ and C. W. LILLEHEI: Renal arteriography during extracorporeal curculation in dogs with a preliminary report upon the effects of low molecular weight dextran. J. Thor. Cardiov. Surg. *41*, 252–262, 1961.

FIRME, C. N., R. ANTHONE, S. ANTHONE and A. E. MACNEILL: Studies with a cellulose membrane oxygenator. J. Thor. Cardiov. Surg. *40*, 253–259, 1960.

FIROR, W. M.: Experiments in cross circulation. Amer. J. Physiol. *96*, 146–152, 1931.

FISHER, B. and E. J. FEDOR: Cardiac temperature gradients during profound hypothermia with extracorporeal perfusion. Proc. Soc. Exp. Biol. Med. *106*, 275–277, 1961.

FISHER, H. W., H. ALBERT, W. L. RIKER and W. J. POTTS: Successful experimental maintenance of life by homologous lungs and mechanical heart. Ann. Surg. *136*, 475–484, 1952.

FISHER, J. H. and B. T. SMYTH: Experimental prolonged partial whole body perfusion. Surg. Forum *10*, 602–604, 1960.

FISHER, L. M. and L. B. JACQUES: An evaluation of siliclad, a new silicone material. J. Appl. Physiol. *13*, 527–528, 1958.

FITCH, E. A. and C. P. BAILEY: Obturators for extracorporeal circulation cannulae. J. Thor. Surg. *37*, 660–662, 1959.

FITZGERALD, J. B. and W. G. MALETTE: The physiologic effects of intravascular Antifoam A. School of Aviation Medicine Aerospace Medical Center Publication Nr 61–7, 1960.

FLEISCH, A.: Ein automatisch regulierender Durchblutungsapparat mit fortläufender Registrierung der Durchbkutungsgeschwindigkeit. pp. 1007–1026 *In:* Handbuch der biologischen Arbeitsmethoden. E. Abderhalden (editor), Abt. V, Teil *8*, H. 3, 1935.

——: Une substance vasodilatatrice des érythrocytes. Schweiz. Med. Wschr. *19*, 223–224, 1938.

——: Le métabolisme basal standard et sa détermination au moyen du "Métabocalculator". Helv. Med. Acta *18*, 23–44, 1951.

—— and P. C. FREI: L'emploi de l'oxygène pur dans les oxygénateurs des coeurs-poumons artificiels. Helv. Physiol. Pharmacol. Acta *18*, 464–466, 1960.

—— and R. STAUFFER: Effet d'une tension électrique sur l'adhérence des protéines plasmatiques à des surfaces métalliques. Helv. Physiol. Pharmacol. Acta *19*, 118, 1961.

FLEISCH, A. O.: Toxizität und therapeutische Anwendung des Sauerstoffes. Helv. Med. Acta *25*, 706–726, 1958.

FLEISCH, H.: Der Einfluss von Zitrat und Liquemin auf die Blutkonservation. Thromb. Diathesis Haemorrhagica *4*, 269–274, 1960a.

——: Mesure de l'hémolyse par la détermination dans le plasma de l'hémoglobine, la méthemalbumine et leurs dérivés. Helv. Med. Acta *27*, 383–407, 1960b.

—— and A. FLEISCH: Der Hemoresistometer: Ein Gerät zur Bestimmung der mechanischen Resistenz der Erythrocyten. Schw. Med. Wschr. *90*, 186–190, 1960b.

FLINDLE, A.: Pumps for chemical duties. Manufact. Chem. *32*, 166–169, 1961.

FOLGA, J. and Z. SEMERAU-SIEMIANOWSKI: Artificial heart-lung apparatus; a preliminary report. Polski Tygodnik Lekarski *10*, 497, 1955 *(Pol)*.

FOOTE, A. V., M. TREDE and J. V. MALONEY, JR.: The use of stored Acid-Citrate-Dextrose (ACD) blood for clinical extracorporeal circulation. Surg. Forum *11*, 230–231, 1960.

FORSTER, R. E., F. J. W. ROUGHTON and F. KREUZER: Photocolorimetric determination of rate of uptake of CO and O_2 by reduced human red cell suspensions at 37° C. J. Appl. Physiol. *2*, 260–268, 1957.

FRANK, O.: Theorie und Konstruktion eines optischen Strompendels. Ztschr. f. Biol. *89*, 83–84, 1929.

——: Bemerkungen zur der vorhergehenden Abhandlung von Otto Ranke: Über die

Registrierung der Strömungsgeschwindigkeit usw. Ztschr. f. Biol. *90*, 181–191, 1930.

——: On the dynamics of cardiac muscle. Translated by C. B. Chapman and E. Wasserman. Amer. Heart J. *58*, 282–317, and 467–478, 1959.

FRASER, R. S. and R. E. RESSAL: Acute myocardial injury during cardiopulmonary bypass. Amer. Heart J. *56*, 926–928, 1958.

FREDERICQ, L.: Sur la circulation céphalique croisée ou échange du sang carotidien entre deux animaux. Arch. Biol. Gand & Leipzig *10*, 127–130, 1890.

FREEBURG, B. R. and C. HYMAN: Blood-borne vasodilating agent from ischemic tissues. J. Appl. Physiol. *15*, 1041–1045, 1960.

FREESE, J. W., A. M. LESAGE, W. G. YOUNG JR. and W. C. SEALY: The effect of core induced hypothermia of 25° and 7° C. on dogs with myocardial infarction. Trans. Am. Soc. Art. Int. Organs *6*, 218–226, 1960.

FREI, P. C.: Altération du sang par des matériaux utilisés en circulation extracorporelle. Helv. Physiol. Pharmacol. Acta *18*, 447–463, 1960.

—— and A. FLEISCH: Procédé nouveau permettant de diminuer l'hémolyse du sang conservé. Helv. Physiol. Pharmacol. Acta *19*, C19–C22, 1961.

VON FREY, M. and M. GRUBER: Untersuchungen über den Stoffwechsel isolierter Organe. Ein Respirations-Apparat für isolierte Organe. Virchow's Arch. f. Physiol. *9*, 519–532, 1885.

FRICK, M. H.: Influence of 5-Hydroxytryptamine on renal function in extracorporeal circulation. Nature (London) *187*, 609–610, 1960.

FRIES, C. C., B. LEVOWITZ, S. ADLER, A. W. COOK, K. E. KARLSON and C. DENNIS: Experimental cerebral gas embolism. Ann. Surg. *145*, 461–470, 1957.

FRÖHLICHER, R.: Untersuchungen über die Wirkungen des Acetylcholins auf das elektrisch zum Flimmern gebrachte isolierte Saugetierherz. Helv. Physiol. Pharmacol. Acta *3*, 231–241, 1945.

G

GABRIO, B. W., D. M. DONEHUE, F. M. HUENNEKENS and C. A. FINCH: VII. Acid-citrate dextrose-inosine (ACDI) as a preservative for blood during storage at 4°. J. Clin. Invest. *35*, 657, 1956.

GADBOYS, H. L., J. NOLAN and J. C. DAVILA:

The effect of mechanical trauma on fibrinogen in heparinized blood. Ann. Surg. *151*, 399–402, 1960.

GÄRTNER, G.: Ueber iutravenöse Sauerstoffinfusionen. Wien. klin. Wochenschr. *15*, 691–697 and 727–731, 1902.

GÄRTNER, R. A., J. ISAACS, R. DEVER and J. H. KAY: Coronary and carotid artery perfusion during total bypass of the heart. Surg. Forum. *6*, 194–196, 1956.

GALLETTI, P. M.: Techniques de perfusion pulmonaire controlée. Poumon Coeur *15*, 777–780, 1959.

——: Physiologic principles of partial extracorporeal circulation for mechanical assistance to the failing heart. Am. J. Cardiol. *7*: 227–233, 1961.

—— and G. A. BRECHER: Theoretical considerations concerning "heart-lung bypass" procedures. Fed. Proc. *19*, 90, 1960.

—— and ——: Cardiovascular adaptation to partial heart-lung bypass. Circul. Res. *8*: 609–615, 1960.

—— and M. A. HOPF: Pulmonary blood flow during partial heart-lung bypass in closed-chest dogs. The Physiologist *2*, 44, 1959.

—— and P. F. SALISBURY: Physiological observations during partial extracorporeal circulation in closed-chest dogs. Trans. Amer. Soc. Art. Int. Org. *4*, 157–172, 1958.

—— and ——: Partial extracorporeal circulation in closed-chest dogs. J. Appl. Physiol. *14*, 684–688, 1959.

——, —— and A. RIEBEN: Influence of blood temperature on the pulmonary circulation. Circulat. Res. *6*, 275–282 1958.

——, W. L. NICKERSON and G. A. BRECHER: Cardiovascular adaptation to partial extracorporeal circulation. Trans. Am. Soc. Art. Int. Organs *5*, 191–196, 1959.

——, M. A. HOPF and G. A. BRECHER: Problems associated with long-lasting heart-lung bypass. Trans. Amer. Soc. Art. Int. Organs *6*, 180–188, 1960.

——, G. A. BRECHER, M. A. HOPF and D. E. BRINSFIELD: Venous flow, venous pooling and edema in artificial circulation. Presented before the 4th International Congress of Angiology, Prague 1961.

GAMMELGARD, R. A., E. HUSFELT and F. THERKELSEN: Experimental open-heart surgery using a heart-lung machine with a simple disposable oxygenator. Acta. Chir. Scandin. *112*, 439–442, 1957.

GARCIA ORTIZ, E.: Hipotermia profunda asociada a circulación extracorporea. Estudio clinico y experimental. Rev. Clin. Esp. *76*, 92–97, 1960.

GEBAUER, P. W., S. C. BRAINARD, C. B. MASON and M. CONNER: A temperature control unit for a commercial disc oxygenator. Hawaii Med. J. *19*, 651–653, 1960.

GEHL, H.: Hemodynamische Veränderungen bei Anwendung eines künstlichen Herzstillstandes. Langenbeck Arch. Klin. Chir. *292*, 678–681, 1959.

GENTSCH, T. O., R. K. BOPP, J. H. SIEGEL, M. CEV and W. W. L. GLENN: Experimental and clinical use of a membrane oxygenator. Surgery *47*, 301–313, 1960.

GEOHEGAN, T. and C. R. LAM: The mechanism of death from intracardiac air and its reversibility. Ann. Surg. *138*, 351–359, 1953.

GERBODE, F. and D. G. MELROSE: The use of potassium arrest in open cardiac surgery. Amer. J. Surg. *96*, 221–227, 1958.

——, ——, A. NORMAN, J. J. OSBORN, H. A. PERKINS and D. M. BAER: Extracorporeal circulation in intracardiac surgery: a comparison between two heart-lung machines. Lancet *2*, 284–286, 1958.

——, J. J. OSBORN, M. L. BRAMSON, G. A. HARKINS, J. K. ROSS and B. F. JOHNSTON: Elective hypothermia during extracorporeal circulation with a new heat-exchange filming oxygenator. Indications and results. Amer. J. Surg. *100*, 338–345, 1960a.

——, —— and B. J. JOHNSTON: Experiences with perfusion hypothermia using an improved rotating disc oxygenator. Thorax *15*, 185–192, 1960b.

GERFIN, A. N., R. D. JONES and F. S. CROSS: Cardiac bypass with the pump-oxygenator for circulatory support during cardiac decompensation. Surg. Forum *11*, 216–218, 1960.

GERSCHMAN, R.: Oxygen effects in biological systems. Proc. XXI Intern. Congress Physiol. Sc. Buenos Aires 222–226, 1959.

——, D. L. GILBERT, S. W. NYE, P. DWYER and W. O. FENN: Oxygen poisoning and X-irradiation: a mechanism in common. Science *119*, 623–626, 1954.

GERTZ, K. H. and H. H. LOESCHCKE: Elektrode zur Bestimmung des CO_2-Drucks. Naturwissenschaften *45*, 160–161, 1958.

——, H. E. HOFFMEISTER and H. KREUZER: Beschreibung und Prüfung eines Schwammoxygenators. Thoraxchirurgie *8*, 111–117, 1960.

GESELL, R. A.: On the relation of pulse pressure to renal secretion. Amer. J. Physiol. *32*, 70–93, 1913.

GIAJA, J.: Léthargie obtenue chez le rat par la dépression barométrique. C. R. Acad. Sci. (Paris) *210*, 80–82, 1940.

—— and V. POPOVIC: Sur les échanges des homéothermes refroidis. C. R. Acad. Sci. (Paris) *234*, 1210–1211, 1952.

GIANELLI, S. JR., M. F. MOLTHAN, R. J. BEST, J. A. DULL and C. K. KIRBY: The effects produced by various types of pump-oxygenators during two-hour partial infusions in dogs. J. Thor. Surg. *34*, 563–569, 1957.

——, J. H. ROBINSON, R. J. BEST and C. K. KIRBY: Hemodynamic mechanisms which automatically maintain a relatively constant blood volume during cardio-pulmonary bypass. Surgery *44*, 378–389, 1958.

——, D. R. MAHAJAN, J. R. NAVARRE and G. H. PRATT: Studies of blood volume changes during cardiopulmonary bypass in dogs. Ann. Surg. *152*, 190–196, 1960.

GIBBON, J. H., JR.: Artificial maintenance of circulation during experimental occlusion of pulmonary artery. Arch. Surg. *34*, 1105–1131, 1937.

——: The maintenance of life during experimental occlusion of the pulmonary artery followed by survival. Surg. Gynec. Obstet. *69*, 602–614, 1939a.

——: An oxygenator with a large surface-volume ratio. J. Labor. Clin. Med. *24*, 1192–1198 1939b.

——: Application of a mechanical heart and lung apparatus to cardiac surgery, Minnesota Med., *37*, 171 1954.

——: Chairman's address. Trans. Amer. Soc. Art. Int. Organ *1*, 158–162, 1955.

——: Extracorporeal maintainance of cardiopulmonary function. Harvey Lect. *53*, 186–224, 1959a.

——: Maintenance of cardiorespiratory functions by extracorporeal circulation. Circulation *19*, 646–656, 1959b.

—— and C. W. KRAUL: An efficient oxygenator for blood. J. Lab. Clin. Med. *26*, 1803–1809, 1941.

——, B. J. MILLER, and C. FEINBERG: An improved mechanical heart and lung apparatus. Med. Clin. N. Amer. *37*, 1603–1624, 1953.

——, ——, A. R. DOBELL, H. C. ENGELL and G. B. VOIGT: The closure of interventricular septal defects on dogs during open cardiotomy with the maintenance of the cardio-respiratory functions by a pump oxygenator. J. Thor. Surg. *28*, 235–240, 1954.

GIBBS, O. S.: An artificial heart. J. Pharmacol. Exp. Therap. *38*, 197–215, 1930.

——: An artificial heart for dogs. J. Pharmacol. Exp. Therap. *49*, 181–186, 1933.

GIBSON, J. G. II, S. B. REES, T. J. McMANUS and W. A. SCHEITLIN: A citrate-phosphate-dextrose solution for the preservation of human blood. Amer. J. Clin. Path. *28*, 569–578, 1957.

GILLIGAN, D. A., M. C. ALTSCHULE and E. M. KATERSKY: Studies of hemoglobinemia and hemoglobinuria produced in man by the intravenous infection of hemoglobin solutions. J. Clin. Invest. *20*, 177–187, 1941.

GILMAN, R. A., R. L. RUSSEL, B. G. MUSSER, and W. GEMEINHARDT: An air trap filter for extracorporeal oxygenator systems. Surgery *42*, 993–995, 1957.

GIMBEL, N. S., and J. ENGELBERG: An oxygenator for use in a heart-lung apparatus. Surg. Forum *3*, 154–157, 1953.

—— and ——: Blood oxygenator: theory and studies in design. Surgery *35*, 645–669, 1954.

GLANTS, R. M.: Certain indices of automatic effect of homologous blood transfusion on functional conditions of the nervous system. Biull. eksp. biol. Med. *47*, 46–49, 1959 (*Po.*)

GLENN, R., and G. R. HOLSWADE: Basic requirements for open heart surgery. Surg. Clin. N. Amer. *41*, 349–358, 1961.

GLENN, W. W. L. and W. H. SEWELL: Experimental cardiac surgery. IV. The prevention of air embolism in open heart surgery; repair of interatrial septal defects. Surgery *34*, 195–206, 1953.

——, T. O. GENTSCH, B. K. KUSSEROW and M. HUME: Coronary blood flow during body perfusion. pp.368–385. In: Extracorporeal Circulation, J. G. Allen, (editor), Springfield, Ill.: Thomas 1958.

——, J. A. J. STOLWIJK, H. ANNAMUNTHODO, G. M. RAPP and M. HIMMEL: An integral fin-type blood heat exchanger. Surg. Forum *10*, 574–577, 1960a.

——, A. L. TOOLE, E. LONGO, M. HUME and T. O. GENTSCH: Induced fibrillatory arrest in open-heart surgery. New Engl. J. Med. *262*, 852–855, 1960b.

GODAL, H. C.: Precipitation of human fibrinogen with heparin. Scand. J. Clin. Lab. Invest. *12*, 56–65, 1960.

GOFFRINI, P.: Recenti contributi della fisiopatologia sperimentale alla chirurgia del cuore esangue. Minerva Chir. *12*, 455–483, 1957.

——, E. ZANELLA, E. BOTTI, and A. PERACCHIA: L'asistolia farmacologica nella chirurgia del cuore esangue. Chir. Patol. Sperim. *5*, 209, 1957.

GOLDBERG, L. I.: Effects of hypothermia on contractility of the intact dog heart. Amer. J. Physiol. *194*, 92–98, 1958.

——, R. D. BLOODWELL, E. BRAUNWALD and MORROW, A. G.: The direct effects of norepinephrine, epinephrine, and methoxamine on myocardial contractile force in man. Circulation *22*, 1125–1132, 1960.

GOLDBERG, M., J. C. REDONDO, A. MOYANO, and R. YOFRE: Oxigenador a disco modificado. Prensa Med. Argent *46*, 871–872, 1959.

GOLLAN, F.: Cardiac arrest of one hour duration in dogs during hypothermia of 0°C followed by survival. Fed. Proc., *13*, 57, 1954.

——: Physiological studies with a pump-oxygenator. Trans. Amer. Soc. Artif. Int. Org. *1*, 78–80, 1955.

——: Physiology of cardiac surgery. 96 pp. Chas. C. Thomas Publ., Springfield, Ill. 1959a.

——: Physiology of deep hypothermia by total body perfusion. Ann. N. Y. Acad. Sci. *80*, 301–314, 1959B.

—— and G. R. MENEELY: Prevention of shock during prolonged periods of ventricular fibrillation by artificial circulation and oxygenation. Fed. Proc., *12*, 53, 1953.

—— and I. A. NELSON: Anoxic tolerance of beating and resting heart during perfusion at various temperatures. Proc. Soc. Exp. Biol. Med. *95*, 485–48, 1957.

——, L. C. CLARK and V. B. GUPTA: Prevention of acute anoxia by means of dispersion oxygenation of blood. Amer. J. Med. Sci. *222*, 76–81, 1951.

——, P. BLOS and H. SCHUMAN: Studies on hypothermia by means of a pump oxygenator. Amer. J. Physiol. *171*, 331–340, 1952a.

——, —— and ——: Exclusion of heart and lungs from the circulation in the hypothermic, closed-chest dog by means of a pump oxygenator. J. Appl. Physiol. *5*, 180–190, 1952b.

——, E. C. HAMILTON and G. R. MENEELY: Consecutive survival of open chest hypothermic dogs after prolonged by-pass of heart and lungs by means of a pump oxygenator. Surgery *35*, 88–97, 1954.

——, J. E. HOFFMAN and R. M. JONES: Maintenance of life of dogs below 10°C without hemoglobin. Amer. J. Physiol. *179*, 640, 1954.

——, R. PHILLIPS, J. T. GRACE and R. M. JONES: Open left heart surgery in dogs during hypothermic asystole with and without extracorporeal circulation. J. Thor. Surg. *30*, 626, 1955a.

——, J. T. GRACE, M. W. SCHELL, E. S. TYSINGER and L. B. FEASTER: Left heart surgery in dogs during respiratory and cardiac arrest at body temperatures below 10°C. Surgery *38*, 363–372, 1955b.

——, G. G. RUDOLPH and N. S. OLSEN: Electrolyte transfer during hypothermia and anoxia in dogs. Amer. J. Physiol. *189*, 277, 1957.

GOLLUB, S., H. S. WINCHELL, E. EHRLICH and A. UHLIN: Thrombocytopenia in massive transfusion. Surgery *45*, 366–370, 1959.

GOMEZ, D. M.: Considerations of oxygen-hemoglobin equilibrium in the physiological state. Amer. J. Physiol. *200*, 135–142, 1961.

GOMORI, P. and L. TAKACS: Circulatory regulation and shifting in hypoxia. Amer. Heart J. *59*, 161–165, 1960.

GOODYEAR, A. V. N. and W. W. L. GLENN: Relation of arterial pulse pressure to renal function. Amer. J. Physiol. *167*, 689–697, 1951.

GORDON, A. S., J. C. JONES, L. G. LUDDINGTON and B. W. MEYER: Deep hypothermia for intracardiac surgery. Experimental and clinical use without an oxygenator. Amer. J. Surg. *100*, 332–337, 1960.

GORDON, L. A.; V. RICHARDS and H. A. PERKINS: Studies in regional heparinization. I, The use of simultaneous neutralization with protamine; preliminary studies. N. Engl. J. Med. *255*, 1025–1029, 1956.

——, E. R. SIMON, J. M. RUKES, V. RICHARDS and H. A. PERKINS: Studies in regional heparinization. II. Artificial kidney hemodialysis without systemic heparinization: Preliminary report of a method using simultaneous infusion of heparin and protamine. New Eng. J. Med. *255*, 1063–1066, 1956b.

GOTT, V. L., R. A. DEWALL, M. PANETH, M. N. ZUDHI, W. WEIRICH, R. L. VARCO and C. W. LILLEHEI: A self-contained disposable oxygenator of plastic sheet for intracardiac surgery. Thorax, *12*, 1–9, 1957a.

——, R. D. SELLER, R. A. DEWALL, R. L. VARCO, and C. W. LILLEHEI: A disposable unitized plastic sheet oxygenator for open heart surgery. Dis. Chest *32*, 615–625, 1957b.

——, J. L. GONZALEZ, M. N. ZUHDI, R. L. VARCO and C. W. LILLEHEI: Retrograde perfusion of the coronary sinus for direct vision aortic surgery. Surgery, Gynec. Obstet. *104*, 319–328, 1957c.

——, ——, M. PANETH, R. L. VARCO, R. D. SELLERS and W. C. LILLEHEI: Cardiac retroperfusion with induced asystole for open surgery upon the aortic valve or coronary arteries. Proc. Soc. Exp. Biol. Med., *94*, 689–692, 1957d.

——, M. BARTLETT and J. A. JOHNSON: High energy phosphate metabolism in the myocardium during various techniques of cardiac arrest as determined by cardiac biopsy. Surg. Forum *9*, 281–284, 1958.

——, ——, ——, D. M. LONG and C. W. LILLEHEI: High energy phosphate levels in the human heart during potassium citrate arrest and selective hypothermic arrest. Surg. Forum *10*, 544–547, 1960.

GRAF, K., O. NORLANDER, A. SENNING and G. STROEM: Untersuchungen über Grösse und Verhalten der menschlichen Extremitätendurchblutung während extrakorporaler Zirkulation. Langenbeck Arch Klin. Chir. *292*, 671–678, 1959.

GRAVEL, J. A., M. BEAULIEU and J. P. DECHENE: Chirurgie expérimentale et la circulation extracorporelle. Union méd. Canada *87*, 1495–1499, 1958.

GREEN, H. D.: Venous drainage recorders. Methods in Med. Research, *1*, 68–77, 1948.

—— and J. H. KEPCHAR: Control of peripheral resistance in major systemic vascular beds. Physiol. Rev. *39*, 617–686, 1959.

GREENBERG, J. J., L. H. EDMUNDS and R. B. BROWN: Myocardial metabolism and postarrest function in the cold and chemically arrested heart. Surgery *48*, 32–41, 1960.

GREGG, D. E.: Regulation of the collateral and coronary circulation of the heart. In: Proc. Harvey Tercentenary Cong. London: Blackwell, 1958.

—— and D. E. SABISTON: Current research and problems of the coronary circulation. Circulation *13*, 916–927, 1956.

—— and R. E. SHIPLEY: Augmentation of left coronary inflow with elevation of left ventricular pressure and observations on mechanism for increased coronary inflow with increased cardiac load. Amer. J. Physiol. *142*, 44–51, 1944.

GRIESSER, G.: Über einen neuen Herz-Lungen-Apparat für den extrakorporealen Kreislauf. Langenbeck Arch. Klin. Chirur., *289*, 325–329, 1958a.

——: Über einen neuen Herz-Lungen-Apparat für den extrakorporalen Kreislarf. Der Chirurg *29*, 294–296, 1958b.

——: Über Fortschritte in der Entwicklung des Oxygenators. Thoraxchirurgie *7*, 108–121, 1960.

—— and V. PASSON: Zur Messung des Minuten-Stromvolumens in extracorporealen Kreislauf. Thoraxchirurgie *7*, 325, 1960.

GRODINS, S., H. STUART and R. L. VEENSTRA: Performance characteristics of the right heart bypass preparation. Amer. J. Physiol. *198*, 552–560, 1960.

GROSS, R. and R. HOLEMANS: Fragen der Blutgerinnung bei extrakorporalem Kreislauf mit der Herz-Lungen-Maschine. Klinische Wochenschrift *39*, 165–172, 1961.

——, J. HEUER and K. SOLTH: Quantitative Beziehungen zwischen Heparin und Thrombocyten. Acta haemat. Basle *16*, 147–157, 1956.

GROSS, R. E.: Discussions on pumps. pp. 24–27 In: Extracorporeal circulation, J. G. Allen (editor) Springfield, Ill.: Thomas, 1958.

——: Open-heart surgery for repair of congenital defects. New Engl. J. Med. *260*, 1047–1057, 1959.

——, R. SAUVAGE, G. PONTIUS and E. WATKINS, JR.: Experimental and clinical studies of a siphon-filling disc-oxygenator system for complete cardiopulmonary bypass. Ann. Surg. *151*, 285–302, 1960.

GUSTAVINO, G. N., J. A. WIKINSKI, R. H. ANDRES, J. QUINTERNO and C. DONADEI: An ocular sign useful for experimental surgery with pump-oxygenator. J. Thor. Surg. *36*, 230–232, 1958.

——, ——, ——, C. A. DONADEI and J. E. QUINTERNO: Estudios sobre fisiología y fisiopatología de la circulación extracorporea con el corazón-pulmón artificial. Sem. med. B. Air. *114*, 521–538, 1959a.

——, ——, ——, —— and ——: op. cit. Sem. Med. B. Air. *114*, 592–603, 1959b.

——, ——, ——, —— and ——: op. cit. Sem. med. B. Air. *114*, 691–699, 1959c.

——, ——, ——, —— and ——: op. cit. Sem. Med. B. Air. *114*, 853–872, 1959d.

——, ——, ——, ——, ——, C. BRAILOVSKI and S. MUZZIO: Estudios sobre el comportamiento mecanico de la circulación menor durante la perfusión com bomba oxigenadora. II. Influencía de la presión positiva intrapulmonar sobre las presiones del circuito menor a flujos variables. Rev. Asoc. Méd. Argent. *73*, 268–273, 1959e.

——, ——, ——, —— and ——: Modification of lung compliance during perfusion with pump-oxygenator (experimental). Dis. Chest *38*, 170–178, 1960.

——, ——, ——, —— and ——: A simple method for starting the siphonage of blood from venae cavae during mechanical bypass. J. Thor. Cardiov. Surg. *41*, 279, 1961.

GUENDEL, W. VON: Das künstliche Herz nach Guendel/Kohler. Beitr. Arbeitsbereich Orthop., 1954, 116f.

——: Einfluss der Benetzbarkeit auf den Verlauf der Blutgerinnung und den Gerinnungsbeginn. In Thrombose und Embolie. pp. 157–160. Basel:Benno Schwabe & Co., 1955.

—— and H. KOHLER: Das künstliche Herz nach GUENDEL-KOHLER. Naturwiss. Rdsch. 1955, 75.

——, H. SCHEBITZ and H. KOHLER: Zur Frage der Ausschaltung des Herzens durch ein künstliches Herz. In Thrombose und Embolie. pp. 1185–1186. Basel: Benno Schwabe & Co., 1955.

GURRUCHAGA, J. and F. O. CAMES: Circulacíon extracorporal. Día. Med., B. Air. *30*, 3103–3104, 1958.

GURVICH, A. M.: Modern foreign technic of artificial blood circulation: review of principal foreign literature. Khirurgiia (Moskva) *2*, 73–81, 1955 (*Rus.*).

GUTELIUS, J. R. and A. R. DOBELL: The acid-base status of donor blood as used for extracorporeal circulation. Canad. J. Surg. *3*, 130–133, 1960.

GUYER, A. and E. PETERHANS: Über die Grösse von Gasblasen. I. Entwicklung an Einzelkapillaren Helv. Chem. Act. *26*, 1099–1107, 1943a.

—— and ——: Über die Grösse von Gasblasen. II. Entwicklung an Filterplatten. Helv. Chem. Act. *26*, 1107–1113, 1943b.

GUYTON, A. C.: Textbook of Medical Physiology, 2nd Ed. W. B. Saunders and Co., Philadelphia and London, 1961.

H

HAAB, P. E., M. A. HOPF and P. M. GALLETTI: Alveolar-arterial gas tension equilibrium during partial heart-lung bypass. Trans. Amer. Soc. Art. Int. Organs *6*, 266–274, 1960.

HACKETT, P. R., E. BLAIR and M. HELRICH: A study of deaths associated with intracardial surgery. Anesth. Analg. *40*, 69–74, 1961.

HAGLUND, G. and H. LUNDBERG: Trials with a new heat exchanger for deep hypothermia. Acta Anesth. Scand. *4*, 167–172, 1960.

HAGOPIAN, E., G. HAUPT, J. McKEOWN JR. and J. Y. TEMPLETON III: A study of gas exchange in a stationary vertical screen oxygenator. Trans. Amer. Soc. Art. Int. Organs *7*, 157–161, 1961.

HALE, D. E.: The value of monitors in cardiac surgery. Amer. J. Cardiol. *6*, 756–762, 1960.

——, P. MORACA and C. E. WASMUTH: Elective cardiac arrest during cardiotomy. Anesthesiology, *18*, 378–388, 1957.

HALL, D. P., E. L. BRACKNEY and E. G. ELLISON: An easy method of continuously measuring flow rates in extracorporeal circulation. Surg. Forum *9*, 205–207, 1959.

——, S. A. SINGAL, W. H. MORETZ, E. L. BRACKNEY, W. F. BUTLER, W. C. MALOY, V. BERNSTEIN and R. G. ELLISON: Myocardial metabolism during elective cardiac arrest determined by biochemical analysis of multiple cardiac biopsies. Surg. Forum *10*, 540–543, 1960.

HALL, J. E., P. A. JAMES, B. G. B. LUCAS and D. J. WATERSTON: Some observations on industrial pumps for extracorporeal circulation in man. Thorax, *13*, 34–48, 1958.

——, ——, —— and D. J. WATERSTON: A pump for extracorporeal circulation. Lancet *1*, 347, 1959.

HALLEY, M. M., K. REEMTSMA and O. CREECH JR.: Cerebral blood flow, metabolism, and brain volume in extracorporeal circulation. J. Thor. Surg. *36*, 506–518, 1958.

HALLEY, M. M., D. M. L. ROSENBERG, R. F. RYAN, K. REEMTSMA and O. CREECH, JR.: The experimental and clinical use of a small capacity rapidly available pump oxygenator. Surg. Forum *9*, 196–198, 1960, 1959a.

——, K. REEMTSMA and O. CREECH JR.: Hemodynamics and metabolism of individual organs during extracorporeal circulation. Surgery *46*, 1128–1134, 1959b.

HAM, T. H., S. C. SHEN, E. FLEMING and W. B. CASTLE: Studies on the destruction of red blood cells. IV. Thermal injury: action of heat in causing increased spheroidicity, osmotic and mechanical fragilities and hemolysis of erythrocytes; observation on the mechanisms of destruction of such erythrocytes in dogs and in a patient with a fatal thermal burn. Blood *3*, 373–403, 1948.

HAMEL, G.: Die Bedeutung des Pulses für den Blutstrom. Zeitschr. Biol. *25*, 474–495, 1888.

HAMER, N. A., J. F. DICKSON III and J. W. Dow: The effect of prolonged veno-arterial pumping on the circulation of the dog. J. Thor. Surg. *37*, 190–199, 1959.

HAMILTON, A. S., W. M. PARKINS and F. WALTZER: A comparison of ten infusion fluids in the treatment of moderate and severe hemorrhage in animals. Amer. J Physiol. *150*, 641–653, 1947.

HANQUET, M.: Problèmes biologiques posés par l'emploi des coeurs-poumons artificiels. Rev. Med. Liège, *13*, 850–854, 1958.

HARDING, F. and M. H. KNISELY: Settling of sludge in human patients; a contribution to the biophysics of disease. Angiology, *9*, 317–341, 1958.

HARKEN, D. E.: Assisted circulation. Presented before the 3rd World Congress of Cardiology, Brussels 1958.

HARKINS, H. N. and P. H. HARMON: Embolism by air and oxygen: comparative studies. Proc. Soc. Exp. Biol. Med. *32*, 178–181, 1934.

HARRIS, M., W. E. BERG, D. M. WHITAKER, V. C. TWITTY and R. L. BLINKS: Carbon dioxide as a facilitating agent in the initiation and growth of bubbles in animals decompressed to simulated altitudes. J. Gen. Physiol. *28*, 225–240, 1945.

HARRISON, D. and L. S. LEUNG: Bubble formation at an orifice in a fluidized bed. Nature (London) *190*, 433–434, 1961.

HARSHBARGER, H. G., J. W. KIRKLIN and D. E. DONALD: Studies in extracorporeal circulation. IV. Surgical techniques. Surg. Gynec. Obstet. *106*, 111–118, 1958.

HARTMANN, A. F. JR., A. ROOS and D. GOLDRING: Acid-base abnormalities in humans associated with the use of the Gibbon-Mayo pump. Flow rates of 2 to 2.4 liters per square meter of body surface per minute. J. Pediat. *56*, 454–464, 1960.

HARTRIDGE, H. and F. J. W. ROUGHTON: The rate of distribution of dissolved gases between the red blood corpuscle and its fluid environment. J. Physiol. (London) *62*, 232–242, 1927.

HARVEY, E. N., D. D. K. BARNES, W. B. McELROY, A. H. WHITELY, D. C. PEASE and K. W. COOPER: Bubble formation in animals. I. Physical factors. J. Cell. Comp. Physiol. *24*, 1–22, 1944a.

——, A. H. WHITELY, W. B. McELROY, D. C. PEASE and D. K. BARNES: Bubble formation in animals. II. Gas nuclei and their distribution in blood tissue. J. Cell. Comp. Physiol. *24*, 23–34, 1944b.

——, W. D. McELROY, A. M. WHITELY, G. M. WARREN and D. C. PEASE: Bubble formation in animals: analysis of gas tension and hydrostatic pressure in cats. J. Cell. Physiol. *24*, 117–132, 1944c.

HASSLER, G. L.: Plastics. IRE Trans. Med. Electronics *6*, 52–53, 1959.

HAYES, E. W., D. P. MORSE, W. L. JAMISON and C. P. BAILEY: A nylon cloth oxygenator for extracorporeal circulation. Proc. Soc. Exp. Biol. Med. *89*, 413–415, 1955.

HEAD, L. R., J. P. COENEN, E. ANGOLA, C. NOGUEIRA, D. MENDELSOHN and E. B. KAY: Operation of the roller pump for extracorporeal circulation. J. Thor. Cardiov. Surg. *39*, 210–220, 1960.

HEADRICK, J. R., D. W. STAYHORN, A. J. MUNOZ and J. E. ADAMS: A method of safely prolonging induced cardioplegia. Surg. Forum, *10*, 509–514, 1960.

HEDON, E.: Expérience de transfusion réciproque par circulation carotidienne croisée entre chiens diabétiques et chiens normaux; leurs résultats. C. R. Soc. Biol. *66*, 699–701, 1909.

——: Transfusion sanguine réciproque entre deux animaux par anastomose carotidienne. C. R. Soc. Biol. *68*, 341–343; 650–653, 1910.

HEINRICH, G. and W. HART: Probleme der extracorporalen Zirkulation mit künstlichem Herz-Lungen-System. Aerztl. Wschr. *14*, 453–457, 1959.

HEIMBECKER, R. C.: Discussion on air embolism. pp. 312–314. In: Extracorporeal Circulation. J. G. Allen, editor. Springfield, Ill.: Thomas, 1958.

——: An improved caval catheter for cardiac bypass. J. Thor. Cardiov. Surg. *40*, 278, 1960.

HELMSWORTH, J. A., L. C. CLARK JR., S. KAPLAN and C. FORD: A new method for the drainage of blood from the open heart during total bypass of the heart and lungs. Surg. Forum, *5*, 35–39, 1955.

——, ——, ——, T. LARGEN and R. T. SHERMAN: Artificial oxygenation and circulation during complete bypass of the heart. J. Thor. Surg. *24*, 117–133 and 151–153, 1952a.

——, ——, ——, R. T. SHERMAN and T. LARGEN: Clinical use of extracorporeal oxygenation with oxygenator pump. J. A. M. A. *150*, 451–453, 1952b.

——, ——, ——, R. T. SHERMAN and T. LARGEN: A discussion of an oxygenator-pump used in total bypass of the heart and lungs in dogs. Surg. Forum *3*, 158–165, 1953a.

——, ——, ——, ——: An oxygenator pump for use in total bypass of heart and lungs. J. Thor. Surg. *26*, 617–631, 1953b.

——, ——, R. T. SHERMAN, S. KAPLAN and T. LARGEN: A method for complete drainage of the superior and inferior vena cava into extracorporeal circuits. Surgery *33*, 835–840, 1953c.

——, R. W. SHABETAI and J. MARGOLIAN: An investigation of cardiac arrest produced by injection of potassium citrate into the coronary circulation. J. Thor. Surg. *36*, 214–219, 1958a.

——, ——, J. E. ALBERS, and P. J. WOZENCRAFT: The local effect of potassium citrate solution in atrial pouches of dogs. J. Thor. Surg. *36*, 221–226, 1958b.

——, S. KAPLAN, L. C. CLARK, A. J. McADAMS, E. C. MATTHEWS and F. K. EDWARDS: Myocardial injury associated with asystole induced with potassium citrate. Ann. Surg. *149*, 200–206, 1959.

HEMINWAY, A.: Some observations on the perfusion of the isolated kidney by a pump. J. Physiol. (London) *71*, 201–213, 1931.

HEMMINGSEN, E. and P. F. SCHOLANDER: Specific transport of oxygen through hemoglobin solutions. Science *132*, 1379–1381, 1960.

HENNEMAN, D. H., J. P. BUNKER and W. R. BREWSTER: The immediate metabolic response to hypothermia in man. J. Appl. Physiol. *12*, 164–168, 1958.

HENROTIN, E., R. VEROFT, G. PRIMO, A. GELIN and J. DUBOIS-PRIMO: Observations expérimentales sur la circulation extracorporelle chez le chien. Acta Chir. Belg. *57*, 428–441, 1958.

HENRY, L. and P. JOUVELET: Appareil à transfusion du sang. Bull. Acad. Med. (Paris) *111*, 312–319, 1934.

HERBST, M., W. GROHMANN, A. GLASER, D. MICHEL and O. HARTLEB: Künstlicher Herzstillstand mit Adenosin-Mono-Phosphorsaure (AMP). Langenbeck Arch. Klin. Chir. *289*, 304–306, 1958a.

——, D. MICHEL, O. HARTLEB, W. GROHMANN and A. GLASER: Beobachtungen bei Injektion von Adenosin-monophosphorsäure und Acetylcholin in verschiedenen Mischungen in die Coronarien am ausgeschalteten Herzen in Hypothermie. Acta Biol. Med. Germ. *1*, 652–657, 1958b.

HERRON, P. W., J. E. JESSEPH and K. A. MERENDINO: An experimental study indidicating the relationship between blood volume and available venous return during extracorporeal circulation. Surg. Forum, *8*, 410–412, 1958a.

——, —— and ——: The effects of arterenol on blood pressure and venous return during extracorporeal circulation. Surgery *44*, 398–401, 1958b.

HEUPEL, H. W. and J. J. WILD: Design of an artificial lung using polyvinyl formal sponge. Lancet *2* 1246–1247, 1956.

HEWITT, W. C., JR., I. W. BROWN, JR., G. S. EADIE, W. W. SMITH and W. C. SEALY: The ultimate in vivo survival of erythrocytes which have circulated through a pump-oxygenator. Surg. Forum *7*, 271–274, 1957.

HEYMANS, C. and E. NEIL: Reflexogenic Areas of the Cardiovascular system. Boston: Little, 1958.

——, J. J. BOUCKAERT, F. JOURDAN, S. J. G. NOVAK and S. PARBER: Survival and revival of nerve centers following acute anemia. Arch. Neurol. Psych. *38*, 304–307, 1937.

HEYMANS, J. F.: Iso-hyper and hypothermisation des mammifères par calorification et frigorification du sang de la circulation carotido-jugulaire anastomosée. Arch. Int. Pharmacodyn. *25*, 1–215, 1921.

HILGER, H. H. and H. BRECHTELSBAUER: Erfahrungen über Stromungsmessung mit verschiedenen Typen elektrisch registrierender Rotameter. Pflüger Arch. ges. Physiol. *263*, 615–627, 1957.

HIRSCH, H., K. H. EULER and M. SCHNEIDER: Über die Erholung und Wiederbelebung des Gehirns nach Ischämie bei Normothermie. Pflüger Arch. ges. Physiol. *265*, 281–313, 1957a.

——, D. KOCH, W. KRENKEL and F. SCHNELLBACHER: Über die Bedeutung des Abtransportes nach Metaboliten (Spülfunktion des Blutes) für die Erholung nach Ischämie. Pflüger Arch. ges Physiol. *265*, 337–341, 1957b.

HIRSCHBOECK, J. S.: Delayed blood coagulation in methyl methacrylate (boilable "lucite") vessels. Proc. Soc. Exp. Biol. Med. *47*, 311–312, 1941.

HODGES, P. C. JR., R. CARDOZO, A. THEVENET and C. W. LILLEHEI: Comparison of rela-tive merits of occlusive and nonocclusive pumps for open-heart surgery; together with description of simple flowmetering method for clinical use. J. Thor. Surg. *36*, 470–478, 1958a.

——, R. D. SELLERS, J. L. STORY, P. H. STANLEY, F. TORRES and C. W. LILLEHEI: The effects of total cardiopulmonary bypass procedures upon cerebral function evaluated by the electro-encephalogram and a blood brain barrier test. pp. 279–294, in Extracorporeal Circulation. J. G. Allen, ed. Springfield, Ill., Thomas, 1958.

HOEKSEMA, T. D. D., J. F. MUSTARD and W. T. MUSTARD: A study of some coagulation factor changes occurring in blood during extracorporeal circulation. Trans. Am. Soc. Art. Int. Organs *5*, 225–232, 1959.

HOFFMAN, E. G. and D. M. CALKINS: Design factors effecting selection of pumps for chemical service. Indust. Engin. Chem. *52*, 561–565, 1960.

HOFFMEISTER, H. E., H. KREUZER and W. SCHOEPPE: Der Sauerstoffverbrauch des stillstehenden, des leerschlagenden und des flimmerden Herzens. Pflüger Arch. ges. Physiol. *269*, 194–206, 1959.

HOFSTRA, P. C., A. A. CRESCENZI, F. SUDAK and P. COOPER: Membrane oxygenator—exposed type. Trans. Am. Soc. Art. Int. Organs *6*, 62–67, 1960.

HOLEMANS, R.: Survey on the problem of blood coagulation in extracorporeal circulation using a heart-lung machine. Belg. T. Geneesk *16*, 371–389, 1960.

——, A. AMERY and M. VERSTRAETE: Clotting deviations during complete cardiac bypass in dogs with a heart-lung apparatus Craford-Senning. Cardiologia, *37*, 193–205, 1960a.

——, C. VERMYLEN and M. VERSTRAETE: Etudes expérimentales de quelques problèmes de la coagulation sanguine en rapport avec la circulation extracorporelle. Med. Exp. *2*, 294–302, 1960b.

HOLLE, F., G. HEINRICH, F. BECKER, M. KOHFAHL and F. ESSLINGER: Cardioplegie durch Acetylcholin und deren sofortige, wirksame Aufhebung durch künstliche Acetylcholinesterase. Thoraxchirurgie *6*, 524–534, 1959.

HOLT, J. P.: The collapse factor in the measurement of venous pressure. Am. J. Physiol. *134*, 292–299, 1941.

HOLT, M., F. MACALALAD and F. J. LEWIS: Autogenous oxygenation with cardiac bypass, hypothermia and an atrioventricular clamp. J. Thor. Cardiov. Surg. *40*, 536–548, 1960.

HOOKER, D. R.: A study of the isolated kidney: The influence of pulse pressure upon renal function. Amer. J. Physiol. 27, 24–44, 1910.

——: The perfusion of the mammalian medulla—the effect of calcium and potassium on the respiratory and cardiac centers. Am. J. Physiol. *38*, 200–208, 1915.

HOPF, M. A. and P. M. GALLETTI: Pulmonary gas exchange partial heart-lung bypass. Submitted for publication in J. Appl-Physiol. 1962.

——, —— and L. GOLDSTEIN: Electroencephalographic observations during long-term partial heart lung bypass. Trans. Am. Soc. Art. Int. Organs *7*, 231–236, 1961.

VON HÖSSLIN, H.: Über die Ursache der scheinbaren Abhängigkeit des Umsatzes von der Grösse der Körperoberfläche. Arch. Path. (Leipzig), pp. 332–379, 1888.

HOTTINGER, G. C. ,R. F. RYAN, J. P. DELGADO and K. REEMTSMA: Physiology of extracorporeal circulation: studies of blood flow, oxygen consumption and metabolism in the isolated and perfused extremity. Surg. Forum *10*, 80–82, 1960.

HOUGIE, C.: Practical considerations in the control of bleeding associated with extracorporeal circulation. Acta Haemat. *24*, 130–134, 1960.

HOUSTON, C. S., T. AKUTSU and W. J. KOLFF: Pendulum type of artificial heart within the chest: preliminary report. Am. Heart J. *59*, 723–730, 1960.

HOWELL, W. H. and E. HOLT: Two new factors in blood coagulation-heparin and pro-antithrombin. Am. J. Physiol. *47*, 328–341, 1918.

HUBBARD, T. F., D. D. NEIS and J. L. BARMORE: Severe citrate intoxication during cardiovascular surgery. J.A.M.A. *162*, 1534–1535, 1956.

HUCKABEE, W. E.: Relationships of pyruvate and lactate during anaerobic metabolism. I. Effects of infusion of pyruvate or glucose and of hyperventilation. J. Clin. Invest. *37*, 244–254, 1958.

HUDSON, W. A.: The electroencephalogram in in experimental cardiopulmonary bypass. Proc. Roy. Soc. Med. *51*, 591–592, 1958.

——: The physiological aspects of extracorporeal circulation. Brit. J. Anaesth. *31*, 378–392, 1959.

HUFNAGEL, C. A.: Blood pumps, conduits and valves. IRE Trans. Med. Electronics *6*, 13–17, 1959.

——, J. D. MCALINDON, A. VARDAR, N. DE VENCIA and L. REED: A simplified extracorporeal pumping system. Trans. Am. Soc. Art. Int. Organs *4*, 60–66, 1958.

——, —— and ——: A simplified extracorporeal pump oxygenating system. Am. Surg. *25*, 314–320, 1959.

——, J. F. SCHABNO, R. PIFARRE, P. A. CONRAD and C. HEWSON: A versatile heat exchanger for use in extracorporeal bypass systems. J. Cardiov. Surg. *2*, 158–164, 1961a.

——, P. A. CONRAD, J. SCHANNO and R. PIFARRE: Profound cardiac hypothermia. Ann. Surg. *153*, 790–796, 1961b.

HUFNER, G.: Über die Bestimmung der Diffusions-Coefficiente einiger Gase für Wasser. Wied. Ann. Physik *60*, 134–168, 1897.

HURT, R., H. A. PERKINS, J. J. OSBORN and F. GERBODE: Neutralization of heparin by protamine in extracorporeal circulation. J. Thor. Surg. *32*, 612–619, 1956.

HURTHLE, K.: Über pulsatorische elektrische Erscheinungen an Arterien. Skand. Arch. Physiol. *29*, 100–113, 1913.

HUTTON, A. M., D. M. CARNEGIE, D. C. HODGSON and C. BISHOP: Anaesthesia for total cardiopulmonary bypass. Guys Hosp. Rep. *108*, 210–217, 1959.

HYMAN, E. S.: A method of introducing blood into a reservoir. Trans. Am. Soc. Art. Int. Organs *5*, 238–239, 1959a.

——: Cause of failure of the artificial heartlung. Trans. Am. Soc. Art. Int. Organs *5*, 257–264, 1959b.

——, D. ROSENBERG, A. L. HYMAN, S. SAYEGH and R. KAHLE: A simple artificial heart-lung: an approach to open heart surgery, Preliminary report. J. Louisiana St. Med. Soc. *108*, 134–136, 1956.

I

IANKOVSKII, V. D.: Compensation and restoration of several functions in animals revived with the aid of the autojector of S. S. Brukhonenko after clinical death. Tez. doklad. 2–1 Vses. konf. patofiziol. Kiev, 131 132, 1956 (*Rus*).

——: Method of artificial blood circulation for the study of the brain in restoration of cardiac activity. Tez. doklad. 2–1 Vses. konf. patofiziol. Kiev, 433, 1956 (*Rus*).

——, A. F. REKASHEVA and A. D. LOMOVITS-

KAIA: On the use of artificial lung apparatus for the revival of organisms. Fiziol. zhurnal SSSR *27*, 499–505, 1939 (*Rus*).

IBRING, G.: Extracorporeal circulation and postoperative erythrocyte destruction; studies based on the endogenous formation of carbon monoxide. Acta Chir. Scand. *116*, 79–89, 1959.

IKINS, P. M., D. M. EMERSON and C. B. MUELLER: Myocardial metabolism during prolonged asytole and cardiopulmonary bypass. Surg. Forum *9*, 180–184, 1959.

ILLING, G.: Circolazione extracorporea mediante dispositivo ad iperpressione di ossigeno. Arch. Ital. Chir. *83*, 221–226, 1958.

ISSEKUTZ, B. V.: Beiträge zur Wirkung des Insulins. II. Insulin-Adrenalin Antagonismus. Biochem. Ztschr. *183*, 283–297, 1927.

ITO, I., W. R. FAULKNER and W. J. KOLFF: Metabolic acidosis and its correlation in patients undergoing open-heart operations. Cleveland Clin. Quart. *24*, 193–203, 1957.

——, W. J. KOLFF and D. B. EFFLER: Prevention of overoxygenation during treatment with a heart-lung machine in cardiac operations. Cleveland Clin. Quart. *25*, 9–17, 1958.

IVANOVA, L. N.: Studies of the pulse, blood pressure and electrocardiogram in experimental artificial circulation. Eksp. Khir. *3*, 20–26, 1958 (*Rus*).

J

JACKSON, R. W.: Formation of gas bubbles from orifices, Part I. The Industr. Chemist *28*, 346–351, 1952a.

——: Formation of gas bubbles from orifices, Part II. The Industr. Chemist *28*, 391–398, 1952a.

JACOBJ, C.: Apparat zur Durchblutung isolirter überlebender Organe. Arch. Exp. Path. (Leipzig). *26*, 388–400, 1890.

——: Ein Beitrag zur Technik der künstlichen Durchblutung überlebender Organe. Arch. Exp. Path. (Leipzig) *31*, 330–348, 1895.

JAMISON, W. L., W. GEMEINHARDT, J. ALAI, A. COIA and C. P. BAILEY: Intracardiac surgery by left ventricular bypass with Gemeinhardt pump. Arch. Surg. *70*, 83–86, 1955.

JACQUES, L. B.: The effect of intravenous injections of heparin in the dog. Am. J. Physiol. *125*, 98–107, 1939.

——, A. F. CHARLES and C. H. BEST: Administration of heparin. Acta Med. Scand. *90*, 190–207, 1938.

——, E. FIDLAR, E. T. FELTSTED and A. G. MACDONALD: Silicones and blood coagulation. Canad. M. Ass. J. *55*, 26–31, 1946.

JEAN, E.: Circulation extracorporelle: le coeur-poumon artificiel d'André Thomas (Les conditions de la chirurgie cardiaque exsangue) Thèse, Fac. Méd. Marseille, 1954.

JERVELL, O.: Investigation of the concentration of lactic acid in blood and urine under physiologic and pathologic conditions. Acta Med. Scand. *68* (Suppl. 24), 1–135, 1928.

JESSEPH, J. E., P. W. HERRON, L. C. WINTERSCHEID, R. R. VETTO and K. A. MERENDINO: Carbohydrate metabolism of the isolated perfused dog heart. Surg. Forum *8*, 290–294, 1958.

JICHA, J., J. PROCHAZKA and M. VRANA: Certain biochemical changes during extracorporeal circulation. Cas. Lek. Cesk. *98*, 1327–1322, 1959 (*Cze*).

JONES, J. E., D. E. DONALD, H. J. C. SWAN, H. G. HARSHBARGER, J. W. KIRKLIN and E. H. WOOD: Apparatus of the Gibbon type for mechanical bypass of the heart and lungs: preliminary report. Proc. Mayo Clin. *30*, 105–113, 1955.

JONES, R. M., E. B. KAY, S. S. HUDACK and F. S. CROSSE: Suggested modifications in the application of the Sigmamotor pump to the technique of controlled cross circulation. J. Thor. Surg. *29*, 408–412, 1955.

JONES, T. W., R. R. VETTO, L. C. WINTERSCHEID, D. H. DILLARD and K. A. MERENDINO: Arterial complications incident to cannulation in open-heart surgery: with special reference to the femoral artery. Ann. Surg. *152*, 969–974, 1960.

JONGBLOED, J.: The mechanical heart-lung system. Surg. Gynec. Obstet. *89*, 684–691, 1949.

——: Observations on dogs with mechanically sustained circulation and respiration. J. Appl. Physiol. *3*, 642–648, 1951.

——: A closed oxygenating system for our heart-lung machine. Proc. Kon. Med. Akad. Wet. (Amst.) Ser. c, *55*, 221–224, 1952.

——: Experiences avec notre appareil coeur-poumon artificiel. J. Physiol. (Paris) *45*, 477–489, 1953.

——: La fixation de l'oxygène sur l'hémoglobine dans notre appareil coeur-poumon artificiel. J. Physiol. (Paris) *46*, 701–703, 1954.

JONTZ, J., G. BOUNOUS, I. HEIMBURGER, S. TERAMOTO, H. B. SHUMAKER JR. and M. ONNIS: Renal and portal blood flow under normothermic and hypothermic conditions during extracorporeal circulation. J. Thor. Cardiov. Surg. *39*, 781–787, 1960.

JORDAN, P. JR., G. E. TOLSTEDT and F. F. BERETTA: A stainless steel bubble oxygenator. J. Thor. Surg. *35*, 411–415, 1958a.

——, —— and ——: Microbubble formation in artificial oxygenation. Surgery *43*, 2, 266–269, 1958b.

JORPES, E., P. EDMAN and T. THANING: Neutralization of action of heparin by protamine. Lancet *2*, 975, 1939.

JOUVELET, P. and L. HENRY: Appareil à transfusion sanguine de Henry et Jouvelet. Bull. Soc. Med. Hop. Paris *50*, 537–539, 1934.

JOYSEY, V. C.: The relation between animal and human blood groups. Brit. M. Bull. *15*, 158–164, 1959.

JUDE, J. R., J. P. FAUTEUX and L. M. HAROUTUNIAN: Differential cardiac warming during hypothermia. Surg. Forum *7*, 294–297, 1956.

JULIAN, O. C., M. LOPEZ-BELIO, W. S. DYE, H. DAVID and W. J. CROVE: The median sternal incision in intracardiac surgery with extracorporeal circulation: a general evaluation of its use in heart surgery. Surgery *42*, 753–761, 1957.

JUST, O., W. NUSSGEN and E. BECK: Anaesthesie bei Herzoperationen mit extrakorporaler Zirkulation. Anaesthesist *8*, 65–70, 1959.

JUVENELLE, A., J. LIND and C. WEGELIUS: Quelques possibilités offertes par l'hypothermie générale profonde provoquée. Presse Méd. *60*, 973–978, 1952.

——, ——, and ——: A new method of extracorporeal circulation. Am. Heart J. *47*, 692–736, 1954.

K

KABAT, H.: The greater resistance of very young animals to arrest of the brain circulation. Am. J. Physiol. *130*, 588–589, 1940.

—— and C. DENNIS: The resistance of young dogs to acute arrest of the cephalic circulation. Proc. Soc. Exp. Biol. Med. *42*, 534–537, 1939.

——, —— and A. B. BAKER: Functional recovery after arrest of the brain circulation. Am. J. Physiol. *132*, 737–747, 1941.

KAMM, L. G.: The Convair heart-lung machine. Trans. Am. Soc. Art. Int. Organs *5*, 180–187, 1959.

KAMMERMEYER, K.: Silicone rubber as a selective barrier. Indust. Engin. Chem. *49*, 1685–1686, 1957.

KANTROWITZ, A. and A. KANTROWITZ: Experimental left heart to permit surgical exposure of the mitral valve in cats. Proc. Soc. Exp. Biol. Med. *74*, 193–198, 1950.

——, E. HURWITT and ——: Experimental artificial left heart for exposure of the mitral area. Arch. Surg. *63*, 604–611, 1951.

——, S. REINER and D. ABELSON: An automatically controlled inexpensive pump-oxygenator. J. Thor. Cardiov. Surg. *38*, 586–593, 1959.

KAPLAN, A. and B. FISHER: Study of the cardioplegic action of potassium ion during normothermia and hypothermia. Ann. Surg. *150*, 833–840, 1959.

—— and ——: Potassium ion as a cardioplegic agent in total cardiac bypass and dur-hypothermia with coronary perfusion. J. Thor. Cardiov. Surg. *39*, 468–477, 1960.

——, M. LEVINE and ——: The fate of potassium as a cardioplegic agent in normothermic animals. Surg. Forum *9*, 272–277, 1959.

KAPLAN, S., L. C. CLARK, E. C. MATTHEWS, F. K. EDWARDS, L. SCHWAB and J. A. HELMSWORTH: A comparison of the results of total body perfusion in dogs during potassium citrate cardiac arrest. sinus rhythm, and induced ventricular fibrillation. Surgery *43*, 14–23, 1958.

——, F. K. EDWARDS, J. A. HELMSWORTH and L. C. CLARK: Blood volume during and after total extracorporeal circulation. Arch. Surg. *80*, 31–37, 1960.

KARLSON, K. E.: The problem of construction of a pump oxygenator to replace the heart and lungs for brief periods. Ph.D. Thesis, U. of Minn., 1952.

——, C. DENNIS and D. E. WESTOVER: Blood oxygenation. I. The Kolff apparatus. II. Multiple horizontal rotating cylinders. Proc. Soc. Exp. Biol. Med. *70*, 223–22, 1949a.

——, —— and ——: Blood oxygenation. III. The vertical revolving cylinder. IV. The vertical revolving cone. Proc. Soc. Exp. Biol. Med. *70*, 225–226, 1949b.

——, ——, D. SANDERSON and C. U. CULMER: An oxygenator with increased capacity: multiple vertical revolving cylinders. Proc. Soc. Exp. Biol. Med. *71*, 204–20, 1949c.

——, ——, D. E. WESTOVER and D. SANDER-SON: Pump-oxygenator to supplant the heart and lungs for brief periods. I. Evaluation of oxygenator techniques; an efficient oxygenator. Surgery *29*, 678–696, 1951.

KASHCHEVSKAIA, L. A.: Biochemical changes in the blood of dogs during artificial blood circulation. Eksp. Khir. *3*, 27–35, 1958. *(Rus)*.

KATZ, A. M., L. N. KATZ and F. L. WILLIAMS: Regulation of the coronary flow. Am. J. Physiol. *180*, 392–402, 1955.

VON KAULIA, K. N. and W. HENKEL: Heparin Adsorption durch Erythrocyten. Schweiz. Med. Wschr. *82*, 1128–11, 1952.

—— and H. SWANN: Clotting deviations during cardiac by-pass: Fibrinolysis and circulating anticoagulant. J. Thor. Surg. *36*, 519–530, 1958a.

—— and ——: Clotting deviations in man associated with open-heart surgery during hypothermia. J. Thor. Surg. *36*, 857–868, 1958b.

——, —— and E. VON KAULLA: Beobachtungen an Gerinnung und Fibrinolyse während chirurgischer Eingriffe am menschlichem Herzen in Unterkühlung oder mittels extrakorporalen Kreislaufes. Klin. Wschr. *36*, 1050–1056, 1958c.

——, —— and B. PATON: Variations of the thrombin time in certain patients under going open-heart surgery; discussion of its prognostic significance. J. Thor. Cardiov. Surg. *40*, 260–270, 1960.

KAVAN, E. M., V. L. BRECHNER, R. D. WALTER and J. V. MALONEY: Electroencephalographic patterns during intracardiac surgery using cardiopulmonary bypass; a comparison of two anesthetic agents. Arch. Surg. *78*, 151–156, 1959a.

——, ——, —— and L. M. LINDE: Electroencephalographic and electrocardiographic patterns during open-heart surgery with the use of cardiopulmonary bypass. Canad. Anesth. Soc. J. *6*, 356–364, 1959b.

KAWASAKI, K.: Study of wettability of polymers by sliding of water drop. J. Colloid Sc. *15*, 402–407, 1960.

KAY, E. B. and F. S. CROSS: Direct vision repair of intracardiac defects utilizing a rotating disc reservoir oxygenator. Surg. Gynec. Obstet. *104*, 701–716, 1957.

——, H. A. ZIMMERMAN, R. M. BERNE, Y. HIROSE, R. D. JONES and F. S. CROSS: Certain clinical aspects of use of pump-oxygenator. J.A.M.A. *162*, 639–641, 1956.

——, J. E. GALAJDA, A. LUX and F. S. CROSS:

The use of convoluted discs in the rotating Surg. *36*, 268–273, 1958a.

——, L. R. HEAD and C. NOGUEIRA: Direct coronary artery perfusion for aortic valve surgery. J.A.M.A *168*, 1767–1768, 1958b.

KAY, J. H. and R. M. ANDERSON: The development of open-heart surgery. U.S.C. M. Bull. *10*, 5–12, 1957.

—— and ——: An autoclavable stationary screen pump-oxygenator with filmer. J. Thor. Surg. *36*, 463–469, 1959.

—— and R. A. GAERTNER: A simplified pump-oxygenator with flow equal to normal cardiac output. Surg. Forum *7*, 267–271, 1957.

KEATS, A. S., Y. KUROSU, J. TELFORD and D. COOLEY: Anesthetic problems in cardiopulmonary bypass for open-heart surgery: Experiences with 200 patients. Anesthesiology *19*, 501–514, 1958.

——, D. A. COOLEY and J. TELFORD: Relative anti-heparin potency of polybrene and protamine in patients undergoing extracorporeal circulation. J. Thor. Cardiov. Surg. *38*, 362–368, 1959.

KEITH, H. R., W. L. FELTON and G. S. CAMPBELL: Extracorporeal circulation in consecutive open-heart surgery patients. Arch. Surg. *81*, 969–970, 1960.

——, E. GINN, G. R. WILLIAMS and G. S. CAMPBELL: Massive hemolysis in extracorporeal circulation. J. Thor. Cardiov. Surg. *41*, 404–407, 1961.

KELLOGG, H. B. JR., L. D. HILL and G. H. LAWRENCE: Problems of animal experimentation with the pump-oxygenator. Bull. Mason Clin. *13*, 43–55, 1959.

KENYON, J. R.: Experimental deep hypothermia. Brit. M. Bull. *17*, 43–47, 1961.

—— and LUBBROOK, J.: Hypothermia below 10°C. in dogs with cardiac recovery on rewarming. Lancet *2*, 171–173, 1957.

KENYON, N. M., R. S. LITWAK, H. J. BECK, R. J. SLONIM, H. C. SPEAR and Y. SHIBOTA: Preliminary observations in isolated hypothermic cardiac asystole. Surg. Forum *10*, 567–570, 1960.

KEOWN, K. K., R. A. GILMAN and C. P. BAILEY: Open-heart surgery. J.A.M.A. *165*, 781–787, 1957.

KERR, E., C. DAVIS, J. WOOLSEY JR., O. GRIMES, H. G. STEPHENS, R. BYRON JR. and H. J. McCORKLE: The maintenance of circulation by cross-transfusion during experimental operations on the open-heart. Surg. Forum *2*, 222–229, 1952.

KEVORKIAN, J.: Rapid and accurate ophtalmoscopic determination of circulatory arrest. J.A.M.A. *164*, 1660–1664, 1957.

KHAIRALLAH, P. A. and I. H. PAGE: A vasopressor lipid in incubated plasma. Am. J. Physiol. *199*, 341–345, 1960.

KHARNAS, S. SH.: On the AIK apparatus for extracorporeal circulation under experimental and clinical conditions. Eks. Khir. *6*, 24–34, 1960, (*Rus*).

——, R. S. VINITSKAIIA and YU. D. VOLINSKII: On the mechanism of acute dilatation of the heart during extracorporeal circulation. Eks. Khir. Anesthes. *1*, 19–21, 1961. (*Rus*).

KHAYUTIN, V. M.: The recording of vascular tone by an autoperfusion method. Sechenov Physiol. J. USSR *44*, 605–613, 1958.

——: Autoperfusion and vascular reactivity. Fiziol. zh. SSSR *45*, 440–447, 1959. (*Rus*).

KIMOTO, S.: Further experiences with brain cooling by irrigation and with the pump-oxygenator. Surg. Gynec. Obstet. *68*, 244–246, 1960.

——, S. SUGIE and K. ASANO: Open-heart surgery under direct vision with the aid of brain cooling by irrigation. Surgery *39*, 592–603, 1956.

KIRBY, C. K.: Discussions on blood changes. pp. 264–266 In: Extracorporeal circulation, J. G. Allen, Ed., Springfield, Ill., Thomas, 1958.

——: Factors affecting blood volume control during open-heart operations. Surg. Clin. N. Amer. *40*, 1561–1568, 1960.

——, S. GIANELLI JR., H. MCMICHAEL, J. C. SCHUDER, J. S. MCCAUGHAN and J. JOHNSON: Simple automatic method of blood volume control during cardiac bypass for open-heart surgery. Arch. Surg. *78*, 193–196, 1959.

KIRKLIN, J. W. and W. S. LYONS: Arterial cannulation for extracorporeal circulation utilizing the external or common iliac artery. Surgery *47*, 648–650, 1960.

——, J. W. DUSHANE, R. T. PATRICK, D. D. DONALD, P. S. HETZEL, H. G. HARSHBERGER and E. H. WOOD: Intracardiac surgery with the aid of a mechanical pump-oxygenator system (Gibbon-type). Report of eight cases. Proc. Mayo Clin. *30*, 201–206, 1955.

——, D. D. DONALD, H. B. HARSHBARGER, P. S. HETZEL, R. T. PATRICK, H. J. C. SWAN and E. H. WOOD: Studies in extracorporeal circulation. I. Applicability of Gibbon-type pump-oxygenator to human intracardiac surgery; 40 cases. Ann. Surg. *144*, 2–8, 1956.

——, R. T. PATRICK and R. A. THEYE:

Theory and practice in the use of a pump-oxygenator for open intracardiac surgery. Thorax *12*, 93–98, 1957.

——, R. A. THEYE and R. T. PATRICK: The stationary vertical screen oxygenator. pp. 57–66 in Extracorporeal circulation. J. G. Allen, ed., Springfield Ill., Thomas, 1958a.

——, D. C. MCGOON, R. T. PATRICK and R. A. THEYE: What is adequate perfusion? pp. 125–138, in Extracorporeal circulation. J. G. Allen, ed., Springfield, Ill., Thomas, 1958b.

KITTLE, C. F. and R. EILERS: Edglugate-Mg as a blood preservative for extracorporeal circulation. Arch. Surg. *81*, 179–185, 1960.

——, W. A. REED, D. M. SPENCER and P. J. WAGNER: Regulation of regional blood flow during extracorporeal perfusion. Surgery *49*, 88–97, 1961.

KIETSCHKA, H. D., E. A. MASSULO and T. A. SCHULKINS: An improved method of obtaining donor blood for experimental heart-lung machine. U. S. Armed Forces Med. J. *10*, 578–581, 1959.

KLOPSTOCK, R., H. H. LEVEEN and P. I. LEVITIAN: Instantaneous blood loss determination during thoracic surgery. J. Thor. Cardiovasc. Surg. *38*, 746–757, 1959.

KNISELY, M. H., T. S. ELIOT and E. H. BLOCH: Sludged blood in traumatic shock. I. Microscopic observations of the precipitation and agglutination of blood flowing through vessels in crushed tissues. Arch. Surg. *51*, 220–236, 1945.

KNOCK, F. E.: Disposable pump-oxygenator for perfusion in small animals. Arch. Surg. *81*, 668–670, 1960.

KNOWLTON, F. P. and E. H. STARLING: The influence of variations in temperature and blood pressure on the performance of the isolated mammalian heart. J. Physiol. (London) *44*, 206–219, 1912.

KOCH, E.: Neuere Apparate zur Künstlichen Durchströmung überlebender Organe. In: Handbuch der biologischen Arbeitsmethoden, E. Abderhalden, ed. Sect. V, pt. *1*, he. *4*, 1927.

KODAMA, J. K., R. J. GUZMAN and C. H. HINE: Some effects of epoxy compounds on the blood. Arch. Environmental Health *2*, 50–61, 1961.

KOLFF, W. J.: Mock circulation to test pumps designed for permanent replacement of damaged hearts. Cleveland Clin. Quart. *26*, 223–226, 1959.

—— and H. T. J. BERK: Artificial kidney: dialyzer with great area. Acta. Med. Scand. 117, 121–134, 1944.

—— and R. BALZER: The artificial coil lung. Trans. Am. Soc. Art. Int. Organs 1, 39–42, 1955.

——, C. P. DUBBELMAN and J. DEGROOT: An artificial heart. Geneesk. Gids. 1, 3–12, 1949. (Dut).

——, D. B. EFFLER, L. K. GROVES, G. PEEREBOOM and P. P. MORACA: Disposable membrane oxygenator (heart-lung machine) and its use in experimental surgery. Cleveland Clin. Quart. 23, 69–97, 1956a.

——, ——, ——, ——, S. AOYAMA and F. M. SONES: Elective cardiac arrest by the Melrose technic: potassium asystole for experimental cardiac surgery. Cleveland Clin. Quart. 23, 98–114, 1956b.

——, ——, —— and P. P. MORACA: Elective cardiac arrest with potassium citrate during open-heart operations: report of 37 cases. J.A.M.A. 164, 1653–1660, 1957a.

——, P. P. MORACA, D. E. HALE and W. L. PROUDFIT: A demonstration of the role of potassium and citrate ions under the conditions of elective cardiac arrest for open-heart operations. Cleveland Clin. Quart. 24, 128–132, 1957b.

——, D. B. EFFLER, L. K. GROVES, C. R. HUGHES and L. J. McCORMACK: Pulmonary complications of open-heart operations: Their pathogenesis and avoidance. Cleveland Clin. Quart. 25, 65–83, 1958.

——, —— and ——: A review of four dreaded complications of open-heart operations. Brit. M. J. 2, 1149–1152, 1960.

KOLIADITSKAIIA, E. A. and E. A. KRUSHEVA: Hematological data during cardiac surgery with extracorporeal circulation. Eks. Khir. Anesthesiol. 1, 22–26, 1961. (Rus).

KOO, K. S., K. J. CHOU and C. PIAN: Experimental extracorporeal circulation. Chin. M. J. 77, 20–26, 1958.

KOTTMEIER, P. K., J. ADAMSONS, J. H. STUCKEY, M. M. NEWMAN and C. DENNIS: Pathological changes after partial and total cardiopulmonary bypass in human animals. Surg. Forum 9, 184–189, 1959.

KOVANOV, V. V. and B. A. KONSTANTINOV: Experimental study of hypothermia, cavopulmonary anastomosis and extracorporeal circulation with regard to open-heart surgery. Eks. Khir. Anesthesiol. 1, 12–18, 1961. (Rus).

KRASNA, I. H., L. STEINFELD, I. KREEL and I. D. BARONOFSKY: Prolonged veno-venous perfusion with oxygenation in experimental

hypoxia of respiratory origin. Surg. Forum 11, 218–220, 1960.

KREEL, I., L. I. ZAROFF, I. H. KRASNA and I. D. BARONOFSKY: A syndrome following total body perfusion. Surg. Gynec. Obstet. 111, 317–321, 1960.

KREUZER, F.: Modellversuche zum Problem der Sauerstoffdiffusion in den Lungen. Helv. Physiol. Pharmacol. 11, (Suppl. 9), 1953.

—— and W. Z. YAHR: Influence of red cell membrane on diffusion of oxygen. J. Appl. Physiol. 15, 1117–1122, 1960.

KROGH, A.: The rate of diffusion of gases through animal tissues, with some remarks on the coefficient of invasion. J. Physiol. (London) 52, 391–408, 1919.

KUDRIASHOV, B. A. and T. M. KALISHEVSKAIA: On the neurohumoral nature of the physiological anticoagulating system. Doklady Acad. Nautz. SSSR 131, 213–216, 1960. (Rus).

KUHN, L. A., F. L. GRUBER, A. FRANKEL and S. KUPFER: The use of closed chest extracorporeal circulation without oxygenation in acute myocardial infarction with shock. Surg. Forum 10, 616–621, 1960a.

——, ——, —— and ——: Hemodynamic effects of extracorporeal circulation in closed-chest normal animals and in those with myocardial infarction with shock. Circul. Res. 8, 199–206, 1960b.

——, —— and ——: Hemodynamic effects of balloon obstruction of the abdominal aorta and superior vena caval-distal aortic shunting in dogs with myocardial infarction and shock. Am. J. Cardiol. 7, 218–226, 1961.

KUNA, S. A. J. GORDON, B. S. MORSE, F. B. LANE III and H. A. CHARIPPER: Bone marrow function in perfused isolated hindlegs of rats. Am. J. Physiol. 196, 769–774, 1959.

KUNKLER, A. and H. KING: Comparison of air, oxygen and carbon dioxide embolization. Ann. Surg. 149, 95–99, 1959.

KUNLIN, J.: Sur l'autoperfusion cardioencéphlique pendant l'exclusion de la circulation intracardiaque en vue de la chirurgie des cavités du coeur. C. R. Acad. Sci. Paris 226, 357–359, 1948a.

——: Exploration chirurgicale des cavités du coeur gauche avec circulation coronaro-encéphalique artificielle chez le chien. C. R. Acad. Sci. Paris 226, 1863–1864, 1948b.

——: Expériences de perfusions supradiaphragmatiques et de circulation extracorporelle totale chez le chien en vue de la chirurgie intracardiaque au moyen d'un coeur et d'un poumon artificiel. Rev. Chir. Paris *71*, 237–264, 1952.

——, S. RICHARD and A. C. BENITTE: Essais favorables de réanimation cardiaque après embolie gazeuse coronarienne expérimentale. C. R. Soc. Biol. *152*, 1687–1688, 1958.

KUSSEROW, B. K.: A mechanical heart-lung apparatus with gas dispersion centrifugal aerator. Proc. Soc. Exp. Biol. Med. *88*, 161–165, 1955.

KUSUNOKI, T., H. C. CHENG, H. H. McGUIRE and L. H. BOSHER: Myocardial dysfunction after cardioplegia. J. Thor. Cardiovasc. Surg. *40*, 813, 1960.

KYLSTRA, J. A., S. D. MOULOPOULOS and W. J. KOLFF: Further development of an ultrathin teflon membrane gas exchanger. Trans. Am. Soc. Art. Int. Organs *7*, 355–360, 1961.

L

LAEWEN, A. and R. SIEVERS: Experimentelle Untersuchungen über die Wirkung von künstlicher Atmung, Herzmassage, Strophanthin und Adrenalin auf den Herzstillstand nach temporärem Verschluss der Aorta und Arteria pulmonalis unter Bezugnahme auf die Lungenembolieoperation nach Trendelenburg. Deutsche Ztschr. f. Chir. (Leipz.) *105*, 174–256, 1910.

LAM, C. R., T. GEOGHEGAN and A. LEPORE: Induced cardiac arrest for intracardiac surgical procedures. J. Thor. Surg. *30*, 620–625, 1955.

——, T. GAHAGAN, C. SERGEANT and E. GREEN: Clinical experiences with induced cardiac arrest during intracardiac surgical procedures. Ann. Surg. *146*, 439–449, 1957a.

——, ——, —— and ——: Experiences in the use of cardioplegia (induced cardiac arrest) in the repair of interventricular septal defects. J. Thor. Surg. *34*, 509–520, 1957b.

——, ——, C. MOTA and E. GREEN: Induced cardiac arrest (cardioplegia) in open-heart surgical procedures. Surgery *43*, 7–13, 1958.

LAMBERTSEN, C. J., J. H. EWING, R. H. KOUGH, R. GOULD and M. W. STROUD: Oxygen toxicity. Arterial and internal jugular blood gas composition in man during inhalation of air, 100% O_2 and 2% CO_2 in O_2 at 3.5 atmosphere ambient pressure. J. Appl. Physiol. *8*, 255–263, 1955/1956.

LAMPERT, H.: Die physikalische Seite des Blutgerinnungsproblem. Leipzig, Georg Thieme, 1931.

LANDEW, M., L. T. BOWLES, S. GELMAN, A. B. LOWENFELS, R. TEPPER and J. W. LORD, JR.: Effects of intra-arterial microbubbles. Am. J. Physiol. *199*, 485–490, 1960.

LARY, G. G.: Experimental maintenance of life by intravenous oxygen: preliminary report. Surg. Forum *2*, 30–35, 1952.

LASKA, J.: Principle of substitute cardiac function and the technical possibilities of such a solution. Cas. Lek. Cesk. *94*, 681–684, 1955, (*Cze*).

LASSEN, N. A.: Cerebral blood flow and oxygen consumption in man. Physiol. Rev. *39*, 183–238, 1959.

LATHEM, W. and W. E. WORLEY: The distribution of extracorpuscular hemoglobin in circulating plasma. J. Clin. Invest. *38*, 474–483, 1959.

LAURENT, D., J. L. CHEVRIER, J. DECAUDAVEINE and M. VALON: Hypothermie et circulation extracorporelle (étude expérimentale en vue de circulation extracorporelle prolongée). Path. Biol. *7*, 95–110, 1959a.

——, ——, S. GAUDEAU, M. VALON and J. LEROY: Étude expérimentale de l'action de la L. Noradrenaline sur le flux coronaire et le métabolisme cardiaque sous circulation extracorporelle. Rev. Fr. Clin. Biol. *4*, 242–254, 1959b.

LAWRENCE, G. H. and R. M. PAINE: Experimental and clinical studies employing a disc oxygenator for complete cardiopulmonary bypass. West. J. Surg. Obstet. Gynec. *68*, 359–364, 1960.

LEE, W. H., JR., T. D. DARBY, J. D. ASHMORE and E. F. PARKER: Myocardial contractile force as a measure of cardiac function during cardiopulmonary bypass procedures. Surg. Forum *8*, 398–402, 1958.

LEEDS, S. E.: A cannula for simultaneous drainage of both cavae in artificial heart experiments. Proc. Soc. Exp. Biol. Med. *75*, 468–469, 1950.

——, N. N. GRAY and O. S. COOK: Prolongation of occlusion of the cavae in dogs by diversion of the circulation. Surg. Gynec. Obstet. *91*, 399–404, 1950.

——, L. PUZISS and P. SIEGEL: The shunting of blood from the right heart by means of a pump with operation on the interior of the heart. Surg. Forum *1*, 265, 1951.

LEGALLOIS, J. J. C.: Expériences sur le principe de la vie. Paris; D'Hautel, 1812.

——: Experiments on the principle of life

(tr. by N. C. and J. C. Nancrede) Philadephia, M. Thomas, 1813.

LEIGH, M. D., J. C. JONES and H. L. MOTLEY: The expired carbon dioxide as a continuous guide of the pulmonary and circulatory systems during anesthesia and surgery. J. Thor. Cardiov. Surg. *41*, 597–610, 1961.

LENFANT, C.: Système pompe-oxygénateur de Lillehei-DeWall. Thèse, Paris 1956.

——, M. WEISS and CH. DUBOST: A propos d'un nouveau filtre sanguin à grand débit. Presse Méd. *64*, 382–383, 1956a.

——, ——, J. ROUANET and CH. DUBOST: Élargissement des limites du système pompe-oxygénateur de Lillehei-DeWall pour chirurgie cardiaque exsangue. Presse Méd. *64*, 1162–1164, 1956b.

——, ——, CH. DUBOST and L. SPROVIERI: Contribution a l'étude du débit coronaire et métabolisme cardiaque sous circulation extracorporelle. Sem. Hop. Paris *33*, 2195–2202, 1957.

LEONARD, E. F. and L. W. BLUEMLE, JR.: The permeability concept as applied to dialysis. Trans. Am. Soc. Art. Int. Organs *6*, 33–37, 1960.

LEONARDS, J. R.: Effective instrument sterilization with a new ethylene oxide technique. Armamentarium, vol. 2, no. IX, 1, Chicago, Ill.: V. Mueller and Co., 1957.

—— and J. L. ANKENEY: A completely occlusive nonhemolytic roller tubing blood pump. Trans. Am. Soc. Art. Int. Organs *4*, 69–73, 1958.

LEPORE, A. A. and F. MORIN: Experimental circulatory arrest and electrical activity of the brain. J. Thor. Cardiovasc. Surg. *41*, 212–224, 1961.

LEROY, G. V., B. HALPERN and R. E. DOLKART: Indirect quantitative method for estimation of heparin activity in vitro: heparin protamine titration test. J. Lab. Clin. Med. *35*, 446–458, 1950.

LESAGE, A. M., W. C. SEALY, I. W. BROWN JR. and W. G. YOUNG JR.: Hypothermia and extracorporeal circulation; experimental studies of profound hypothermia of 10 to 20°C. Arch. Surg. *79*, 607–613, 1959.

——, J. M. LEE, A. OTTOLENGHI, W. G. YOUNG, JR. and W. C. SEALY: Central nervous system injury following deep hypothermia and circulatory arrest. Trans. Am. Soc. Art. Int. Organs *7*, 261–268, 1961.

LETAC, R. and S. LETAC: La circulation extracardiaque avec oxygénation par le poumon du sujet. Marseille Chir. *11*, 128–130, 1959.

LEVEEN, H. H., B. SCHATMAN and G. FALK: Cardiac arrest produced by massive transfusions. Surg. Gynec. Obstet. *109*, 502–508, 1959.

LEVIN, M. B., R. A. THEYE, W. S. FOWLER and J. W. KIRKLIN: Performance of the stationary vertical screen oxygenator (Mayo-Gibbon) J. Thor. Cardiovasc. Surg. *39*, 417–426, 1960.

LEVITSKAYA, L. A.: On methods of control of hemorrhage following operations on the dry heart with an apparatus for extracorporeal circulation. Eksp. Khir. *6*, 34–38, 1960 (*Rus*).

——, I. D. SHISHKINA, N. S. KONDRAT'EVA and N. S. SUPKO: Hematologic factors in artificial blood circulation using the apparatus of artificial blood circulation AIK. Eksp. Khir. *3*, 42–47, 1958 (*Rus*).

LEVOWITZ, B. S., M. M. NEWMAN, J. H. STUCKEY, M. C. KERNAN, H. N. ITICOVICI and C. DENNIS: A mechanical pump-oxygenator for direct vision repair of artrial septal defects. J. Thor. Surg. *32*, 647–660, 1956.

——, M. KENAN and R. MONSEES: Central venous pressures during total cardiac bypass. Surg. Forum *8*, 402–406, 1958.

LEVY, S. E. and A. BLALOCK; Fractionation of the output of the heart and of the oxygen consumption of normal unanesthetized dogs. Am. J. Physiol. *118*, 368–378, 1937.

LEWIN, R. L., C. E. CROSS, P. A. RIEBEN and P. F. SALISBURY: Influence of decreased vascular pressures on mechanics of ventilation in dogs. Am. J. Physiol. *198*, 873–876, 1960.

LEWIS, F. J., R. BENVENUTO and N. DEMETRAKOPOULOS: A new pump oxygenator employing polyethylene membranes. Quart. Bull. Northwest Univ. Med. School *32*, 262–267, 1958.

LIEBAU, G.: Über ein ventilloses Pumpprinzip. Naturwissenschaften *41*, 327, 1954.

——: Prinzipien kombinierter ventilloser Pumpen, abgeleitet vom menschlichen Blutkreislauf. Naturwissenschaften, *42*, 339, 1955.

LICHTY, J. A., JR., W. H. HAVILL and G. H. WHIPPLE: Renal thresholds for hemoglobin in dogs. Depression of renal threshold due to frequent hemoglobin injections and recovery during rest periods. J. Exp. Med. *55*, 603–615, 1932.

LILLEHEI, C. W.: Controlled cross circulation for direct-vision intracardiac surgery; correction of ventricular septal defects, atrioventricularis communis and tetralogy of Fallot. Post. Grad. Med. *17*, 388–396, 1955.

—— and R. H. CARDOZO: Use of median sternotomy with femoral artery cannulation in open cardiac surgery. Surg. Gynec. Obstet. *108*, 707–714, 1959.

——, M. COHEN, H. E. WARDEN and R. L. VARCO: The direct vision intracardiac correction of congenital anomalies by controlled cross circulation. Surgery *38*, 11–29, 1955a.

——, ——, ——, N. R. ZIEGLER and R. L. VARCO: The results of direct vision closure of ventricular septal defects in eight patients by means of controlled cross circulation. Surg. Gynec. Obstet. *101*, 446–466, 1955b.

——, ——, ——, R. C. READ, J. B. AUST, R. A. DEWALL and R. L. VARCO: Direct vision intracardiac surgical correction of tetralogy of Fallot, pentalogy of Fallot and pulmonary atresia defects. Report of first ten cases. Ann. Surg. *142*, 418–445, 1955c.

——, R. A. DEWALL, R. C. READ, H. E. WARDEN and R. L. VARCO: Direct vision intracardiac surgery in man using a simple, disposable artificial oxygenator. Dis. Chest. *29*, 1–8, 1956a.

——, ——, V. L. GOTT and R. L. VARCO: The direct vision correction of calcific aortic stenosis by means of a pump oxygenator and retrograde coronary sinus perfusion. Dis. Chest *30*, 123–132, 1956b.

——, J. L. GOTT, R. A. DEWALL and R. L. VARCO: The surgical treatment of stenotic or regurgitant lesions of the mitral and aortic valves by direct vision utilizing a pump oxygenator. J. Thor. Surg. *35*, 154–190 1958.

——, H. E. WARDEN, R. A. DEWALL, P. STANLEY and R. L. VARCO: Cardiopulmonary bypass in surgical treatment of congenital or acquired cardiac disease. Arch. Surg. *75*, 928–929, 1959.

——, D. M. LONG and D. LEPLEY: Comparative study of polybrene and protamine for heparin-neutralization in open heart surgery. Ann. Surg. *151*, 11–16, 1960.

LIM, R. A., K. REHDER, R. A. HARP, B. DAWSON and J. W. KIRKLIN: Circulatory arrest during profound hypothermia induced by direct blood stream cooling, an experimental study. Surgery *49*, 367–374, 1961.

LINDBERGH, C. A.: An apparatus for the culture of whole organs. J. Exp. Med. *62*, 409–431, 1935.

LINDBERGH, E. F.: The relationship between perfusion blood temperature and available venous return during extracorporeal circulation. J. Thor. Surg. *37*, 663–672, 1959.

LINDERHOLM, H. and O. NORLANDER: Carbon dioxide tension and bicarbonate content of arterial blood in relation to anesthesia and surgery. Acta Anaesth. Scand. *2*, 1–14, 1958.

LITTLE, J. M., H. D. GREEN and J. E. HAWKINS JR.: Evidence from cross-transfusion experiments that the diminished urine flow accompanying ischemic compression shock is not due to humoral factors. Am. J. Physiol. *151*, 554–563, 1947.

LITTLEFIELD, J. B., J. F. DAMMANN, P. R. INGRAM and W. H. MULLER JR.: Changes in pulmonary artery pressure during cardiopulmonary bypass. J. Thor. Surg. *36*, 604–615, 1958a.

——, P. R. INGRAM, F. S. BLANTON, JR., J. F. DAMMANN and W. H. MULLER JR.: Bronchial artery left auricular blood flow: its relation to pulmonary damage in extracorporeal circulation. Surg. Forum *8*, 428–432, 1958b.

——, E. M. LOWICKI and W. H. MULLER JR.: Experimental left coronary artery perfusion through an aortotomy during cardiopulmonary bypass. J. Thor. Cardiov. Surg. *40*, 685–691, 1960.

LITWAK, R. S., A. J. GILSON, R. SLONIM, C. C. McCUNE, I. KIEM and H. L. GADBOYS: Alterations in blood volume following "normovolemic" total body perfusion. Accepted for publication in J. Thor. Cardiov. Surg. 1962.

LITWIN, M. S., F. G. PANICO, C. RUBINI, D. E. HARKEN and F. D. MOORE: Acidosis and lacticacidemia in extracorporeal circulation: the significance of perfusion flow rate and the relation to perfusion respiratory alkalosis. Ann. Surg. *149*, 188–199, 1959.

LOBPREIS, E. L.: The danger of hypoglycemia during cardiopulmonary bypass. J. Thor. Surg. *37*, 334–341, 1959.

——, E. RASCHKE, Y. WATANABE and J. V. MALONEY: A clinical evaluation of fresh and stored heparinized blood for use in extracorporeal circulation. Ann. Surg. *152*, 947–953, 1960.

LÖCHNER, W.: Stoffwechselvorgange in der Lunge. Beitr.z.Silikoseforschung *49*, 1–74, 1957.

——, J. PIIPER, E. SCHURMEYER and R. BOSTROEM: Ueber die Grosse eines Milchsäureschwundes in der Lunge narkotisierter

Hunde. Pflüger Arch. ges. Physiol *264*, 549–560, 1957.

LOEBELL, C. E.: De conditionibus quibus secretiones in glandulis perficiuntur. Diss., Marburg, 1849.

LOESCHKE, H. H.: Fortläufende Messungen während extracorporaler Zirkulation. Thoraxchirurgie *7*, 439–455, 1960.

——, K. H. GERTZ and E. S. BUCHERL: Gaswechsel und Säurebasengleichgewicht bei Variation von Ventilation und Perfusion an mit einer Herzlungenmaschine perfundierten Hunden. Mit einem Anhang: Zur Theorie eines Oxygenators. Pflüger Arch. ges. Physiol., *270*, 121–146, 1959.

LOFSTROM, B.: Intravascular aggregation and oxygen consumption: aggregation of red blood cells produced by high molecular weight dextran or by hypothermia. Acta Anaesth. Scand. *3*, 41–51, 1959.

——: Induced hypothermia and intravascular aggregation. Acta Anaesth. Scand. *3*, (Suppl. 3) 1–19, 1959.

——, and B. ZEDERFELDT: Effect of heparin on intravascular aggregation in induced hypothermia. Acta Chir. Scand. *116*, 163–166, 1959.

LÖHR, B.: Uber Pumpen, Schläuche und Kanülen in heute gebrauchlichen Herz-Lungen-Maschinen. Thoraxchirurgie *6*, 302–311, 1959.

——: Über die Arbeitsweise des Mayo-Gibbon Pumpoxygenators. Langenbeck Arch. Klin. Chir. *292*, 701–704, 1959.

——: Induzierter Herztillstand bei intracardialen Eingriffen mit künstlichem Kreislauf. Thoraxchirurgie *7*, 123–129, 1960.

——, H. MEESSEN and R. POCHE; Elektronenmikroskopische Untersuchungen des Herzmuskels vom Hund bei experimentellem Herzstillstand durch Kaliumcitrat und Anoxie. Arch. für Kreislaufforsch. *33*, 108–137, 1960.

LONG, J. A.: Pulsating perfusing apparatus. Science *103*, 170, 1946.

——: A pulsating perfusion apparatus. J. Lab. Clin. Med. *32*, 300–303, 1947.

LOPEZ-BELIO, M. and O. C. JULIAN: High output bubble oxygenator with variable oxygenating chamber for cardiac bypass. Surgery *47*, 772–783, 1960.

——, H. H. SU and O. C. JULIAN: The effect of a non-oxygenated coronaropulmonary flow in certain phases of cardiac bypass. Surg. Forum *8*, 424–428, 1958.

——, R. C. BALAGOT, S. EL ISSA, A. LIMA, I. SANCHEZ, F. GOMEZ, G. TASAKI and O. C.

JULIAN: Effect of acute changes in peripheral resistance during cardiopulmonary bypass. Surg. Forum *10*, 592–597, 1960.

——, G. TASAKI, R. BALAGOT, I. SANCHEZ, F. GOMEZ and O. C. JULIAN: Effect of hypothermia during cardiopulmonary bypass on peripheral resistance. Alteration by dilute blood perfusate and by chlorpromazine. Arch. Surg. *81*, 283–290, 1960.

LORD, J. W., JR., E. CORYLLOS, A. B. LOWENFELS, R. DYSART, C. G. NEWMANN and J. W. HINTON: Evaluation of operations for revascularization of the myocardium by the study of coronary blood flow using extracorporeal circulation. Surgery *43*, 203–213, 1958.

LOVAT-EVANS, C., F. GRANDE and F. Y. HSU: Two simple heart-oxygenators circuits for blood-fed hearts. Quart. J. Exp. Physiol. *24*, 283–286, 1934.

LUDBROOK, J. and V. WYNN: Citrate intoxication; a clinical and experimental study. Brit. M. J. *2*, 523–528, 1958.

LUDWIG, C. and A. SCHMIDT: Das Verhalten der Gase, welche mit dem Blut durch den reizbaren Säugethiermuskel strömen. Leipzig Berichte, *20*, 12–72, 1868.

LUKAC, F. and M. PRCIC; Heart-lung apparatus (artificial heart) and its use in extracorporeal circulation. Med. Arhiv. *13*, 71–80, 1959 (*Se*).

LÜSCHER, E. F.: Blood platelets - their relationship to the blood clotting system and to hemostasis. A review. Vox Sanguinis *5*, 259–271, 1960.

LYNCH. H. F. and E. F. ADOLPH: Blood flow in small blood vessels during deep hypothermia. J. Appl. Physiol. *11*, 192–196, 1957.

LYONS, W. S., J. W. DUSHANE and J. W. KIRKLIN: Post-operative care after whole body perfusion and open intracardiac operations: use of Mayo-Gibbon pump-oxygenator and Browns-Emmons heat exchanger. J.A.M.A. *173*, 625–630, 1960.

M

MacNEILL, A. E., J. E. DOYLE, R. ANTHONE and S. ANTHONE: Technic with parallel flow, straight tube blood dialyzer. N. Y. St. J. Med. *59*, 4137–4148, 1959.

McCABE, S.: Pump for replacement of the heart. Trans. Am. Soc. Art. Int. Organs *5*, 289–292, 1959.

McCAUGHAN, J. S. JR., H. McMICHAEL, J. C.

SCHUDER and C. K. KIRBY: An evaluation of various devices for intracardiac suction. Trans. Am. Soc. Art. Int. Organs 4, 130–142, 1958a.

——, ——, —— and ——: The use of a totally occlusive pump as a flowmeter with observations on hemolysis caused by occlusive and nonocclusive pumps and other pump-oxygenator components. Surgery 44, 210–219, 1958b.

——, ——, —— and ——: Ethylene oxide sterilization of a completely assembled vertical screen pump-oxygenator. Surgery 45, 648–654, 1959.

——, R. WEEDER, J. C. SCHUDER and W. S. BLAKEMORE: Evaluation of new non-wettable macroporous membranes with high permeability coefficients for possible use in a membrane oxygenator. J. Thor. Cardiovasc. Surg. 40, 574–581, 1960.

McFARLAND, J. A., L. B. THOMAS, J. W. GILBERT and A. G. MORROW: Myocardial necrosis following elective cardiac arrest induced with potassium citrate. J. Thor. Cardiovasc. Surg. 40, 200–208, 1960.

McGOON, D. C., E. A. MOFFITT, R. A. THEYE and J. W. KIRKLIN: Physiologic studies during high flow, normothermic, whole body perfusion. J. Thor. Cardiovasc. Surg. 39, 275–287, 1960.

McGREGOR, R. R.: Silicones and their uses. New York, McGraw-Hill Book Co., 1954.

——: Silicone rubber. IRE Trans Med. Electronics 6, 51, 1959.

——: Silicones defoamers in blood oxygenators. Bull Dow Corning Center f. Aid Med. Res. 2, 6, 1960.

McGUIRE, H. H., JR., L. H. BOSHER, JR. and R. W. RAMSEY: Exploration into narcosis for surgical cardioplegia. Trans. Am. Soc. Art. Int. Organs 6, 323–328, 1960.

McKEEVER, W. P., D. E. GREGG and P. C. CANNEY: Oxygen uptake of the non-working left ventricle. Circulat. Res. 6, 612–623, 1958.

McKENZIE, M. B. and C. N. BARNARD: Experimental studies in extracorporeal circulation using the helix reservoir bubble oxygenator. S. Afr. M. J. 32, 1145–1151, 1958.

—— and ——: A note on priming the DeWall oxygenator. S. Afr. M. J. 34, 108, 1960.

McLAUGHLIN, E. D., T. F. NEALON, and J. H. GIBBON, JR.: Treatment of bank blood by resins. J. Thor. Cardiov. Surg. 40, 602–610, 1960.

McLEAN, J.: The thromboplastic action of cephalin. Amer. J. Physiol. 41, 250–257, 1916.

McMILLAN, I. K. R.: Flow meters, pp. 139–149, in: Extracorporeal Circulation, J. G. Allen, ed., Springfield, Ill., Thomas, 1958.

MAGENDIE, M.: Lectures on the blood and on the changes which it undergoes during disease. Lecture III. Lancet 1, 105–109, 1838.

——: Les phénomènes physiques de la vie., vol. 2, Paris, J. B. Baillière, 1842.

R. MAGNUS: Die Thätigkeit des überlebenden Säugethierherzens bei Durchströmung mit Gasen. Arch. Exp. Path. Pharmacol. 47, 200–208, 1902.

MAGOVERN, G. J., R. S. CARTWRIGHT, J. F. NEVILLE and E. M. KENT: Metabolic acidosis and the dissociation curve of hemoglobin during extracorporeal circulation. J. Thor. Cardiov. Surg. 38, 561–572, 1959.

MAHER, F. T., J. V. YOUNG, L. C. WATKINS and J. L. BOLLMAN: Laboratory experences with the Skeggs-Leonards artificial kidney. Proc. Mayo Clin. 31, 350–356, 1956.

——, L. C. WATKINS JR., J. C. BROADBENT and J. L. BOLLMAN: Significance of homologous donor blood to the toxic reaction in dogs. Circulat. Res. 6, 47–54, 1958.

MAHONEY, E. B., J. A. DE WEESE, T. I. JONES and J. A. MANNING: Coronary artery perfusion with oxygenated whole blood in open cardiac surgery under hypothermia. Bull. Soc. Int. Chir. 17, 34–40, 1958.

MAIER, C. G.: Producing small bubbles of gas in liquids by submerged orifices. In: O. C. Ralston: The ferric sulfate-sulphuric acid progress. U. S. Dept. of Comm., Bur. of Mines, Bull. 260, 1927.

MAJER, A.: personal communication, 1958.

MALETTE, W. G.: Cerebral anoxia resulting from hyperventilation. Surg. Forum 9, 208–211, 1958.

——, J. B. FITZGERALD and E. KOEGEL: A low volume oxygenator for regional perfusion. Publ. 61–16, School of Aviation Medicine, USAF Aerospace. Med. Center, Brooks A. F. Base, Texas, 1960.

MALMEJAC, J.: Controlled hypothermia: physiological bases for bloodless heart surgery at 15°-20°C. J. Cardiov. Surg. 1, 155–168, 1960.

—— and C. MALMEJAC: Chirurgie cardiaque expérimentale à 16°-18°C. Intérêt de la notion de "lavage" myocardique et cérébral. Algérie Med. 64, 49–66, 1960.

MALONEY, J. V., JR., W. L. LONGMIRE JR., K. J. SCHMUTZER, S. A. MARABLE, E. RASCHKE and J. E. Arzouman: An experimental and clinical comparison of the bubble dispersion and stationary screen pump oxygenators. Surg. Gynec. Obstet. *107*, 577–587, 1958.

Maluf, N. S. R.: Factors inducing renal shutdown from lysed erythrocytes: an experimental study. Ann. Surg. *130*, 49–67, 1949.

Maraist, F. B. and W. W. L. Glenn: Experimental cardiac surgery. III. Caval blood flow as measured directly with the caval venous return shunted past the right heart. Surgery *31*, 146–160, 1952.

Margaglia, F., F. Caluzzi and E. Ciocatto: Il cuore-polmone artificiale attualmente in uso presso la Clinica Chirurgica di Torino. Atti. Soc. Ital. Cardiol. *21*, Communicazioni 194–196, 1959.

Margraff, W.: Die Einwirkung einer O_2-Durchströmung auf menschliches Blut. Langenbeck Arch. Klin. Chir. *289*, 716–719, 1958.

Margulis, M. S.: On the optimal artificial blood flow in extracorporeal circulation. Eksp. Khir. *4*, 58–60, 1959 (*Rus*).

———: Effectiveness of extracorporeal blood circulation in experimental conditions with the use of various forms of artificial circulation. Eksp. Khir. *5*, 12–18, 1960 (*Rus*).

——— and V. Yu. Ostrovsky: Electroencephalographic observations during extracorporeal circulation under experimental conditions. Eksp. Khir. *6*, 42–46, 1960 (*Rus*).

Marinesku, V., D. Setlacheck, E. Malitski, G. Litarchek and B. Fotiade: Certain aspects of our experiences with cardiac surgery. Khirurgiia (Sofia) *12*, 929–944, 1959 (*Rus*).

Marion, P., J. Gounot, S. Estanove, J. F. Estanove, R. Cosson, A. Jeunet and R. Gounot: Remarques sur les facteurs d'hémolyse en circulation extracorporelle. Lyon Chir. *54*, 894–899, 1958.

Martin, H. N.: A new method of studying the mammalian heart. Studies from the biological Laboratory, Johns Hopkins University, *2*, 119–130, 1881.

Martin, M. V., S. Paladino, F. J. Sime, S. Quaresma, S. Singer, R. de G. Santos, L. G. D'Oliveira and H. J. Felipozzi: Pré e pósoperatório na cirurgia intracardíaca com emprêgo do coração-pulmáo artificial. Med. Cir. Farm. (Rio) *270*, 460–470, 1958.

Martinez-Bordiu, C., F. Serrano Munoz and C. Rubio-Martinez: Nuestra experiencia en circulatión extracorporea. Bol. Cult. Cons. ges. Coll. Med. España *22*, 15–22, 1959.

Marx, T. I., M. Litman, D. R. Miller, F. F. Albritten Jr. and M. R. Klein: The impingement oxygenator. Experimentation in the study of a new method of blood oxygenation. Surgery *45*, 992–1004, 1959.

———, W. E. Snyder, A. D. St John and C. E. Moeller: Diffusion of oxygen into a film of whole blood. J. Appl. Physiol. *15*, 1123–1129, 1960.

Massimo, C. and L. Boffi: La perfusione coronaria come complemento dell' ipotermia nella chirurgia a cuore esangue; perfusione coronarica retrograda per l'aggressione dell'aorta ascendente. Minerva Cardioangiol. *6*, 408–411, 1958.

———, ——— and L. Pozzi: Sinusal standstill with ventricular automatism during retrograde perfusion of the coronary sinus under hypothermia for direct surgical approach to the artic valves (an experimental study). J. Thor. Surg. *36*, 227–229, 1958.

Matthews, E. C., L. C. Clark, F. K. Edwards, S. Kaplan and J. A. Helmsworth: Studies during the immediate postoperative period following total body perfusion. Arch. Surg. *77*, 313–318, 1958.

Matthews, J. H., J. J. Buckley and F. H. Van Bergen: Acute effect of low-flow extracorporeal circulation on cerebral physiology. Anesthesiology *18*, 169–170, 1957.

Mavor, G. E., R. K. McEvoy, R. A. Harder and E. B. Mahoney: Ressuscitation of the K-arrested hypothermic heart (an experimental study). Brit. J. Surg. *44*, 521–529, 1957.

Mazzoni, P. and F. Baisi: Una nuova tecnica per determinare una "ipotermia profonda" nell'animale: la perfrigerazione extracorporea del sangue. Arch. Chir. Tor. *9*, 175–186, 1954.

Melnick, D., E. Burack and G. R. Cowgill: Development of incompatibilities in dogs by repeated infusions of red blood cells. Proc. Soc. Exp. Biol. Med. *33*, 616–621, 1936.

——— and G. R. Cowgill: Differentiation of blood groups in the dogs based on antigenic complexes present in the erythrocytes. Proc. Soc. Exp. Biol. Med. *36*, 697–700, 1937.

Melrose, D. G.: A heart-lung machine for use in man. J. Physiol. (London) *127*, 51–53, 1955.

———: The principles of heart-lung machines.

Lect. Sci. Basis Med. (London) *6*, 85–89, 1958.

——: Pumping and oxygenating systems. Brit. J. Anaesth. *31*, 393–400, 1959.

——, and I. AIRD: A mechanical heart-lung for use in man. Brit. M. J. *2*, 57–62, 1953.

——, J. W. BASSETT, P. BEACONSFIELD, I. G. GRABER and R. SHACKMAN: Experimental physiology of a heart lung machine in parallel with normal circulation. Brit. M. J. *2*, 62–66, 1953.

——, B. DREYER, H. H. BENTALL and J. B. E. BAKER: Elective cardiac arrest: preliminary communication. Lancet *2*, 21–22, 1955.

——, M. L. BRAMSON, J. J. OSBORN and F. GERBODE: The membrane oxygenator. Some aspects of oxygen and carbon dioxide transport across polyethylene film. Lancet *1*, 1050–1051, 1958.

MENDELSOHN, D., JR., T. N. MACKRELL, M. A. MACLACHLAN, F. S. CROSS and E. B. KAY: Experiences using the pump oxygenator for open cardiac surgery in man. Anesthesiology *18*, 223–235, 1957.

——, ——, D. W. MACDONALD, C. NOGUEKIA, L. R. HEAD, JR. and E. B. KAY: Management of the patient during open heart surgery. Surgery *45*, 949–965, 1959.

MENDLOWITZ, M.: The specific heat of blood. Science *107*, 97–98, 1948.

MENGES, G. and L. RULAND: Gas-Sterilisator zur Trockensterilisation von Herz-Lungen-Maschinen. Chirurg *30*, 192, 1959.

MERCHANT, R. C. and V. G. RANADE: Effects of acetylcholine, potassium chloride, adrenaline and pilocarpine on cooled heart. Ind. J. M. Sci. *13*, 431–435, 1959.

MERCKER, H.: Sauerstoff-Perflation. Ein neuer Weg zur Erhaltung der Funktion von Organen. Deutsche Med. Wschr. *84*, 1745–1746, 1959.

MEREDITH, J. H., J. H. ARTESANI and J. H. MAMLIN: Temperature compensated self-calibrated oxygen monitoring device. J. Thor. Cardiov. Surg. *40*, 582–587, 1960.

MERENDINO, K. A., W. E. QUINTON, G. I. THOMAS, J. E. JESSEPH, P. W. HERRON, R. E. TREMBLAY, R. X. MAGUIRE and R. R. VETTO: Description of a modified bubble-type pump-oxygenator. Surgery *42*, 996–1001, 1957.

MERRIT, D. H., W. C. SEALY, W. G. YOUNG JR. and J. S. HARRIS: Potassium, magnesium and nostigmine for controlled cardioplegia: evaluation with isolated perfused cat heart. Arch. Surg. *76*, 365–371, 1958.

MEYER-WEGENER, H.: Die Herabsetzung der Hämolyse in Herz-Lungen-Maschinen und Blutkonserven durch Vorbehandlung der Spender mit α-tocopherol. Klin. Wschschr. *38*, 407–408, 1960.

——and H. R. NEY: Eine einfache Herz-Lungen-Maschine mit neuem Filmoxygenator. Chirurg *31*, 4–7, 1960.

MEYLER, F. L. and D. DURRER: The influence of poly-vinyl-chloride tubing on the isolated perfused rat's heart: preliminary communication. Vox Sang. *4*, 239–242, 1959.

——, A. F. WILLBRANDS and D. DURRER: Influence of polyvinyl chloride tubing on the isolated perfused rat's heart. Circulat. Res. *8*, 44–46, 1960.

MICHAELS, A. S. and R. B. PARKER JR.: Sorption and flow of gases in polyethylene. J. Polymer Sci. *41*, 53–72, 1959.

MICHAL, G., S. NAEGLE, W. H. DANFORTH, F. B. BALLARD and R. J. BING: Metabolic changes in heart muscle during anoxia. Am. J. Physiol. *197*, 1147–1151, 1959.

MICOZZI, P., CORTESINI, G. PEZZOLI and A. PASANISI: La perfusione retrograda del circolo coronario con sangue a bassa temperatura nella chirurgia sperimentale della valvola aortica in circolazione extracorporea. Arch. Chir. Tor. *13*, 429–447, 1959a.

——, N. MOGAVERO, G. NOVELLI, A. PASANISI and A. VENTURINI: L'arresto cardiaco farmacologico nella chirurgia a cuore aperto. Arch. Chir. Tor. *16*, 191–204, 1959b.

——, G. P. NOVELLI and R. CORTESINI: Caratteristiche techniche e modalità d'impiego di un ossigenatore di superficie a dischi ruotanti. Arch. Chir. Tor. *17*, 13–35, 1960a.

——, G. PEZZOLI, F. TRANI and R. CORTESINI: Il ruolo del circolo bronchiale in chirurgia cardiaca. Arch. Chir. Tor. *17*, 53–67, 1960b.

MIDDELDORF, F. H.: Konstruktionsmerkmale und Anwendungsmöglichkeiten von Chemie-Pumpen. Chemie-Ingenieur Technik *33*, 31–36, 1961.

MILLER, B. J., J. H. GIBBON, JR. and M. H. GIBBON: Recent advances in the development of a mechanical heart and lung apparatus. Ann. Surg. *134*, 694–708, 1951.

——, —— and C. FINEBERG: An improved mechanical heart and lung apparatus; its use during open cardiotomy in experimental animals. Med. Clin. N. Amer. *37*, 1603–1624, 1953a.

——, ——, V. F. GRECO, B. A. SMITH, C. H. COHEN and F. F. ALLBRITTEN: The production and repair of interarterial septal defects under direct vision with the assistance of an extracorporeal pump-oxygenator circuit. J. Thor. Surg. *26*, 598–616, 1953b.

——, ——, ——, C. H. COHEN and F. F. ALLBRITTEN: The use of a vent for the left ventricle as a means of avoiding air embolism to the systemic circulation during open cardiotomy with the maintenance of the cardio-respiratory function of animals by a pump-oxygenator. Surg. Forum *4*, 29–33, 1954.

MILLER, D. R. and F. F. ALLBRITTEN: "Coronary suction" as a source of air embolism: an experimental study using the Kay-Cross oxygenator. Ann. Surg. *151*, 75–84, 1960.

MILLER, J. H.: A mechanical heart and turbulence oxygenator. Circulat. Res. *3*, 159–164, 1955.

MILNES, R. F. and R. VANDERWOUDE: A stainless disc oxygenator for cardiac bypass. Univ. Mich. Med. Bull. *23*, 166–171, 1957.

——, J. D. MORRIS, R. VANDERWOUDE, J. BURGE and H. SLOAN: Observations on the use of a simple bubble-type oxygenator for open cardiotomy. Univ. Mich. Med. Bull. *23*, 33–40. 1957a.

——, R. VANDERWOUDE, J. D. MORRIS and H. SLOAN: Problems related to a bubble oxygenator system. Surgery *42*, 986–992, 1957b.

——, ——, H. SLOAN and J. D. MORRIS: Extended asystole. Arch. Surg. *77*, 13–17, 1958.

MIRABEL, J., G. ARFEL and N. DU BOUCHET: Manifestations encéphalographiques d'anoxie cérébrale au cours de la chirurgie cardiaque. Anesthésie (Paris) *14*, 518–543, 1957.

DEL MISSIER, P. A., A. A. ANGRIST, L. C. REID and J. W. HINTON: The relation of the specific tissue to the common muscle in the heart. Surg. Forum *8*, 311–313, 1958.

MITTELMAN, A., R. BEALS, S. BHONSLAY, R. A. DETERLING, JR. and H. G. BARKER: Changes in steroid metabolism associated with extracorporeal circulation. Trans. Am. Soc. Art. Int. Organs *5*, 283–287, 1959.

MOCCHI, N. and A. CASCONE: Sulla diversa azione dell'eparina a piccole ed alte dosi sull'agglutinabilità piastrinica. Haematologica (Pavia) *43*, 397–406, 1958.

MOERSCH, R. N. and D. E. DONALD: A study of circulation in the lung following pulmonary artery occlusion. Surg. Forum *9*, 378–382, 1959.

MOFFITT, E. A. and R. A. THEYE: Management of anesthesia, perfusion and support-ive care during open-intracardiac operations and extracorporeal circulation. Brit. J. Anaesth. *31*, 411–416, 1959.

——, R. T. PATRICK, H. J. C. SWAN and D. E. DONALD: A study of blood flow, venous blood oxygen saturation, blood pressure and peripheral resistance during total body perfusion. Anesthesiology *20*, 18–26, 1959.

MOLL, M. and H. BARTEIS: Ein kritische Prüfung der offenen und der geschlossenen Methode zur Bestimmung des Sauerstauffverbrauchs nach Veränderung des inspiratorischen Sauerstoffkonzentration. Pflüger Arch. ges. Physiol. *271*, 583–594, 1960.

MONDINI, P.: Pneumectonia totale bilaterale con sporavvivenza dell'animale mediante l'uso d'un nuovo ossigenatore del sangue. Acta Chir. Patavina *4*, 3, 1948.

——: Nuovi indirizzi nel campo dell'ossigenoterapia extrapolmonare: possibilità di sostituire temporaneamente la funzione polmonare dell'animale "in toto" mediante l'uso di un nuovo apparecchio ossigenatore. G. Ital. Chir. *5*, 703–781, 1949.

—— and P. ZILIOTTO: Sulla emorragia a nappo dopo ossigenazione e circolazione extracorporea. Minerva Chir. *13*, 163–167, 1958.

——, C. ZACCARINI, A. PORRO, P. ZILIOTTO and L. CAVALLONI: Arresto farmacologico del cuore per la chirurgia cardiaca a cielo scoperto. Acta Chir. Ital. *12*, 43, 1956.

MONKHOUSE, F. C., R. L. McMILLAN and K. W. G. BROWN: The relation between heparin blood levels and blood coagulation times. J. Lab. Clin. Med. *42*, 92–97, 1953.

MONROE, R. G. and G. FRENCH: Ventricular pressure-volume relationships and oxygen consumption in fibrillation and arrest. Circulat. Res. *8*, 260–266, 1960.

——, —— and J. L. WHITTENBERGER: Effects of hypocapnia and hypercapnia on myocardial contractility. Am. J. Physiol. *199*, 1121–1124, 1960.

MONTGOMERY, V.: Respiratory characteristics of extracorporeal pump-oxygenators. J. Thor. Cardiovasc. Surg. *39*, 288–304, 1960.

——, B. C. PATON, J. LUCERO and H. SWAN: The design of monitoring devices for use with a pump-oxygenator. J. Thor. Cardiov. Surg. *39*, 225–228, 1960.

MOORE, R. F., T. H. LEHMAN and C. V. HODGES: Treatment of acute hyperkalemia utilizing extracorporeal perfusion of blood through cation exchange resin columns. Surg. Gynec. Obstet. *112*, 67–74, 1961.

DE MORAIS, D. J., C. S. LEITE, W. JASBIK and S. FRANCO: Estudo metabólico e hemodinâmico na circulação extracorpórea com exclusão cardiopulmonar. Hospital (Rio) 57, 201–223, 1960a.

——, S. A. FRANCO, W. JASBIK and J. SADER: Circulação extracorpórea prolongada com hemolise minima (Uso de plasma no oxygenador em substituição ao sángue). Rev. Bras. Cir. 39, 129–132, 1960.

MORGENSTERN, L., P. F. SALISBURY, M. M. HYMAN and D. STATE: Open heart surgery with the aid of a pump oxygenator. Calif. Med. 86, 29–31, 1957.

MORIN, G. and H. METRAS: Étude critique des méthodes d'exclusion des cavités cardiaques pour l'abord chirurgical de celles-ci. Arch. Mal. Coeur. 41, 739–744, 1948.

MORRIS, G. C., R. R. WITT, D. A. COOLEY, J. H. MOYER and M. E. DEBAKEY: Alterations in renal hemodynamics during controlled extracorporeal circulation in the surgical treatment of aortic aneurism. J. Thor. Surg. 34, 590–598, 1957.

——, W. C. AWE, H. W. BENDER, D. A. COOLEY and M. E. DEBAKEY: Effects of extracorporeal circulation on renal function, pp. 315–326. In: Extracorporeal Circulation, J. G. Allen, ed., Springfield, Ill., Thomas, 1958.

MORROW, A. G., J. W. GILBERT, E. SHARP, J. ROSS and C. S. WELDON: Experimental use of the Melrose pump oxygenator. Trans. Am. Soc. Art. Int. Organs 3, 46–48, 1957.

MORSE, D. P.: Open heart surgery in 1960—"A many splendour'd thing". Dis. Chest 38, 533–549, 1960.

MORTENSEN, J. D., S. M. SMITH and G. HILL: Bacterial contamination of oxygen used in cardiopulmonary bypass. J. Thor. Cardiov. Surg. 41, 675–679, 1961.

MOULDER, P. V., R. G. THOMPSON, C. A. SMITH, B. L. SIEGEL and W. E. ADAMS: Cardiac surgery with hypothermia and acetylcholine arrest. J. Thor. Surg. 32, 360–370, 1956.

MÜLLER, A.: Über den Sauerstofftransport durch dünne Schichten von Wasser und Hämoglobinlösungen. Helv. Physiol. Pharmacol. Acta 6, 21–41, 1948.

——, L. LASZT and L. PIRCHER: Über die Verwendung des Pitot-Rohres zur Geschwindigkeitsmessung. Helv. Physiol. Pharmacol. Acta 12, 98–111, 1954a.

——, —— and ——: Über die Verwendung des Castelli-Prinzipes zur Geschwindigkeitsmessung. Helv. Physiol. Pharmacol. Acta 12, 300–315, 1954b.

MÜLLER, F.: Allgemeine Methodik zur Untersuchung überlebender Organe. Handbuch d. biol. Arbeitsmeth. Abderhaldens Sect. V, pt. I, no. I, pt. 23, 1921.

MÜLLER, P. B.: Durchströmungsapparatur für Stoffwechselversuche am isolierten Organ. Schw. Med. Wschr. 69, 1087–1090, 1939.

MULLER, W. H. JR., J. B. LITTLEFIELD and J. F. DAMMANN: Pulmonary parenchymal changes associated with cardiopulmonary bypass, pp. 336–341. In: Extracorporeal Circulation, J. G. Allen, ed., Springfield, Ill.: Thomas, 1958.

MURDOCK, C. E. JR.: Auriculovenous hemodialysis. Arch. Surg. 81, 53–57, 1960.

MURPHY, W. P., JR.: The cardiac programmer to trigger an arterial pump. Trans. Am. Soc. Art. Int. Organs 7, 361–366, 1961.

MUSICANT, W. W., R. R. LEWIS, B. S. MUSICANT, R. M. ANDERSON and J. H. KAY: Hypothermic analgesia for open heart surgery with the heart lung machine. J. Thor. Surg. 37, 184–189, 1959.

MUSTARD, W. T.: Clinical and experimental experience with homologous and heterologous lung perfusion. Trans. Am. Soc. Art. Int. Organs 1, 94–95, 1955.

—— and A. L. CHUTE: Experimental intracardiac surgery with extracorporeal circulation. Surgery 30, 684–688, 1951.

——, —— and E. H. SIMMONS: Further observations on experimental extracorporeal circulation. Surgery 32, 803–810, 1952.

——, ——, J. D. KEITH, A. SERIK, R. D. ROWE and P. VLAD: A surgical approach to transposition of the great vessels with extracorporeal circuit. Surgery 36, 39–51, 1954.

——, W. SAPIRSTEIN and D. PAV: Cardiac bypass without artificial oxygenation. J. Thor. Surg. 36, 479–487, 1958.

MUTO, R., R. J. WALTHER and H. S. SISE: A new cannula for bypass of left ventricle using autogenous lung oxygenation and a closed pumping system. J. Thor. Cardiov. Surg. 41, 635–642, 1961.

N

NAKAMOTO, S.: Removal of edema fluid by ultrafiltration with the disposable twin coil artificial kidney—report of two cases. Cleveland Clin. Quart. 28, 10–15, 1961.

NARBONA, A. B., J. L. BARCIA SALORIO, P. CARBONELL, M. GUANTER and A. DELTORS:

Factor acigos, circulación extracorporal y hipotermia: estudio experimental; communicacion previa. Med. españ. *37*, 505-523, 1957.

NASHAT, F. S., A. K. YASSIN and S. SUBHIYAH: The effect of CO_2 on the preservation of blood. Arch. Int. Pharmacodyn. *130*, 86-95, 1961.

NEGRE, E., J. DU CAILAR, H. PUJOL, A. THEVENET and M. ATTISSO: Arrêt circulatoire en hypothermie profonde—étude expérimentale. Anesth. Analg. (Paris) *16*, 465-474, 1959.

NELSON, R. M., H. H. HECHT, R. W. HARDY, D. G. McQUARRIE and J. BURGE: Extracorporeal circulation for open heart surgery. J. Thor. Surg. *32*, 638-646, 1956.

NEPTUNE, W. B., J. A. BOUGAS and F. G. PANICO: Open-heart surgery without the need for donor-blood priming in the pump-oxygenator. New Eng. J. Med. *263*, 111-115, 1960.

NEUBAUER, O. and H. LAMPERT: Ein neuer Bluttransfusionsapparat. Zugleich ein Beitrag zur Kenntnis der thrombagogen Eigenschaften fester Stoffe. Münch. Med. Wschr. *77*, 582-586, 1930.

NEVILLE, W. E., S. KAMEYA, M. OZ, B. BLOOR and G. H. A. CLOWES, JR.: Profound hypothermia and complete circulation interruption. Arch. Surg. *82*, 108-119, 1961.

NEWMAN, M. M.: A self-regulating diaphragm pump. Trans. Am. Soc. Art. Int. Organs *4*, 75-79, 1958.

——, J. H. STUCKEY, B. S. LEVOWITZ, L. A. YOUNG, C. DENNIS, C. FRIES, E. J. GORAYER, M. ZUHDI, K. E. KARISON, S. ADLER and M. GLIEDMAN: Complete and partial perfusion of animal and human subjects with the pump-oxygenator. Surgery *38*, 30-37, 1955.

NICHOLS, H. T., D. P. MORSE and T. HIROSE: Coronary and other air embolization occuring during open cardiac surgery. Surgery, *43*, 236-244, 1958.

NIEDNER, F. F.: Grundprinzipien des künstlichen Herzens und der Herz-Lungen-Apparatur. Dtsch. Med. Wschr. *78*, 1233-1234, 1953.

NIESEL, W., G. THEWS and D. LUBBERS: Die Messung des zeitlichen Verlaufes der O_2-Aufsättigung und—Entsättigung menschlicher Erythrocyten mit dem Kurzzeit Spektralanalysator. Pflüger Arch. ges. Physiol. *268*, 296-307, 1959.

NILSSON, I. M. and J. SWEDBERG: Coagulation studies in cardiac surgery with extra-corporeal circulation using a bubble oxygenator. Acta. Chir. Scandin. *117*, 47-54, 1959.

NIXON, P. G.: A pump for use in open heart surgery. Lancet *1*, 1074-1075, 1959a.

——: A simple flowmeter and safety device for the extracorporeal circulation. Lancet *2*, 830, 1959b.

NIXON, F. G. F., V. A. GRIMSHAW, L. A. CATCHPOLE, H. M. SNOW and K. LAWRENCE: Clinical experience with the Melrose oxygenator at normal and reduced temperatures. Thorax *15*, 193-197. 1960.

NOBLE, T. C. and J. ABBOTT: Hemolysis of stored blood mixed with isotonic dextrose-containing solutions in transfusion apparatus. Brit. Med. J. *2*, 865-866, 1959.

NOELL, W. and M. SCHNEIDER: Quantitative Angaben über Durchblutung und Sauerstoffversorgung des Gehirns. Pflüger Arch. ges. Physiol. *250*, 35-41, 1948.

NONOYAMA, A.: Hemodynamic studies on extracorporeal circulation with pulsatile and non-pulsatile blood flows. Arch. Japan. Chir. *29*, 1381-1406, 1960.

NORBERG, B. and A. SENNING: A study of serum enzymes during and after open heart surgery with the Crafoord-Senning heart-lung machine. Acta Chir. Scandin. *245*, 275-282, 1959.

NORLANDER, O.: Anesthesiologische Erfahrungen aus der intracardialen Chirurgie mit der Crafoord-Senning Herz-Lungen-Maschine. Thoraxchirurgie *7*, 149-162, 1960.

——, S. PITZELE, I. EDLING, B. NORBERG, C. CRAFOORD and A. SENNING: Anesthesiological experience from intracardiac surgery with the Crafoord-Senning heart-lung machine. Acta Anaesthes. Scandin. *2*, 181-210, 1958.

NOSSOVA, E. A.: High-energy phosphate content of the brain of dogs during "clinical death" and revival in hypothermia. Voprosy Med. Khimii 6, 260-263, 1960 (*Rus*).

NOVELLI, G., P. MICOZZI, E. SCRASCIA and N. MOGAVERO: L'associazione dell'ipotermia alla circulazione extracorporea nella chirurgia a cuore aperto. Arch. Chir. Torace *13*, 449-465, 1959.

NUÑEZ, L. E. and C. P. BAILEY: New method for systemic arterial perfusion in extracorporeal circulation. J. Thor. Surg. *37*, 707-710, 1959.

NUNN, D. D., C. A. BELISLE, W. H. LEE, JR. and E. F. PARKER: A comparative study of aortic occlusion alone and of potassium citrate arrest during cardiopulmonary bypass. Surgery *45*, 848–851, 1959.

NYHUS, L.: Discussion on blood changes, p. 266. In: Extracorporeal Circulation, J. G. Allen, ed. Springfield, Ill., Thomas, 1958.

NYIRI, W.: Experimentelle Untersuchungen über gekreuzte Bluttransfusion bei Urämie. Arch. Exp. Pathol. Pharmacol. *166*, 3–4, 1926.

NYSTEN, P. H.: Recherches de physiologie et de chimie pathologique, pour faire suite à celles de Bichat sur la vie et la mort. Paris, J. A. Brosson, 1811.

O

O'BRIEN, L. J. and M. M. GUEST: Functional reactivation of the hypothermic heart after potassium arrest. Amer. J. Physiol. *196*, 961–965, 1959.

OECONOMOS, N.: Acquisitions récentes en chirurgie cardiaque; la circulation extracorporelle associée à l'arrêt cardiaque provoqué. Rev. Méd. Moyen Orient *15*, 498–502, 1958.

OGATA, T., Y. IDA, J. TAKEDA, A. NONOYAMA and H. SAKAKI: Experimental studies on the extracorporeal circulation by use of our pulsatile arterial pump. Lung (Japan) *6*, 381, 1959.

——, ——, A. NONOYAMA, J. TAKEDA and H. SASAKI: A comparitive study of the effectiveness of pulsatile and nonpulsatile blood flow in extracorporeal circulation. Arch. Japan. Chir. *29*, 59–65, 1960.

OHLWILER, D. A. and E. B. MAHONEY: Regional heparinization and heparin inactivation by erythrocytes. Surg. Gynec. Obstet. *107*, 353–358, 1958.

OINUMA, S.: The relative rates of oxidation and reduction of blood. J. Physiol. (London) *43*, 364–373, 1911.

OLIVER, T. and D. MURPHY: Influenzal pneumonia: The intravenous injection of hydrogen peroxide. Lancet *1*, 432–433, 1920.

OLMSTED, F., W. J. KOLFF and D. B. EFFLER: Three safety devices for the heart-lung machine. Cleveland Clin. Quart. *25*, 169–176, 1958.

OLSON, R. E. and D. A. PIATNEK: Conservation of energy in cardiac muscle. Ann. N. Y. Acad. Sci. *72*, 466–479, 1959.

OLSSON, P., G. WILLIAM-OLSSON and H. LAGERGREN: The elimination rate of heparin from plasma on normothermic and hypo-thermic dogs. Acta Chir. Scandin. *245*, 359–362, 1959.

OPITZ, E. and F. PALME: Darstellung der Höhenanpassung im Gebirge durch Sauerstoffmangel. III. Graduierung der Höhenkrankheit durch das Elektroencephalogramm. Pflüger Arch. ges. Physiol. *248*, 330–375, 1944.

—— and M. SCHNEIDER: Über die Sauerstoffversorgung des Gehirns und den Mechanismus von Mangelwirkungen. Ergebn. Physiol. *46*, 127–260, 1950.

OPPENHEIMER, M. J., J. M. STAUFFER, L. A. SOLOFF and T. M. DURANT: Physiological effects of carbon dioxide gas introduced into coronary arteries. Am. J. Physiol. *196*, 1308–1311, 1959.

ORTON, R. H. and K. N. MORRIS: Deliberate circulatory arrest; the use of halothane and heparin for direct-vision intracardiac surgery. Thorax *14*, 39–47, 1959.

OSBORNE, J. J.: A blood pump for whole blood without anticoagulants. Science *117*, 537–538, 1953.

——: Experience with an air-driven pump-oxygenator with special reference to blood coagulation. Trans. Amer. Soc. Artif. Int. Org. *1*, 81–83, 1955.

——, R. MACKENZIE, A. SHAW, H. PERKINS, R. HUNT and F. GERBODE: Cause and prevention of hemorrhage following extracorporeal circulation. Surg. Forum *6*, 97–100, 1956a.

——, F. GERBODE, H. A. PERKINS and R. HURT: The technic of heart-lung bypass with a pump oxygenator. Am. J. Surg. *92*, 287–291, 1956b.

——, ——, ——, M. BRAIMBRIDGE, D. MELROSE and P. KAHN: A disposable filming pump-oxygenator. Experimental and clinical use in 70 patients. J. Thor. Surg. *37*, 472–481, 1959.

——, M. L. BRAMSON and F. GERBODE: A rotating disc blood oxygenator and integral heat exchanger of improved inherent efficiency. J. Thor. Cardiov. Surg. *39*, 427–437, 1960.

OSBURN, J. O. and K. KAMMERMEYER: Separation of gases by plastic membranes. New diffusion cell design. Indust. Engin. Chem. *46*, 739–742, 1954.

OSELLADORE, G., A. BENCINI and P. L. PAROLA: Le nostre ricerche sperimentali sul problema della circolazione extracorporea. Minerva Med. *12*, 1–15, 1957.

O'SHAUGHNESSY, L.: The future of cardiac surgery. Lancet *2*, 969–971, 1939.

OTHMER, D. F. and C. J. FROHLICH: Correlating permeability constants gases through plastic membranes. Indust. Engin. Chem. *47*, 1034–1040, 1955.

OTTENBERG, R. and C. L. FOX, JR.: Rate of removal of hemoglobin from circulation and its renal threshold in human beings. Am. J. Physiol. *123*, 516–525, 1938.

OTTOLENGHI, R. and G. D. DRAGO: Funzionalità renale durante circolazione extracorporea. Minerva chir. *13*, 1474–1475, 1958.

OVERBECK, W., K. WIEMERS, G. RICHTER and E. G. KANIAK: On the combination of extracorporeal circulation with deep hypothermia. Bull. Soc. Int. Chir. *19*, 78–86, 1960.

OWENS, G., L. SAWYERS and J. W. WARD: Electroencephalographic responses in dogs during reduced blood flow. Surg. Forum *6*, 506–510, 1956.

——, J. E. ADAMS, R. E. DAWSON, E. M. LANCE, J. L. SAWYERS and H. W. SCOTT, JR.: Observed central nervous system responses during experimental employment of various pump-oxygenators. Surgery *44*, 240–253, 1958.

OWENS, G., J. E. ADAMS, F. M. McELHANNON and R. W. YOUNGBLOOD: Experimental alterations of certain colloidal properties of blood during cardiopulmonary bypass. J. Appl. Physiol. *14*, 947–948, 1959.

OZ, M., S. KAMEYA, W. NEVILLE and G. H. A. CLOWES, JR.: The relationship of blood volume, systemic peripheral resistance, and flow rate during profound hypothermia. Trans. Am. Soc. Art. Int. Organs *6*, 204–213, 1960.

P

PADHI, R. K., E. S. KO, R. L. G. RAINBOW and R. B. LYNN: Some observations on deep hypothermia using extracorporeal circulation. Angiology *12*, 12–16, 1961.

PAINTER, F. G., W. G. MALETTE, W. B. SUMMERS and K. R. McKENZIE: A simplified bubble pump-oxygenator. Angiology *8*, 348–351, 1957.

PALADINO, S., J. S. PERFEITO, R. G. SANTOS, L. G. D'OLIVEIRA and H. J. FELIPOZZI: Aspectos fisiólogicos das intervenções cardíacas com o emprégo do conjunto coração-pulmão artificial. (*1*) Observaçaos sobre o equilibrio acido-basico. Revista Paulista de Medicina *53*, 224–233, 1958.

PANETH, M., R. SELLERS, V. L. GOTT, W.

WEIRICH, P. ALLEN, R. C. READ and W. C. LILLEHEI: Physiologic studies upon prolonged cardiopulmonary bypass with the pump oxygenator with particular reference to (1) acid-base balance, (2) syphon caval drainage. J. Thor. Surg. *34*, 570–579, 1957.

PANICO, F. G.: An extracorporeal pump-oxygenator for organ perfusion. J. Appl. Physiol. *15*, 757–758, 1960.

—— and W. B. NEPTUNE: A mechanism to eliminate the donor blood prime from the pump-oxygenator. Surg. Forum *10*, 605–609, 1960.

PANUM, P. L.: Experimentelle Untersuchungen über die Transfusion, Transplantation oder Substitution des Blutes in theoretischer und practischer Beziehung. Virchow Arch. pathol. Anat. *27*, 240–295 & 443–459, 1864.

PAPADOPOULOS, C. N. and A. S. KEATS: The metabolic acidosis of hyperventilation produced by controlled respiration. Anesthesiol. *20*, 156–161, 1959.

PARKIN, T. W. and W. F. KVALE: Neutralization of heparin and protamine. J. Lab. Clin. Med. *32*, 1396, 1947.

—— and ——: Neutralization of anticoagulant effects of heparin with protamine. Amer. Heart J. *37*, 333–342, 1949.

PARKINS, W. M., J. M. JENSEN and H. M. VARS: Brain cooling in the prevention of brain damage during periods of circulatory occlusion in dogs. Ann. Surg. *140*, 284–287, 1954.

PAROLA, P. L. and A. BEUCIM: Ein neue Methode zur extracorporallen Blutsauerstoffversorgung; der Schwamm Sauerstoffversorger. Thoraxchirurgie *5*, 159–163, 1957.

——, ——, G. BOSELLI, A. AMBROSINI and D. GALMARINI: Variazioni delle componenti morfologiche e di alcune costanti biochimiche del sangue dopo periodi di circolazione extracorporea con l'apparecchio Bencini-Parola. Minerva Chir. *13*, 1478–1482, 1958a.

——, ——, P. FERRABOSHI, G. TIBERIO and T. LONGO: Vantaggi e svantaggi dei diversi sistemi di incannulazione venosa ed arteriosa attuabili per l'esclusione del cuore e dei polmoni a mezzo della circolazione extracorporea del sangue. Minerva Chir. *13*, 1482–1485, 1958b.

——, ——, T. LONGO and P. FERRABOSCHI: Pompe e valvole negli apparecchi per circolazione extracorporea del sangue; sistemi di regolazione automatica del flusso e sistemi di sicurezza. Minerva Chir. *13*, 1485–1488, 1958c.

PATRICK, R. T.: Anaesthesie von Patienten für intrakardiale Operationen. Langenbeck Arch. klin. Chir. *289*, 250–257, 1958.

——, R. A. THEYE and E. A. MOFITT: Studies in extracorporeal circulation. V. Anesthesia and supportive care during intracardiac surgery with the Gibbon-type pump oxygenator. Anesthesiol. *18*, 673–685, 1957.

PATON, B., W. C. PEARCY and H. SWAN: The importance of the electroencephalogram during open cardiac surgery with particular reference to superior vena caval obstruction. Surg. Gynec. Obstet. *111*, 197–202, 1960.

PATON, B. C., V. MONTGOMERY and H. SWAN: Methods for the control of extracorporeal circulation. Arch. Surg. *82*, 405–416, 1961.

PATT, H. H., J. V. CLIFT, P. B. LOH, J. C. ROA, J. WEXLER and A. M. SELIGMAN: Veno-arterial pumping in normal dogs and dogs with coronary occlusion. J. Thor. Cardiov. Surg. *39*, 464–467, 1960.

PATTLE, R. E.: The cause of the stability of bubbles derived from the lung. Phys. Med. Biol. *5*, 11–26, 1960.

PAYR, E.: Beiträge zur Technik der Blutgefäss—und Nervennaht, nebst Mitteilungen über die Verwendung eines resorbirbaren Metalles in der Chirurgie. Langenbeck Arch. klin. Chir. *62*, 67–93, 1900.

PEDEN, J. C., JR. and J. A. McFARLAND: Use of the plasma thrombin time to assess the adequacy of in vivo neutralization of heparin: comparative studies following operations employing extracorporeal circulation. Blood *14*, 1230–1236, 1959.

PEDERSON, D. and O. SECHER: Halothane anaesthesia in cardiac surgery. Act. Anesth. Scan. *2*, 169–179, 1958.

PEIRCE, E. C., II: The value of a low flow pump-oxygenator combined with hypothermia. Trans. Am. Soc. Art. Int. Organs *2*, 28, 1956.

——: Regulation of blood volume and venous pressure during partial and total cardiopulmonary bypass. Trans. Am. Soc. Art. Int. Organs *4*, 80–84, 1958a.

——: Diffusion of oxygen and carbon dioxide through teflon membranes. Arch. Surg. *77*, 938–943, 1958b.

——: A modification of the Clowes membrane lung. J. Thor. Cardiov. Surg. *39*, 438–448, 1960a.

——: Further development of a simplified method for determining metabolic and respiratory pH factors. Trans. Am. Soc. Art. Int. Organs *6*, 240–246, 1960b.

——: A simplified heat exchanger for perfusion hypothermia. Accepted for publication in Arch. Surgery, 1961a.

——: Measurement of organ blood flow during blood stream cooling and warming. Trans. Am. Soc. Art. Int. Organs *7*, 252–260, 1961b.

—— and C. H. DABBS: Metabolic acidosis and oxygen consumption before, during and following total cardiopulmonary bypass with and without hypothermia. Surg. Forum *10*, 597–601, 1960.

—— and V. B. POLLEY: Differential hypothermia for intracardiac surgery—preliminary report of a pump-oxygenator incorporating a heat exchanger. Arch. Surg. *67*, 521–525, 1953.

—— and J. L. SOUTHWORTH: Pump circuit for experimental intracardiac surgery of the left heart. Arch. Surg. *66*, 218–225, 1953.

——, C. H. DABBS, W. K. ROGERS and F. L. RAWSON: A practical method of differential hypothermia to permit use of a low pump oxygenator flow. Trans. Am. Soc. Art. Int. Organs *4*, 123–129, 1958a.

——, ——, ——, —— and R. TOMPKINS: Reduced metabolism by means of hypothermia and the low flow pump oxygenator. Surg. Gynec. Obstet. *107*, 339–352, 1958b.

——, ——, —— and ——: A new method for open heart surgery. J. Tenn. St. M. A. *52*, 39–44, 1959.

——, W. K. ROGERS, C. H. DABBS and F. L. RAWSON: Clinical experience with membrane lung in conjunction with hypothermia. J. Tenn. St. M. A. *54*, 39–45, 1961.

PEMBERTON, A. H., M. M. BORTIN and B. G. NARODICK: A stainless steel Y connector with valves for use in extracorporeal perfusion with a rotating disc oxygenator. J. Thor. Cardiov. Surg. *41*, 274–278, 1961.

PENICK, G. D., H. E. AVERETTE, JR., R. M. PETERS and K. M. BRINKHOUS: Hemorrhagic syndrome complicating extracorporeal shunting of blood: An experimental study of its pathogenesis. Thromb. Diathesis Haemorrhagica *2*, 218, 1958a.

——, H. R. ROBERTS, W. P. WEBSTER and K. M. BRINKHOUS: Hemorrhagic states secondary to intravascular clotting: an experimental study of their evolution and prevention. Arch. Path. *66*, 708–714, 1958b.

PENIDO, J. R. F., H. J. C. SWAN and J. W. KIRKLIN: Oxygen content of blood arterialized in bubble-type plastic sheet oxygonator (an experimental study). Proc. Mayo Clin. *32*, 389–394, 1957.

PENISTON, H. W. and V. RICHARDS: A simple circulatory bypass system. Proc. Soc. Exp. Biol. Med. *90*, 515–517, 1955.

—— and ——: The experimental use of brain perfusion in open cardiac surgery. Surg. Forum *6*, 176–180, 1956.

PENRY, J. K., A. R. CORDELL, F. R. JOHNSTON and M. G. NETSKY: Experimental cerebral embolism with antifoam A. J. Thor. Surg. *37*, 342–351, 1959.

——, ——, —— and——: Cerebral embolism by antifoam A in bubble oxygenator system: An experimental and clinical study. Surgery *47*, 784–794, 1960.

PERKINS, H. A., J. J. OSBORN, R. HURT and F. GERBODE: Neutralization of heparin in vivo with protamine; a simple method of estimating the required dose. J. Labor. Clin. Med. *48*, 223–226, 1956.

——, —— and F. GERBODE: The effect of heparin on the platelet count in vitro, with particular reference to the collection of blood for extracorporeal circulation. Am. J. Clin. Path. *30*, 397–403, 1958.

——, —— and ——: The management of abnormal bleeding following extracorporeal circulation. Ann. Intern. Med. *51*, 658–667, 1959.

——, —— and ——: A simple technique for the comparison of clotting times of fresh whole blood exposed to various foreign surfaces. J. Cardiov. Surg. *1*, 180–187, 1960.

PETERSON, L. H., R. F. JENSEN and J. PARNELL: Mechanical properties of arteries in vivo. Circulat. Res. *8*, 622–639, 1960.

PETRI, G.: Extracorporeal complete perfusion. Orv. Hetil. *100*, 1425–1431, 1959. (*Hun*).

PETROVSKII, B. V. and G. M. SOLOV'EV: Experimental operations on the heart with cross-circulation. Khirurgiia (Moskva) *4*, 17–24, 1956. (*Rus*).

PEZZOLI, G. and A. PULIN: Problemi di fisiopatologia del circolo polmonare di interesse chirurgico; rapporti fra circulazione bronchiale e polmonare. Attivita riflessogena del piccolo circolo. Minerva Chirurgica *12*, 498–517, 1957.

——, G. DRAGO, P. MICOZZI and R. CORTESINI: Studio del bilancio acidobase durante la circolazione extracorporea. Arch. Chir. Torace *17*, 35–51, 1960.

PIERUCCI, L., JR., G. J. HAUPT and J. Y. TEMPLETON, III: Studies in profound hypothermia. Trans. Am. Soc. Art. Int. Organs *6*, 197–203, 1960.

PISKORZ, A., J. ZAWILSKI, I. BOWBELSKA and S. DROZDOWSKI: Experimentelle Untersuchungen über induzierte Unterbrechungen der Herztätigkeit. Thoraxchirurgie *6*, 384–389, 1959.

——, ——, —— and ——: Experimental investigations on temporary arrest of cardiac function. Polski prezgl. chir. *31*, 165–170, 1959. (*Pol*).

PIWNICA, A., M. WEISS, C. LENFANT and C. DUBOST: Circulatory arrest and deep hypothermia induced with a pump oxygenator system and a heat exchanger. J. Cardiov. Surg. *1*, 74–84, 1960a.

——, ——, L. SPROVIERI, C. LENFANT and C. DUBOST: Présentation d'un échangeur thermique pour circulation extracorporelle. Ann. Chir. (Paris) *14*, 693–700, 1960b.

PONFICK, E.: Experimentelle Beiträge zur Lehre von der Transfusion. Virchow Arch. pathol. Anat. *62*, 273–335, 1875.

PONTIUS, R. G., E. WATKINS, B. S. MANHEIM, R. G. ALLEN, L. R. SAUVAGE and R. E. GROSS: Studies of acid-base derangement during total cardiac bypass. Surg. Forum *8*, 393–397, 1958.

PORTELA, A.: Personal communication, 1961.

POTH, E. J.: Discussions on oxygenators. pp. 112–113. In: Extracorporeal Circulation, J. G. Allen, ed., Springfield, Ill., Thomas, 1958.

POTTS, W. J., W. L. RIKER and R. DeBORD: An experimental study of respiration maintained by homologous lungs. J. Labor. Clin. Med. *38*, 281–285, 1951.

——, ——, —— and C. E. ANDREWS: Maintenance of life by homologous lungs and mechanical circulation. Surgery *31*, 161–166, 1952.

PRADOS, J. W. and E. C. PEIRCE, II: The influence of membrane permeability and of design on gas exchange in the membrane lung. Trans. Am. Soc. Art. Int. Organs *6*, 52–61, 1960.

PRESTON, F. W. and R. P. PARKER: New antiheparin agent "Polybrene": effect in peptone shock and experimental radiation injury. Arch. Surg. *66*, 545–550, 1953.

——, R. HOHF and O. TRIPPEL: Neutralization of heparin with Polybrene. Quart. Bull. Northw. Univ. Med. School, *30*, 138–143, 1956.

PREVOST, J. L. and J. A. DUMAS: Examen du sang et de son action dans les divers phénomènes de la vie. Ann. Chimie Physique *18*, 280–296, 1821.

PROVENZALE, L. and L. TONELLI: Chirurgia

intracardiaca sperimentale a cielo scoperto. L'esclusione dal circolo delle cavità destre. Arch. Chir. Torace 8, 31–35, 1951.

—— and ——: Chirurgia intracardiaca sperimentale a cielo scoperto—l'esclusione dal circolo delle cavità sinistre. Arch. Chir. Torace 8, 17–29, 1951.

Q

QUINTERO, M., Y. SHIBOTA, W. E. NEVILLE and G. H. A. CLOWES JR.: Acute portal hypertension and congestion as a cause for unexplained arterial hypotension and blood loss from the circuit during perfusion in dogs. Trans. Am. Soc. Art. Int. Organs 5, 248–253, 1959.

R

DE RABAGO, G. M. URQUIA, H. MEDINA, A. ESQUIVEL and M. SOKOLOWSKI: Circulacion extracorporea experimental con el pulmon corazon artificial de Kay-Cross. Rev. Clin. Esp. 71, 303–312, 1958.

RACE, D. and J. W. W. THOMPSON: Control and degrees of oxygenation during total body perfusion. Brit. M. J. 2, 1058–1059 1960.

RADERECHT, H. J.: Austauschtransfusion als physiologisuch-chemische Arbeitsmethode. I. Theoretieche Grundlagen und Methodik. Acta Biol. Med. Germ. 1, 173–187, 1958a.

——: Zur Anwendung der Austauschtransfusion als physiologisch-chemische Arbeitsmethode. III. Über das Verhalten des Fibrinogenspiegels. Acta Biol. Med. Germ. 1, 432–443, 1958b.

RAHN, H.: The role of N_2 gas in various biological processes with particular reference to the lung. Harvey Lect. 55, 173–200, 1960.

RAIKO, Z. A., I. R. PETROVIR and T. E. KUDRITSKAIA: Phosphorus compounds and lactic acid in the tissues of the brain and heart in hypothermic animals during temporary cardiac arrest and restoration of the general circulation by a combination of therapeutic measures. Fiziol. Zh. SSSR 45, 1489–1496, 1959 (Rus).

RANDALL, J. E. and R. W. STACY: Pulsatile and steady pressure-flow relations in the vascular bed of the hindleg of the dog. Am. J. Physiol. 185, 351–354, 1956.

READ, R, C., V. P. GEORGE, M. COHEN and

C. W. LILLEHEI: Cardiac bypass using autogenous lung for oxygenation. With particular reference to open gravity drainage of the pulmonary venous return. Surgery 40, 849–846, 1956.

——, J. A. JOHNSON and H. KUIDA: Systemic and coronary pressure-flow relationships during total body perfusion in the dog. Am. J. Physiol. 190, 49–53, 1957a.

——, H. KUIDA and J. A. JOHNSON: Effect of alterations in vasomotor tone on pressure-flow relationships in the totally perfused dog. Circulat. Res. 6, 676–682, 1957b.

——, —— and ——: Venous pressure and total peripheral resistance in the dog. Am. J. Physiol. 192, 609–612, 1958.

REDO, S. F.: The effects of intra-arterial air injection on the electroencephalogram, electrocardiogram, arterial and venous blood pressure. Surg. Forum 9, 166–171, 1959.

——: An evaluation of various cardioplegic methods utilizing perfused guinea pigs heart. Surg. Gynec. Obstet. 108, 211–222, 1959.

—— and B. Y. PORTER: The role of the lack of oxygen in irreversible cardiac arrest. Surg. Gynec. Obstet. 109, 431–444, 1959.

—— and L. I. ARDITI: The causes and treatment of arterial hypotension, circulatory collapse and shock following cardiovascular operations. Surg. Clin. N. Amer. 41, 309–313, 1961.

REED, W. A. and C. F. KITTLE: Physiologic changes and survival rate in prolonged oxygenation perfusion with complete cardiopulmonary bypass. Surg. Forum 8, 420–423, 1958a.

—— and ——: Survival rate and metabolic acidosis after prolonged extracorporeal circulation with total cardiopulmonary bypass. Ann. Surg. 148, 219–225, 1958b.

—— and ——: Observations on toxicity and use of antifoam. Arch. Surg. 78, 220–225, 1959.

REEMTSMA, K., M. M. HALLEY, W. H. LETSON, W. E. GIBSON III, P. HANLEY III and O. CREECH, JR.: Studies of organ flow and metabolism during extracorporeal circulation. Surg. Forum 9, 154–156, 1959a.

——, R. F. RYAN, R. T. KREMENTZ and O. CREECH, JR.: Treatment of selected adenocarcinomas by perfusion techniques. Arch. Surg. 78, 724–727, 1959b.

REPOGLE, R. L. and R. E. GROSS: Renal circulatory response to cardiopulmonary bypass. Surg. Forum 11, 224–225, 1960.

REYNOLDS, S. R. M., F. W. LIGHT, JR., G. M.

ARDRAN and M. M. L. PRICHARD: The qualitative nature of pulsatile flow in umbilical blood vessels, with observations on flow in the aorta. Bull. Johns Hopkins *91*, 83–104, 1952.

——, M. KIRSCH and R. J. BING: Functional capillary beds in the beating KCl-arrested and KCl-arrested perfused myocardium of the dog. Circulat. Res. *6*, 600–611, 1958.

RIBERI, A. and H. B. SHUMACKER: Elective cardiac arrest under moderate hypothermia. Ann. Surg. *148*, 21–31, 1958.

RICHARDS, A. N. and C. K. DRINKER: An apparatus for the perfusion of isolated organs. J. Pharmacol. Exp. Therap. *7*, 467–483, 1915.

RIJLANT, P.: L'activité électrique des artères. C. R. Soc. Biol. (Paris) *110*, 587–589, 1932.

RINGER, S.: Further contribution regarding influence of different constituents of blood on contraction of heart. J. Physiol. (London) *4*, 29–42, 1882.

RITTER, E. R.: Pressure-flow relations in kidney: alleged effects of pulse pressure. Am. J. Physiol. *168*, 480–489, 1952.

ROBICSEK, F.: Orifice plate flowmeter for extracorporeal circuit. IRE Trans. Med. Electronics. ME-6, 249, 1959a.

——, P. W. SANGER and F. H. TAYLOR: A blood flowmeter for extracorporeal surgery. Surgery *46*, 396–399, 1959b.

——, ——, —— and F. KOLONITS: The measurement of blood flow through extracorporeal circuits. J. Thor. Cardiov. Surg. *41*, 395–403, 1961.

ROCHLIN, D. B., T. R. TALBOT, R. O. GORSON and W. S. BLAKEMORE: A method for the continuous or repeated determination of blood volume. Surgery *42*, 659–663, 1957.

ROCHOW, E. G.: An introduction to the chemistry of the silicones. 2nd ed., New York, John Wiley & Sons, Inc. 1951.

RÖCKEMANN, W.: Eine durch Pressluft betriebene Kreislaufpumpe. Pflüger Arch. ges. Physiol. *266*, 671–673, 1958.

ROE, B. B.: A simple device to facilitate coronary artery perfusion. Surgery *44*, 554–555, 1958.

——, W. L. WEIRICH, D. MOORE and B. SWENSON: An efficient, low volume semidisposable screen oxygenator. Surg. Forum *11*, 232–233, 1960.

ROHDE, E.: Untersuchungen am überlebenden Warmblüterherzen—zur Physiologie des Herztoffwchsels. Ztschr. Physiol. Chem *68*, 181–235, 1910.

ROSE, J. C. and H. P. BROIDA: Effects of plas-

tic and steel surfaces on clotting time of human blood. Proc. Soc. Exp. Biol. Med. *86*, 384–386, 1954.

——, E. J. LAZARO and H. P. BROIDA: Dynamics of complete right ventricular failure in dogs maintained with an extracorporeal left ventricle. Circulat. Res. *4*, 173–181, 1956.

ROSS, D. N.: Hypothermia, pt. I. A technique of blood stream cooling. Guy Hosp. Rep. *103*, 97–115, 1954a.

——: op. cit., pt. II. Physiological observations during hypothermia. Guy Hosp. Rep. *103*, 116–138, 1954b.

——: Practical applications of hypothermia. Brit. Med. Bull. *11*, 226–228, 1955.

——: The techniques of veno-venous cooling and rewarming. Guy Hosp. Rep. *108*, 245–251, 1959a.

——: Some experimental observations on selective hypothermia. Guy Hosp. Rep. *108*, 252–257, 1959b.

——: Hypothermia and the heart-lung machine. Brit. M. J. *2*, 571–572, 1960.

——: A heart-lung machine for infants and young children. Lancet *2*, 1064–1065, 1960.

ROSS, J. JR.: Factors influencing the formation of bubbles in blood. Trans. Am. Soc. Art. Int. Organs *5*, 140–144, 1959.

——, J. W. GILBERT, JR., E. H. SHARP and A. G. MORROW: Elective cardiac arrest during total body perfusion: the relationship of elevated intracardiac pressures during arrest to subsequent myocardial function and pathologic pulmonary changes. J. Thor. Surg. *36*, 534–542, 1958.

——, C. J. FRAHM and E. BRAUNWALD: Influence of the carotid baroreceptors and of vasoactive drugs on systemic vascular volume and venous distensibility. Circulat. Res. *9*, 75–82, 1961a.

——, C. J. FRAHM and E. BRAUNWALD: The influence of intracardiac baroceptors on venous return, systemic vascular volume and peripheral resistance. J. Clin. Invest. *40*, 563–572, 1961b.

ROTELLAR, E.: A blood pump which minimizes hemolysis. Lancet *1*, 197, 1958.

ROTHNIE, N. G. and J. B. KINMONTH: Bleeding after perfusion for open heart surgery. Importance of un-neutralized heparin and its proper correction. Brit. Med. J. *1*, 73–77 1960a.

—— and ——: Neutralization of heparin after perfusion. Brit. Med. J. *2*, 1194–1196. 1960b.

——, A. G. NORMAN, M. STEELE and J. B.

KINMONTH: Changes in blood-coagulation due to perfusion for cardiac surgery. Brit. J. Surg. *48*, 272–281, 1960.

ROUGHTON, F. J. W.: Average time spent by blood in human lung capillary and its relation to rates of CO uptake and elimination in man. Am. J. Physiol. *143*, 621–633, 1945.

—— and R. E. FORSTER: Relative importance of diffusion and chemical reaction rates in determining rate of exchange of gases in the human lung, with special reference to true diffusing capacity of pulmonary membrane and volume of blood in the lung capillaries. J. Appl. Physiol. *2*, 290–302, 1957.

—— and J. C. RUPP: Problems concerning the kinetics of the reactions of oxygen, carbon monoxide and carbon dioxide in the intact red cell. Ann. N. Y. Acad. Sci. *75*, 156–166, 1958.

ROWEN, H., P. VILES and J. L. ANKENEY: The effect of total body perfusion upon cardiac output and vascular resistance. J. Thor. Cardiov. Surg. *40*, 529–535, 1960.

RUBINI, J. R., R. R. BECKER and M. A. STAHMAN: Effect of synthetic lysine polypeptides on rabbit blood coagulation. Proc. Soc. Exp. Biol. Med. *82*, 231–233, 1953.

RUBINSTEIN, D., S. KASHKET and O. F. DENSTEDT: Studies on the preservation of blood. VI. The influence of adenosine and inosine on the metabolism of the erythrocyte. Canad. J. Biochem. Physiol. *36*, 1269–1276, 1958.

——, ——, R. BLOSTEIN and O. F. DENSTEDT: Studies on the preservation of blood. VII. The influence of inosine on the metabolic behavior of the erythrocyte during the preservation of blood in the cold. Canad. J. Biochem. Physiol. *37*, 69–79, 1959.

RUCH, T. C. and J. F. FULTON: Medical physiology and biophysics. Philadelphia and London: W. B. Saunders Co., 1960.

RUEDI, B. and A. FLEISCH: Vitesse du courant sanguin et hémolyse. Helv. Physiol. Parmacol. Acta *18*, 90–91, 1960.

RUTHERFORD, R. B. and H. SWAN: Experimental partial perfusion. Surg. Forum *11*, 212–214, 1960.

RYGG, I. H.: Personal communication, 1958.

—— and E. KYVSGAARD: A disposable polyethylene oxygenator system applied in a heart-lung machine. Acta Chir. Scand. *112*, 433–437, 1956.

—— and ——: Further developement of the heart-lung machine with Rygg-Kyvsgaard plastic bag oxygenator. Minerva Chir. *13*, 1402–1404, 1958.

——, H. C. HENGELL and ——: A heart-lung with a disposable polyethylene oxygenator system. Danish Med. Bull. *3*, 200–202, 1956.

S

SABISTON, D. C. JR., J. L. TALBERT, L. H. RILEY and A. BLALOCK: Maintenance of the heart beat by perfusion of the coronary circulation with gaseous oxygen. Ann. Surg. *150*, 361–370, 1959.

SAEGESSER, F., CH. HAHN, J. PETTAVEL and J. J. LIVO: Traitements de certains cancers par perfusion régionale de chimothérapiques au moyen de la machine coeur-poumon artificiel de Rygg-Kyvsgaard. Schweiz. Med. Wschr. *90*, 11–14, 1960.

SAKAKIBARA, S.: Intracardiac surgery under direct vision. Bull. Heart Inst. Japan *1*, 1–8, 1957.

——, H. ORIHATA and K. HASE: Heart-lung machine for use of intracardiac surgery apparatus and clinical experience. Bull. Heart Inst. Japan *1*, 126–132, 1957.

——, ——, ——, T. KAMMA, K. TAKAHASHI, A. ISIHARA, T. BEPPU, S. YAMAGUTI, K. KURODA, G. MATSUMURA and H. ARAKI: Hypothermia and low flow rate extracorporeal circulation with oxygenator for open-heart surgery. Bull. Heart. Inst. Japan *2*, 213–250, 1958.

——, ——, A. ISIHARA and T. KURODA: Intracardiac operation under direct vision. Bull. Heart Inst. Japan *3*, 1–10, 1959.

SALISBURY, P. F.: Apparatus for cross-transfusion. Proc. Soc. Exp. Biol. Med. *71*, 604–607, 1949.

——: Artificial internal organs. Sci. Am. *191*, 23–28, 1954.

——: Blood pump gas exchange system ("artificial heart-lung machine") of large flow capacity. J. Appl. Physiol. *9*, 487–491, 1956a.

——: Extracorporeal circulation as an aid to cardiac surgery. pp. 695 sqq. in: Handbuch der Thoraxchirurgie, Derra ed., Düsseldorf, 1956b.

—— and J. H. MILLER: Cross transfusion. II. Therapeutic effect in acute mercury nephrosis. Proc. Soc. Exp. Biol. Med. *74*, 16–19, 1950.

——, A. A. BOLOMEY and J. H. MILLER: Cross transfusion. III. Clinical experiences with 6 cases. Am. J. Med. Sci. *223*, 151–167, 1952.

——, L. MORGENSTERN, M. M. HYMAN, J. M. SHORE and D. STATE: Physiological factors in the use of the pump oxygenator. Trans. Am. Soc. Art. Int. Organs *1*, 68–77, 1955.

——, ——, M. M. HYMAN and D. STATE: Prolonged surgical exposure of the aortic valve with perfusion of the systemic circulation; with or without retrograde and antegrade perfusion of the myocardium. Trans. Am. Soc. Art. Int. Organs *2*, 58–65, 1956.

——, P. WEIL and D. STATE: Factors influencing collateral blood flow to the dog's lung. Circulat. Res. *5*, 303–309, 1957.

——, N. BOR, R. J. LEWIN and P. A. RIEBEN: Effects of partial and of total heart-lung bypass on the heart. J. Appl.Physiol. *14*, 458–463, 1959a.

——, ——, ——, —— and C. E. CROSS: Effects of partial and of total heart-lung bypass on the circulation. Trans. Am. Soc. Art. Int. Organs *5*, 197–209, 1959b.

——, P. M. GALLETTI, R. J. LEWIN and A. RIEBEN: Stretch reflexes from the dog's lungs to the systemic circulation. Circulat. Res. *7*, 62–67, 1959c.

——, C. E. CROSS, P. A. RIEBEN and R. J. LEWIN: Comparison of two types of mechanical assistance in experimental heart failure. Circulat. Res. *8*, 431–439, 1960a.

——, ——, —— and ——: Physiological mechanisms which explain the effects of veno-arterial pumping and of left ventricular by-pass in experimental heart failure. Trans. Am. Soc. Art. Int. Organs *6*, 176–179, 1960b.

——, ——, K. KATSUHARA and P. A. RIEBEN: Factors which initiate or influence edema in the isolated dog's heart. Circulat. Res. *9*, 601–606, 1961.

SALTZMAN, A. and S. S. ROSENAK: Design of a pump suitable for blood. J. Labor. Clin. Med. *34*, 1561–1563, 1949.

SANGER, P. W., F. H. TAYLOR, F. ROBICSEK and H. J. DVORAK: Some problems in open heart surgery. Am. Surg. *25*, 578–584, 1959.

——, F. ROBICSEK, F. H. TAYLOR, T. T. REES and R. STAM: Vasomotor regulation during extracorporeal circulation and open-heart surgery. J. Thor. Cardiov. Surg. *40*, 355–371, 1960.

SARAJAS, H. S. S. and L. SAURE: Renal affection resulting from blood trauma in extracorporeal circuits. Nature (London) *185*, 768–769, 1960.

——, R. KRISTOFFERSON and M. H. FRICK: Release of 5-hydroxytryptamine and adenosine triphosphate in extracorporeal circulatory systems as a result of corpuscular blood trauma. Am. J. Physiol. *197*, 1195–1198, 1959.

SARKAR, T., I. E. ROEKEL and T. F. McDERMOTT: Use of five per cent dextrose in water with citrated blood. Am. Surg. *25*, 273–277, 1959.

SATTER, P.: Heparin and protamine in the extracorporeal circulation. German Med. Monthly *6*, 79–80, 1961.

SAXTON, G. A. JR. and C. B. ANDREWS: An ideal heart pump with hydrodynamic characteristics analogous to the mammalian heart. Trans. Am. Soc. Art. Int. Organs *6*, 288–291, 1960.

SCHEBITZ, H., H. KOHLER and W. GUENDEL: Zur Frage der Ausschaltung des Herzens durch ein künstliches Herz. Zbl. Vet. Med. *1*, 215–231, 1954.

SCHERMER, S.: Die Blutmorphologie der Laboratoriumstiere. Leipzig, Johann Ambrosius Barth, 1958.

SCHIMERT, G.: A simple bubble type of pump oxygenator for intracardiac surgery. Surgery *40*, 1018–1022, 1956.

——, P. C. HODGES, R. D. SELLERS and C. W. LILLEHEI: A rotating drum film oxygenator. Surg. Gynec. Obstet. *107*, 527–531, 1958.

SCHMIDT, A.: Die Athmung innerhalb des Blutes. Arbeiten aus der Physiologischen Anstalt zu Leipzig. Zweiter Jahrg. 1867, pp. 99–130.

SCHMIDT-MENDE, M.: Extra- und intrazellulare Electrolytverschiebungen im Zusammenhang mit der extrakorporalen Zirkulation. Langenbeck Arch. Klin. Chir. *292*, 681–685, 1959.

SCHMITT, H. and H. A. SCHMIDT: Vergleichende Untersuchungen über die Verwendbarkeit von ACD-und ACDI Stabilisatoren zur Blutkonservierung. Ärztl. Wschr. *14*, 172–174, 1959.

SCHMUTZER, K. J.: Intra-und postoperative Probleme bei der Anwendung des extrakorporalen Kreislaufes. Langenbeck Arch. Klin. Chir. *292*, 66–671, 1959.

——, S. A. MARABLE, E. RASCHKE, J. V. MALONEY, JR. and W. P. LONGMIRE JR.: Zur Problematik des extrakorporalen Kreislaufes. Langenbeck Arch. Klin. Chir. *290*, 64–85, 1958.

SCHNEIDER, M.: Durchblutung und Sauerstoffversorgung des Gehirns. Verh. dtsch. Ges. Kreisl.-Forsch. *19*, 3–25, 1953.

——: Über die Wiederbelebung nach Kreislaufunterbrechung. Thoraxchirurgie *6*, 95–106, 1959.

SCHOLANDER, P. F.: Oxygen transport through hemoglobin solutions: How does the presence of hemoglobin in wet membrane mediate an eightfold increase in oxygen passage? Science *131*, 585–589, 1960.

SCHÖNBACH, G., W. THORBAN, H. L. L'ALLEMAND and E. WAGNER: Der Einfluss von Minutenvolumenänderungen auf die Durchströmung lebenswichtiger Organe bei Anwendung der Herz-Lungen-Maschine. Langenbeck Arch. Klin. Chir. *289*, 714–716, 1958.

——, W. THORBAN, R. VOSS, H. L'ALLEMAND and E. WAGNER: Über den Einfluss des sogenannten "low flow" auf die Organstrukturen bei Anwendung der Herz-Lungen-Maschine. Thoraxchirurgie *6*, 516–524, 1959.

SCHRAMEL, R. J., R. CAMERON, M. M. ZISKIND and O. CREECH, JR.: Studies of pulmonary diffusion after open heart surgery. J. Thor. Cardiov. Surg. *38*, 281–291, 1959.

VON SCHRÖDER, W.: Über die Bildungsstätte des Harnstoffs. Arch. Exp. Path. Pharmacol. *15*, 364–402, 1882.

SCHWARTZ, S. I., J. A. DEWEESE, F. N. NIGUADULA, P. V. GABEL and E. B. MAHONEY: Tissue oxygen "tension" at various flow rates of extracorporeal circulation. Surg. Forum *9*, 151–154, 1959.

VON SCHWARZ, H. F. and N. P. MALLICK: Herzstillstand durch kalte Koronarperfusion beim normal warmen Tier. Schweiz. Med. Wschr. *91*, 447–450, 1961.

SCOTT, V. F.: Fluid control in heart-lung bypass operations in open heart surgery. S. Afr. Med. J. *34*, 249–252, 1960.

SCRIBNER, B. H., J. E. Z. CANER, R. BURI and W. QUINTON: The technique of continuous hemodialysis. Trans. Am. Soc. Art. Int. Organs *6*, 88 103, 1960.

SCURR, C. F.: Cardio-pulmonary bypass: physiological considerations. Proc. Roy. Soc. Med. *51*, 581–589, 1958.

SEALY, W. C., I. W. BROWN, JR., W. G. YOUNG JR., C. R. STEPHEN, J. S. HARRIS and D. MERRITT: Hypothermia, low flow extracorporeal circulation and controlled cardiac arrest for open heart surgery. Surg. Gynec. Obstet. *104*, 441–451, 1957a.

——, W. G. YOUNG JR., J. S. HARRIS and D. H. MERRITT: Potassium, magnesium, prostigmine solution for induced cardiac arrest; laboratory and clinical observations on this method during extracorporeal circulation and hypothermia. Trans. Am. Soc. Art. Int. Organs, *3*, 19–22, 1957b.

——, I. W. BROWN JR. and W. G. YOUNG JR.: Report on the use of both extracorporeal circulation and hypothermia for open heart surgery. Ann. Surg. *147*, 603–613, 1958a.

——, W. G. YOUNG, JR., I. W. BROWN, JR., A. LESAGE, H. A. CALLAWAY, J. S. HARRIS and D. H. MERRITT: Potassium, magnesium and neostigmine for controlled cardioplegia. Arch. Surg. *77*, 33–38, 1958b.

——, I. W. BROWN, JR., W. G. YOUNG, JR., W. W. SMITH and A. M. LESAGE: Hypothermia and extracorporeal circulation for open-heart surgery. Its simplification with a heat exchanger for rapid cooling and rewarming. Ann. Surg. *150*, 627–638, 1959a.

——, A. M. LESAGE and W. G. YOUNG, JR.: Tolerance of the profoundly hypothermic dog to complete circulatory standstill. Proc. Soc. Exp. Biol. Med. *102*, 691, 1959b.

——, W. G. YOUNG JR., I. W. BROWN JR., W. W. SMITH and A. M. LESAGE: Profound hypothermia combined with extracorporeal circulation for open heart surgery. Surgery *48*, 432–438, 1960.

——, ——, A. M. LESAGE and I. W. BROWN, JR.: Observations on heart action during hypothermia induced and controlled by a pump oxygenator. Ann. Surg. *153*, 797–812, 1961.

SEGMULLER, G.: Der Oxygenator im extrakorporellen Kreislauf. Helvet. Chir. Acta *27*, 181–195, 1960.

SELKURT, E. E.: Effect of pulse pressure and mean arterial pressure modification on renal hemodynamics and electrolytes and water excretion. Circulation *4*, 541–551, 1951.

SEMB, G.: Some experimental results with a bubble type heart–lung machine. Acta Chir. Scand. *117*, 1959a.

——: Some results regarding the gaseous exchange in a bubble oxygenator. Acta Chir. Scand. *117*, 39–40, 1959b.

SEMERAU-SIEMIANOWSKI, Z. and J. M. FOLGA: Experiments with the new apparatus for extracorporeal circulation and oxygenation constructed by Z. Semerau-Siemianowski and J. M. Folga. Polski Tygodnik Lekarski *13*, 2028–2035, 1958 (*Pol*).

SENNING, A.: Ventricular fibrillation during extracorporeal circulation. Acta Chir. Scand. (Suppl.) *171*, 1–79, 1952.

——: Extracorporeal circulation combined

with hypothermia. Acta Chir. Scand. *107*, 516–524, 1954.

——: The risk of rapid and large citrated blood transfusions in experimental hemorraghic shock. Acta Chir. Scand. *109*, 394–402, 1955a.

——: Ventricular fibrillation during hypothermia, used as a method to facilitate intracardiac operation. Acta Chir. Scand. *109*, 303–309, 1955b.

——: Plasma heparin concentration in extracorporeal circulation. Acta Chir. Scand. 55–59, 1959a.

——: Erfahrungen in der Herzchirurgie mit der Herz-Lungen-Maschine. Thoraxchirurgie *6*, 483–505, 1959b.

——, J. ANDRES, P. BORNSTEIN, B. NORBERG and M. ANDERSON: Renal function during extracorporeal circulation at high and low flow rates: experimental studies in dogs. Ann. Surg. *151*, 63–70, 1960.

SERGEANT, C. K., T. GEOGHEGAN and C. R. LAM: Further studies in induced cardiac arrest using the agent acetylcholine. Surg. Forum *7*, 254–257, 1957.

SERVELLE, M., J. ROUGEULLE, G. DELAHAYE, P. H. BONNEL, P. VERNANT, C. CORNU, H. PERROT, P. LAURENS, J. MONTAGNE and H. TEILLEUX: Un nouveau coeur artificiel. Arch. Mal. Coeur *51*, 558–572, 1958.

——, ——, H. PERROT, C. CORNU, B. MAUPIN, G. DELAHAYE and J. MONTAIGNE: Coeur-poumon artificiel. Oxygénation par bullage et par étalement. Arch. Mal. Coeur *53*, 635–643, 1960.

SERVIN, E. J., JR. and R. R. RHODES: Pump theory. Indust. Engin. Chem. *52*, 557–560, 1960.

SEVERINGHAUS, J. W.: Respiration and hypothermia. Ann. N. Y. Acad. Sci. *80*, 384–394, 1959.

——: Temperature gradients during hypothermia. Ann. N. Y. Acad. Sci. *80*, 515–521, 1959.

—— and A. F. BRADLEY: Electrodes for blood pO_2 and pCO_2 determination. J. Appl. Physiol. *13*, 515–520, 1958.

SEWELL, W. H. and W. W. L. GLENN: Observations on the action of a pump designed to shunt venous blood past the right heart directly into the pulmonary artery. Surgery *28*, 474–494, 1950.

—— and ——: Experimental cardiac surgery. II. Further observations on the development of a perfusion pump for the purpose of shunting the venous return directly into the pulmonary artery. Surg. Forum *1*, 265, 1951.

SHABETAI, R.: Cardiac bypass without artificial lung. Am. Heart J. *60*, 482–483, 1960.

SHANG, TY: Continuous perfusion with arterialized blood under hypothermia. Zhong Waike *7*, 1175–1177, 1959 (*Chin*).

SHAW, K. M., R. M. PIGGOTT, F. ACHESON, N. BURTON, T. CHAPMAN, R. M. FRY, R. BENSON, S. DAWSON, O. MURPHY and D. HOGAN: Cardiopulmonary bypass using the Mono pump: an experimantal study. J. Irish Med. Ass. *47*, 12–17, 1960.

SHAW, R. S. and M. GROVE-RASMUSSEN: A rotary transfusion pump. Studies on hemolysis. Ann. Surg. *138*, 928–931, 1953.

SHELLITO, J. G., B. H. BUCK, E. P. CARREAU, R. H. ROBINSON and A. AYTAC: The use of citrated blood in extracorporeal circulation. Am. Surg. *25*, 796–800, 1959.

SHEN, S. C., W. B. CASTLE and E. M. FLEMING: Experimental and clinical observations on increased mechanical fragility of erythrocytes. Science *100*, 387–389, 1944.

SHEN, T. C., T. G. NI, C. T. LOO and R. K. S. LIM: The gas metabolism of the mechanically perfused stomach. Chin. J. Physiol. *5*, 103–114, 1931.

SHIELDS, T. W. and F. J. LEWIS: Rapid cooling and surgery at temperatures below 20°C. Surgery *46*, 164–174, 1959.

SHIH, M. H., T. H. WAN, Y. S. LAW, H. S. LING, C. Y. JEN and C. S. HUANG: Studies in extracorporeal circulation: the stationary screen oxygenator. Zhong Waike *28*, 211–213, 1960 (*Chin*).

SHIMAMOTO, T., H. YAMAZAKI, M. INOUE, T. FUJITA, N. SAGAWA, T. ISHOKA and T. SUNAGA: Effect of adrenaline and noradrenaline on "silicone like property" of blood vessels. Proc. Jap. Acad. *36*, 234–239, 1960a.

——, ——, ——, ——, ——, T. SUNAGA and T. ISHIOKA: Discovery of antithromboembolic effect of nialamid. Protection of "silicone like property" of blood vessels by nialamide. Proc. Jap. Acad. *36*, 240–245, 1960b.

SHIMOMURA, S., E. ANDREAE, A. L. LOOMISBELL and H. F. FITZPATRICK: Pressure-flow relationships of the sigmamotor pump as used in cardiac bypass. J. Thor. Surg. *35*, 747–750, 1958.

SHIPLEY, R. E. and C. WILSON: An improved recording rotameter. Proc. Soc. Exp. Biol. Med. *78*, 724–728, 1951.

—— and ——: A simplified recording rotameter. Meth. in Med. Res. *8*, 346–351, 1960.

SHUMACKER, H. B., JR.: Comments on the distribution of blood flow. Surgery *47*, 1–16, 1960.

SHUMWAY, N. E.: A classification of elective cardiac arrest for open heart surgery. Dis. Chest *36*, 315–318, 1959a.

——: Forward versus retrograde coronary perfusion for direct vision surgery of acquired aortic valvular disease. J. Thor. Cardiov. Surg. *38*, 75–80, 1959b.

—— and R. R. LOWER: Topical cardiac hypothermia for extended periods of anoxic arrest. Surg. Forum *10*, 563–566, 1960.

——, M. L. GLIEDMAN and F. J. LEWIS: Coronary perfusion for longer periods of cardiac occlusion under hypothermia. J. Thor. Surg. *30*, 598–606, 1955.

——, —— and ——: A mechanical pump-oxygenator for successful cardio-pulmonary bypass. Surgery *40*, 831–839, 1956.

——, R. R. LOWER and C. STOFER: Selective hypothermia of the heart in anoxic cardiac arrest. Surg. Gynec. Obstet. *109*, 750–754, 1959.

SIMKOVIC, I., J. BOLF, K. SHISKA, M. GUPKA, V. SMRECHANSKY, M. SHNORRER and P. ZIMA: A Czechoslovakian apparatus for extracorporeal circulation. Eksp. Khir. *6*, 16–22, 1960 (*Rus*).

SINGH, I.: Intravenous injection of oxygen with the animal under ordinary and increased atmospheric pressure. J. Physiol. (London) *84*, 315–322, 1935.

——: Life without breathing. Arch. Int. Pharmacodyn. *129*, 239–243, 1960.

—— and M. J. SHAH: Intravenous injection of oxygen under normal atmospheric pressure. Lancet *1*, 922–923, 1940.

SIRAK, H. D., R. H. ELLISON and R. M. ZOLLINGER: Cardiotomy into an empty left ventricle. Surgery *28*, 225–233, 1950.

VON SKRAMLIK, E.: Ein Apparat zur Durchströmung der Leber. Pflüger Arch. ges. Physiol. *180*, 1–24, 1920.

SLOAN, H., J. D. MORRIS, R. VANDERWOUDE, H. HEWITT and G. LONG: Clinical experience with a rotating disc oxygenator. Surgery *45*, 139–148, 1959.

SMITH, H. L., L. H. BOSHER, S. VASLI, J. A. SMITH and W. E. HIRD: A study of the efficiency of a new type multiple stage droplet oxygenator. Trans. Am. Soc. Art. Int. Organs *3*, 63–66, 1957.

SMITH, P. K., A. W. WINKLER and H. E. HOFF: Electrocardiographic changes and concentration of magnesium in serum following intravenous injection of magnesium salts. Am. J. Physiol. *126*, 720–730, 1939.

SMITH, W. T.: Cerebral lesions due to emboli of silicone antifoam in dogs subjected to cardiopulmonary bypass. J. Path. Bact. *80*, 9–18, 1960.

SMITH, W. W.: An efficient blood heat exchanger for use with extracorporeal circulation. IRE Trans Med. Electronics *6*, 34–36, 1959.

——, I. W. BROWN JR., W. G. YOUNG, JR. and W. C. SEALY: Studies of edglugate-Mg: a new donor blood anticoagulant-preservative mixture for extracorporeal circulation. J. Thor. Cardiov. Surg. *38*, 573–585, 1959.

SNOW, H. M. and A. COULSON: Reduction of haemolysis during perfusion. Lancet *2*, 154, 1960.

SNYDER, D. D., C. N. BARNARD, R. L. VARCO and C. W. LILLEHEI: Serum transaminase patterns following intracardiac surgery. Surgery *44*, 1083–1091, 1958.

——, G. R. WILLIAMS and G. S. CAMPBELL: Open versus closed left artrial drainage during crossclamping of the thoracic aorta. J. Thor. Cardiov. Surg. *39*, 634–639, 1960.

SONES, F. M. JR.: Results of open-heart surgery with elective cardiac arrest by potassium citrate in patients with congenital and acquired heart disease. Dis. Chest *34*, 299–316, 1958.

SORENSEN, A. H.: New, pulse-giving, hydraulic pump for extracorporeal circulation. Lancet *1*, 959–960, 1960.

SOULIER, J. P.: Les modifications du Ca^{++} dans les transfusions massives et la circulation extracorporelle utilisant du sang citraté. Rev. Hemat. Paris *13*, 437–444, 1958.

SOUTHWORTH, J. L. and E. C. PEIRCE, II: Cross-circulation for intracardiac surgery. Arch. Surgery *64*, 58–63, 1952.

——, ——, T. TYSON and R. L. BOWMAN: Diaphragm pump for artificial circulation. (Tyson Bowman pump). Arch. Surg. *66*, 53–59, 1953.

SPATARU, T. and I. NICODIUM: Modell eines elektrischen, automatischen Transfusionapparates für verschiedene Seren. Zbl. Chir. *84*, 736–739, 1959.

SPENCER, M. P. and A. B. DENISON, JR.: Square-wave electromagnetic flowmeter for surgical and experimental application. Meth. Med. in Res. *8*, 321–341, 1960.

SPENCER, F. C. and H. T. BAHNSON: The use of ethylene oxide for gas sterilization of a pump oxygenator. Bull. Johns Hopkins Hosp. *102*, 241–244, 1958.

SPOHN, K.: Der gegenwärtige Stand der Probleme des extracorporalen Kreislaufes bei Operationen am bluttrocknen Herzen, unter besonderer Berücksichtigung der Herz-Lungen-Maschine von Crafoord-Senning. Ann. Univ. saraviensis, Med. *6*, 292–294, 1958.

——, E. KOLB, R. FREY and J. HEINZEL: Der gagenwärtige Stand der Operation am bluttrockenen Herzen mit Hilfe von Herz-Lungen-Maschinen und artifiziellem Herzstillstand. Münch. Med. Wschr. *100*, 523–528, 1958.

——, ——, J. HEINZEL, A. KRATZERT, W. WENZ, W. WOERNER, H. G. LASCH, H. H. SESSNER, W. RAULE, U. GOTTSTEIN, E. KUHN and K. SCHREIER: Ergebnisse von Tierversuchen mit der Herz-Lungen-Maschine nach Craoford-Senning. Langenbeck Arch. Klin. Chir. *289*, 705–713, 1958.

SPRENG, D. S., JR., C. DENNIS, L. A. YOUNG, G. E. NELSON, K. E. KARLSON and C. PEREYMA: Acute metabolic changes associated with employment of a pump-oxygenator to supplant the heart and lungs. Surg. Forum *8*, 165–171, 1953.

SPROVIERI, L., D. LAURENT, P. STURLESE, P. BLONDEAU and C. DUBOST: Dispositif de circulation extracorporelle avec possibilité d'hypothermie associée. Modifications de l'appareil de Lillehei-DeWall. Presse Méd. *68*, 1141–1142, 1960.

STANNET, V. and M. SZWARC: The permeability of polymer films to gases. A simple relationship. J. Polymer Sci. *16*, 89–91, 1955.

STARR, A.: Oxygen consumption during cardiopulmonary bypass. J. Thor. Cardiov. Surg. *38*, 46–56, 1959.

STAUB, H.: Methode zur fortlaufenden Bestimmung des Gaswchsels isoliert durchströmter Organe im geschlossenen System. Arch. Exp. Path. Pharmakol. *162*, 420–427, 1929.

STEELE, D. E.: Letter to the editor. Lancet *1*, 419, 1959.

STEPHEN, C. R., M. BOURGEOIS-GAVARDIN, S. DENT, I. W. BROWN, Jr. and W. C. SEALY: Anesthestic management in open heart surgery: electroencephalographic and metabolic findings in 81 patients. Anesth. Analg. *38*, 198–205, 1959.

——, S. J. DENT, W. C. SEALY and K. D. HALL: Anesthetic and metabolic factors associated with combined extracorporeal circulation and hypothermia. Am. J. Cardiol. *6*, 737–746, 1960.

STEPHENSON, S. E., JR., J. L. SAWYERS, G. L. HOLCOMB, F. GOLLAN, R. A. DANIEL JR. and H. W. SCOTT: Metabolic changes associated with the use of the micro-bubble type pump-oxygenator under normothermic and hypothermic conditions. Surg. Forum *7*, 257–261, 1957.

STEWART, E., J. J. OSBORN and F. GERBODE: Instrumentation and monitoring during open-heart surgery. Arch. Surg. *80*, 677–684, 1960.

STEWART, J. W. and M. F. STURRIDGE: Hemolysis caused by tubing in extracorporeal circulation. Lancet *1*, 340–342, 1959.

STIRLING, G. R., P. H. STANLEY and C. W. LILLEHEI: The effects of cardiac bypass and ventriculotomy upon right ventricular function (with report of successful closure of ventricular septal defect by use of atriotomy). Surg. Forum *8*, 433–437, 1958.

STODDART, J. C.: Nickel sensitivity as a cause of infusion reactions. Lancet *2*, 741–742, 1960.

STOKES, T. L. and J. B. FLICK: An improved vertical cylinder oxygenator. Proc. Soc. Exp. Biol. Med. *73*, 528–529, 1950.

—— and J. H. GIBBON, JR.: Experimental maintenance of life by a mechanical heart and lung during occlusion of the venae cavae followed by survival. Surg. Gynec. Obstet. *91*, 138–150, 1950.

STORLI, E. A., J. E. CONNOLLY, M. B. BACANER and D. L. BRUNS: The relationship of coronary blood flow to the effectiveness of mechanical support of the circulation in acute heart failure. Surg. Forum *11*, 214–216, 1960.

STORY, J. L., P. HODGES and L. A. FRENCH: Effect of total cardiopulmonary bypass on cerebrovascular permeability. Univ. Minn. Bull. *29*, 287–293, 1958.

STRUMIA, M. M., L. S. COLWELL and A. DUGAN: The preservation of blood for transfusion. III. Mechanisms of action of containers on red blood cells. J. Lab. Clin. M. *53*, 106–116, 1959.

STUCKEY, J. H., M. M. NEWMAN, B. S. LEVOWITZ, K. KARLSON, S. ADLER, E. J. GOYAREB and L. A. YOUNG: The creation and repair of interventricular septal defects in dogs using the heart-lung machine. Trans. Am. Soc. Art. Int. Organs *1*, 63–64, 1955.

——, ——, C. DENNIS, B. S. LEVOWITZ, H. N. ITICOVICI, E. J. GOYAREB, M. KERNAN and L. A. YOUNG: The creation and repair of interventricular septal defects in dogs utilizing the heart-lung machine. J. Thor. Surg. *32*, 410–416, 1956.

——, ——, ——, ——, ——, ——, —— and ——: The artificial heart-lung apparatus—experimental creation and repair of interventricular septal defects. Surg. Forum *6*, 185–189, 1956.

——, ——, ——, E. H. BERG, S. E. GOODMAN, C. C. FRIES, K. E. KARLSON, M. BLUMENFIELD, S. W. WEITZNER, L. S. BINDER and A. WINSTON: The use of the heart-lung machine in selected cases of acute myocardial infraction. Surg. Forum *8*, 342–344, 1958.

——, B. F. HOFFMAN, P. K. KOTTMEIER and H. FISHBONE: Electrode identification of the conduction system during open-heart surgery. Surg. Forum *9*, 202–204, 1959.

——, ——, N. S. AMER, P. F. CRANEFIELD, R. R. CAPELLETTI and R. T. DOMINGO: Localization of the bundle of His with a surface electrode during cardiotomy. Surg. Forum *10*, 551–554, 1960.

STURTZ, G. S., J. W. KIRKLIN, E. C. BURKE and M. H. POWER: Water metabolism after cardiac operations involving a Gibbon-type pump-oxygenator: I. Daily water metabolism, obligatory water losses and requirements. Circulation *16*, 988–1000, 1957a.

——, ——, —— and ——: Water metabolism after cardiac operations involving a Gibbon-type pump-oxygenator: II. Benign forms of water loss. Circulation *16*, 1000–1003, 1957b.

SU, C. S., R. HARDIN and H. KING: The use of hypothermia with cardiopulmonary bypass for open heart surgery (an experimental study). Surgery *44*, 1079–1082, 1958.

SUGARMAN, H. J., S. A. WESOLOWSKI, J. ANZOLA and C. S. WELSH: The use of an isolated homologous lung as a donor oxygenator. Bull. New Engl. Med. Cent. *13*, 107–113, 1951.

SULLIVAN, S. L., JR. and C. D. HOLLAND: Double pipe heat exchangers. Indust. Engin. Chem. *53*, 285–288, 1961.

SWAN, H. J. C.: Factors in the control of the circulation which may be modified during total body perfusion. IRE Trans. Med. Electronics *6*, 32–33, 1959.

——, V. MONTGOMERY, D. JENKINS and T. L. MARCHIORO: A method for the continuous measurement of plasma volume in the dog. Ann. Surg. *151*, 319–329, 1960.

—— and B. PATON: The combined use of hypothermia and extracorporeal circulation in cardiac surgery. J. Cardiov. Surg. *1*, 169–175, 1960.

——, —— and V. MONTGOMERY: The relationships between respiratory and blood gases in the control of total body perfusion. Bull. Soc. Int. Chir. *19*, 69–77, 1960.

SWEDBERG, J. and S. C. NETTELBLAD: Extracorporeal circulation: experimental and clinical results. Acta Chir. Scand. *117*, 60–68, 1959.

L. SZEKERES, G. LICHNER and F. VARGA: Über die verschiedene Empfindlichkeit der rechten und linken Herzkammermuskulatur gegenüber Hypoxie. Arch. Kreislaufforsch. *28*, 125–135, 1958.

T

TABER, R. E. and L. A. TOMATIS: Operation of a bubble-type pump oxygenator. Surg. Clin. N. Amer. *39*, 1539–1551, 1959.

TADDEI, C., P. MOSETTI and G. B. GEMMA: Studio dei fenomeni che accompagnano l'ipothermia generale ottenuta con la circolazione e refrigerazione extracorporea del sangue, in animali normali ed in animali neuroplegizzati. Minerva Chir. *9*, 116–1125, 1954.

TAILBY, S. R. and S. PORTALSKI: The hydrodynamics of liquid films flowing on a vertical plate. Trans. Inst. Chem. Engineers *38*, 324–330, 1960.

TAINTER, M. L.: Use of the Gibbs artificial heart in the study of circulatory phenomena, with descriptions of improvements in the device and of responses to some drugs. Arch. Int. Pharmacodyn. *42*, 186–199, 1932.

TAKEDA, J.: Experimental study on peripheral circulation during peripheral circulation, with a special reference to a comparison of pulsatile flow with non-pulsatile flow. Arch. Japan. Chir. *29*, 1407–1430, 1960.

TALBERT, J. T., L. H. RILEY, JR., D. C. SABISTON JR. and A. BLALOCK: Retrograde perfusion of the coronary sinus with gaseous oxygen. Am. Surg. *26*, 189–192, 1960.

TAUX, W. N. and T. B. MAGATH: Blood banking for intracardiac surgery. J.A.M.A. *166*, 2136–2139, 1958.

TAYLOR, A. C. (consulting editor): Hypothermia. Ann. N. Y. Acad. Sci. *80*, 285–549, 1959.

TAYLOR, D. G.: Clinical perfusion technique. Guy Hosp. Rep. *108*, 194–202, 1959.

TAYLOR, H. P., W. J. KLOFF, P. S. SINDELAR and J. J. CAHILL: Attempts to make an "artificial uterus". pt. I. The adaptation of blood pumps and oxygenator for this purpose. Am. J. Obstet. Gynec. *77*, 1295–1300, 1959.

TAYLOR, R.: A mechanical heart-lung apparatus. I.B.M. J. Res. Develop. *1*, 330–340, 1957.

TEMPLETON, J. Y., III: Characteristics of an ideal oxygenator., pp. 67–68., In: Extracorporeal Circulation. J. G. Allen, ed., Springfield, Ill., Thomas, 1958.

TEPPER, R.: A method of detecting microbubbles resulting from the passage of blood through heart-lung machines. Trans. Am. Soc. Art. Int. Organs *4*, 118–120, 1958.

——, S. GELMAN, A. B. LOWENFELS and J. F. LORD JR.: A method for the detection of micro-bubbles resulting from the passage of blood through heart-lung machines. Surg. Forum *9*, 171–174, 1959.

TEREBINSKII, N. N.: Contribution to the study of open access to the atrioventricular valves of the heart. Medgiz, Moskva, 1940 (*Rus*).

——, M. K. MARTSINKEVICH and T. T. SHERBAKOVA: The possibility of using a complete artificial blood circulation in experimental intracardial operations. Khirurgiia (Moskva) *1*, 8–10, 1950 (*Rus*).

TERESCHENKO, O. YA.: Blood proteins as affected by cerebral injury or a severe anemic condition of the central nervous system in dogs. Voprosy Med. Khimii *6*, 351–357, 1960 (*Rus*).

THALIMER, W., D. Y. SOLANDT and C. H. BEST: Experimental exchange transfusion using purified heparin. Lancet *2*, 554–556, 1938.

THEWS, G.: Untersuchung der Sauerstoffaufnahme und -abgabe sehr dünner Blutlamellen. Pflüger Arch. ges. Physiol. *268*, 308–317, 1959.

——: Die Sauerstoffdiffusion im Gehirn. Ein Beitrag zur Frage der Sauerstoffversorgung der Organe. Pflüger Arch. ges. Physiol. *271*, 197–226, 1960.

—— and W. NIESEL: Zur Theorie der Sauerstoffdiffusion im Erythrocyten. Pflüger Arch. ges. Physiol. *268*, 318–333, 1959.

THEYE, R. A., R. T. PATRICK and J. W. KIRKLIN: The electroencephalogram in patients undergoing open intracardiac operations with the aid of extracorporeal circulation. J. Thor. Surg. *34*, 709–716, 1957.

THIEBLOT, L., P. FOURRIER and DUCHENE-MARULLAZ: Etude expérimentale des effets de l'injection intra-artérielle de sang à contre-courant. Lyon Chir. *55*, 42–45, 1959.

THOMAS, J. A.: Nouveaux procédés de perfusion physiologique et aseptique permettant la survie prolongée d'organes ou d'organismes pesant plusieurs kilogrammes. J. Physiol. (Paris) *40*, 123–146, 1948.

——: Coeur-poumon à membrane pulmonaire artificielle. C. R. Acad. Sci. Paris *246*, 1084–1088, 1958a.

——: Über eine Herz-Lungen-Maschine mit künstlicher Alveolar-Membran. Langenbeck Arch. Klin. Chir. *289*, 286–294, 1958b.

——: Physiologie du coeur-poumon à membrane pulmonaire artificielle. C. R. Acad. Sci. Paris, *248*, 291–294, 1959.

—— and P. BEAUDOIN: Groupe cardio-pulmonaire artificiel destiné à la perfusion aseptique au sang du corps humain. C. R. Acad. Sci. Paris, *231*, 390–392, 1950.

—— and ——: Caractéristiques du coeur-poumon artificiel pour la perfusion au sang du corps humain. J. Physiol. (Paris) *43*, 311–327, 1951.

——, J. VAYSSE, C. D'ALLAINES, D. LAURENT J. L. CHEVRIER, G. RICORDEAU, B. JAULMES, N. DU BOUCHET, J. MIRABEL, B. I. LATSCHA, G. ARFEL, M. VALLON and J. D'ALLAINES: Le coeur-poumon à membrane pulmonaire artificielle. Premiers résultats chirurgicaux. Arch. Mal. Coeur (Paris) *51*, 801–811, 1958.

——, L. SALOMON and L. SALOMON: La survie des grands foetus des mammifères perfusés aseptiquement. J. Physiol. (Paris) *40*, 233–250, 1948.

THOMASSEN, R. W., J. P. HOWBERT, D. F. WINN, JR. and S. W. THOMPSON: The occurence and characterization of emboli associated with the use of a silicone antifoaming agent. J. Thor. Cardiov. Surg. *41*, 611–622, 1961.

THROWER, W. B., F. J. VEITH, S. LUNZER and D. E. HARKEN: The effect of partial extracorporeal bypass on sodium excretion in normal dogs and in those with heart failure. Surg. Gynec. Obstet *110*, 19–26, 1960.

TOCANTINS, L. M.: Cephalin, protamine and the anti-thromboplastic activity or normal and hemophilic plasma. Proc. Exp. Biol. Med. *54*, 94–97, 1943.

TOMATIS, L. A., R. E. TABER, C. R. LAM and E. W. GREEN: Experimental studies with low oxygen flow rates in the bubble oxygenator. Henry Ford Hosp. Med. Bull. *6*, 341–344, 1958.

TOMIN, R., A. KONTAXIS, B. WITTELS, R. GRIGGS, W. E. NEVILLE and G. H. A. CLOWES, JR.: Pulmonary changes secondary to prolonged perfusion. Trans. Am. Soc. Art. Int. Organs *7*, 187–194, 1961.

TORRES, F., G. S. FRANK, M. M. COHEN, C. W. LILLEHEI and N. KASPAR: Neurologic and electroencephalographic studies in open heart surgery. Neurology *9*, 174–183, 1959.

TOSATTI, E.: La macchina cardio-polmonare. Atti Mem. Soc. Romana Chir. *6*, 3, 1949.

——: Ulteriori studi sulla macchina cardio-polmonare. Atti Mem. Soc. Romana Chir. *7*, 1–12, 1950.

——: Il cuore artificiale. Milano: Istituto Sieroterapico Milanese S. Belfanti 1951.

TOUNTAS, C., S. MOULPOULOS, M. FRANGOPOULOS and D. GEORGIADOU: Experimental observations on cardiac arrest induced by anoxia or potassium citrate injection. Bull. Soc. Int. Chir. *19*, 10–20, 1960.

TREDE, M., S. KUBICKI and O. JUST: Über EEG-Beobachtungen bei Herzoperationen mit dem extrakorporalen Kreislauf. Anaesthesist, *8*, 76–82, 1959.

TRUBETSKOY, A. V.: Construction and function of a perfusion apparatus with a bubble oxygenator. Eksp. Khir. *6*, 22–24, 1960 (*Rus*).

TUCCI, G., F. TOMAI and N. MOTOLESE: Problemi ematologici nella circolazione cardiopolmonare extracorporea. Arch. Chir. Torace *16*, 15–28, 1959.

TUFFIER, T.: Discussion of the future of cardiac surgery. In: Congrès Soc. Int. Chir. p. 5, 1920.

TULLIS, J. L.: Physicochemical effects of extracorporeal circulation. pp. 77–84. In: Conference on blood problems in extracorporeal circulation and massive transfusions, Washington, 1958.

—— and E. G. ROCHOW: Non-wettable surfaces. Blood *7*, 850–853, 1952.

TURNER, M. D., W. A. NEELY and W. O. BARNETT: The effects of temporary arterial, venous and arteriovenous occlusion upon intestinal blood flow. Surg. Gynec. Obstet. *108*, 347–350, 1959.

TYRER, J. H.: The peripheral action of digoxin on venous pressure: a study using sheep with an "artificial heart." Med. J. Austral. *1*, 497–502, 1952.

U

UNDERWOOD, J., C. ROTH and A. STARR: The influence of anesthetic technique on oxygen consumption during total cardiopulmonary bypass. Anesthesiol. *21*, 263–268, 1960.

UNGAR, I., J. EGLAJS, T. BUHL, R. LESCOE, J. COPE, H. COLEMAN and E. DONAT: A study of three methods of inducting cardiac arrest in dogs maintained on total body perfusion by means of a pump-oxygenator; namely localized hypothermia, potassium and anoxia. Trans. Am. Soc. Art. Int. Organs *7*, 237–250, 1961.

URSCHELL, H. C. and J. J. GREENBERG: Differential hypothermic cardioplegia. Surg. Forum *10*, 506–509, 1960a.

—— and ——: Differential cardiac hypothermia for elective cardioplegia. Ann. Surg. *152*, 845–855, 1960b.

——, —— and C. A. HUFNAGEL: Elective cardioplegia by local cardiac hypothermia. New Engl. J. Med. *261*, 1330–1332, 1959.

——, —— and E. J. ROTH: Rapid hypothermia: An improved extracorporeal method. J. Thor. Cardiov. *39*, 318–329, 1960.

V

VADOT, L.: La viscosité et la perte de charge du sang dans les canalisations utilisées en chirurgie cardio-vasculaire. Path. Biol. *7*, 1887–1892, 1959.

——: Essai de détermination de la résistance des hématies à l'hémolyse traumatique— Application à la construction d'une pompe occlusive pour circulation extra-corporelle. Path. Biol. *8*, 1167–1174, 1960.

VAINRIB, E. A., G. A. EFRES, and E. A. FRID: Some problems in the theory of the mechanical heart. Med. Promyshlennost SSSR *10*, 14–19, 1956 (*Rus*).

——, E. A. FRID, L. N. MARTYNOV, M. G. ANANEV, S. A. MUSHEGIAN and L. A. LEVITSKAIA: Apparatus for artificial blood circulation. Med. Promyshlennost SSSR *11*, 50–55, 1957 (*Rus*).

—— and ——: Some theoretical questions in connection with the apparatus for artificial circulation. Eksp. Khir. *3*, 9–14, 1958 (*Rus*).

—— and A. D. KHAZAN: Apparatus for artificial blood circulation Voen. Med. Zh. (Moskva) *1*, 44–49, 1959 (*Rus*).

——, E. A. FRID, YU. G. KOSLOV, L. N. MARTYNOV, S. A. MUSHEGIAN and L.

A. LEVITSKAIA: A clinical model of apparatus for artificial circulation. Method of preparation and handling of the apparatus. Eksp. Khir. *3*, 15–24, 1958 (*Rus*).

VAN ECK, C. R. R.: Der Gasstoffwechsel während des extracorporalen Kreislaufs. Thoraxchirurgie *7*, 173–178, 1960.

VANPEPERSTRAETE, F. and G. D. ARDENNE: Circulation extracorporelle; présentation d'un coeur-poumon artificiel basé sur les principes de la récolte du sang par gravité et de l'oxygénation par bullage. C. R. Soc. Biol. (Paris) *152*, 685–687, 1958.

VAN ROOD, J. J. and J. VAN DER SLUYS VEER: Blutspenderprobleme bei Anwendung der Herz-Lungen-Maschine. Thoraxchirurgie *7*, 131–139, 1960.

VARCO, R. L., C. BARNARD, R. A. DEWALL and C. W. LILLEHEI: Studies on varying rates of perfusion for intracardiac surgery using the helix-reservoir oxygenator. pp. 167–178. In: Extracorporeal Circulation, J. G. Allen, ed. Springfield, Ill., Thomas, 1958.

VASLI, S., H. L. SMITH, JR. and L. H. BOSHER, JR.: A multiple stage droplet oxygenator. J. Appl. Physiol. *14*, 470–472, 1959.

VAUGHAN, B. E. and E. A. BOLING: Rapid assay procedure for tritium labelled water in body fluids. J. Lab. Clin. Med. *57*, 159–164, 1961.

VAYSSE, J.: Le coeur poumon à membrane pulmonaire artificielle de J. André Thomas. Sem. Hop. Paris *35*, 722–736, 1959.

VAYSSE, P., J. P. BINET and N. OECONOMOS: Coeur artificiel et dérivation circulatoire. Presse Méd. *60*, 1474–1478, 1952.

VECCHIETTI, G.: La trasfusione crociata. Quad. Clin. Obstet. Ginec. *3*, 251, 1948.

——: Therapeutic possibilities of cross-transfusion. Obst. Gynec. *1*, 402–417, 1953.

VEITH, F. J. and W. B. THROWER: Studies of assisted circulation in heart failure: method of producing heart failure in the dog and the effect of partial extracorporeal bypass on normal dogs and those with heart failure. Surg. Forum *10*, 622–625, 1960.

DE VERNEJOUL, R., H. DE METRAS, P. OTTAVIOLI, E. JEAN and R. COURBIER: Circulation extracorporelle; les conditions de chirurgie intracardiaque exsangue. Marseille Chir. *6*, 334–345, 1954.

VETTO, R. R., L. C. WINTERSCHEID and K. A. MERENDINO: Studies in the physiology of oxygen consumption during cardiopulmonary bypass. Surg. Forum *9*, 163–166, 1959.

VILES, P. H., J. L. ANKENEY and L. M. COX: The effect of 2% carbon dioxide on pH and pCO_2 during extracorporeal circulation. J. Thor. Cardiov. Surg. *39*, 619–623, 1960.

VINITSKAYA, R. S. and YU. D. VOLINSKY: The dependance of the tissue oxygen consumption on the minute blood volume and the arterial blood pressure during the extracorporeal circulation. Eksp. Khir. *6*, 47–53, 1960 (*Rus*).

VISHNEVSKII, A. A. and M. G. ANANEV: Artificial blood circulation and its perspectives of application. Eksp. Khir. *3*, 3–9, 1958 (*Rus*).

——, T. M. DARBINIAN, V. F. PORTNOV, T. N. PROMTOVA and S. SH. KHARNAS: Coronary and carotid perfusion in extracorporeal circulation associated with hypothermia. Eksp. Khir. *6*, 6–16, 1960 (*Rus*).

VOGEL, H.: Die Geschwindigkeit des Blutes in den Lungenkapillaren. Helv. Physiol. Pharmacol. Acta *5*, 105–121, 1947.

VOLLBRECHT, I. H., H. W. OBERSTEDT and I. K. KLAMROTH: Rohrenwärme-Austauscher mit Verdrängerkörpern. Chemie-Ingenieur-Technik *33*, 19–22, 1961.

VOWLES, K. D. J., C. M. COUVES and J. M. HOWARD: Excision of the aortic arch using a mechanical left heart bypass: a study of the problems. Surg. Forum *8*, 442–445, 1958.

W

WAACK, R., N. H. ALEX, H. L. FRISCH, V. STANNETT and M. SZWARC: Permeability of polymer films to gases and vapors. Indust. Engin. Chem. *47*, 2524–2527, 1955.

WADE, W. H. and R. VICKERS: The use of dextran sulfate as an anticoagulant for open-heart surgery. Surg. Forum *9*, 143–145, 1959.

WAGNER, E., G. SCHOENBACH, W. THORBAN and H. L'ALLEMAND: E.K.G.Veränderungen nach hypoxämischem Herzstillstand bei Anwendung der Herz-Lungen-Maschine. Langenbeck Arch. Klin. Chir. *292*, 685–691, 1959.

WALDHAUSEN, J. A., R. C. WEBB, F. C. SPENCER and H. T. BAHNSON: Study of the canine lung as an oxygenator of human and canine blood in extracorporeal circulation. Surgery *42*, 726–733, 1957.

——, C. R. LOMBARDO, J. A. McFARLAND, W. P. CORNELL and A. G. MORROW: Studies of hepatic blood flow and oxygen consumption during total cardiopulmonary bypass. Surgery *46*, 1118–1127, 1959a.

——, J. Ross, Jr., C. R. Lombardo, T. Cooper, J. W. Gilbert and A. G. Morrow: Flow and volume regulation during cardiopulmonary bypass: the use of an electromagnetic flowmeter and a device for automatic control of oxygenator volume. Trans. Am. Soc. Art. Int. Organs *5*, 172–176, 1959b.

——, N. S. Braunwald, R. D. Bloodwell, W. P. Cornell and A. G. Morrow: Left ventricular function following elective cardiac arrest. J. Thor. Cardiov. Surg. *39*, 799–807, 1960.

Wallace, H. W.: Cardiac metabolism. N. Eng. J. Med. *261*, 1322–1324, 1959.

——, H. J. Sugarman and H. F. Rheinlander: The effect of extracorporeal circulation on myocardial metabolism. Trans. Am. Soc. Art. Int. Organs *6*, 282–286, 1960a.

——, —— and ——: Myocardial metabolism during cardiopulmonary bypass. Bull. Tufts N. Engl. M. Cent. *6*, 16–17, 1960b.

——, H. F. Rheinlander and H. J. Sugarman: Cardiac metabolism during extracorporeal circulation. Arch. Surg. *82*, 138–146, 1961.

Walter, R. D., E. M. Kavan, V. L. Brechner and J. V. Maloney, Jr.: E. E. G. changes during cardiac surgery with cardiopulmonary bypass. Electroencephalog. Clin. Neurophysiol. *10*, 180–181, 1958.

Warden, H. E., M. Cohen, R. C. Read and C. W. Lillei. ··: Controlled cross-circulation for open intracardiac surgery. J. Thor. Surg. *28*, 331–343, 1954.

——, R. A. DeWall, R. C. Read, J. B. Aust, M. Cohen, R. L. Varco and C. W. Lillehei: Total cardiac bypass utilizing continuous perfusion from reservoir of oxygenated blood. Proc. Soc. Exp. Biol. Med. *90*, 246–250, 1955a.

——, R. C. Read, R. A. DeWall, J. B. Aust, M. Cohen, N. R. Zeigler, R. L. Varco and C. W. Lillehei: Direct vision intracardiac surgery by means of a reservoir of "arterialized venous" blood. J. Thor. Surg. *30*, 649–657, 1955b.

——, M. Cohen, R. A. DeWall, E. A. Sqmw+m, J. J. Buckley, R. C. Read and C. W. Lillehei: Experimental closure of interventricular septal defects and further physiologic studies on controlled cross circulation. Surg. Forum *5*, 22–28, 1955c.

Warren, R. and A. Wysocki: Assay of heparin in blood: a critique. Surgery *44*, 435–441, 1958.

Wasserman, F., M. W. Wolcott, C. G. Wherry and L. Brodsky: Comparative effect of 15% potassium chloride and 30% potassium citrate in resuscitation from ventricular fibrillation following acute myocardial infarction; an experimental study. J. Thor. Cardiov. Surg. *38*, 30–39, 1959.

Watkins, D. H. and E. R. Duchesne: Postsystolic myocardial augmentation. Developmental consideration and technique. Arch. Surg. *82*, 839–855, 1961.

Watkins, E.: Discussion of effects on renal function. p. 326. In: Extracorporeal Circulation, J. G. Allen ed., Springfield, Ill., Thomas, 1958.

—— and A. C. Hering: A suction apparatus for use during open cardiotomy. Arch. Surg. *79*, 35–39, 1959.

——, —— and H. D. Adams: Design and use of a pump oxygenator. Surg. Clin. N. Amer. *40*, 609–632, 1960.

Waud, R. A.: A mechanical heart and lung. Canad. J. M. Sci. *30*, 130–135, 1952.

——: The use of the artificial heart-lung in pharmacology. Trans. Am. Soc. Art. Int. Organs *1*, 87–93, 1955a.

——, A. M. Lansing and R. A. Lewis: The effects of veratrum, dibenzyline and hexamethonium on blood pressure as studied with an artificial heart-lung. J. Pharm. Exp. Ther. *114*, 271–278, 1955b.

Weil, M. H., L. D. MacLean, M. B. Visscher and W. W. Spink: Studies on the circulatory changes in the dog produced by endotoxin from gram-negative micro-organisms. J. Clin Invest. *35*, 1191–1198, 1956.

Weil, P., P. F. Salisbury and D. State: Physiological factors influencing pulmonary artery pressure during separate perfusion of the systemic and pulmonary circulations in the dog. Am. J. Physiol. *191*, 453–460, 1957.

Weirich, W. L., R..W. Jones and M. F. Burke: The effect of elective cardiac arrest induced by potassium citrate and acetylcholine on ventricular function. Surg. Forum *10*, 528–532, 1960.

Weiss, M. and L. Sprovieri: Contribution à l'étude des dérivations circulatoires pour chirurgie cardiaque; à propos d'un nouveau procédé de récupération atraumatique du sang intra-cardiaque. Maroc Méd. *37*, 1281–1289, 1958.

——, C. Lenfant, J. Rouanet-Weiss, Ch.

Dubost, L. Sprovieri, G. Pintos and R. Cianciarulo: L'arrêt cardiaque provoqué sous circulation extracorporelle. Etude expérimentale. I. De la méthode de Melrose appliquée à l'abord chirurgical du ventricule droit. II. Du comportement cardiaque. Presse Méd. 1649–1652 and 1726–1729, 1957.

——, A. Piwnica, C. Lenfant, L. Sprovieri, D. Laurent, Ph. Blondeau and Ch. Dubost: Deep hypothermia with total circulatory arrest. Trans. Am. Soc. Art. Int. Organs 6, 227–234, 1960a.

——, C. Tardieu, A. Piwnica, P. Finetti, M. C. Blayo and J. J. Pocidalo: Effets d'une circulation extracorporelle partielle sur le débit cardiaque du chien rachianesthésié. J.Physiol (Paris) 52, 245–247, 1960b.

Weiss, W. A. and C. P. Bailey: Extracorporeal circulation in cardiac surgery. Anesth. Analg. 39, 438–450, 1960.

——, J. S. Gilman, A. J. Catenacci and A. E. Osterberg: Heparin neutralization with Polybrene administered intravenously. J.A.M.A. 166, 338–348, 1958.

Weiss-Berg, E.: Probleme des Gasaustausches in der Lunge. Helv. Physiol. Acta 17, 338–348, 1959.

Wennemark, J. R., R. Benvenuto and F. J. Lewis: Destruction of the specialized conduction tissue in the live canine heart with iodine. J. Thor. Cardiov. Surg. 39, 137–143, 1960.

Wesolowski, S. A.: Extracorporeal circulation; continuous controlled variation of the frequency, volume, and systolic rise time of the pulse. J. Appl. Physiol. 6, 809–814, 1954.

——: The role of the pulse in the maintenance of the systemic circulation during heartlung bypass. Trans. Am. Soc. Art. Int. Organs 1, 84–86, 1955.

—— and C. S. Welch: A pump mechanism for artificial maintenance of the circulation. Surg. Forum 1, 226–233, 1951.

—— and ——: Experimental maintenance of the circulation by mechanical pumps. Surgery 31, 769–793, 1952.

——, H. H. Miller, A. E. Halkett and C. S. Welch: Experimental replacement of the heart by a mechanical extracorporeal pump. Bull. N. Engl. M. Center 12, 41–50, 1950.

——, J. H. Fisher and C. S. Welch: Heart-lung bypass using pumps and isolated homologous lungs. Surg. Gynec. Obstet. 95, 762–771, 1952.

——, ——, J. F. Hennessey, R. Cubiles and

C. S. Welch: Recovery of the dog's heart after varying periods of acute ischemia. Surg. Forum 3, 270–277, 1953a.

——, —— and C. S. Welch: Perfusion of the pulmonary circulation by nonpulsatile flow. Surgery 33, 370–375, 1953b.

——, L. R. Sauvage and R. D. Pinc: Extracorporeal circulation. The role of the pulse in maintenance of the systemic circulation during heart-lung bypass. Surgery 37, 663–682, 1955.

Westin, B., R. Nyberg and G. Enhorning: A technique for perfusion of the previable human fetus. Acta paediat. Upps. 47, 339–349, 1958.

——, J. A. Miller, Jr., R. Nyberg and E. Wedenberg: Neonatal asphyxia pallida treated with hypothermia alone or with hypothermia and transfusion of oxygenated blood. Surgery 45, 868–875, 1959.

Wiggers, C. J.: Physiology in health disease. Philadelphia, Lea and Febiger, 1949.

——: Cross-circulation; pp. 386–387, in Physiology of Shock. New York, Commonwealth Fund, 1950.

——, and A. B. Maltby: Further observations on experimental aortic insufficiency. IV. Hemodynamic factors determining the characteristic changes in aortic and ventricular pressure pulses. Am. J. Physiol. 97, 689, 1931.

Wilkens, J. H.: Vibration pump-foam oxygenator with a maximal capacity of 2 liters per minute. Acta Physiol. Pharmacol. Neerl. 4, 300, 1955.

Wilkinson, J. F., G. G. Freeman, N. New and R. B. Noad: Silicone rubber tubing in blood transfusion work. Lancet 2, 621–624, 1956.

Williams, J. A. and J. Fine: Measurement of blood volume with a new apparatus. N. Engl. J. Med. 264, 842–848, 1961.

Willman, V. L., P. Zafiracopoulos and C. R. Hanlon: Air embolism; pp. 295–302; in Extracorporeal Circulation, J. G. Allen, ed., Springfield, Ill., Thomas, 1958a.

——, E. C. Neville and C. R. Hanlon: Cardiac metabolism under conditions associated with open-heart operations. I. Coronary sinus flow and myocardial oxygen consumption. Surg. Forum 8, 287–290, 1958b.

——, T. Cooper, P. Zafiracopoulos and C. R. Hanlon: Depression of ventricular function following elective cardiac arrest with potassium citrate. Surgery 46, 792–796, 1959.

——, ——, —— and ——: Measures to limit myocardial depression associated with elective cardiac arrest. Surg. Forum *10*, 514–517, 1960a.

——, —— and C. R. HANLON: Prophylactic and therapeutic use of digitalis in open-heart operation. Arch. Surg. *80*, 860–863, 1960b.

——, H. S. HOWARD, T. COOPER and C. R. HANLON: Ventricular function after hypothermic cardiac arrest. Arch. Surg. *82*, 120–138, 1961a.

——, T. COOPER, A. RIBERI and C. R. HANLON: Cardiac assistance by diastolic augmentation. Trans. Amr. Soc. Art. Int. Organs *7*, 198–201, 1961b.

WILSON, M. and K. VOWLES: A disposable rotating oxygenator capable of being sterilized by heat for a heart-lung machine. Thorax *15*, 181–184, 1960.

WINCKLER, A. W., H. E. HOFF and P. K. SMITH: Electrocardiographic changes and concentration of potassium in serum following intravenous injection of potassium chloride. Am. J. Physiol. *124*, 478–483, 1938.

WINTERSCHEID, L. C., R. R. VETTO and K. A. MERENDINO: Myocardial carbohydrate metabolism during induced cardiac arrest and post-arrest perfusion. Ann. Surg. *148*, 481–487, 1958.

——, R. R. VETTO, J. B. BLUMBERG and K. A. MERINDINO: A coronary sinus system for use during cardiopulmonary bypass. Surgery *48*, 785–795, 1960.

WOOD, E. H., W. F. SHUTTERER and D. E. DONALD: The monitoring and recording of physiologic variables during closure of ventricular septal defects using extracorporeal circulation. Bibl. Cardiol. *9*, 61–74, 1959.

WRIGHT, I. S.: The discovery and early development of anticoagulant: a historical symposium. Circulation *19*, 73–134, 1959.

WRIGHT, S.: Applied Physiology, rev. by Keele, C. A. and E. Neil, London, Oxford University Press, 1961.

WRIGHT, T. A., J. M. DARTE and W. T. MUSTARD: Apparent increase in blood prothrombin during extracorporeal bypass and during slow coagulation in siliconed containers. Lancet *1*, 1157–1158, 1958.

——, —— and ——: Postoperative bleeding after extracorporeal circulation. Canad. J. Surg. *2*, 142–146, 1959.

WU, Y. K.: Recent progress in cardiovascular surgery in China. China Med. J. *80*, 415–416, 1960 (*Chin*).

WULFF, H. B., I. M. NILSSON and J. SWEDBERG: Bekämpfung der postoperative Blutungsgefhar bei Anwendung einer Herz-Lungen- Maschine. Thoraxchirurgie *7*, 140–147, 1959.

WYMAN, M. G., M. H. WEIL and J. V. BLANKENHORN: Partial cardiopulmonary bypass utilizing selective veno-arterial perfusion. J. Clin. Invest. *38*, 1056–1057, 1959.

Y

YASARGIL, E. C.: Ein neues Prinzip der Durchführung des extracorporellen Kreislaufs. Thoraxchirurgie *7*, 304–325, 1960.

YATES, P. O., A. B. CASSIE, J. F. DARK, G. D. JACK and A. G. RIDDELL: The detection of antifoam emboli following perfusion with a heart-lung machine. Lancet *1*, 130, 1959.

YOUNG, L. E., W. O'BRIEN, S. N. SWISHER, G. MILLER and C. L. YUILE: Blood groups in dogs. Their significance to the veterinarian. Am. J. Vet. Med. *13*, 107–213, 1952.

YOUNG, W. G., W. C. SEALY, I. W. BROWN, W. C. HEWITT, H. A. CALLAWAY, D. H. MERRITT and J. S. HARRIS: A method for controlled cardiac arrest as an adjunct to open-heart surgery. J. Thor. Surg. *32*, 604–611, 1956.

——, ——, ——, W. W. SMITH, H. A. CALLAWAY and J. S. HARRIS: Metabolic and physiologic observations on patients undergoing extracorporeal circulation in conjunction with hypothermia. Surgery *46*, 175–184, 1959.

Z

ZACOUTO, F.: Circulation extra-corporelle permettant chez le chien une hypothermie régionale rapide, intense et prolongée. C. R. Soc. Biol. (Paris) *152*, 257–259, 1958.

—— and E. CORABOEUF: Entretien de l'hématose chez le chien par un système de circulation croisée et de pompes intermédiaires. C. R. Soc. Biol. (Paris) *149*, 1212–1214, 1955.

ZAROFF, L. I., I. KREEL, D. J. KAVEE and I. D. BARONOFSKY: Mechanical failure during extracorporeal circulation. A method for prevention. Surgery *45*, 645–647, 1959.

ZELLER, O.: Versuche zur Wiederbelebung von Tieren mittelst arterieller Durchströmung des Herzens und der venösen Zentral-vorgänge. Dtsch. Ztschr. Chir. *95*, 488–559, 1908.

ZENKER, R., G. HERBERER, H. GEHL, H. BORST, R. BEER and Y. H. YEH: Zur Auf-rechthaltung der Organfunktionen und des Stoffwechsels im extrakorporalen Kreis-lauf. Langenbeck Arch. Klin. Chir. *289*, 294–302, 1958.

ZIEGLER, E. E.: The intravenous administra-tion of oxygen. J. Lab. Clin. Med. *27*, 223–232, 1941.

ZIESKE, H. JR. and M. N. LEVY: A self-adjust-ing perfusion pump controller. J. Appl. Phy-siol. *14*, 1059–1060, 1959.

ZIMMERMAN, H. A., J. MARTINS DE OLIV-EIRA, C. NOGUEIRA, D. MENDELSOHN and E. B. KAY: The electrocardiogram in open-heart surgery. J. Thor. Surg. *36*, 12–22, 1958.

ZUHDI, N., W. JOELL, J. CAREY, M. L. FAG-ELLA and A. GREER: Cerebral changes dur-ing cardiorespiratory bypass using the he-lix reservoir bubble oxygenator. J. Thor. Surg. *37*, 703–706, 1959.

——, G. KIMMELL, J. CAREY and A. GREER: Vacuum regulator for cardiotomy return and chest drainage systems. J. Thor. Cardiov. Surg. *39*, 221–224, 1960a.

——, ——, J. MONTROY, J. CAREY and A. GREER: A system for hypothermic perfu-sions. J. Thor. Cardiov. Surg. *39*, 629–633, 1960b.

——, B. McCOLLOUGH, J. CAREY and A. GREER: The use of citrated banked blood for open-heart surgery. Anesthesiology *21*, 496–501, 1960c.

——, B. McCOLLOUGH, J. CAREY and A. GREER: Double-helical reservoir heart-lung machine. Arch. Surg. *82*, 320–325, 1961.

Index

Page numbers in **boldface type** indicate main reference.